A TEXT-BOOK

OF THE

PRACTICE OF EQUINE MEDICINE.

BY

WILLIAM ROBERTSON, F.R.C.V S., &c,

PRINCIPAL AND PROFESSOR OF HIPPOPATHOLOGY IN THE ROYAL
VETERINARY COLLEGE, LONDON

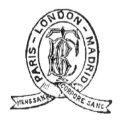

LONDON:

BAILLIÈRE, TINDALL AND COX,
20, KING WILLIAM STREET, STRAND.
NEW YORK. JENKINS.

PREFACE.

———◆◆———

THE present attempt to exhibit in a concise form a detailed account of the principal diseases to which the horse is liable, and the modes of their management in accordance with what are known as the recognised general principles of medicine, has been undertaken chiefly with the view of providing for my students the means of following more easily and intelligibly the teaching which is given in the course of Hippopathology carried out in this institution

I have not touched upon that part of the study of medicine recognised as the theory or science, but have restricted myself to the subject-matter of the class-work

The former has been in text-books, and is now in lectures in a systematic form, more ably dealt with than might be carried through by one who has continuously devoted his attention more to the practical details than to the speculative or experimental inquiries of professional work

To the busy practitioner of veterinary medicine, knowing how much isolation is apt to dwarf or egotize him, I am not without hope that this digest of the practice of equine medicine may prove useful, by recalling to his recollection facts and conditions liable to be forgotten, and by giving him the views and conclusions of another regarding conditions which are daily engaging his attention, and often taxing his resources

The plan of the text-book is laid out in three sections The two earlier, which are exceedingly brief, direct attention to the objects which engage the energies of the practitioner of animal medicine, the methods by which he may gather information in and for the prosecution of the practice of his work ; together with a notice of the classification adopted in attempting to systematize that knowledge The last, comprising the greater portion of the book, is devoted to a detailed description of the chief diseases to which the horse in our country is liable

This section is arranged in two divisions, the first embracing general and constitutional diseases, the other those which we usually regard as local, and which are examined in groups in accordance with the situations or localities where their diagnostic lesions are chiefly met with.

Of the several chapters comprising this section the ones on ' Bursattee ' and ' Surra ' have been compiled from information obtainable regarding these affections, scattered throughout our periodical professional literature, or received personally from other sources They give, I believe, a fair and condensed account of what is known up to the present time of these diseases affecting the horses of our Eastern Empire

To my colleague, Mr. Penberthy, I would here desire to express my thanks for assistance rendered in correcting the proofs of the sheets as they passed through the press.

ROYAL VETERINARY COLLEGE, LONDON,
July, 1883

CONTENTS.

———◇———

SECTION I

SECTION II.

SECTION III.

I. GENERAL DISEASES

A. IDIOPATHIC FEVERS, AND ALLIED DISEASES CHIEFLY OF AN EXOGENOUS ORIGIN.

CONTENTS

PRACTICE OF EQUINE MEDICINE.

———⟩∘⟨———

SECTION I

CHAPTER I

INTRODUCTION.—OBJECTS OF STUDY

In dealing with the disturbances of animal activities which we recognise under the term of *disease,* the abnormal conditions are usually regarded under two lights—either grouped as particular phenomena which within certain limits manifest themselves with a wonderful similarity as changes of a generic nature in all animals, or as individual exhibitions of altered activities in particular animals

Under the first of these considerations or modes of dealing with unnatural activities, the subject-matter of GENERAL PATHOLOGY, cognizance is taken of all pertaining to those abnormal phenomena which are ordinarily found associated with, or together make up every, or nearly every, unnatural, *i e. diseased* condition or perverted organic action which demands our attention in animal bodies, including such morbid phenomena as are known by the names ' CONGESTION,' ' INFLAMMATION,' ' DEGENERATION,' etc, and which are more or less constantly associated and found in connection with every disease

Under the second, SPECIAL PATHOLOGY, attention is directed to all matters and influences connected with the manifestations of particular and individual diseases as exhibited in particular animals

Although, in the systematic teaching of medicine, it is

1

generally considered necessary to begin with, or certainly at
least to carry on contemporaneously with, the study of the
practice of medicine and surgery, i e the study of special diseases, that of GENERAL PATHOLOGY—a consideration of those
general truths arrived at from comparison of many diseases or
of particular diseases with each other, truths which have been
established by observation and experiment—yet it ought never
to be forgotten that the first of these divisions, the one which
it is proposed specially to consider, comes first in the order of
nature   It is from this, the study of special diseases, the
phenomena which they exhibit, their causation, modes of development, termination, and the textural changes which are the
result of their existence, as also from their relationship to
each other in all pertaining to their individuality, that we
approach the study of the more extensive and general truths
relative to disease in general, known by the term of GENERAL
PATHOLOGY

While thus merely directing attention to the necessity which
exists for a knowledge of the subject and matters embraced in
the province of GENERAL PATHOLOGY, with its many associated
branches and subjects of human knowledge, it is neither intended, nor considered necessary in the further prosecution of
this particular section of SPECIAL PATHOLOGY—'The Practice of
Equine Medicine,' to which it is purposed giving a rational
and concise consideration—that, either introductory to or
mingled with this special pathological teaching, any special
treatment or investigation shall be carried out on matters pertaining to the peculiar province of GENERAL PATHOLOGY, those
great truths, leading facts, and acknowledged inferences drawn
from observation and experiment

For this reason there shall be left untouched the consideration both of those complex vital processes whose phenomena,
more or less combined, constitute disease, as 'IRRITATION,' 'CON-
GESTION,' 'INFLAMMATION,' 'HYPERTROPHY,' 'ATROPHY,' 'DE-
GENERATION,' etc, and the examination in any minute manner
of the varied products and changed elemental structures which
are met with as the special results of disease, matters pertaining
specially to the department of pathological histology and
chemistry

CHAPTER II.

METHODS BY WHICH DISEASE MAY BE ELUCIDATED AND UNDERSTOOD.

FOR a correct and comprehensive appreciation of those subjects which together form the department of the practice of medicine, human or veterinary, for a solution of such problems as are presented for our consideration—for problems they often are—there is one, and only one, way of attainment, viz, through the correct cultivation of our powers of observation We may all of us be observers, we must all of us be observers, if we are successfully to cultivate the practice of veterinary medicine

For although I can scarcely acquiesce in the opinion entertained by some that to be an observer requires as great a range of faculties as to make a speculative thinker, that to note facts is as lofty a range of intellect as to conceive thought, still there is little doubt that in the science of medicine it is not easy to overestimate the importance of correct observation, seeing it is by pure induction, by the observation of individual facts, that we rise to those general inferences which are to us the most comprehensive expressions of attainable truth

No doubt facts are of themselves of little worth until associated with mind, they must be registered and collated, and except as indices of particular functional or organic changes, and the exact relation which they bear to these, are of comparatively trifling practical value in advancing the study of clinical or systematic medicine.

In this study of the 'Practice of Veterinary Medicine,' embracing, as it does, the CAUSATION, HISTORY, PHENOMENAL EXHIBITIONS, and TREATMENT of special diseases and disturbed states of the system, these present themselves for our consideration in two somewhat different characters or aspects

1 As these diseases offer themselves to our notice in separate, distinct, and individual cases or animals—the so-called CLINICAL study ;

2 As they form, or constitute, or are gathered or grouped into particular classes or genera of diseases—the SYSTEMATIC study.

Although in the prosecution of the study of special pathology in any department, it is quite possible, without much special theoretical knowledge, to attain a creditable amount of information and manipulatory dexterity, it is yet certain that this theoretical knowledge renders the attainment, when opportunity offers, of sound practical information much easier, and clears the way of many difficulties for the student's advancement

Still it must never be forgotten that the practice of medicine, human or veterinary, can only be learnt by actual contact with, and personal examination of, the diseased, both as this disease is exhibited in the living animal and laid out for our inspection in the organs and tissues in which the unnatural action seems specially located In every instance our most fertile field for obtaining information is that of practical everyday work, while to assist and utilize the contact every advantage must be taken of all means to obtain and systematize fact, and by the special education of all our senses

In whatever character or aspect, whether clinically or according to any system of medical classification, we, as students or practitioners, make examinations of disease, there is always the certainty that a wonderful similarity of subjects or problems will be placed before us for consideration

The greater number of these may be grouped under—

I The CAUSATION, or ÆTIOLOGY, embracing the origin, or rather the agents through the action of which derangement or disease is produced.

II SYMPTOMATOLOGY, or SEMIOLOGY, a consideration of the morbid phenomena or symptoms by which we become aware that derangement has occurred in the system

III. The NATURE, LOCALITY, FORMS, and course of development of disease.

IV The TEXTURAL ALTERATIONS discoverable in the body before and after death as the results of disease

V THERAPEUTICS, including the entire management, medicinally and dietetically, of animals suffering from disease.

I.—ÆTIOLOGY, OR CAUSATION OF DISEASE

Due attention to this is always of the utmost importance, seeing that in comprehending it we are materially assisted in

forming our DIAGNOSIS and PROGNOSIS, as well as directed in
the selection of our PROPHYLACTICS and special THERAPEUTICS
ÆTIOLOGY not only tells us of the general causes which induce
disturbance, but also of the special causes of special diseases
and the modes of their operation The same causes, we can
understand, may produce different diseases, and different
causes may develop the same diseases Still in practice we
find that the different classes of diseases arise from a limited
number of causes When diseases only arise from certain
determinate or specific causes, they are spoken of as specific
diseases

Various terms have been employed to group or comprehend
what are designated as causes of disease; but for all useful
purposes, to regard them as *remote* and *proximate* is sufficient
The latter is in reality the condition or conditions of the parts
diseased upon which the symptoms depend. The *remote* are
further regarded as *predisposing* and *exciting* *Predisposing*
causes are those which confer upon the individual or part a
greater susceptibility to be acted upon by the exciting than
others differently circumstanced *Exciting* causes are such as
directly produce the textural changes or disturbances.
Neither of these, however, have anything distinctly and un-
alterably connected with them which certainly and in all
conditions compels them to action in this and no other
way.

Causes are also spoken of as *intrinsic* or *extrinsic, endogenous* or *exogenous.* The *intrinsic* or *endogenous* are all
such which in operation owe their existence to inherited or
acquired power or potentialities residing in the animal itself.
Extrinsic or *exogenous* include all which act upon the animal
from without.

1. Under INTRINSIC or ENDOGENOUS causes of disease may
be ranked

a Heredity, such as appear to be capable of propagation
from parent to progeny, by which we do not mean that the
actual diseased condition is necessarily propagated; it may be
so, but more often it is a tendency or disposition under trifling
influences to develop some particular disease or one like it.

Of some of these conditions we are certain, of others not
so They may be general or systemic diseases, or only local

changes or disturbances. Of diseases which seem to owe their existence to this are

(i) Certain constitutional or blood diseases, as rheumatism

(ii) Many exhibitions of arthritic disease, not rheumatic, largely affecting bone tissue, as spavin and the peculiar joint disease of young animals

(iii) Early degeneration of organs and particular tissues, generally appearing as local diseases.

(iv) Anatomical malformations and some diseases of special sensation

(v.) Some affections of the nervous system, as epilepsy and the so-called chorea

(vi) Probably certain skin diseases, as some forms of eczema.

b. Age —Many diseases are more apt to attack animals before they reach maturity; and special organs in particular states of development, as well as particular states of certain structures dependent on their age, predispose to disease

c. General or Constitutional Vigour —This depending on the state of activity and robustness of the whole system, its general tone, and probably also its relation to present states, dependent on previous disease

d. Breed or Variety —Certain races of animals are doubtless more susceptible of particular diseases than others.

e. Temperament —This influence with the horse may not be so well made out as with some other animals; but there are fairly reasonable grounds for believing that it does exist.

f. Idiosyncrasy or Medical Constitution —By this is meant to be indicated that some animals are, apart from obvious causes, more liable to be acted upon by adverse agencies than others.

2. EXTRINSIC OR EXOGENOUS INFLUENCES. *a. Atmospheric.* —The respirable air with which animals are surrounded ever exercises a certain amount of influence, even when uncontaminated, through its moisture or dryness, but more particularly when impregnated with noxious emanations from living animals or material given off from decaying organic matter or other unwholesome gases Its electrical condition, probably, and its excess or deficiency in ozone may also tend to induce an action of a predisposing or exciting character

b. Temperature—Excess of heat or the opposite, and more certainly sudden alternations from the one to the other, act both systemically and locally

c. Telluric—This acts variously, as through the character of the materials of the food-supply grown from particular soils, by the nature of its geological formation as to its capability of retaining or discharging moisture, its reception and treatment of the sun's rays, or the amount of organic matter which it holds undergoing decay. The breaking up of soils has a marked and often peculiar influence in determining the appearance of serious maladies amongst animals

d. Dietetic. Food and Water—The food may be wrong as to quantity or quality, or given at improper intervals, and under unfavourable conditions of animal health and work. Water, either in excess or deficiency, but most frequently from its contamination with poisons, mineral or vegetable, or organic germs, may act injuriously

e. Work—This operates both in respect of its amount, or its amount in relation to other conditions of health and adaptability, and when thus operating, may do so both constitutionally and locally, more often in the latter direction

f. Defective Sanitary Conditions—Of these the chief are defective ventilation, imperfect light, bad drainage, and want of cleanliness of body.

g. Mechanical Causes—Under this head may be placed improperly fitting harness, continued pressure from other external objects, bad shoeing, all probably operating in inducing local injury rather than direct constitutional disease

Besides these, there are other causes which operate in inducing altered states of healthy activities, and which usually act in a definite and determinate manner. A large class of these are the so-called poisons, mineral and vegetable; but in addition there are others not usually ranked as such. These latter may be roughly grouped. 1st, as originating within the animal itself, developed within the organism through faulty digestion and perversion of assimilation; 2nd, agencies connected with the vegetable kingdom, as parasitic plants developed in both external and internal parts of the body; 3rd, such as belong truly to the animal kingdom, including (*a*) all poisons of a purely animal material, (*b*) animal parasites, and (c) the specific results following inoculation by specific animal virus, in whatever form transmitted from animal to animal

II SEMIOLOGY, OR SYMPTOMATOLOGY.

Whatever may be the nature or extent of the significance which we may attach severally to the terms *symptom* and *sign* of disease, whether we regard them as simply every occurrence or circumstance taking place or happening in the diseased body, which is capable of being perceived or appreciated as indicating a state of disease, or as something in addition, as, in fact, a part of the disease itself, and as virtually a constituent of its existence and identity as any specific lesion or structural change, we must remember that for the proper collection of these symptoms appropriate means and methods must be employed, and when possession of these is obtained, much thought and reflection is needful for their correct interpretation Symptom must be weighed against symptom, the relation of one to the other, and of the whole to each, considered, in this way only can we arrive at any just conclusion as to the nature of the disease, the probability of its course and termination, or of the treatment requisite

Symptoms are spoken of as *general* when they affect, to a greater or less extent, the whole system, *local*, when confined to a particular part or organ, *premonitory*, when they precede the full appearance of the diseased action, *positive*, or *direct*, when consisting of phenomena actually present or connected with the diseased part, *indirect*, when such phenomena are absent or developed in some situation remote from the seat of the disease, *characteristic*, when seen in the same or a similar disease, *commemorative*, when developed during the course of the disease

They are also spoken of as *diagnostic* when they lead us to distinguish one disease from another, *pathognomic*, when peculiar to some particular disease; *prognostic*, when they enable us to predict the course of the disease

In following out this study of the practice of equine medicine, which is in reality the recognition of veterinary medicine as an art, inasmuch as it is directed to observe and to ascertain as far as possible the causes, the nature, the means of cure or of alleviation, and the most successful modes of the prevention of disease in the horse, it will be for our advantage, at this particular stage, to recognise and examine those large and general sources of information, those channels through which symptoms of derangement are exhibited and from which signs of disease are collected, and by which we are led better to understand the causes or factors which may have induced this disease, and the localities and textures specially the seats of morbid changes, all of which are needed to qualify us for giving a place to any diseased process or condition in whatever system of nosology we may choose to adopt, as also to form a *prognosis* of the case or to direct our treatment.

Symptoms are valuable, but we must know how, or the manner in which, these are to be gathered We must have some system or method in conducting the clinical examination of our patients, so as to abstract from them the information they are able to yield.

No doubt the experienced practitioner can gain his knowledge of a case of disease in any or in many ways, and probably by the observance of little method, but for all who are only commencing the acquisition of practical knowledge, and who wish to advance, method is all but indispensable.

The *subjective* examination in our patients must of course, if admitted, be a much weaker foundation upon which to build than the objective, which ought in proportion, therefore, to be more thoroughly and carefully carried out And although it may seem a little troublesome and tedious at first, ' case-taking ' in the practice of veterinary medicine will amply repay, both from the immediate benefit and information obtained, as well as from pleasure afforded in after-life by reference to work executed long antecedent.

Many plans have been sketched upon which case-taking has been recommended, and possibly each has something better than the others ; for us, however, it is probable that a combination of regional and physiological examination is that which best serves the purpose

Before, however, proceeding to carry out this in detail, and make note of the facts as they occur, it is generally expedient to carry out some preliminary examination.

(1) Observation must be made of the breed, age, general

appearance of the animal as to bulk and condition, nature of work in which employed, character of food-supply, and location.

(2) History (*a*) of present illness, whether traceable to any particular cause, its length of duration, whether acute or chronic, whether increasing in intensity or the opposite (*b*) Previous state of health, if subject to similar attacks or any other disease, if the ordinary functions of animal life are correctly performed   (*c*) Endeavour to discover if, previous to our inspection, treatment has been adopted, and of what nature, this we know is nearly always a necessary inquiry as respects our patients

In all our interrogations much tact is requisite, particularly when attempting to elucidate the causes which are often patent enough, the attendants so frequently maintaining a careful reserve, for fear they are criminated   Having obtained in this way, by an intelligent and orderly questioning of the animal's attendants, as much information as we may anticipate, we can, by carrying out a systematic individual examination, disclose objective phenomena, physical signs of disease, even more reliable, when considered independently, than those obtained by the former method   Here again method is essential, and much assistance is obtainable from the use of particular instruments

In many acute diseases of the horse, the symptoms are so quickly developed and so distinctly diagnostic, that all our attention is at once directed to the region and organs from which the disturbance proceeds; otherwise, and in less pronounced cases, although much may be learnt from general observation, it is always preferable to make a systematic and thorough examination   This, as already stated, is probably more easily accomplished by dealing with the system regionally and functionally.

1 Of the Head and Cranial Region—Although much may be gathered from the character of the facial expression as a whole, as well as from special central and peripheral indications, particularly when the cranial nerve-centres are disturbed, observation with our patients, and particularly the horse, settles at once on the visible mucous membranes as a source from which a large amount of information may be gained, and probably, in conjunction with the state of the pulse and cardiac action, there is no source to which practical veterinary surgeons more constantly appeal than the visible mucous membranes.

From the character of the epithelium covering the schneiderian and conjunctival membranes, and the mode in which the capillaries are disposed in the submucous layer, not only is any fulness or turgescence of these vessels plainly visible, but in many instances changes, physical as well as chemical, which have occurred in the blood are laid out for our observation The heightening in colour and increased vascularity observed in the mucous membrane of the eyes and nasal chambers from engorgement of the capillaries, whether the direct result of arterial pressure or of venous obstruction, must not in every case be accepted apart from other symptoms and signs as infallibly indicative of inflammation. We are certainly, upon the whole, tolerably safe when we regard the existence of this heightened colour and increased vascularity as indicative of vascular excitement, and not unfrequently as an early accompaniment of congestive and inflammatory action in membranous structures, both of the serous and mucous class Marked injection of the conjunctival membrane is probably rarely, or ever, absent in vascular excitement in connection with the cerebral structures

When from derangement or structural changes in the liver, the bile is either not elaborated from the blood, or, when secreted, is in great part improperly disposed of, much of it again in some form finding its way into the circulation, how rapidly and persistently do the mucous membranes of mouth, nose, and eyes tell us of the disturbance, and continue to maintain their peculiar yellow tinge as long as biliary compounds remain in the blood, and while the diseased condition of the liver continues

When from the operation or many causes the condition of *anæmia* is established, a condition in which the sum-total of the circulating blood is lessened, or the proper balance or equilibrium which ought to exist amongst its several constituent elements is disturbed, early and satisfactory evidence is afforded by the general bloodlessness of the more extensive mucous membranes, and the curiously injected vessels of part of the conjunctiva

In the different forms which the fever of influenza may
assume, a leading feature by which several of these may be
separated from each other is the physical character of these
membranes

Witness the bright pink colour of the conjunctival membrane in that particular form where the connective tissue is
prominently involved, and which has given to it its most commonly employed designation, 'pink-eye' Again, in the bilious
form we have the true hepatic hue spread over the whole
buccal membrane as well as the schneiderian and conjunctival
When degradation of tissue is imminent, and when the blood
is being poisoned by absorption of effete materials consequent
on tissue change, or from noxious emanations received from
without, such necræmic changes as occur to the formed materials of the blood are made plainly visible to our observation
by blood spots, and stellate rays branching from these *petechiæ*
and *vibici*, found on the nasal membrane. While when disease
marked by these features and of such a type as indicated
by these destructive changes is under treatment, the most
noticeable symptom, and one to be depended upon, is the persistence or otherwise of these blood spots , indeed, their disappearance and recurrence on the visible mucous membranes
in these fevers are surely indicative of the subsidence or
otherwise of the other, and what may appear the graver,
symptoms

With these membranes also are associated the characteristic
lesions of some of our most serious and harassing diseases of
animals, as glanders, cattle plague, epizootic aphtha, etc

The information to be obtained from the condition of the
buccal membrane, although not so diagnostic and specially indicative of particular organic changes in the very numerous
disorders of the digestive system to which the horse is so
liable, as in the case of those general or specific fevers to which
we have already referred, is yet ample and explicit, and well
deserving of our closest attention   A furred and pasty condition of the tongue, with a sour and disagreeable smell, is
a sure enough indication of indigestion, gastric or intestinal
An excessively moist state of the mouth from an over-supply
of saliva indicates irritation of the posterior parts of the mouth
or fauces, irregularities of the teeth, or the presence of foreign

bodies in the soft structures, or some disturbance of the vascular or special nervous supply.

2. **Thorax.** *a. Circulatory System*—Here the indications by which we may be directed in forming an estimate either of the nature or extent of disturbance are central as well as peripheral. Attention must be given to the position of the heart, its sounds and impulse, as also to such symptoms as cardiac dyspnœa and palpitation. In our patients, however, it is probable that the peripheral indications—those afforded by the state of the pulse—are more generally depended upon.

Regarding the pulse as the vibration or beating of the arteries from afflux of the blood in response to the contractions of the heart, we find that its different characters or conditions in disease are referable to—(1) the number of pulsations or beats in a given time, (2) to the rapidity or degree of quickness with which each pulsation is accomplished, (3) to the character or volume, hardness or strength of each pulsation, (4) to the equality or inequality either of the pulsations themselves or of the intervals occurring between each (5) to the various impressions each pulsation may produce on the finger.

b. Respiratory System.—While observing and noting the condition of respiratory function, we have to recollect that between the function of respiration and that of circulation, *i.e.* between the entrance and expulsion of atmospheric air from the lungs and the contraction of the heart and propulsion of the blood through its appropriate channels, there is in health a tolerably constant relationship, which relationship is not observed in disease. We may find the cardiac contractions much increased in number without a corresponding relative increase in the respirations. In disease disturbance of the respiration may and does occur, both in respect of the rapidity or frequency with which the act is performed, and also as to the character of the act.

In our clinical examinations and observations of disease, we are particularly required to note the number of the respirations per minute: whether easy, calm, and full-drawn, or difficult, painful, cut short when half accomplished and irregularly carried out. Also it is needful to remember a few cardinal facts in connection with the performance of this act, which, if neglected, even accurate observation may mislead, such as—

(1) That simple numerical increase in the number of the respirations is capable of production by various means, and is
generally in direct proportion to acceleration of the circulation   That the respirations are increased in number to provide for the aeration of a larger amount of blood which by increased circulation is being passed through the lungs, and is
thus not necessarily indicative of disease.   (2) That oppressed
or difficult breathing—*dyspnœa*—is a marked symptom of
many diseases because resulting from various causes   That
difficulty of breathing, although characteristic of serious structural changes in the cavity of the thorax from inflammatory
or other causes, is not a sign of chest disease alone.   That it
may occur as a symptom, merely from the pain induced in the
performance of the respiratory acts, as well as from the results
of inflammatory action, causing obliteration of the air-cells or
adhesions of the otherwise movable portions of the organs of
the thorax ; also that in numerous instances it has a direct
relation with conditions interfering with the due performance
of the natural activities of the nervous centres which regulate
the respiratory act   (3) That the forms of respiration recognised by the terms abdominal breathing and thoracic breathing are accomplished respectively by the muscles and structures of the opposite cavity, those of the other being, from
disease in connection with them, held in abeyance.   (4) That
the so-called irregular breathing, *i.e.* where there is a want of
harmony between the inspiratory and expiratory acts, and
which occasionally terminates by becoming spasmodic in the
expiratory act, is well seen, and largely diagnostic of that
form of disease of the lung-tissue ordinarily recognised under
the name of ' broken-wind '   (5) That snoring, or stertorous
breathing, depending on a relaxed or paralyzed condition of
the soft palate, when encountered is usually indicative of
cerebral mischief of a serious character, and precursive of dis-
solution

In addition to peculiarities connected with the act of respiration properly so called, and deserving of notice, there is
the occurrence of special phenomena or sounds included under
the term 'coughing.' A cough is generally attendant on some
irritation of the lower or upper air-passages, and is the involuntary effort to get rid of the irritation ; the sound is pro-

duced by the forcible expulsion of the air through the closed glottis, generally attendant on direct irritation of the respiratory organs as stated, but not always, seeing we know cough may result from dental or gastric disturbance This cough when existing must not merely be observed, but its character must be noted When moist, it is usually associated with such diseased conditions of the mucous membrane of the air-passages as common catarrh, or some forms of bronchitis or laryngitis, where the secretion of the membrane has been much increased When hard, dry, and painful, the inflammatory action in the air-tubes and passages is of the non-secretory character, as in the earlier stages of the greater number of the diseases affecting these While when accompanying inflammations of the serous membrane of the chest, its short, suppressed, and painful character is very striking, being evidently emitted spasmodically in spite of efforts to suppress it

Besides the careful observance of these symptoms associated with the respiratory function, we must by physical examination, by auscultation and percussion, endeavour to obtain some knowledge of the changes steadily occurring to the central organs and the thorax as a whole.

3 Abdomen —Here the direction of our inquiry and examination is chiefly with the view to discover the state of the great natural secretions and evacuations

In not a few instances, particularly where disease is located in the abdominal cavity and organs contained there, physical changes, visible externally, will arrest our attention and supply us with facts useful for our guidance Chiefly, however, are we to note the state of the functional activities of the organs situated in this region as indices of the natural conditions Besides merely observing phenomena as presented to us, inquiry must be made as to the frequency and character of the intestinal evacuations, and the discharge of urine

Tympany, with or without associated pain, points to indigestion, frequent and moist evacuations are indicative of irritation of the villous surface of the digestive canal, and when excessive, this state in the horse is always a more serious condition than retention of the evacuations Retention of fæcal matter suggests disease of the bowels or liver, with more rarely involvement of the kidneys and other gland-structures

Attention ought to be given to the discharge of urine, so as to determine whether micturition is frequent and painful, or executed at long intervals with restricted discharge

Note is to be taken of the total amount of the urine voided during the twenty-four hours, of its colour, consistency, clearness, density, odour, chemical reaction, and disposition to form a deposit It will require to be examined also as to excess or deficiency of such natural constituents as urea, and such unnatural ones as albumen If a sediment exist after being at rest, note is to be made of its manner of formation, its solubility or otherwise by heat, nitric or acetic acid, or liquor potassæ The presence of such formed materials as blood, pus, epithelial cells, or renal casts must be determined by the microscope

In addition to noting these physical phenomena, we must observe in what manner the functions of these organs are carried out , whether there exists a simple difficulty in micturition, *dysuria*, or a more perfect suppression or retention of the fluid, *ischuria*, both of which conditions point to disease, either of the urinary organs proper, the urine conduits, changes in the secretion itself, or disease of contiguous organs and structures We have to recollect that as frequent micturition indicates an irritable condition of the urine tube, and probably also of the kidneys, so inability to retain the urine points to relaxation of the sphincter vesicæ; and suppression of the secretion to inflammatory and other structural diseases of the kidneys, primarily occurring there, or resulting secondarily and in association with serious textural changes, following some general or even local disease That the last condition is of all others the most serious, seeing that unless relieved the poisoning of the blood by unremoved effete and excrementitious material is sure to terminate fatally

ANIMAL THERMOMETRY.—Besides this collecting of information by observation and questioning of a subjective and objective nature, as indicated in the systematic examination of the different regions and functions of the animal body, there is another source of obtaining certainty in matters of fact, and one which must not be neglected in clinical examination of cases; that is, attention to the temperature or calorific function of the body We require to remember that a generally diffused and equable surface-temperature, with a tolerably soft and pliant condition of the skin, free from excess of scales, 'scurf,' and hair not standing erect, are sufficiently indicative of health , that marked and persistent deviation from one or all of these conditions is generally sufficient to attract attention as indicative of at least functional disturbance

As a sequel of disturbed nervous force, and as accompanying capillary congestion, we have to recollect the occurrence of irregularly distributed surface-temperature—indicated through the touch—either of the body or the extremities , and that this is a feature well enough marked during the course of many diseases, and that accompanied with slight rigor and staring of the coat, it is the chief feature in the greater number of the slighter or more ephemeral febrile attacks

Probably from time immemorial—certainly from a very remote period—it has been recognised that many diseased conditions of the animal body were associated or accompanied with an increase in the animal heat ; it is only in very recent years, however, that instrumental means of measuring this thermal disturbance were adopted in veterinary practice

I am aware that there are some amongst the veterinary surgeons of the present day who, lightly esteeming the aids furnished by the thermometer, are fain to believe that its use has made little progress in veterinary medicine, and that the deductions to be obtained from its readings are misleading and unreliable That it is gradually but steadily becoming more extensively employed as an aid to diagnosis is most certainly known ; and I am satisfied that those who have once adopted it will not willingly dispense with its use It gives confidence to the observant practitioner from stage to stage in the disease , while the variations observed in the temperature are amongst the most significant indications by which he is directed in forming his estimate of the character and development of the disease, and in choosing his remedies with which to meet it, or by which to fortify his patient to pass successfully through it To reap the full benefit, however, from the employment of animal thermometry, it has to be borne in mind that it must be carried through the entire course of the disease with care and scrupulous ·attention. It ought to be employed twice daily, and each day at the same period of the day

2

Here again caution is needed to guard against supposing that the use of the thermometer can ever dispense with the accurate observation and registration of symptoms; the collating of these and their association with mind. We must never forget that the thermometer, like the microscope and other instruments, "are merely instruments of pathological inquiry, each one adapted for the determination of particular classes of facts. They can only elucidate disease when they are brought to bear on physical properties the nature of which they are able to appreciate, and it is only from their combined and appropriate use in connection with general symptoms and signs that our knowledge of the nature of diseases will be advanced."

In addition to its employment as an aid in the diagnosis of existing disease, it is further to be remembered that it possesses a distinctive value as marking for us that exaltation in body temperature which exists during the incubative period of zymotic and contagious diseases. This is a point not to be overlooked, seeing that upon its adoption extensively and with knowledge depends our power oftentimes of circumscribing or eradicating the most serious animal plagues.

In following out the clinical study of any case, particularly in its symptomatology, it is ever to be remembered that wherever possible, we ought carefully to follow it through its entire course, observing and noting any new phenomena and complications which may occur; and if a fatal termination be the result, to see that an after-death examination as methodical and minute is carried out.

Diagnosis.—Having made the examination of our patient in this manner, or in one which may be expected to yield like results, and noted mentally or in our case-book the various facts, the information thus obtained in every case of disease, by intelligent questioning of attendants and by careful examination of our patients, is not to be valued as an ultimate result, but to be at once utilized for further and higher purposes. Mind must be brought into contact with facts, symptoms converted into signs of disease or otherwise explained, a diagnosis of our case has to be made. By this is meant a full and accurate idea of the origin, seat, character, and extent of the disturbance

Symptoms, however accurately noted, are only of use in so far as they lead us to know and understand the morbid state of the parts under review. In forming a diagnosis we have to determine, (1) Whether the disease is acute or chronic—rarely have we in our patients to hesitate as to the reality of illness, (2) Whether it involves the entire system or only some particular organ, (3) If a systemic disease, of what class and whether it is free from complication; if some particular organ or set of organs are only invaded, to what extent? also, is the disturbance one of function merely, or is there evidence of textural change?

The certainty and rapidity with which a diagnosis may be made varies much in some forms of disease; from the prominence of certain clinical phenomena or pathognomic symptoms there may be no difficulty—the abnormal state of parts may be clearly presented for our recognition In others, even after comparing in the mind the relationships which exist amongst various generic affections in the matter of their symptomatology, and the exclusion from our reckoning—because not existing—of others in some degree similar, it may often be a difficult matter to form a correct diagnosis.

In many instances, particularly those which are rather obscure much may be obtained from patiently waiting and watching the disease as it develops itself

Prognosis —In attempting to give a 'prognosis,' or forecast, of the probable termination of any case, having determined from a consideration of its causation and a careful analysis of symptoms its true character, there is always required a good grasp of material collected by observation, with a due appreciation of surrounding and indwelling influences We have first to settle what points are to be determined, and how many of these apply to the case under consideration. Usually there are submitted for solution such questions as—(1) Whether the probabilities of life or death are greater? (2) If these are in favour of recovery, is it likely to be prolonged or readily reached? may it be expected to be complete, with a restoration to full normal functional activity, or only of a partial character, entailing weakened organs or tissues less capable of fulfilling natural activities, or more susceptible of contracting the same or some other disease?

To determine these and many other points it is ever found

that experience with a large grasp of facts and correct interpretation of symptoms is needful. While it is not to be
forgotten if these do not exist, or their interpretation is specially
difficult, that a statement of eventualities may be all which
we are warranted in giving. If, on the contrary, there is
evidence for forming a definite opinion, this ought to be stated
plainly, and with the confidence which the evidence before us
entitles us to do

III. THE NATURE, LOCALITY, FORM, AND COURSE OF DEVELOPMENT OF DISEASE.

Under these considerations we have to regard—

1. The particular and strange activities we call disease, in
their general and particular manifestations and their relations
to normal conditions; not merely their deviations from what
is recognised as health, but the manner of such deviations,
with the probable influences which may result from the operation of such activities

2. The localizations of these disturbances and the structures
invaded, the changes in form or manifestations which these
assume under the varying and diversified influences to which
they are subject, and under which they advance or recede, all
tending to the production of those modifications in diseased
processes known as types or variations.

3. The complications which, although appearing at the same
time, are not necessarily part of the recognised clinical phenomena, and the textural changes and ultimate impairment of
functional activity known as sequelæ

IV. TEXTURAL ALTERATIONS THE RESULT OF DISEASE

Here we learn through examination of the impress left by
the abnormal activities, these modified health processes, more
of the nature and character of the changes we recognise as
disease. Under the examination of the result of these activities,
the anatomy of disease, are grouped all which we may learn by
macroscopic, microscopic, or chemical examination of their
conditions and change. While by pathological histology we
take cognizance of the growth, development, decline, or change
of those elementary structures which these unnatural activities

have produced These two fields of work, morbid anatomy and histology, have done much to advance our knowledge of diseased processes , and in conjunction with the cultivation of the science of physiology in its widest sense, must be depended upon for the elucidation of many of the yet unsolved problems of disease which we regard as merely modifications of normal activities.

V. THERAPEUTICS

Whatever estimate we may place upon the careful noting and consideration of the matters already detailed, we find that all must converge to the ultimate point—and are only valuable in so far as they elucidate this—of furnishing indications for management of the individual case, the regulation of its therapeutic treatment—the ultimate object of all medical study

One great reason why directions have been pointed out rather minutely, as to the correct gathering of information respecting individual diseases, is to guard against falling into the common error of indulging in merely routine practice , the treating of diseases by name, and according to the class to which we believe they belong , the merely acting upon the inferences, deductions, and experience of others forgetting that each case ought to furnish a separate study, as likely to exhibit individuality of features and phenomena, and to be benefited by, or to necessitate, an individuality of treatment

In order to avoid such mistakes, and secure all possible advantage and benefit, it is needful that we should keep in our recollection those objects we purpose achieving

1 We must ever recollect that in many instances of general disease there is the danger of its extending, and that our first duty is to take such steps as shall secure to the best of our ability the immunity of those as yet unaffected The exercise of these preventive or prophylactic therapeutics is in veterinary medicine of the utmost importance, from the association and close contact which our patients so often hold with each other

By the proper application of remedies of a like class, it is not to be forgotten that in the individual we may exercise an influence whereby certain maladies of a recurring character may be diminished this will be particularly seen if we consider the numerous affections of the digestive organs to which the horse is liable And it is more through a careful and rational exercise of the principles of prophylactics or preventives than aught else that we may assert our right and capacity of acting as sanitary officers in warding off and reducing to the minimum the harassing and destructive epizootics to which our animals are liable

2 In managing the actually diseased, if we may not be able to cure—that is, to arrest and remove disordered activities when they arise—we should remember that much may be done to confer upon the animal sufficient power whereby it may be safely guided through the course of the disease without materially damaging its future usefulness, and leaving as a legacy such conditions as will render it at some future time more susceptible of the same or some other disorder.

Also that although as a rule wrong in principle to treat symptoms irrespective of morbid conditions, upon which they evidently depend, yet much benefit may result from judicious attempts at their alleviation Such palliative measures always recommend themselves to the careful practitioner, both from the immediate benefit to the suffering, and the chance that they will tend to obviate evil results and render recovery more perfect

The lines of our treatment are laid down for us in the nature, causes, and seat of the disease, together with agencies which are operating intrinsically and extrinsically, and the stage of the diseased process at which our intervention takes place

The exact forms in which our treatment comes into operation are—(a) The purely medicinal, comprising the employment, systemically and locally, of such medicinal agents and topical manipulatory interference as observation and experiment have indicated are likely to be productive of benefit (b) All measures of a dietetic and hygienic character which a just appreciation of the disease and its surroundings indicate, including a judicious arranging, not merely of the food and water, but also of the clothing, general treatment, and sanitary conditions of the location By these often more may be accomplished than through the use of drugs All must by the professional attendant be ordered and strictly indicated in detail.

SECTION II.

UNDER this section it is proposed to glance at some topics which may with equal propriety be regarded as belonging to the 'Theory or Science of Medicine' as to the 'Practice,' but a slight knowledge of which is very necessary ere the detailed description of disease is entered upon

CHAPTER I

NOSOLOGY, OR, THE DEFINITION, NOMENCLATURE, AND CLASSIFICATION OF DISEASE.

IN following out the limited but large subject, the 'PRACTICE OF EQUINE MEDICINE,' it will be found necessary both for the systematizing of our knowledge, and for the concentration of our facts and observation, as also as a ready means of access to what we have obtained, that we should follow to some extent at least the ordinarily recognised lines and principles upon which is constructed the '**Nosology**' of the present day

The diseases which engage the veterinarian's attention require to be defined and distinguished, both individually and as associated in groups They must be named, so that both as individuals and divisions they may be recognised and distinguished from other individuals and groups, and they require for convenience' sake, at least in their examination, to be relegated in classes, orders, and species

The defining, naming, and classifying of diseases, embracing and making up the department of nosology, have been carried out at different periods of the history of medicine on very varying and different principles

The idea enunciated by Sydenham and carried out by Sauvages, that diseases, like animals and plants, might be most satisfactorily studied and arranged, as zoologists and botanists have catalogued, in classes, orders, and genera, animals and plants, each class, order, and species marked off from every other by the exhibition of characteristic phenomena, has not sufficient attraction or usefulness to cause it to be carried out, and in our day has given place to one which, if less strict and methodical, is regarded as more natural

Our presently received and generally adopted system of defining disease is certainly what may be termed an artificial one, and takes for its essential or starting-point, in the definition and distinction of particular diseases, the possession or occurrence of the same symptoms or phenomena, either as they occur individually or are linked together in successively developed groups   In this way certainly some of the benefits of a definition are obtained, and each disease is by a short enumeration of leading features distinguished and marked off from every other

There is, however, much difference amongst pathologists, whether any attempted definition of disease ought to be drawn from a consideration of those outward signs and phenomena exhibited during the course of the disease, or from the internal pathological conditions upon which these phenomena are believed to depend

It is probably better, considering the changing character which by experimental investigation and by clinical observation is liable to be conferred on what we now regard as the proximate causes of disease, that the distinction and definition of it be conducted upon principles as far as possible removed from theory and the region of speculation   If we may not be able to give such a definition of any diseased condition as to include all its characteristics, and so accurately define and separate it from all others, that it shall for all time remain and prominently stand forth as a distinct and circumscribed and isolated thing, we may at least be able sufficiently to describe its exhibitional features and phenomena, that those who desire it may be able to identify it with accuracy sufficient for practical work and treatment

In the *nomenclature* or *naming* of disease there is encountered not only difficulty, but also much which is amusing, if not instructive.

The name of a disease, it has been well said, ought to be of such a nature that, as in the science of chemistry, anyone knowing only moderately well the principles of the science ought at once on hearing it to have a not unjust idea of its nature and character—that the name, in short, ought to be an epitome of the definition

This of course may also be objected to, seeing that the definition of disease drawn from an appreciation of certain proximate causes is ever, with a change of views regarding such cause, liable to express what would be considered an error

From the earliest times when men have observed diseases, names have been given to these expressive of very different ideas, and drawn from very various sources. Some have been named from the parts affected, some from the leading or characteristic feature or features, some from a peculiar physical character of the results of the local diseased action, and some from the situations or localities where first observed or most usually encountered.

There is no doubt that the nomenclature of disease will change as knowledge of disease becomes more precise and definite, but merely to change a name because we fancy that it has hitherto incorrectly had attached to it a certain assemblage of symptoms which we now believe are the result of some cause other than the one formerly credited with their production is unwise, seeing our knowledge of these matters is liable to change

As has been justly said, no one has a call to change an old name when this has been largely recognised, certainly to a new disease, as to a new object, he who indicates its existence is rightfully entitled to give it a name

Classification—Having described and defined our disease, as also given to it a name, it is of advantage to arrange these diseases, which we now look upon as veritable entities, in groups and orders

No doubt there are good and sufficient grounds to be urged by those who have propounded and who support the very different principles upon which the classification of diseases has been based. Being, in the majority of instances, a matter of convenience and facility for carrying out certain definite purposes, and for the attainment of certain definite ends, it is easily understood that, as a means to the accomplishment of these ends, this mere classification will vary in accordance with the dissimilarity or variety of the ultimate object in view. The greater number of the systems of classification adopted are artificial. Some few, indeed, make an approach to what may with some consistency be regarded as natural; in these there is an attempt to bring together diseases which have natural relations or affinities with each other.

It is scarcely our province, nor is it probable that a detailed account of the various principles upon which classifications of disease have been made will to us in our present study be fraught with much benefit. Still we may notice, as showing the extent of ground and the diversity of its character which has been travelled over in formulating these different classifications, that they have been based upon—

(a) *Nature and ascertained, or supposed, causes of disease;*

(b) *The pathological conditions accompanying disease,*

(c) *The symptoms or characteristic phenomena resulting from the morbid condition,*

(d) *From a consideration of the general nature and locality of the diseased conditions;* and many others

If it be true what has been said with respect to human medicine, that the time has not yet come for the formulating of a classification of diseases on a basis comprehensive enough, having the details of its plan to agree in every respect with the facts as they exist in nature, simply because the material does not exist, " and that attempts to make so-called natural systems of arrangement must end in disappointment, on account of the uncertain and fluctuating data on which they must be based "—if this be true as respects that grand division of medical science, compared with which our special province is but a child of yesterday as regards its association with science and liberal knowledge, we need scarcely wonder that we are compelled to confess, nor need we be ashamed to do so, that veterinary nosology is yet in an infantile state, and that the classification of the diseases of animals is not only difficult but defective and imperfectly understood. While it is quite evident that until pathologies, human and veterinary, are cultivated side by side in their true and reciprocal bearing, no real advance in this particular direction in either field of inquiry, of a philosophical and comprehensive character, can be expected to be made.

And although practical medicine will never suffer to be bound by strict and rigid classification, description, or nomenclature, still, in studying it systematically, a distinct and understood system of classification of the subjects to be treated is of decided advantage.

The arrangement or classification of equine diseases which seems most easily comprehended, and which for practical purposes seems as efficient as any other, and which I shall endeavour to adhere to as closely as possible in further describing these in detail, is that which regards diseases as forming two great groups.

GROUP I.—GENERAL, OR SYSTEMIC DISEASES : diseases which seem to affect the entire system, or at least the greater part of it, at the same time, and in which the entire functions of the animal body are simultaneously disturbed.

GROUP II.—LOCAL DISEASES · usually sporadic diseases, in which special organs or systems are primarily disturbed, and in the course of which lesions tend to be localized

The first group is divided into two classes .

Class A —**Fevers** and some other affections, chiefly *exogenous* diseases, depending for their development upon the operation of agencies acting from without the animal body.

Class B —**Constitutional** diseases, such as appear to depend upon an indwelling disposition or *cachexia ;* although chiefly *endogenous*, they may result from the entrance of agencies from without

The second group, local diseases characterized by the existence of particular local morbid processes, is divided into many classes corresponding to the system of organs affected.

In the first group, that of general or systemic diseases, there are included diseases infectious or contagious, propagable by intercourse of one animal with another, or by inoculation, diseases known as *epizoötic* or *enzootic*, and diseases recognised as constitutional. With the exception of the last class, the others are often grouped and spoken of as diseases of the *zymotic* class.

The *exogenous* class, then, of general or systemic diseases, comprehends and includes all of the principal diseases of our animals which are spoken of as *epizootic, enzoötic, infectious, contagious,* or *specific* · all those which we believe due to peculiar telluric or meteorological conditions, to the noxious emanations from decaying animal or vegetable matter, and those depending upon specific disease poisons, whatever these may be, capable of passage and of propagation from one living organism to another, and in that passage and propagation capable of infinite multiplication, and communicable by direct contact, or indirectly through various channels of communication and association, contaminating food supplies and drinking water or infecting the an

---

CHAPTER II

OF EXOGENOUS AGENCIES, SPECIFIC AND CONTAGIOUS DISEASES, AND ENZOOTIC AND EPIZOOTIC INFLUENCES

SEEING that in the course of the consideration of the details pertaining to the practice of equine medicine there must of necessity be frequent cause for the employment of the terms 'contagious' and 'infectious,' so generally employed with reference to diseases of all animals, before entering upon the study of these affections in order and individually, it will be useful to give a little attention to those terms *contagion* and *contagious* diseases, *enzootic* and *epizootic* influences, so often in our mouths

A contagious, otherwise specific, disease, may be defined as an unnatural or morbid state of an animal body, owing its existence to the reception from without of certain living entities which have been developed in connection with an animal previously in a similar diseased condition

The implantation of the virus or specific poison of a contagious disease may take place directly or indirectly, by inoculation, by contact, or by emanations proceeding from the diseased

It seems highly probable that many circumstances, operating both in the diseased and the healthy, extrinsically and intrinsically, have an influence in determining the extent or virulence, so to speak, of the specific infecting virus. It is also highly probable that no specific or contagious disease ever originates *de novo*. This was not always the opinion, nor even now are all agreed upon the certainty of it.

Whether contagious diseases are in every instance of their appearance to be regarded as originating from the reception and development in those affected of the germs of the particular malady—it matters not whether this fructifying element be specific organisms, living and particulate, which by virtue of their inherent life-energy originate this particular diseased action, or are merely the bearers of the more inappreciable and occult agent, the specific contagium—it is at least certain that these disease-producing germs, when received, whether animate contagia or not, comport themselves in the production of the morbid conditions and phenomena which follow their reception into the animal body in a manner analogous to ordinary poisons, or medicinal agents given in poisonous doses, and that they are regulated by general laws applicable to both classes of agents.

But although specific disease-germs, or poisons, are, like ordinary poisonous agents, possessed of certain common properties, and yield obedience to several laws of general applicability, there are still many points of divergence or peculiarity in the actions of animal poisons inducing contagious or specific disease, which peculiarities account for much that is specific in the natural history of these maladies.

They resemble ordinary poisons in that when received into an animal body they are followed by the exhibition of certain phenomena or specific actions; they also, like poisons, preserve between their entrance and development of symptoms a varying period of repose; and further, the phenomena resulting from the reception of both may vary in accordance with the quantity received, and the power or capacity of the recipient.

Morbid poisons differ from ordinary poisonous agents most markedly in that when received into the animal body there is conferred upon them the power of indefinite increase or multiplication. The most minute quantity of the virus of glanders will, when introduced into the system of the horse, contaminate the whole circulating fluid and much of the secretions, and produce material sufficient to infect many hundreds of animals

Another remarkable difference between these specific contagia or poisons, and other toxic agents, is that many of them, when received into the animal body, possess the property of exhausting the constitution of its susceptibility, or at least greatly lessening it, to another successful inoculation with the same virus.

In addition to this analogy between the laws regulating the action of ordinary and specific animal poisons, experimental research has taught us that the modes of their operation are likewise very much the same, in so far as, being absorbed by the veins, they, like ordinary poisonous or medicinal agents, enter the circulation, produce upon the constituents of the blood a peculiar or specific action, pass through the blood, and ultimately produce their specific local results in specific elemental tissue changes or otherwise, in certain determinate parts or tissues, between which and these specific implanted agents there is a particular affinity.

Nature of the Contagium of Contagious Diseases — The disease-producing agent or material developed and elaborated in the animal body, which, when implanted into another animal organism, induces a similar disease, is known by the name of *contagium, specific virus*, or *materies morbi*. It has been variously regarded as consisting of noxious gases, palludial or animal effluvia, organic molecules, or germs which have been in existence with, and are now detached from, living animal matter. Certainly the direction in which present pathological experimental research seems to point is that of regarding all contagious and specific diseases as the result of the introduction into the animal body of distinct particulate and living organisms—true animate contagia—which have not been the result of, or developed or elaborated from, degraded or degenerating proto or bioplasm, but are the descendants of similarly endowed and organized forms, living entities, proceeding from, and tending to, the generation or development of similar living entities

This latest view of the origin of infectious and specific diseases, as consisting in individual living organisms, although not universally believed, is yet extensively endorsed and acquiesced in by a very large section of the most able observers, and investigators in the science of biology. While when adopted and acted upon in its entirety, and to the full extent of its bearings, by us as practical veterinary surgeons and as sanitary inspectors, or conservators of animal and public health, it wonderfully simplifies our actions, and strengthens our hands in dealing with those terribly destructive and harassing scourges which from time to time have devastated communities and nations.

Arguments have been adduced to prove that at least certain inoculable, contagious, and specific diseases of animals, as *glanders* in the horse, *rabies* in the dog, and *anthrax* in cattle, may be developed spontaneously, and that in these instances, instead of accepting the theory or view of animate contagia as the actively operating cause, we must turn to our knowledge of the laws of chemistry and physiology for an explanation of their origin

The greater and more weighty part of the evidence in favour of the spontaneous enzootic origin of the contagious or specific diseases of animals is undoubtedly negative in character, *i e* to say that cases are occasionally met with in which it is impossible to trace the origin of the particular disease to the individual originating source   This is easily understood when we remember the many and unseen modes by which may be conveyed the active agent of propagation.   Cases of zymotic pleuro-pneumonia, or of the contagious mouth-and-foot fever of cattle, regularly occur, in which it is impossible to trace the individual infecting animal, yet the whole history of these diseases militates against the idea of their being propagated by any other agency than specific contagion, and if for contagious lung-fever and zymotic aphtha, so for others of the same class

Enzootic and Epizootic Influences.—Although it may be perfectly true, as stated, that contagious diseases must ever be regarded as originating in the action of specific agencies acting from without, whether these consist of malarial emanations, germinal matter separated from previously living animals, or individual living entities, there is at the same time no doubt that, as to their time of appearance, the severity of their indi-

vidual manifestation, and the extent of the outbreak, they are
largely influenced—the whole class of the zymotic, contagious,
and specific diseases in animals—by surrounding local conditions
and circumstances, such operating causes constituting the so-
called *enzootic* influences, and any diseases so originating are
recognised as *enzootic* diseases. The moulding, determining,
or enzootic influences are such as may be peculiar to the
physical nature or character of the district, its geological
formation, its altitude, nature of soil, character of the water-
supply, variations of temperature, etc , also such influences as
operate through medium of food, character of the location
or stabling, ventilation and sanitary conditions, nature and
amount of the work they are engaged in, and the age of the
animals.

When these same diseases so originating rapidly extend
from the foci of their origin and attack great numbers of
animals, at the same time and at varying intervals of time,
they are spoken of as *epizootic* diseases, or *panzootic* diseases .
and the influences determining the expansion or spread of
such diseases are termed *epizootic* or *panzootic* influences

The conditions which favour the passing into active operation of the enzootic influences are many, chief of which are
associated with the specific morbid virus itself, and the facilities
offered by the living soil in which it is to be implanted The
specific disease material upon which all these diseases exist,
and without which they would cease to be, although not always,
in a state of activity, is never entirely and absolutely destroyed,
but is ever ready, from some centre where it exists, to develop
and extend itself, and become epizootic when surrounding
conditions are favourable.

The entire history of these specific diseases gives us the
same information . the constancy of the one persisting element,
the infecting virus, their irregular alternations of active development and recurring quietude.

It also tells us of the undiminished power or virulence of
the *materies morbi*, its unvarying modes of development, its
unvarying issue in similar organic changes in the animal body,
and its production with no variation of the same identical
specific virus or contagious entity by which it has been propagated from age to age.

Of the influences which determine these contagious diseases to move on from the centres of development or appearance, and spread in somewhat erratic manner until large numbers of animals are seriously affected, much has been said, but comparatively little determined.

With truth it may be said that the whole which can be affirmed with certainty regarding *epizootics* is that which has been remarked of *epidemics*, "That there must be some distempered condition of circumstances around us, some secret power that is operating injuriously upon our system, and to this we give the name of *epidemic influence*, or constitution."

From the study and observation of the phenomena presented during the course of both epidemics and epizootics, there appears a certain feasibility—to give the results of observation, as far as they have been carried, no higher appellation—in viewing this influence as regulated by certain laws, which no doubt with more extended and accurate observation may yet be formulated somewhat in conformity with the importance of the subject. However, we may even now assert that this epizootic influence, whatever it may be, amongst other laws which seem to regulate its operations and modes of manifestations, is evidently possessed of a special determining influence, not only disposing to disease, independently of any other known cause, but also conferring greater virulence on ordinary recognised causes of particular diseases. It seems also to give evidence of its existence by variation in form and type of particular disease—at one time *sthenic*, at another *asthenic*. To this prevailing form or type, diseases of a very different class seem to conform themselves; for during the prevalence of a well-marked epizootic, other diseases which may occur are inclined to exhibit features somewhat akin to the speciality of symptoms characteristic of the prevailing epizootic. It is also to be observed that epizootic influences are most marked and powerful at the outset of an outbreak, becoming milder towards the termination: that during the prevalence of epizootics, particularly if of a virulent character, common diseases in the human subject, when affecting a class or system of organs similar to that upon which the existing epizootic has particularly seized, are inclined to show marked deviations from the usual lines of recognised symptoms and character, with a tendency to imitate the prevailing epizootic

While it is also deserving of notice that during the continuance of severe epizootics, ordinary wounds, either received accidentally or inflicted in the course of surgical practice, are more inclined to show tardiness in healing, with an unhealthy condition of granulating tissue, than wounds of the same character during seasons when such influences do not prevail

SECTION III.

DETAILED DESCRIPTION OF GENERAL DISEASES.

A. IDIOPATHIC FEVERS AND OTHER DISEASES CHIEFLY OF AN EXOGENOUS ORIGIN.

CHAPTER I.

SIMPLE FEVER —CONTINUED FEVER —FEBRICULA.

Definition —*A simple functional disturbance of comparatively short but variable duration, characterized and accompanied by rigors, elevation of temperature, frequent pulse and respirations*

What is intended to direct attention to now is not that complex morbid state which more or less constantly accompanies many diseases as part of their phenomena, and is modified and shaped, so to speak, by the nature and character of the disease of which it is a prominent symptom This fever, or pyrexial condition, we speak of invariably with an accompanying or qualifying word or term indicative of the organ or system of organs invaded, from the lesions of which the disease, of which the fever is merely a symptom, derives its name Thus we speak of the fever of pneumonia, or the fever of enteritis, etc. Nor yet is it of that febrile state which, to the surgeon, is so important in connection both with his operative interference and injuries accidentally received, and variously termed inflammatory, irritative, hectic, or typhoid But it is to fever *per se* as a distinct and independent diseased condition, unconnected with any appreciable lesion or structural change, a condition possessing all the essential characters of the true febrile state, but arising independently of any antecedent disease, and terminating without the production of further morbid complications It is to that diseased condition in which the

3—2

febrile symptoms constitute the prominent or only features, which runs a more or less definite course without the necessary development of any distinct local lesion, to fever as a *primary* or *idiopathic* condition, and not to fever plus other local changes, which is appropriately regarded as fever *secondary*, or *symptomatic*

Ætiology —Although in the present state of our knowledge it may be impossible to state, in such a manner as to be perfectly free from objection, the ultimate or true causes of fever, and to give the rationale of the mode of their operation so as to construct a perfect theory of the pyrexial state, although we may not be able to tell what are the exact relations of pyrexia and tissue-disintegration, whether they are cause and effect or are both the result of a common cause, whether the production or discharge of the animal heat be primarily or chiefly affected, we are nevertheless in a position to observe that many causes by which animals and ourselves are surrounded and acted upon have a wondrous influence upon the textures of the living body, and that apparently very trifling influences are productive of very great and important changes in these bodies

Judging from a rather extensive collection of facts, it seems highly probable that many cases of febricula owe their origin to the entrance of some of the contagia of the specific fevers, that this is only prevented from fully developing by certain conditions operating intrinsically and extrinsically, and by the amount of the poison received It is also not uncommon to find what seems simple fever developing into some more determinate and distinct form

In the horse, simple continued fever is, however, encountered most frequently in cases where animals, hitherto in a comparatively natural condition of life, have been suddenly subjected to the influence of conditions which, compared with those they have previously experienced, may not inaptly be designated artificial   These may be largely classed as sudden variations in the temperature surrounding them, exhaustion, and fatigue

It is particularly a disorder affecting the horses of dealers, or those who regularly receive consignments of animals from districts or individuals where previously they have enjoyed greater liberty and more freedom of location Rarely are horses in any numbers brought from markets or the country, and placed in stables in cities, without a considerable proportion of these exhibiting symptoms, more or less marked, of fever

Exposure to wet, fatigue, and exhaustion induced by travelling or imperfect and irregular dieting, or, where these causes may not be blamed, simple transference from the open air and unrestrained exercise to confinement in stables, are evidently the agents which to ordinary observers are the most potent factors in the production of this disordered condition

Whether these are to be regarded as the disturbers of the nervous centres controlling the discharge of the animal heat, and by the retention of this heat causing elevation of body-temperature and ultimate disorder of the functions of animal nutrition, or whether the whole chain of phenomena should be regarded as proceeding from and inseparably linked to original textural changes as the originating cause, it is for us, in the application of preventive measures, at least sufficient to know that certain recognisable and controllable agencies are obviously capable of thus operating in an injurious manner on the animal body

Nature and Symptoms—In ordinary cases, and free from complications, simple fever is a comparatively mild and benign disease, disposed to run a definite course, and to terminate favourably in from two to eight days It is essentially a disturbed or perturbed state of all, or nearly all, the chief functions of the animal body

Derangement of the functions of enervation is indicated by disturbed or perverted sensation, by pain and general prostration, the circulatory and respiratory functions are affected, as indicated by the frequency and altered character of the pulse and by the embarrassed or accelerated breathing, digestion is in abeyance and the secretory functions perverted or impaired, while the chemical changes always in operation in the animal body are in the febrile state particularly active, as evidenced by the marked and rapid wasting of muscular tissue

The two great central points in this condition of pyrexia, as in fever, when occurring as a complex morbid process in association with distinct or recognised structural changes, where it is superadded to other recognised diseased states, are disintegration of tissue and disturbance of temperature

The relation which these two phenomena bear to each other, as also their connection, severally and combined, with the existence and maintenance of the pyrexial state, are questions which even yet require further elucidation by comparison of facts derived from observation and experiment.

According to investigations it has been found that in the early stages of fever there is a slight increase of the discharge of carbonic acid, but a constant and distinct increase in the elimination of urea. Towards the termination of the fever the loss of weight has been stated to be most marked, and to be chiefly through that of water and carbonic acid.

The question may be asked, Whence comes this excess of nitrogen? Not from the food, we know, for little or none may be taken. It must come from the tissues, from the albumen of their formed elements or the fluids; probably the former. This is believed from the fact that the salt secreted in fever is potass, not soda, thus the source of the nitrogen must contain potass. But blood-plasma possesses chiefly sodium salts, while the formed materials of the blood— the globules and the sarcos elements of muscular tissue— contain salts of the other base. Consequently urea, the nitrogen compound, is probably the result of disintegration of these tissues.

As regards the production and discharge of heat in the pyrexial state, there is much difficulty; nor will it, in all probability, be determined until more progress has been made in our knowledge of the relations in health between temperature and heat-production. It is well known that the production of heat may be much increased in the animal body without any elevation of temperature, and that a high temperature may exist without increased production.

The results of the measurement of the actual amount of heat discharged in fever has led to rather different and somewhat conflicting views, by different observers, as to the extent of heat-production taking place.

Whatever may be the relation of the textural changes and disintegration of tissue to the febrile state, whether the heat-production or the heat-distribution, or discharge, is primarily or chiefly disturbed, it seems most probable that the ultimate cause must be looked for in the changes which occur in the textural elements of the tissues rather than in disturbed nerve force, which operating on the discharge of the superabundant heat produced, retaining it within the body, elevates the temperature and so disturbs nutrition.

In observing the course and development of simple fever in the horse, there is little difficulty in marking it in its entirety into the three stages of *attack*, *development*, and *decline*.

The *attack* is not, as a rule, insidious, but is delivered at once; it is ushered in by a distinct rigor, or shivering-fit, or, in less severe cases, by a simple staring of the coat, which may persistently maintain this condition or may exhibit alternate smoothness and elevation, the temperature of the surface of the body seems at this time lowered, with an unequal distribution of warmth in the extremities.

Muscular pain is shown by the disinclination to move, and by the alternate resting of different limbs; enforced movement is evidently painful, while the impression conveyed by simply looking at the animal is that he is suffering from languor and weariness, and very uncomfortable. The pulse at this stage is frequent, probably seventy per minute, and rather small in volume; it may be hard—that is, feel as if the tonicity of the arterial coats had increased—or it may be the opposite, the respirations merely slightly accelerated, not altered in character, internal temperature, as indicated by the thermometer, 102° to 106° F, or even higher; there is little or no appetite, but thirst is not marked.

Following this stage, in a few hours, we have the second, the perfect *development* of the febrile condition. The surface-temperature is increased, no staring coat, rigors gone; pulse increased in volume from the now established condition of reaction; appetite the same, with thirst most probably. The bowels are now seen to be confined, and the urinary secretion lessened in amount, while, if observed, it may give evidence of alteration in character by change in colour and consistence; it contains less water, more urea and colouring matter than in health; this diminution of the amount of water is most marked at the outset of the febrile state.

Throughout the continuance of the fever the perverted con-

dition of the secretions will be obvious, the skin maintaining
a rather harsh and dry character, the bowels inclined to be
confined, and the urine limited in amount The temperature
will remain high for some days until defervescence occurs
there will most probably be occasional slight exacerbation of
the febrile symptoms, indicated by the elevation of temperature towards night, with remission in the morning One
feature characteristic of the temperature in simple continued
fever deserves notice , it is the great rapidity or suddenness
with which it reaches a very high elevation, and its correspondingly rapid decline to one moderately high At its very
outset the temperature will probably be 106° F., while the fall
within a few hours may be 4°, the extreme height not being
again reached during the disease

Although, considering the character of its entire course,
simple fever in the horse may safely be regarded as continued
fever, there are cases where it exhibits characters of the remittent type , i e that although the febrile symptoms are, as a
rule, continuous and steadily persistent until a marked change
occurs, we yet meet with cases where these symptoms suffer
abatement during the progress of the disease, to be again distinctly marked by a return to their former severity

Some cases move so rapidly through the various phases of
invasion, full development, and decline, that the pyrexial condition has disappeared in two or three days, and the only trace
of its existence may be a trifling amount of debility, indicated
by an absence of the usual vivacity and energy of movement.
In more persistent examples, however, the change from the
second stage of full development of the pyrexial symptoms to
subsidence or decline of the fever is obvious enough Here
we find the skin assumes a moist and pliant condition ; it may
be bedewed with sensible perspiration, and accompanied with
an increased discharge of urine Such cases, however, where
the moist condition of the skin is so visibly marked in the
horse, I have found are usually such as seem inclined to pass
rapidly through their different stages, and are not unfrequently
those, also, where we find indications of the true remittent
type of the fever

At the outset of this condition of pyrexia, the animal may
seem seriously ill , the pulse increased in frequency to seventy

per minute, small in volume and tense, the respirations hurried, rigors, or even shivering, either largely distributed over the body, or more probably confined to the large extensor muscles of the arm and those of the haunch and thigh these rigors may even be accompanied—generally followed—by the occurrence of local and patchy perspirations Succeeding these conditions, in a few hours the temperature may fall considerably, the surface of the body assume a more natural condition, and altogether, the horse seems much improved ; he may even be disposed to look for food. These favourable conditions, however, do not continue, or at least are only of limited duration, and are followed by a return of the former pyrexial symptoms, usually not so violent as at first, but neither so disposed to remit, and are likely to persist until a more gradual and steady decline is ushered in

The subsidence or decline of the pyrexial symptoms, notably the lowering of the elevated temperature in fever, is spoken of under the term of *defervescence* , when this decline, or lowering of temperature, takes place suddenly—at a bound, as it were— it is called a *crisis* ; when it is accomplished steadily but gradually, a *lysis*

In simple fever in the horse, the defervescence as a rule—at least the severe cases—occurs in neither of these manners, but rather through a combination of both There is first of all, as already noticed, a rather sudden and marked decline in the temperature, which having reached the point marked by this first break, or fall, does not decline further by sudden or spasmodic jerks, but is characterized by a gradual subsidence

The fall in the temperature and abatement of the other pyrexial symptoms is accompanied by a return of appetite, and usually by an increase of the water eliminated through the kidneys It is, however, to be remembered that in all cases of simple fever, should an animal suffer from some previous debility or structural change of any organ, there is the probability that diseased activities may be there re-established, and complications result

Treatment —Simple continued fever in the horse, as in every other animal, is a benign affection not disposed to terminate in serious complications, and inclined of itself to run a natural course, terminating in restoration to health

To ordinary observers it appears a more serious affair than many others which are attended with dangerous complications, and hence the aid of skilled assistance is oftener invoked than would be were its true nature understood Being, from its nature, disposed to run a certain and determinate course, and issue in a favourable termination, it is in all cases inexpedient to make any attempts to cut this course short by what is termed a cure. Pitcairn has well said: " I do not like fever curers. You may guide a fever; you cannot cure it. What would you think of a pilot who attempted to quell a storm ? Either position is equally absurd In the storm you steer the ship as well as you can, and in the fever you can only employ patience and judicious measures to meet the difficulties of the case "

Following these indications, the points which demand our attention are—(1) Moderation of the pyrexial symptoms, as vascular excitement, respiratory disturbance, and elevation of temperature, at least where these are excessive. (2) Following the subsidence of them, to assist the system, when depressed, to establish a reaction. (3) To combat symptoms, untoward or unexpected, as they occur

The first of these is best secured by at once, if it is possible, placing the animal in a moderately warm loose box, clean, well lighted, and capable of being well ventilated , while even if the box at our command is not possessed of all these sanitary requirements, which few are, it is generally to be preferred to an ordinary stall During the cold stage it is advisable to make an attempt to equalize the surface-temperature by good hand-rubbing and moderate clothing, not, however, troubling the horse with overmuch handling, rather resting contented with the application of a light woollen rug, and, in certain animals, with placing a set of bandages on the limbs

In the employment of medicinal agents I have found much benefit from salines, as chlorate of potass or nitrate of potass alone, or combined with sweet spirits of nitre and camphor A very good formula, and one which I have employed with much benefit for many years in simple fever, as well as in other complicated and more serious disturbances where fever is present as a constant and marked feature of the disease, is—

℞ Potass Chloras vel Potass Nit. ʒiii ; Spir Æther. Nit fl ʒi ; Liq Ammon Acet. fl. ʒiv.; Aquæ ad oj. M fiat haustus This may be given twice, or, if needful, thrice daily If this draught is given only twice daily, it will be good to allow chlorate of potass, either alone or combined with nitrate of potass, from two to six drachms of each of the salts, during the day, in the drinking water, which, when thirst is a prominent feature, is seldom refused Unless the weather is very cold, I am not aware that any benefit is derived from compelling the animal to drink tepid water, or at least water raised above the temperature of the surrounding atmosphere.

In moderate cases the draught mentioned, continued for two days, will produce very favourable results, and when discontinued, the salines, as chlorate and nitrate of potass, may be continued for one or two days longer

As soon as the excessive pyrexial symptoms become mitigated, the animal will most probably be inclined to take some food, which should, however, be allowed only in moderation, and of such a character as to keep the bowels in a good and moist condition. Grass, when it can be got, is preferable to aught else, succeeding this, good sweet hay, probably damped, a few steamed oats, with bran or a few carrots

During the course of the fever, it is of advantage to remove the clothing and bandages from the body and limbs once or twice daily, and gently to damp or sponge the body-surface previous to replacing the covering. Should the bowels continue confined, it is rarely advisable to give aloes or any purge during the course of the disturbance. If given at all, let it be when recovery is sufficiently pronounced, when good may result from the exhibition of a mild laxative, by which effete material, which may have resulted from the continued disturbance, may be passed off by the increased action of the bowels.

Confirmed constipation during the continuance of the fever ought to be combated by the dieting or the use of tepid water enemata.

CHAPTER II

INFLUENZA —EPIZOOTIC OR PANZOOTIC CATARRHAL FEVER

Synonyms—Epizootic catarrh, Horse sickness, Horse distemper, Febris catarrhalis, etc.

Definition—*A peculiar or probably a specific febrile disease of the horse, generally appearing as an epizootic, in which the organs of respiration and circulation are most uniformly involved, attended with marked lassitude and prostration, with in many cases complications arising from implication of those of digestion and locomotion.*

Historical Notice.—Although from very early—even the most remote—periods, it is perfectly evident, when we peruse the records of the past, that men have paid attention to diseases which have originated in the supposed action of extraordinary telluric and meteorological influences, and which from centres of origin have spread over extensive territories and kingdoms, devastating and impoverishing by their destruction of men as well as animals, there is not, as far as we are aware, any credible notice of the existence of influenza in either animals or men previous to the tenth century. It is nearly the opening of the fourteenth century (1299) ere there is evidence indicative of the occurrence of this panzootic catarrhal fever in horses. At this date Larentius Rusius speaks of it as a certain fever which broke out amongst horses at Seville, marked by want of appetite, drooping head, weeping eyes, and hurried beating at the flanks. He says "The malady was epidemical, and more than one thousand horses died." In 1648 Solleysel, a celebrated French veterinarian, describes an outbreak of an epizooty amongst the horses of the French army in Germany. It began by fever, great prostration and running from the eyes, and there was an abundant mucous discharge of a greenish colour from the nostrils. The horses also experienced loss of appetite, and their ears were cold. Few of those attacked recovered. The treatment adopted was with a view to neutralize the malignity of the poison, and to fortify nature, for it was a poison, says this author, which gave rise to the disorder, and was the cause of the fever (Fleming's "Animal Plagues"). The year 1688 is marked by a visit of epidemic catarrhal fever all over Europe, spreading from east to west. In this catarrh horses also participated, being, it was remarked, attacked first. In 1693 a similar attack is also recorded, at first appearing amongst horses, to be followed by a similar fever in man. In 1699 we have notice of a widespread visit of this catarrhal fever both in Europe and America, while Ruthly, in his history of the weather and seasons, mentions that in 1727-28, over the greater part of England and Ireland, and also in the remote parts of the kingdom, horses were seized with cough, sore throat, and shortness of breath, and that many died

In 1732 Gibson, of London, gives a very interesting and full account of a severe horse distemper, which broke out amongst the horses of the metropolis and over the country

In this notice of the epizooty of 1732, Gibson mentions that although not fatal, he believed it to be very catching, seeing that where any horse was seized with it, those on each side were very generally infected as soon as he began to run at the nose

This epidemic, or epizootic catarrh, appears to have had a most universal distribution, and to have produced universal alarm, both Old and New World being visited by it, travelling in both apparently from north to south.

From 1732 to 1767 there is only notice of a moderate amount of epidemic or epizootic fevers. Huxham, in "Observations on the Air and Epidemical Diseases, London, 1758," notices that in 1743 many horses suffered from illness and emaciation, the result of colds and sore throats While in the latter year influenza again spread over both America and Europe, affecting first animals, and afterwards men, being particularly virulent in London and over England.

The prevalence of this catarrhal disease was again, by those chronicling its ravages, connected with meteorological and telluric disturbances.

Since the beginning of the present century influenza has in this country appeared amongst our horses in a markedly epizootic form on several occasions, certainly in 1850, 1863, 1864, and in 1871 and 1872. In America, under the name of "Horse Disease," there was in 1872 and 1873 a very widely distributed—and although not very fatal, nevertheless, from the number of animals affected, an extremely harassing and expensive—outbreak of influenza.

Starting from Toronto, where it appeared about the 1st of October, and where in little more than a week by far the larger number of the horses in that city were invalided, it had before the end of the month distributed itself, and appeared at the chief centres of population, not only in the Dominion, but also over a large area of several of the states of the Union.

Nature of the Disease.—The name "Influenza" is, like many others in medical nosology, much abused, and where most carefully and guardedly employed, is rather ambiguous. It is often a convenient term under which to shroud our doubt or ignorance, and when employed by one man it often conveys to another a different impression from that which it was intended to do.

It is not invariable in its forms of development, nor strictly uniform in its symptoms. The fever of one season or district will present considerable variations both in symptoms and lesions from that occurring in a different locality or at another time. These variations, it may be, can to a certain extent be accounted for by the consideration of many extrinsic influences which may be brought to bear on the animal constitution. However, there are forms where none of these influences seem sufficient to account for the differences exhibited in its development during life, nor for the dissimilarity of the lesions observable after death in only variations of one and the same malady.

It seems to originate under favourable surrounding conditions through the reception into the animal body, and its development there, of what is probably a specific animal virus or reproductive agent whereby the circulating life-fluid, the blood, is first vitiated, and after a varying period of latency, inducing disturbed enervation, resulting in prostration, great debility, and fever. The peculiar or specific action of the contagium, whether this be unwholesome gases generated by decay and putrefaction of animal or vegetable matter, plasmic or bioplasmic spores or granules emanating from already diseased animal textures or living particulate organisms, issuing from antecedent and similar organisms, and passing on to the production of corresponding organic entities, it is for our present purpose sufficient to know that these are as yet undetermined, the specific action, it would appear, is exhibited, developed, or brought to maturity in connection with particular organs, structures, and tissues As to the frequency of its location and apparent severity of action, this specific poison shows marked and steadily distinctive preferences

The mucous membrane of the nasal passages, the eyes, throat, and upper air passages, are the situations and structures most frequently and regularly invaded Following these in susceptibility, we notice the bronchi, the textures of the lungs, and the pleuræ, and in a smaller number of cases the mucous membrane and structures of the alimentary canal and its associated glands and secretory organs; while in some manifestations the force of the disease seems expended on another class of structures—the serous and fibro-serous

When the agent or factor immediately acting in the production of the disease is sufficiently potent to issue in the full development of the pyrexial state, it will be found that in all such well-marked accompanying fevers the type is inclined to be remittent, with daily, or rather evening, exacerbations These exacerbations are maintained throughout the course of the disease, which in the ordinary catarrhal form is of very variable duration, until perfect defervescence is established, which is usually not suddenly, but gradually by lysis.

From the mode in which influenza is spread and developed over vast tracts of countries, as also from the forms of seizures observed in men and animals, together with the organs and textures specially involved, and the symptoms which all animals exhibit, it has been concluded that in its intrinsic nature influenza is closely allied, if not identical, in men and animals; however, the differences in the structural changes occurring during the progress of the disease in the horse, as also the general severity of the symptoms, and the larger percentage of fatal results, seem to indicate that this particular blood-contamination in this animal is not identical with that which is encountered in man It is indeed highly probable that the organisms, if we accept the immediately inducing agencies as of this nature, possess in each individual species an individuality and specific distinctness for each

species, and that this diseased condition owes its existence in
each species to the reception of its own particular specific
poison, and to no other   As so far corroborative of this is the
fact, that whatever may be the type of the epizootic in any
particular outbreak, this is in the greater number of the cases
maintained throughout the period of its existence in the
district

ÆTIOLOGY AND MODES OF PROPAGATION

Generally, in all well-marked outbreaks of influenza, the
seizures amongst the horses of a large district of country have
been so universal, neither age, sex, breed, nor condition
either of physical strength or sanitary location apparently
influencing its spread, that at a first and casual view causes
or determining influences seem to be completely beyond our
discerning   More carefully considered, however, we find that
influenza, like other epizootic, zymotic, and contagious disease, is largely aided in its dissemination over countries and
districts, and in its maturation of development in individuals,
by predisposing or favouring influences, consisting of, or
owing their existence to, certain surrounding conditions
which environ the animal, or under which its life and life
functions are carried out

So largely do these favouring, determining, or predisposing
influences operate in the distribution and development of
influenza, that it is highly probable that the severity of
individual cases, as also the rapidity of its dissemination, is
more to be attributed to the condition in which the disease
finds the patient than to any inherent power of the poison
itself

Although the exact nature of the epizootic influences which
give rise to influenza is unknown save in so far as we may
be able to observe that, like all other epizootics, it seems, as
regards its appearance, virulence, and spread, to be regulated
by certain laws, the more potent of these factors or influences
which operate in determining or predisposing to its appearance
are cognizable by every ordinary observer

All exhausting and debilitating influences overwork, bad
feeding, unwholesome sanitary conditions—as defective ventilation, darkness, dampness, and filth—tend to excessive waste of
the component structures of the animal body, as well as pre-

vent the natural elimination and removal of the worn-out and impure tissue elements, thereby deteriorating and degrading that upon which all structures rely for their sustenance and power, the blood, and rendering it a convenient medium and soil for the reception and growth of organic poisons

Influenza, although it may occur at any season of the year, is more common during late spring and autumn than at other seasons   At these particular periods horses, from the activity of the skin incident to the change of their hairy covering, are very susceptible to adverse atmospheric influences   violent and extreme alternations of temperature, undue exposure to extremes of heat and cold, are at this time more likely to act injuriously upon them   Add to this confinement in damp, warm, and close stables, and we can easily comprehend that ordinary coughs or colds, induced by atmospheric influences, are more likely to pass on to bronchitis and pneumonia, or bad forms of influenza to occur if this epizootic is prevailing

We know well enough that with darkness in stables is usually associated dampness and filth , these, with the other debilitating and poisonous influences of animal malaria and emanations arising from decomposing vegetable refuse and animal excreta, brought to bear on animal bodies already debilitated by overwork, for which no amount of food is a sufficient recompense, are the conditions most inimical to animal life and health ; and when diseases of common and ordinary types, or of specific and epizootic characters, appear amongst animals so circumstanced they are intensified, in their characters, and rendered more fatal in their results

There seems, however, strong reason to doubt that even under such an assemblage of adverse influences as these, the specific contagious diseases—of which, in all probability, influenza in horses is one—are capable of being produced, unless the specific poison on which they are dependent for their existence is already present.   Such conditions as these exogenous and endogenous, debilitating and impoverishing influences are always in some situations at work , but influenza is only an occasional visitant, and at irregular intervals

Other and different agencies, farther-reaching in their influence and more subtle in their operation, have at different times been advanced as the causes which, directly and

indirectly, tend to induce influenza these are the influences
or agencies meteorological and telluric Probably less in our
day than in previous periods, when the causes of epidemic and
epizootic diseases were more matters of speculation and imagination, and not as now subjects of experimental inquiry, and to
be demonstrated and made patent to the senses by the evidence
of fact and observation, is this class of agencies viewed with
favour and accepted as sufficient to explain the appearance of
these diseases. It is found to prevail under the most opposite
of atmospheric conditions of heat and cold, dryness and
moisture, high and low barometric pressure, and of varying
and opposite electrical conditions Neither in its distribution
does it seem influenced by geological formations nor varying
conditions of soil or cultivation, and as little by astronomical
influences or terrestrial movements.

It has been said, and with much truth, by Professor J. Law,
in his article on 'The Horse-Disease' in America, that 'Much
of the confusion in which the subject of causation is involved
would be cleared away could we decide as to whether the
disease is contagious In other words, if the introduction of a
sick animal into a healthy district well out of the former area
of the disease lead to a speedy diffusion of the malady in this
new locality, we must conclude that there exists a specific
poison capable of being carried in the diseased body, and probably capable of increasing indefinitely there. If these
conditions can be brought into extensive operation in a new
locality by the mere arrival of a sick or infected animal—if it
can be shown that the malady is communicated from one
animal to another—and that it will spread rapidly in a new
locality from a newly imported sick animal as a centre—we
can only conclude that the malady is caused by a specific
poison, of which the diseased system is at once the storehouse
and the field for its fertile reproduction'—*The Veterinarian*, 1873

There is little doubt that both the contagious and non-contagious views of the origin and propagation of influenza in the
horse may be supported by evidence which is often very difficult, if not impossible, to controvert It seems to appear
amongst a number of horses previously healthy, and where, as
far as we are able to discover, no contact, either by direct or

indirect means, can be discovered. Or its appearance may even have been suddenly more extensive; it may, instead of attacking one or two animals in a particular stud, have made a simultaneous invasion of several studs over a considerable extent of country. Knowing, however, the great difficulty there often is in tracing from their source of origin to a fresh and new field of development even undoubted and incontrovertibly contagious diseases, as in the case of epizoötic pleuro-pneumonia and rinderpest, we are disposed to consider of greater value a few well-authenticated cases of origin from direct contact of diseased with previously healthy animals, than many recorded instances of attacks or invasions, where the most that can be said is that, as far as we know, contagion has had no share in the appearance and development of the disease.

That influenza may not be propagated by inoculation requires further proof, while what has already been done in this direction is susceptible of a different interpretation. From my own experience of this disease, an experience pretty extensive and particularly bearing upon the question of its propagation, I am disposed to regard it as contagious, and capable of transmission from the actually suffering to the healthy animal.

There undoubtedly does appear to be a difference as to its powers of propagation in different phases or developments of the disease, the mildest and most benign manifestations evidently possessing this power in a much less degree than those more decided and malignant types of the fever.

I have for many years had opportunities of observing that the occurrence of influenza amongst agricultural horses, when the disease existed—for it is not every season that this fever is met with in an epizoötic form—has borne a direct relation to the numbers of imported animals, i.e. animals brought by dealers from a distance into the district of which I speak—the border counties of England and Scotland.

Now this is exactly what was experienced in the same district in the case of epizoötic pleuro-pneumonia in cattle, when that disease was infinitely more common than it is now. Being in reality a feeding, not a breeding, district, there was the periodical necessity for an importation of fresh stock; and as surely as this fresh supply entered the district, so surely

4—2

was there a more or less pronounced outbreak of the contagious lung fever of cattle

The imported horses to which I have referred come from a distance, collected at fairs or markets, or from other dealers; they are, on their arrival at the stables of the dealers, often delayed in their distribution over the district by the appearance of influenza fever, and, when not disposed of before its outbreak, are rarely retained until perfectly recovered, but sold as early as possible   The advent of these strange horses amongst those of the district is followed by the occurrence of the fever in very many of the stables to which they have been consigned, and it rarely exhausts itself until the greater number have shown more or less of the disease   These phenomena are of regular occurrence, and upon their recurrence horse-keepers can with tolerable certainty calculate

The evidence which I have been able to collect, on the occasion of several special invasions of influenza, points in the same direction   Although not so conclusive as that to which I have alluded, the facts connected with its dissemination in those instances were—(1) That the disease showed itself earlier at those places where animals were brought largely into contact with others, centres of local trade, than at other points where these conditions were reversed   (2) That from these centres of contact it could be traced as propagating itself to more isolated localities   These facts seem to point to the presence in the diseased animal of a specific poison or contagium, which is capable of transference to other and healthy animals ; and that, when received by them, is capable in them of producing a like diseased condition to that existing in the animal from which this infecting agent proceeded ; also that in the contaminated animal it is further capable of increase or augmentation, and of transference again to another suitable host

Of the causes which operate in the production of epizootic influenza, in so far as preparing a suitable soil or habitat upon which the morbific influences may operate, we know something—causes which seem to have a determining influence in the appearance of all contagious or zymotic diseases   These have been noticed as intrinsic and extrinsic, debilitating and degrading forces   Of the exact nature of direct or epizootic influences, which determine the appearance of the fever, we know little.

While if proved to be contagious—capable of propagation from one animal to another—the exact nature of the contagium has not in the present state of our knowledge been determined. Whether it is to be regarded, as the views of Hallier and others indicate, as consisting of the microscopic spores of fungi or other low forms of vegetable life, or as minute, granular matter floating in the air, and derived from living but diseased animal tissue, opinion is divided.

The theory propounded by Dr Beale, and one which in our time has received a large amount of support, is that the contagium of these specific diseases ought to be regarded as either consisting of, or contained in, the nuclear or granular plasmic material, of varying form, size, and structure, which, separated from the living diseased animal, is capable, when gaining access to the body of one susceptible, of growing and increasing at the expense of the elements of that body, and of inducing some form of specific disease. And that in cases of increased body-temperature this living, germinal, or bioplasmic material is capable of wondrous and rapid increase.

Experimental research, however, seems to tell us that these specific contagious diseases are more correctly regarded as originating through the implantation in the healthy animal of individual living organisms or their germs, that these living contagia have proceeded from previously living organisms, and are proceeding to other and like living organisms. Further, that it is probable that each specific disease owes its existence to the presence and activity of a specific and individually distinct living organism.

SYMPTOMS, COURSE, AND COMPLICATIONS.

To give a colour to this universal, convertible, and convenient name 'influenza,' divisions and groupings of it have been attempted, and their character indicated by such terms as *catarrhal influenza, typhoid pneumonia, typhoid pleuro-pneumonia, rheumatic influenza, catarrho-rheumatic,* etc. Certainly we do in actual practice encounter various forms and

manifestations of this fever, and, although objections may be
urged against such an artificial nomenclature, there is no
doubt that, merely as a matter of convenience, it is advisable
to regard the phenomenal exhibitions as they are presented to
our consideration in groups having some natural affinities

For this reason it will be better to view the symptoms as
observed in—1. The simple uncomplicated or catarrhal form
2 The pulmonary or thoracic form 3 The abdominal enteric
or intestinal catarrhal form 4 The rheumatic form

Now, although these different manifestations may possess
much in common thus to associate and group them under the
common designation of *influenza* or *distemper*, they yet
possess differences great and distinctive

The great distinguishing peculiarities and features, which in
all the differing forms pervade or accompany the disease, are
the pyrexial symptoms invariably of a more or less marked
adynamic or typhoid type, great prostration and debility, with a
greater or smaller amount of inflammatory action of a catarrhal
character of the respiratory, and less often of the other mucous,
membranes It is thus that we find the true catarrhal form
generally accompanying every development of influenza, only
having the other phenomena superadded

1 Of the Uncomplicated Respiratory Catarrhal Form—In
this manifestation of the fever the constitutional symptoms
are in many cases only slightly marked, the rigors or shivering-fits may escape observation, the animal even continuing
to partake of its ordinary diet, although not so greedily
There is usually sneezing, a short, troublesome cough and a
somewhat dry or staring condition of the coat Examination
of the animal will probably disclose irregular distribution of
the surface-temperature; probably a little swelling over the
larynx, and tenderness of the throat on manipulation The
conjunctival membrane is suffused, with it may be tears
trickling over the face, redness and dryness of the schneiderian membrane, with varying elevation of internal temperature, pulse frequent, and possessed of little force or volume,
with marked dulness and disinclination to move. For a few
days these symptoms steadily increase in severity, particularly
the prostration and debility, the cough deeper and more painful in the act, which is generally paroxysmal The animal

keeps his head depressed and nose protruded, while the soreness of the throat is indicated by the violent fits of coughing
induced by handling the parts, or on attempting to swallow
food, or even water in some instances this difficulty to swallow
cannot be overcome, and masticated food and water may be
ejected by the nose

The nasal membrane, at first dry, is now moistened with a
thin serous discharge, sometimes mingled with a little flaky
mucus; the mouth feels hot and clammy, and thirst is
marked The pulse becomes more frequent and feeble, number-
ing from seventy to eighty beats per minute, and the internal
temperature may reach 107° F The respiration not much
altered in character, but increased in frequency, probably less
deep and extensive; auscultation over the trachea at its lower
portion may detect the harsh or rough sounds, indicative of a
certain amount of inflammation of the larger bronchi.

In these early stages the condition of the secretions is much
altered the bowels torpid, faeces dry, pellety, and coated with
mucus, the urine scanty — little water being eliminated,
although much is taken into the system—it is tinged with
pigmentary matter, and often loaded with urates

In a few days, more probably about the end of the first week
from the onset of the fever or appearance of the cough, the
discharge from the nose will increase in amount, and change
from the thin serous to the thicker cellular character; the
cough is rather moister, and not so distressing The pulse
is less frequent, and of more volume, the impulse of the
heart against the left side, which at the outset was so marked,
becomes less manifest, the temperature declines steadily, the
animal regains his appetite, and a more natural condition of
the secretions ensues

Should this favourable turn continue, the general prostration, disinclination to move, and marked debility, which have
all through been so prominent symptoms, begin to disappear,
and convalescence may be established in fourteen days from
the commencement of the attack

Frequently, however, even in this simplest form of distemper,
the recovery is at this point retarded The swelling in the
region of the throat, from the implication of the glandular
structures there, and infiltration of the connective tissue, be-

comes more tense and defined, ultimately terminating in suppuration in the submaxillary or parotid gland and surrounding tissue. This condition, when it does occur, is usually preceded by return of the pyrexial symptoms, as elevation of temperature and capricious appetite.

One manifestation of this catarrhal type of influenza—occasionally prevalent in certain seasons and in particular localities
—has been, during late years, so distinctly marked and possessed of leading features so striking, notably the colour of the
conjunctival membrane, that it has by many been regarded
and spoken of as a distinct and separate affection under the
name of *pink-eye*, or *epizootic cellulitis*. This, however, is
probably better regarded as merely a modification of the
simplest form of the fever we are now examining, than as an
affection differing essentially from it.

In this particular manifestation of influenza the force of the
poison seems directed to, and expended upon, those organs
and tissues, chiefly external, of the fibrous or fibro-serous
order; while where fatal results occur, the structural changes,
when any are visible, are principally in connection with internal structures of the same fibrous or fibro-serous character.
Here the constitutional disturbance is sometimes a very marked
feature: the temperature is elevated, probably 105° F., there
is a cough, not marked by much involvement of the lower air-
passages; and the pulse is generally possessed of more volume
and tonicity than where the mucous membrane of the respiratory tract is markedly affected.

The conjunctiva is of a clear pink colour, hence the name
pink-eye, and, when looked at carefully, will show in many
cases infiltration of the subjacent connective tissue, giving the
appearance of conjunctival œdema.

The invasion of the subcutaneous connective tissue is very
attractive in swelling of the limbs of an anasarcous nature and
consequent stiffness: this swelling and stiffness—the result
of infiltration into the cellular tissue, which is largely distributed amongst muscles and tendons, and which occurs as the
basement structure of the serous membranes of the joints—is
not unfrequently critical in its appearance: seeing that where
much pain existed in early stages of the disturbance, it is
largely mitigated when such swellings are developed: the

animal may still be stiff, and have difficulty in moving, but restlessness and pain are less marked

A somewhat similar condition of the evacuations and more important secretions exists here to what we find in other modifications, where a preference of selection in the specific action of the poison is shown in the direction of the respiratory membrane proper

It has been noticed that in this type of catarrhal distemper there is a more marked tendency to sudden and unexpected death of the patient than in any other, and that this unexpected and fatal termination is to be attributed to the presence of thrombi in the cavities of the heart This disposition to form thrombi has been attributed to the excess in the blood of the fibrinogenous—fibrine-forming—materials, characteristic of this type of the disease Probably this condition, when it does occur, may have an influence in the production of these clots, still we must not shut our eyes to the fact that another and equally probable cause, and quite demonstrable, may also exist, viz, the participation by the valvular structures and appendages of the cardiac cavities in the specific action of the invading virus We know that anatomically these are composed of tissue analogous to that which seems specially implicated in this manifestation of the fever Nor must we forget that thrombi may form, in certain conditions of cardiac action, rather rapidly

2 **Of the Thoracic or Pulmonary Form**—As already stated, the catarrhal form of the fever, in its varied manifestations, may justly be regarded as the simplest, and it has usually so far expended its force that the affected animal is in fourteen days fairly convalescent

Complications, evidencing involvement of the thoracic viscera, may, however, at any stage retard the recovery they generally show themselves rather early than late, they may, indeed, be present from the commencement of the attack

These thoracic complications naturally arrange themselves in several distinctive groups, chief of which are—a *Capillary bronchitis*; b *Bronchitis, with cardiac disease*, c *Pneumonia*, or rather *Pleuro-pneumonia*

a. *Capillary Bronchitis*—At any stage of the initiatory fever chest symptoms may become distinctly marked the respira-

tions are quickened, more so than the pulse, the animal has a
pinched and anxious expression of the face; the nostrils are
dilated, dyspnœa is marked, or it may be distressing, the
sides heave, and the patient is disposed to place his head in
the direction where fresh air is most likely to be encountered
The appearance of the visible mucous membrane is entirely
different from what is met with in the simple uncomplicated
form   The colour of the nasal membrane will vary from a
bright purple to that of a dull leaden hue, and as the disease
advances, it will take on a yellowish-purple colour, probably
studded with petechiæ, and streaked with straw-coloured rays
The secretion from the nose is scant, and may be tinged with
blood, the mouth is clammy, and tongue furred, the internal
temperature high—103° F. to 106° F.—while the surface-heat
is irregularly distributed, both as to localities and to time

The animal seems stupid or torpid from the imperfect
aeration of the blood, and shows great disinclination to move;
and, when moved, the weakness and prostration are great—
much greater, indeed, than seems accountable for, considering
the period of continuance or the severity of the disease

Physical examination of the chest by auscultation reveals
roughness of the inspiratory murmur heard over the lower
part of the great air-tube, sibilant or wheezing sounds distributed over more or less of the lung surface, indicative of
inflammation of the smaller bronchi; and crepitation or
crepitant sounds—these last not invariably present, and when
heard not uniformly distributed   This crepitation, when the
bronchial sounds continue persistent, is disposed to pass into
the so-called subcrepitant and mucous rales rather than to be
succeeded by signs of lung consolidation

b *Bronchitis with Cardiac Disease*—When the bronchitis,
which may be regarded as the basis of the thoracic complications, is associated with cardiac or pericardiac disease, the
condition is ordinarily indicated by the peculiar character of
the pulsations and heart's action   This disturbance at both the
centre and periphery of the circulatory system is appreciated
in the condition of the pulse usually termed irregular   In
this there are a certain number—the majority of the beats of
a recognised normal character   These are followed by a few,
generally limited in number, which show a marked departure

from the recognised healthy standard. These interposed beats, so to call them, may as to time be increased in frequency, or they may be of an entirely different character; usually they are possessed of both features, irregular as to relative time, and irregular as compared with the character of the other pulsations.

Accompanying such cardiac complications, there is also, in some instances, particularly those where this complication has existed for some time, a disposition to dropsical swellings in the dependent parts of the body and limbs. Although structural changes in connection with the heart may not be a very common complication of influenza, considering the number of animals affected, functional disturbance to the extent of palpitation and irregular action is very common.

c *Pneumonia or Pleuro-pneumonia*—This manifestation of the thoracic form of the fever is one which, besides being common, is also extremely dangerous. In this form, whether the lung substance or the pleura, or both combined, are invaded, we have exhibited in a most characteristic manner the specificity of the inflammatory action. Although the pleurisy or pneumonia of influenza may bear in some manner comparison with common pleurisy or pneumonia, and although located in the same structures, in its progress, development, and textural results it is in some points distinctive.

In ordinary pleuritis and pleuro-pneumonia the exudation is usually rapid and of a plastic character, and the organizations and organized adhesions are perfect, firm, and well defined.

In the thoracic manifestations of influenza we frequently find effusion, but the material effused is of an entirely different character. It does not seem to possess the same capacities for organization as the other, while as to perfectly formed adhesions, they are not at all frequently met with.

When the true lung structure is implicated, either chiefly or along with the pleura, there is not only marked prostration and muscular debility, as in those instances where adynamic fever is a distinguishing feature, and the upper air-passages only involved, there is also much pain both when a fit of coughing occurs and when an attempt is made to move the animal. The results of the diseased action and the disposal of the products offer little of further special differential characters from those which will be noticed when we come to discuss common inflammatory processes in these same structures

All cases of this character do not terminate favourably by the steady removal of the diseased products, for succeeding a time, probably several days, of not only apparent but actual convalescence, we have in these cases of pulmonic complication a reappearance of pyrexia, which may continue for some time, and is always very liable to terminate fatally. The period of the appearance of this secondary fever seems to coincide with the removal by absorption of the effused and changed products of the inflammatory action, which if not removed from the system by the ordinary processes of secretion and elimination, on retention produce poisoning of the blood, inducing hectic fever, and in some instances disseminated abscesses and pyæmia.

These abscesses are most apt to occur in connection with the lymph glands on the tract of the larger absorbents in the vicinity of organs and particular structures which have been marked as the special seats for the manifestations of the specific action of the infecting virus

3 Abdominal, Intestinal-Catarrhal, or Enteric Form or Complications—The thoracic, or pulmonary form of influenza, which has now been lightly sketched, is very frequently, even from the development of its primary symptoms, more particularly independent of the usual and uncomplicated catarrhal form or fever than any other of its recognised types; that is to say, the illness is in many instances found to start with the positive appearance of chest symptoms, and to persistently exhibit these during the entire course of the disease, no premonitory fever being observable

In the enteric form, or where the abdominal and enteric complications are so marked and occupy such a prominent position and determining influence on the character, course, and termination of the disease as to warrant us in using these as a distinctive appellation, we more rarely find that they appear or are developed in the earliest stages of the disease.

In some seasons, in certain districts and amongst a particular class of horses, the enteric features of the disease are so distinctive and so regular in their appearance, as well as possess such a determining influence on the ultimate results, together with the fact that one of the most noticeable of these enteric symptoms or complications is evidently connected with the special functions of the liver, as to have caused many observers to give the name of *Bilious fever* to this particular form or development of influenza

However, it is probably as well, if not better, instead of considering such a manifestation as a distinctive and separate disease, to regard it as a form or modification of the malady in the same way, and for similar reasons, that we have preferred to regard what some have specialized by the names of *epizootic cellulitis* and *epizootic pleuro-pneumonia* as only forms, modifications, or types of this specific fever of the horse

As already remarked, abdominal complications are found to follow some premonitory catarrhal symptoms, the two continuing in association through the course of the disease, only that the former bear the ascendency, give the affection its speciality or type, and possess the determining influence on the result

The first observable change of symptoms from such as accompany an ordinary catarrhal disturbance is fugitive abdominal pain the horse is restless, inclined to paw, as in colic, and strike at his belly with his hind feet, though not in a violent manner Or these more pronounced manifestations not being present, we may notice that, although previously not disposed to lie down, he is now found repeatedly resting, but evidently not at ease , that when down he turns his head in an anxious manner towards the flank at such times the respirations may be disturbed, and clammy sweats bedew the body in patches

The conjunctival and buccal membranes assume a yellow, or saffron tinge, and the tongue is furred, dry, and shrunken in appearance , the evacuations from the bowels scanty, wanting colour, hard, pellety, and coated with mucus The urine is small in amount, increased in density, and coloured with pigmentary matter and mucus. There is no appetite, but considerable thirst when not actually suffering pain Manipulatory examination over the surface of the body in such cases will often disclose tenderness of the abdomen, markedly in some over the region of the liver The pulse varies from a slight increase in frequency and loss of tone to an increase of

thirty beats per minute, and the possession of a settled wiry
character. Respiration, in the former cases, is not much
altered; but in the latter, where the increase in number is
marked, the respirations are proportionately increased also,
and with both characters of the pulse the nature of the
respirations is abdominal.

When the prostration is great—for in all it is a distinct and
peculiar feature—I have observed that the membrane of the
mouth and tongue is marked with petechiæ, or blood-spots,
often of a considerable size, and that there also exists effusion
and infiltration of a straw-coloured exudate beneath the
buccal membrane on the inferior and lateral sides of the
tongue, while the mouth is filled with ropy saliva, the whole
appearances betokening the application, or at least such as we
would expect to see from the action, on the parts of a smart
rubefacient. The temperature of the body, taken in the rectum,
is not, during the development and continuance of the
abdominal symptoms, so markedly high as in the pulmonic
form of the disease, or even in some stages of the simple
catarrhal. No doubt it is high—102° to 104° F—but rarely
does it pass beyond 105° F; while, like all the other forms, the
fever is not merely simply continued, but truly remittent.

This special form of influenza in the horse I have most
frequently encountered affecting animals performing a fair
amount of work, and enjoying good, rather liberal dieting

One phase of its development where fatal results are rapidly
reached, attended with catarrh and other changes of the
mucous membrane of the bowels, and hæmorrhagic markings
of large extent in the stomach and anterior parts of the
alimentary canal, is found closely associated with imperfect
sanitary conditions and the action of other extrinsic
debilitating influences.

4 **The Rheumatic Form.**—Like the greater number of the
manifestations of this fever, the rheumatic, in its peculiar
diagnostic symptoms, rarely exhibits itself independently of,
but usually as a sequel to, the occurrence of the ordinary
catarrhal, or at least the greater number of such cases are
preceded by or accompanied with the specific inflammation of
the mucous membrane of the upper or lower air-passages so
diagnostic of influenza.

It may be that very early in the appearance of the catarrhal symptoms we recognise the peculiar stiffness, with some crackling of the joints, which betokens the existence of the rheumatic tendency

The serous and fibro-serous textures entering into the formation of the articulations, and connected with the tendons, ligaments, and investing membranes and coverings of these and some particular muscles, seem to be specially selected for developing the action of the poison

The pain in the limbs, and in part the difficulty of executing movement, indicated by the muscular twitchings in these and the repeated lifting of them from the ground, is to be accounted for from the specific inflammation affecting these structures, and from the infiltration of fluid into the subjacent textures the result of this morbid action

Although as a rule the inflammation of these fibrous and fibro-serous connecting and investing structures of joints and capsules is distributed over the greater part of the body, and generally in the limbs, we also find it localized in certain muscles, or sets of muscles, or rather their coverings, indicated by local pain and special lameness Not unfrequently the involvement of the intimate structures of the tendons of muscles and their investing fibrous sheath is very sudden—so sudden that the animal, considered to be progressing satisfactorily enough to-day, may to-morrow be found a cripple, the supposition being common that some injury has been sustained during the night   The structures most commonly affected in this manner are the great tendons of the flexor muscles of the foot, the *perforans* and *perforatus*, and the situation is generally between the knee and fetlock.   When affected in this manner, the structures feel hot, swollen, tense, and exceedingly tender on manipulation , the lameness is also great   This condition of these great tendinous structures is apt to show a decidedly metastatic, or shifting character, attacking, it may be all the limbs in the course of a few days , and it is also apt to persist after all other symptoms of the disease have disappeared, their continuance alone preventing the animal from making a perfect recovery

This form of the disease is said to be of more frequent occurrence in colder latitudes, as North Germany, Denmark,

Norway, and Scotland I have encountered it oftener amongst the coarser breeds of horses, or where the temperament was lymphatic, and where much connective tissue existed in connection with the limbs

When the true rheumatic features become added to the ordinary catarrhal, there is usually an augmentation in the severity of the constitutional disturbance; the pulse becomes more frequent, firm, and incompressible, with tumultuous action of the heart; indeed, cardiac involvement, or complication in the course of the progress of this form, is rather common

Now, although these different manifestations of influenza which have been described, in respect of the chief features and symptoms of their appearance and development, are the usual and prevailing forms or types of the fever, and although each of these may be encountered tolerably free and sufficiently distinct to entitle it to its distinguishing name, as such has been defined and restricted, it ought at the same time to be borne in mind that many outbreaks or manifestations of the disease may be seen where the true character would be best described as a compound of two or more of these.

GENERAL ANATOMICAL CHARACTERS OF INFLUENZA.

The organic lesions visible on making an after-death examination of cases of influenza are always and in every instance of more than merely passing interest Here we have always to deal with the diversity of form or type, and in a less degree with that of individual cases. We must also recollect that it is only from comparison of observations as carried out over a number of individual instances that we are capable of, or in a position to form, generalizations

The organic changes which we meet with on examination after death vary in accordance with the type or form which the fever may have assumed during life, and consequently of the class of organs involved

The extent, characteristic features, and distinctiveness of structural changes, may also vary in accordance with the mere severity of the disease, whatever may have been its form, with the amount or virulence of the infecting or contaminating agent, whatever that may be, and with the time occupied in the production or completion of the lesions observed

Thus it is that in instances where the inducing factor seems the most powerful, where the amount and strength of the virus implanted in the animal seem to have been most potent, seeing it is struck down at the very outset, ere even a good and complete chain of well-developed symptoms is established, we often meet with the least characteristic and distinctly marked morbid lesions understood to be diagnostic of the disease.   It is a fact pretty well established by recorded observation that in other diseases of a similar character, as well as in influenza, the most distinctly marked and characteristic changes, those most typical of the disease in any form, are to be observed, not in the ones which have succumbed at once to the attack, but in such as have steadily passed through its different stages, and have only yielded after a long and determined struggle with the disease

In the greater number of the cases of influenza exhibiting distinct pyrexial features together with more or less implication in the diseased action of the organs of respiration, the most generally exhibited changes are seen in connection with these organs   The fauces, with larynx and pharynx, are much tumefied from infiltration of the submucous tissue, the membrane itself varying in colour from a dark red to a livid gangrenous appearance.   The inner tracheal surface similarly coloured, the markings disposed in streaks or irregularly formed and distributed patches, the bronchi the same, and filled with frothy mucus occasionally of a rusty colour

Within the thorax, the alterations observable are in accordance with the severity of the attack and its partiality for particular structures.

In many instances the intimate lung-tissue is not much involved; and when divided with the knife, nothing abnormal may be noticed with the unaided vision, with the exception that the minute bronchi may be filled with frothy spume, and the general pulmonary tissue somewhat heightened in colour. There may, however, even when the lungs themselves do not exhibit much change, be very distinctive alterations in connection with the covering of these organs and the walls of the chest

Such changes generally range from heightening in colour, the result of engorgement of the vessels of the pleural mem-

5

branes, with a small amount of pale, straw-coloured fluid in
the pleural cavities, to much thickening of the covering membrane, extending to a deposition over more or less of its surface
of a soft, ill-formed, aplastic, yellowish-coloured lymph, so
matted and arranged over the diseased portions as to form
irregular and variously sized loculi, or spaces containing fluid
with a greater amount of effusion in the pleural sacs this
fluid varying in colour according to the amount of blood it
may contain, in which there occasionally float shreds of soft,
ill-formed, and partly adherent lymph

This want of capacity for organization is peculiarly characteristic of the lymph effused in influenza, and indeed in all
inflammatory actions accompanying epizootic diseases. It is
very distinctive when contrasted with the exudation of ordinary
pleuritis or pneumonia Seldom in this epizootic fever have
we the well-marked fibrinous adhesions between the pleural
surfaces so often seen in sporadic inflammation of the membranes of the chest

In other cases, although the animal may have lived for
several days after the chest complications have been fairly
developed, there may be no encrustation of the pleurae with
flocculi of lymph; on the contrary, these membranes may remain
perfectly smooth, only the colour altered to a dark metallic hue,
while the fluid in the cavities is somewhat turbid and of a
fœtid smell

These changes in the pleural membranes, and the effusion
of fluid in the pleural sacs, may occur in a comparatively short
time, and be unaccompanied with much textural change of
lung-tissue. The period of time occupied in the accomplishment of these and other changes of structures within the chest
is a question with which we as practitioners, liable to be cited
in courts of law as skilled witnesses, ought to be conversant
When the lungs are inflamed in their intimate structure, it is
rarely in the entirety of the organs, rather in portions or
sections, often at the inferior or lower portions, and when so
involved, the inflammatory exudate in this true pulmonic
structure is of the same aplastic and undecided character as
respects organization as when occurring in connection with
the pleural membranes On being divided or cut into with a
knife, we do not find that firm and distinct cohesion of parts

and textures such as is encountered in the second or third stage, the red and grey hepatization of ordinary pneumonia, there is always a greater amount of serosity and little well-defined and fibrillated exudation

When manipulated, its parts fall or break up with greater readiness under the same amount of force employed; and often when the cut surface is gently scraped with the knife purulent-looking fluid is gathered from the surface. The composition of both this exudate and that contained in the cavities of the pleural sacs is somewhat different from that which accompanies and is associated with common inflammatory action in the same situation and textures. Occasionally the pulmonic tissue, although changed, is so little solidified that its condition may more correctly be termed carnification. Of a soft, doughy feeling, the infiltrated material never takes on fibrillation, while the colour of the lung itself in such cases partakes of a dull, metallic hue, characteristic of humid gangrene, and it is emphysematous.

The thoracic surface of the diaphragm presents similar appearances as to adhesions and colour with the costal pleura.

The heart and containing membrane the pericardium, in the great majority of cases of *equine distemper* even of a mild form, are evidently, even from the symptoms exhibited during life, considerably involved; while in such as terminate fatally, where the thoracic features are dominant, the lesions of these structures are quite decided.

The pericardium may be simply heightened in colour from the hyperæmic condition of its vessels, and its inner serous membrane merely marked with ecchymosis or blood-spots and contain in the pericardial sac a moderate amount of serous fluid, or it may participate in the altered appearance and condition of the pleural membranes being roughened with flocculi of imperfectly organized lymph, and much thickened in substance, containing a large amount of rather dark-coloured serum, and marked with numerous blood-spots, which seem as if pure blood had been effused in circumscribed patches beneath the serous layer

The muscular tissue of the heart may be unaltered in appearance. At other times it is somewhat blanched and softened, presenting in many instances the same petechial spots or ecchymoses in connection with the endocardium that have been observed as existing beneath the lining membrane of the pericardium

In many cases which have disappointed our expectations of recovery by a rather sudden death, certain textural changes may be looked for, as thrombi, blood-clots in the cavities of the heart, or growths of a fibrous and warty character on the valves, or both   The cases of cardiac thrombi and valvular excrescences are most common when the fever has been of that form in which the fibrous, fibro-serous, and connective tissues of the body have been largely implicated.

In the abdominal form of the disease, in addition to the lesions met with in the respiratory system, the characteristic or peculiar structural changes, evidences of the enteric complications, are to be looked for in connection with the viscera and structures of the peritoneal cavity. The peritoneum is sometimes marked with petechiæ and vibices, blood-spots and blood-rays, while the cavity itself may contain a perceptible increase of the fluid usually present there

In the stomach, duodenum, and other portions of the intestine, we observe a varied arrangement of textural changes. In the first of these situations, in some manifestations of this form, particularly where sanitary and other extrinsic conditions are unhealthful, large, irregularly formed hæmorrhagic spots in connection with the mucous membrane are of common occurrence.

In the intestines, with a general and uniformly swollen state of the entire mucous membrane, much infiltration of the submucous tissue, and a yellowish-coloured gelatinous exudate, there are scattered over the membrane smaller hæmorrhagic patches similar to the larger ones seen in the stomach , while spread over extensive tracts there may be the appearance of much irritation, with denudation and removal of the epithelial structures, the result of the specific catarrhal inflammation

These changes, although encountered more or less extensively throughout the entire bowel, are usually most conspicuous in the *cæcum caput coli*, and where gland-structures are most abundant.

In the urinary bladder a somewhat analogous condition of

the lining membrane, thickened, infiltrated, and marked with petechiæ, is observed.

When yellowness of the visible mucous membranes has been a distinctive feature of the abdominal complications there is generally observed a turgid and full condition, amounting in some instances to marked friability of the liver, incident to the congested state of the viscus and impairment of its functions.

The kidneys and other gland-structures are often changed in character, hyperæmic, and marked with spots of hæmorrhagic effusion, or blanched, soft, and exhibiting elemental tissue changes, the result of hæmal vitiation and malnutrition.

In certain instances, both in this type and in others where aberration of nerve force is a noticeable symptom, we may find in the membranes of the central organ of the cranium and spinal canal vascular arborescence and an extra amount of straw-coloured fluid.

When rheumatic or metastatic inflammation of the limbs and articulations has been exhibited during life, the presence of inflammatory exudation is easily enough demonstrated in the thickening of tendons, the infiltration of the connective tissue around and underlying the fibrous and fibro-serous membranes of joints. Those cases, however, where the rheumatic form or complications are most marked and characteristic do not often, unless developed in connection with some other form, prove fatal.

TREATMENT.—In the treatment of influenza it is needful to remember that the affection is essentially febrile—a specific pyrexial state—and that, like all specific fevers, it has a distinct and regular course, which is pursued from incubation to termination ; that this course may not be cut short in its development, or cured, as we are apt to say ; that our object ought to be the judicious guidance of the animal through the course of the fever, which certainly requires to be carefully watched, and complications treated as they may arise.

In the entire management of this disease the animal physician will require not only to draw upon the resources of pure therapeutics, but will find much benefit—in many cases of the simpler forms probably more benefit—from a correct knowledge of the laws of hygiene, and from a strict enforcement of these

Regarding the collection of phenomena we encounter in this fever as indicative of what is understood as active inflammatory action, and having no regard to the specificity of the conditions and the certainty of a particular blood-contamination, the most potent of remedies in active inflammations, blood-letting, has been too often indiscriminately had recourse to.

We ought not to forget that even allowing that here the blood is contaminated, that we cannot deal with it while in the body, but as a whole; and that supposing it should be established that here or in any other form of inflammatory action certain constituents of the blood are in excess, we have not the power in depletion to remove these morbid constituents, excluding the remaining parts upon which life depends

The principle upon which so many have gone, and that upon which many still continue to act in adopting the system of blood-letting in every inflammatory disease, proceeds from their belief in, or, in cases where no belief is expressed, the adoption of that theory which makes inflammation to consist merely in the excessive determination of blood to the affected part, in which for the time being there is an actual increase of nutrition

Were such really the case, the abstraction of blood would be a rational method of cure

However in the parts where this action is localized all healthy nutrition is suspended; in fact, the perversion of nutrition is the great feature, or one of the great features, of inflammation

Now, although we do find cases of acute inflammation in our patients of such organs as the meninges of the brain the pleura, the peritoneum, the fibrous textures of joints and of the feet, which are cured or benefited by rapid and full depletion, and which, as far as we can observe, do not terminate so favourably when this is neglected, still there seems reason to believe that many types of inflammatory action are only rationally and successfully combated when not only blood-letting is avoided, but when that which seems a diametrically opposite course—stimulation—is pursued

Blood is a peculiar fluid, and its removal from the living

diseased animal a means potent for good or evil, and ought
not to be resorted to indiscriminately Depletion in many
cases of catarrhal influenza, where constitutional disturbance
is not productive of even diminished appetite, may be borne
with impunity, but in the severer and more malignant forms,
as surely as we bleed, so surely will we have a protracted recovery, or, it may be, death.

Cathartics are nearly equally dangerous Here the mucous
membrane is extremely susceptible to be acted upon injuriously by any irritant, and in the existing state of the
animal might acquire an activity not easy of arrestment,
while anything that nauseates is to be carefully avoided as
tending still further to weaken an already depressed system
As well give opiates to a man in a state of coma as active
purgatives to a horse suffering from the adynamic fever of
influenza Should the bowels require aught to facilitate their
action, let it be of the simplest nature or mildest form, particularly while the fever lasts

Along with these two leading systems of treatment, and
one which has gone hand in hand with them and been nearly
as blindly employed, is 'counter-irritation.'

Blister, bleed, and physic was certainly doing something,
although that something was subduing the animal instead of
the disease

The application to external surfaces of agents calculated to
produce an amount of irritation or vesication has more steadily
preserved its position in theory, and many are disposed to
think practically has been productive of more beneficial results
than either of the already mentioned curative agents

By whatever mode, or through whatever channels, they may
produce their action, whether by producing a severe action in
external textures, thereby lessening the dangers attendant on
the internal disease, diverting the morbid action from the
dangerous and uncontrollable to that which is less so and
more immediately under our direction, or whether they produce their beneficial and therapeutic results by reflex action,
removing pain, nerve irritation, and general or local vascular
tension and disordered nutrition, that is by operating on the
peripheral nerve-fibres which convey the impression received
to the nerve-centres, which impression is then modified, trans-

ferred, or transposed, so that both common sensation and nutritive function are modified and altered ; or that by their simple excitant action on the heart, bloodvessels, and absorbents they produce an extra amount of vital energy, and operate by a more active distribution of vital fluid and absorption of the more liquid portions of the material effused, restoring impaired structures to somewhat of their normal functions—in whatever way their action is brought about, they seem less liable to dangerous sequences, even when employed indiscriminately, than the other so-called cardinal remedies, bleeding and purging.

When engaged closely with the details of medicine, we are apt to imagine that no recovery from disease can be secure apart from the employment of medicines ; and in this way physic often reaps a harvest of credit to which it has no just claim Against this tendency all require to be warned, while probably no disease which we are called upon to treat yields better results to a strictly enforced and correct hygienic arrangement than influenza in all its forms For although we place much reliance on the judicious employment of medicinal agents, it is nevertheless tolerably certain that no amount of medicaments will ever supersede or compensate for the want of good careful nursing

At the very outset of the fever, have the horse laid aside from work, if so engaged at the time ; many an animal has been doomed to a protracted recovery, or has ultimately succumbed to the disease, that might have survived and been restored to health had rest been enforced whenever the disease appeared Next to cessation from work, have the animal placed if possible, in a roomy, clean, well-ventilated, light, and dry loose box ; or if compelled to remain in a stall, see that a sufficiency of pure air gains admittance, and scrupulous attention is paid to cleanliness. The advantages of a good loose box are such that, with a sufficient supply of fresh air, we can always regulate the bodily warmth by means of clothing, which ought to consist of a woollen rug and bandages for the legs, with hood or head-cap It is needful to maintain the surface-temperature, thereby preserving the equilibrium of the general circulation and facilitating transpiration and secretion by the skin

This clothing ought to be removed, at least once daily, the body and limbs gently rubbed over, the former with a little tepid water and vinegar; the clothes shaken in the open air, and all replaced

In many of these cases the use of the Roman, otherwise called the Turkish, bath, is deserving of trial. We want facts from which to reason respecting the action of the skin in febrile diseases generally in the horse

As regards food in every form, and all through the disease, although always objectionable to carry its allowance to the extent of cramming the creature, it is advisable to coax his appetite where it is deficient, and it is astonishing what may be done in inducing a sick animal to eat by coaxing Green food, when procurable, is to be preferred, in the absence of this, fresh roots sliced and given from the hand, or a little picked hay, should be offered—anything, in short, the animal seems fond of, always endeavouring to keep it of such a nature that the bowels may not become constipated

Should they become confined, it is better not to give physic or purging medicine, properly so called, endeavour to overcome this condition by enemata of tepid water, or tepid water with oil, while, if taking any mash or steamed oats with a little bran, most animals will readily enough, with a little education, take linseed-oil along with it, in ounce or two-ounce doses It is not necessary that the animal should be compelled to drink nothing but lukewarm water This is a beverage which few animals, unless habituated to it, care for, and, if allowed to stand in the stable for some time, the water will be warm enough Cold linseed-tea, or milk, are both to be recommended as drinks, according to conditions, they are nourishing, and, from their demulcent properties, well suited to the irritated and irritable mucous surfaces

In the employment of medicinal agents we must be largely guided by the nature and severity of the symptoms as they develop themselves The more rational, and, in actual practice, the more satisfactory procedure, is the exhibition of such agents as may act more directly on the constitution of the blood, as tend to allay the considerable systemic irritation shown by the exaltation of body-temperature and rapid tissue-change, to support failing energy and combat complications as they arise.

During the first four or five days of the attack, over which the fever is most marked, benefit will be derived from allowing daily, in the water, from four to eight drachms each of nitrate and chlorate of potass. In addition to this I have found extremely useful the exhibition, twice daily, of the draught composed of these same salts with liquor ammoniæ acetatis and sweet spirits of nitre, recommended in simple fever, or another formula containing, in addition, camphor and belladonna.

> ℞ Pulv. Potass Nit   ʒii
> Pulv. Camphoræ et Extr. Belladon ... aa ʒ ss.
> Spirit _Eth Nit   . fl ʒi —ʒii
> Liq. Ammon. Acetat .... fl. ʒiv
>   Misce ut fiat haustus

In a few days, as the temperature begins to show evidence of subsidence, and the pulse is softer and less frequent, or where the prostration is very marked from the outset, a somewhat more stimulant treatment will be found advisable, such as carbonate of ammonia in bolus, or in solution in cold gruel, or, where expense is not so much an object, and when the fever has perceptibly declined, there is nothing better than port wine with sulphate of quinine.

Probably in those cases where the fibrous or connective-tissue structures are extensively involved, where it is feared that the state of the blood is favourable to the formation of cardiac or cerebral thrombi, the preferable stimulant is ammonia in some form, either the carbonate in bolus or solution, or the aromatic spirit of ammonia, and these are much better given rather often, and in moderate doses, than at long intervals and in full quantities.

They may be given alone, or added to the fubrifuge draught already mentioned, which may be lessened in amount and given thrice, instead of twice, daily.

In all cases where deglutition is performed with difficulty, or where there is a troublesome cough, the medicinal agents are best administered in the form of electuary, the menstruum being treacle.

℞ Pulv Camphoræ   ℥iv
   Pulv Myrrhæ et Pulv Potass Nit   aa   ℥viii
   Extr Belladon.   .   ℥ii
   Pulv Glycirh Rad.....   .   ..   ..   ℥viii
   Theriacæ . .   ..   q s.
               Misce fiat electuar

This, in small portions, is smeared over the tongue and
buccal membrane, or placed, by means of a piece of wood,
between the molar teeth several times daily; it thus becomes
liquefied gradually, and, in being swallowed, has a beneficial
action on the membrane and structures of the pharynx and
throat This internal local treatment may also be supplemented by an occasional gargling with a solution of nitrate or
chlorate of potass, or diluted sulphurous acid In many instances where the condition of the throat has been bad, the
membranes tumefied from submucous infiltration, and of a
livid character, I have fancied that good has resulted from
fumigation with sulphurous acid gas generated by the burning
of sulphur This is particularly applicable when a number of
animals are affected at the same time, as also with a view to
arrest the progress of the disease, and recommends itself from
the ease with which it may be accomplished and carried to any
extent

Both during the dry stage of the inflammation of the membrane of the upper air-passages, and also when this has been
succeeded by the moist stage of increased secretion, when
there is much cellular discharge from the nostrils, the inhalation of the vapour of hot water has a soothing and grateful
effect; this is accomplished in different ways, usually by means
of scalded bran or chopped hay, placed in an ordinary nose-
bag, and held to the horse's nose In addition, the material in
the nosebag may be medicated, by which means not only
local but also systemic irritation is sometimes considerably
alleviated The agents employed in this medication are usually
preparations of opium, sulphurous acid, iodine, turpentine, or
belladonna.

In addition to this internal treatment of the laryngeal and
pharyngeal symptoms in most of the influenza cases, it is often

advisable, particularly where the cough and irritation are troublesome, or even prior to and in lieu of these measures, to employ, externally, heat and moisture This is done by swathing the throat in woollen cloths or bandages wrung from hot water, and retained in position and warmth for some hours continuously Where there are many animals affected, or where from other causes, as individual peculiarities, this is inapplicable, similar results, viz relieving tension and local irritability, may be obtained through the use of sinapisms, ammonia liniment, or mild cantharides liniment

During the progress of all the more serious cases of influenza, and where the thoracic complications are evident or dreaded, the condition of the chest and the contained organs must be carefully watched. The internal temperature, nature of the respirations, condition of the heart's action and of the pulse, ought to be noted, where possible, once daily—certainly at each visit of our patient. The involvement of the lower air-passages, the pleura and lungs, as also the heart, must ever be present to our minds as a possible condition of all cases, however simple they may at first appear.

When, from the signs and characteristic features of the diseased action, which have already been detailed, the evidence derived from auscultation, the distressed and catching breathing, the marked ridge along the margin of the ribs, etc., we are satisfied that pulmonary and pleural structures are inflamed, it will be for us to consider whether by external agencies we may be able to afford relief to the animal

This without doubt may be successfully done by the employment of means similar to what has been indicated as applicable to the same condition in the upper air-passages

Where pain is a less obvious feature in the course of the development of the thoracic complications, but where we are satisfied that effusion is taking place into the pulmonary structure, and consolidation is the result, experience and observation seem to indicate that the application of a smart cantharides liniment over the chest is productive of more lasting benefit than the treatment by means of the hot-water blankets Cantharides liniment I prefer to mustard for many reasons; amongst others, that it is less likely to produce irritation and pain I am aware that my experience in the use of this agent is not corroborated by all, indeed by many able veterinarians, who, advocating the use of a vesicant, in these cases prefer mustard applied as directed for the throat, while not a few are opposed to the use of these agents in any form. By such their use is opposed on various grounds. They cannot and do not remove or mitigate the inflammatory action, either in these cases of pulmonic inflammation or any other similar action, we are told: and post-mortem examinations, it is said, confirm this. Certainly, it is allowed that such treatment has not had this desirable result in fatal cases—those only in which the evidence of structural change has been obtained, but we ought to remember that a certain amount of caution is required in drawing conclusions from cases examined after death, as contrasted with such as have recovered. For aught we know, it may be that structural conditions might be very different if viewed where improvement was evident after the application of a blister.

Again, it is asserted that they ought not to be applied, as their application increases the pain and fever. Such may be the case in certain instances—probably those which terminate fatally, that they do so in every case, or even in the majority, I cannot from experience allow.

The general or frequent result of the application of a cantharides liniment to the sides in very many instances where inflammatory action has been progressing in the lung-tissue is that in six or twelve hours the general febrile symptoms are subdued. I have observed in that time that the temperature has fallen 2° or 3° F., the pulse become less frequent by ten beats per minute, and the respirations lessened nearly one-third in number, and changed from the catching abdominal character to a regularity certainly not normal, but much improved from the condition existing previous to the application of the vesicant

Indiscriminate blistering of the chest in pleuro-pulmonic inflammation is at all times to be condemned, but when judiciously and moderately employed in the pulmonic inflammation attendant on certain forms of influenza fever in the horse, does not deserve to be stigmatized in every case as worse than useless. In actual practice, I am satisfied that much good has resulted from its employment.

In those forms where the abdominal complications are prominent features, the horse inclined to be restless, and occasionally lying down and rising again, as if suffering from colic, with a confined condition of the bowels, it will be needful to give our attention to relieve this restlessness and pain ; enemata of tepid water or tepid water and oil, with the application to the abdomen of woollen cloths wrung from pretty warm water, are often sufficient to attain the end desired.

Where the pain is more persistent, or where the confined state of the bowels is accompanied with a distinct yellow condition of the visible mucous membranes, it will most probably be needful to exhibit a moderate dose of linseed oil, to which has been added one or two ounces of tincture of opium, or from ten to fifteen drops of Fleming's tincture of aconite while the hot-water applications to the abdomen may be supplemented with smart friction with soap or ammonia liniment, while where pain is the prominent feature, and not accompanied by marked constipation, it is readily enough relieved by subcutaneous injection of the solutio morphia hypodermica B P

When both pain and constipation have continued more or less troublesome for some days, with a foul condition of the mouth and tongue, the animal all the time continuing to partake occasionally of a little mash, an endeavour ought to be made to induce it to take along with the mash a certain quantity of linseed oil, or a rather full allowance of sulphate of soda In such cases, the exhibition twice daily in bolus of half a drachm of opium and twenty grains of calomel, together with the oil, will prove efficacious in removing or relieving the pain and confined condition of the bowels

In those manifestations of the enteric type where there is not much obvious pain, but in which the lesions are largely exhibited in connection with the mucous membrane of the alimentary canal, and where circumscribed hæmorrhagic effusions are apt to occur, good has been observed to follow the combination of the simple salines with full and frequent doses of salicylic acid, followed after a few days by the addition of one of the mineral acids In these cases where collapse seems imminent, a free use of alcohol is often demanded

The rheumatoid symptoms accompanying certain forms of

influenza and ordinarily developed after the fever has existed some days, and marked by much pain, fugitive swelling of the tendons of the muscles of the limbs, and infiltration in connection with the fibrous textures of the joints, are most successfully combated by warm-water applications, through means of bandages or warm poultices both water and poultices may, when the pain is excessive, be medicated with tincture of opium

Even after the animal has well recovered from the fever, and in all other respects apparently reinstated in health, the results of this peculiar inflammation of the tendons may remain in the form of permanent thickenings and swellings, either of the substances of the tendons themselves, or of fibrous textures closely connected with them These alterations of structure are best treated by blistering with ungt. cantharides, or a compound of ungt. cantharides and ungt. hydrarg biniodid , this may require to be repeated Or in many cases the preferable treatment is the actual cautery, and a lengthened period of rest Internally in such troublesome cases, iodide of potassium or Donovan's solution seems the best alterative ; and either may be continued for some weeks, unless counter-indicated by dyspepsia following its lengthened exhibition

The great majority of what may be called ordinary cases of influenza in the horse when placed under treatment sufficiently early are decidedly benign in character, and usually amenable to judicious treatment, the cardinal principles of which, sanctioned both by science and practice, are to avoid everything which weakens or debilitates the system, especially eschewing purging and bleeding , allow plenty of cool, pure air , clothe the body to keep the skin warm and promote secretions , keep the bowels moist by the diet, or, if needful, by some mild laxative give saline medicine with anodynes and mild stimulants to counteract in some degree the degraded condition of the blood and relieve the distressing symptoms as they arise.

Following the subsidence of the fever, and during the period of convalescence, much may be done both by dieting and otherwise to strengthen debilitated organs, and generally to improve the functional health and vigour of the whole system Dyspepsia or indigestion, is best met by allowing in the drinking water carbonate of soda, or placing chalk in the manger, changing the diet and exhibiting mild vegetable tonics. These latter, when not producing the desired effect, ought to be changed or alternated with others, as sulphate of iron or liquor arsenicalis. The latter is a good tonic, and readily taken in the food or drinking water.

Sequelæ—Although the larger percentage of the cases of influenza terminate favourably, and leave no permanent functional disturbance or structural change, all are not thus clear of obnoxious and damaging sequelæ

The untoward and damaging results which follow an attack of influenza in the horse are chiefly encountered in connection with the principal organ of circulation—the heart, and with these of respiration, the lungs and air tubes, great and small, or with the tendons and sheaths of the great flexor muscles of the limbs. In a less number we have changes in connection with the great nerve-centres; these, however, are more likely to develop themselves during the height of the fever than after its defervescence

The changes which thus result from the diseased action in the upper portion of the air-tube and in the region of the larynx are the most common, and tend, by their interference with the free passage of air to and from the lungs, to produce varying abnormal sounds. The structural changes thus resulting in defective performance of function are various, as thickening of laryngeal lining membrane, enlargements in connection with the vocal cords, disease of muscular structures connected with the sections or cartilages of the larynx whereby these cartilages are imperfectly maintained in their natural position and relation to each other, thereby altering the calibre and form of the entrance to the great air-tube

In the lower air-passages, the smaller air-tubes and air-cells, the defective functional activity incident to change of structure is less marked, unless the horse is caused to make rapid exertion, when the deficient pulmonic aerating surface will most probably induce some amount of dyspnœa or embarrassment in breathing

When the heart and its appendages are the seats of change incident to previous disease, the consequences are much more serious than where the respiratory organs proper are involved

In the vast majority of the former cases the animals so affected are unfit for even a moderate amount of work Effusion into the cavity or sac of the pericardium, hydropericardium, with thickening of its texture from organization of the effusion resulting from the inflammatory action, are the chief changes obviously resulting from an attack of influenza, in which the covering of the heart immediately participates

In connection with the heart itself, we may have defective muscular contractility, the result of certain peculiar changes which have occurred in the intimate structure of the muscular fibres, or there may be thrombi in the great cavities, and stretching into the large bloodvessels ; or more frequently there exists a diseased condition consisting in deposition, thickening, or adventitious growth of a fibrous or warty character on the valves of the heart, by which their perfect efficiency is interfered with and materially lessened

These cardiac lesions again are, as a rule, the fruitful and immediate cause of local dropsical swellings over the inferior parts of the body and of the limbs

When thickening of the tendons or tendinous sheaths of the great flexor muscles of the limbs remain as the effect of an attack of this fever, the usefulness of the animal may be impaired for a lengthened period, or permanently destroyed.

Besides these, but of less frequent occurrence, and always of a doubtful and dangerous character, are certain peculiar renal disturbances, consequent upon blood-changes and contaminations.

CHAPTER III

STRANGLES—FEBRIS PYOGENICA EQUI, COLT ILL, ETC.

Definition.—*A specific febrile disease of the horse, probably under certain conditions contagious, in which the pyrexial symptoms are not invariably well marked, and characterized in those cases which take a regular course by the eruption of one or more abscesses amongst the connective tissue associated with the gland-structures between the branches of the lower jaw, which on reaching maturity discharge pus.*

Pathology. *a—Nature of the Disease*.—Pre-eminently an equine disease, it has from the earliest periods been recognised and described by the term now given it, 'Strangles' In some districts of our country probably as well known by the name 'Colt Ill'

Gervase Markham (1648) calls it 'a great and hard swelling between the horse's nether chaps upon the roots of his tongue and about his throat, which swelling, if it be not prevented, will stop the horse's windpipe, and so strangle or choke him, from which effect, and none other, the name of this disease took its derivation'

It is probably more truly a disease of youth, adolescence, or colt-hood, although it is equally certain that horses of all ages, and, in our islands at least, of every breed and under every condition of surroundings and of food-supply, are liable to become affected with this fever.

Although it has been under observation for such a lengthened period, and the amount of facts and observation collected with regard to strangles is very extensive and wonderfully precise, we are not yet perfectly agreed as to its nature or causes of production.

Some veterinarians, British as well as foreign, prefer to consider it as in no respect differing from ordinary catarrh either in its origin, development, or results Others again seem disposed to view it as akin to such malignant diseases as 'Scrofula,' or 'Glanders.' By some it has been named Adenitis Scrofulosa Æquorum, while yet another class regard this fever as merely the natural outcome, development, or maturation of the peculiarly distinctive or fermentative action of some exogenous agencies, variable, it may be, as to their origin, or of some constituent of the blood which exists congenitally in all horses, but to a greater extent in some than others.

It is certainly in many respects different from common catarrh, for although invading textures and organs many of which are ordinarily the seat or locality for the exhibition of the symptoms of catarrh, it does so in a somewhat different manner, and with different results.

Common catarrh attacks animals of the different species with little apparent partiality, and animals of the same species in a similar manner. Strangles is peculiar to the equine species, and particularly prone to seize upon those which have not yet reached maturity. Common catarrh has no disposition to develop during any period of its course any peculiar or distinctive eruption. Strangles is characterized in its truly typical forms by the development of specific furunculoid abscesses. An animal which has suffered from or passed through one well-marked attack of catarrh is in nowise protected from further invasions of the same; an animal which has passed through a well-marked and typical attack of strangles is so far protected, that although it may again be seized, it is undoubtedly not so liable as others of the same age which have never suffered from an attack of the fever.

From scrofula, or scrofulous inflammation of the gland-structures, it is entirely different, the only likeness being that certain of the gland-structures in different parts of the body are localities where occasionally both diseases may exhibit themselves. Scrofulous inflammation in connection with adenoid tissue is not as a rule, even when carried well through, characterized as being followed by a visible manifestation of increased vigour, by an impulse being given to the healthy growth and development of the animal so affected. Strangles, when passing favourably through its different stages of febrile development, formation, and maturation of eruption or boil, is very often followed by a visible impetus or start in healthy functional activity and growth.

There is much in the nature and development of strangles, as also in the nature of the influence produced on the animal which has once been affected with this disease, to induce us to

6—2

regard it as truly an eruptive febrile disease of the horse
Like the entire class of the eruptive fevers, the so-called
greater *exanthemata*, whether in man or animals, it has certain
class features which serve to form a bond of union amongst
these, giving them a community of character and interest.
1 All these fevers are characterized by more or less well-developed pyrexial symptoms which run a definite course 2 They
are all identified by an eruption, which passes through a regular
series of changes from its appearance to its maturation and
decline. 3 They sometimes appear as epidemics or epizootics
4 They attack all, or the greater number of individuals
5 They are only disposed to attack an individual once in a
lifetime 6 They are disposed to run a definite course, and
are dangerous mainly when checked in their course, they are
best treated by simply guiding this course 7 They may be
all propagated by contagion

Now if we carefully consider the nature or character of
strangles, by examining it a little in detail upon these several
leading features which have been mentioned as characteristic
of the specific eruptive fevers, we may be able to see in how
much it agrees with these, and where also it may be regarded
as differing

1 *All these fevers are marked by more or less well-developed
pyrexial symptoms, which run a definite course*—None, I
suppose, will deny that fever, distinct and definite in character,
is a distinguishing feature of strangles Although probably
not the essential or diagnostic feature of the disease, it is nevertheless nearly invariably present In its character it is steady
and continued, sometimes remittent, in rare cases intermittent,
and when of the intermittent type, it is always indicative of
the same grave lesions The relation of the fever to the
eruption is always the same When the abscess moves steadily
through its different stages, from the infiltration of the connective tissue, softening of exudate, appearance of pus, thinning
of the cutaneous tissues and discharge of the contained fluid,
the fever preserves a similar steady and gradual advance, then
a quiet but regular defervescence When, however, the maturation of the phlegmon is in any way arrested, or, the abscess
having been discharged, a change in constitutional symptoms
shows itself, the general lymphatic gland system seems speci-

ally affected, and disseminated abscesses appear, in such cases the pyrexial symptoms change, with fever of a different type ushering them in

2. *All these specific eruptive fevers are identified by an eruption which passes through a regular series of changes, from its appearance to development and decline* —In strangles the diagnostic feature, conjoined with the fever, is the appearance of an eruption in the form and character of a more or less extensive pustule or abscess For although there is a considerable difference in character and appearance between the abscess of strangles and the rash of scarlatina, it is yet as truly an eruption in the former case as the pustules of variola in man or sheep

3 *These fevers sometimes appear as epidemics, or epizootics.* —Strangles sometimes appears as an epizootic, and, when so appearing, is apparently regulated by those laws which possess a determining and guiding influence over epidemics and epizootics generally Such determining influence, whatever that may be, seemingly operates in the production of disease independent of ordinary recognised causes, also by giving increased energy and power in the production of particular diseases This fever may, as other epizootics frequently are, by such an influence be modified and altered in its essential character and form of development.

4 *They attack all, or the greater number of, individuals* — Ordinary inflammatory diseases of any organ, or set of organs, do not affect large numbers of animals Comparatively few horses suffer from common laryngitis, or even catarrh ; very few horses escape being affected with strangles

5 *These diseases are only disposed to attack an individual once in a lifetime*—Although this is not absolutely true of strangles, it is as true of it as of any other of the same class of diseases with which we are comparing it

6 *They are disposed to run a definite course, and are dangerous when checked or interfered with in this course* — Strangles, as a true febrile disease, is always disposed to follow a distinct course , is only successfully treated when the natural development of the fever is not interfered with, but correctly guided to its natural termination

7 *They may all be propagated by contagion*—So, under certain conditions, may strangles be propagated

It may be perfectly true that irrefragable proof cannot be adduced to demonstrate that strangles is in every case, and in all manifestations, contagious No more can it be proved that other well-established contagious diseases are in all cases transmitted by contagion When appearing amongst horses where the evil and deteriorating influences incident to over-crowding, imperfect dietetic and generally bad sanitary conditions are not brought into operation, strangles does not so often-manifest that low or typhoid form in which it mainly exhibits its contagious properties

When appearing simultaneously amongst a number of animals, its origin is usually attributed, by those who deny its contagious character, to the 'something in the air' theory, to occult and inappreciable atmospheric influences, or, it may be, to the general operation of the same depressing and vitiating influences which have developed it in the first.

It should never be forgotten that even diseases which are certainly contagious are only surely transmitted in this way when other conditions in those to be acted upon are favourable for the reception and development of the contagium or vitiating element , while at the same time evidence can be adduced to satisfy most minds that it is highly probable, to place the statement in the mildest form, that in certain instances strangles is capable of transmission from the diseased to the healthy

Most veterinarians who have practised in the country and in breeding districts can call to mind many instances where strangles has been introduced to studs of horses, and amongst these propagated, by the purchase of a fresh animal labouring under the disease

I have also observed that, when strangles breaks out amongst young horses, they generally become affected in greater numbers within a given time, when they are in actual contact or close proximity, than when they are kept at different parts of the same homestead, or where they have greater liberty and are less restricted to close company with the others suffering from the disease I have, moreover, found that not only has an imported diseased animal brought the affection amongst others previously healthy, but further, that previously healthy colts, placed in stables where diseased ones had recently been located, have also contracted the disease Without admitting the influence of contagion in these cases, it seems difficult to explain why disease should break forth amongst the previously healthy on the introduction to their company of an animal already ill, or why horses, previously free from strangles, should at once exhibit and develop the fever on being placed in stables where contaminated animals had recently been located

As corroborative of the statement that strangles is non-contagious, it has been stated that it may not be propagated by inoculation That this statement is correct we are not certain, rather would it appear that experimentation is needed to settle the point

No doubt many cases of the disease are easily or only satisfactorily accounted for apart from the idea of contagion altogether

The opinion of the older observers, that there existed, ready formed in the blood of the young animal, some special material or arrangement of constituent materials which, when acted upon by agencies from without, resulted in the development of the fever and production of the abscess, and that this maturation and discharge of purulent matter was the means through which the animal body discharged itself of this deleterious agent, or rectified the abnormal arrangement of the constituent elements, and was thus the indication and assurance that a more healthful and vigorous growth and development of organs and functions was certain to follow, is not very widely separated from what may be regarded as the presently entertained idea of the nature of this disease, and its mode of development, when the origin by contagion is denied

The source of this poison may, it is held by those who advocate the non-communicable nature of the disease, be traced to the effete or worn-out materials of the body, which have through some fault failed to be thrown off, and which may further have undergone decomposition or chemical changes, these, it is thought, being sufficient of themselves to induce ulterior changes in healthy tissue, or such changes may only be assisted by this retention, and may be chiefly dependent for their production on the reception into the system of the results of the putrefaction

and changes of animal excreta or other noxious materials, resulting from the decomposition of other animal or vegetable
matter. No doubt, in many instances this seems, and in
reality is, a good and sufficient explanation of the phenomena
which attend upon or constitute the specific fever, and it may
be the mode through which, in numerous instances, strangles
is induced.

There are, however, many cases and particular outbreaks of
the disease, chiefly those which partake of a malignant type
and are associated with a low form of fever, where the evidence and facts in connection with its appearance and spread
all point to specific contagium as the origin of the outbreak
and the medium through which it is propagated.

However potent or hurtful may be the action of effete and
changing animal tissue, either when retained within the
animal body or after its ejection from the economy, there seems
as much reason to believe in the disease-producing agency of
poisonous material, particulate living contagia, circulating in
the blood of the actually diseased and given off by the
excretion of the skin and lungs, as well as in the morbid
material and changed tissue elements from the local eruptions
or pustules.

This poisonous and disease-producing material will remain
floating in the atmosphere, and unless ventilation is sufficient
to ensure its dispersion or dilution to the point of innocuous-
ness, will find an entrance into the animal body through the
respiratory tract, and in this way may produce the disease.

b. Causation.—It has been said that this is peculiarly a
disease of domestication, and that the true causes are inseparably connected with a forced confinement in stables. It is
certainly true that horses located in stables are more largely
the subjects of strangles than others differently circumstanced.
This is as it must always be in a country such as ours, where
horses of necessity, both from climatic and utilitarian considerations, must in greater numbers be stabled than roaming
at large. That, however, it is a disease peculiarly owing its
origin to enforced confinement experience will not endorse,
as it is tolerably well known that very large numbers of
animals so affected have never been housed.

Dentition has occasionally been looked upon as an immediate inducing factor Still although the fever does largely manifest itself in animals during the period of life when the inception of teeth is being actively carried on there does not seem any sufficient reason why we ought to regard this act as an active developing agent in the production of strangles

The more rational views to take of its causes and modes of propagation seem to be those already noticed when remarking on the question of its contagious or non-contagious character

1 To regard it as resulting from a species of zymosis induced by the absorption into and addition to the circulating fluids and blood of some peculiar noxious agents, the product of chemical changes on organic matter extrinsic to the animal, which on entering the circulation either of themselves or in conjunction with other deleterious materials which have been retained unnaturally in the body, and which are rendered possible of augmentation, are capable of producing certain specific changes in the blood, these changes exhibiting themselves in the local eruption and suppurative action

The highly susceptible state of the system of young and growing horses, those in which we observe this disease most extensively, together with the operation of those causes which induce imperfect elimination of waste and degraded tissue, and the conditions with which young and fresh animals are so often surrounded, seem to point to this infringement of the laws of hygiene and dietetics as a very probable source of the origin of strangles

2 To regard strangles as capable of being propagated by contagion That any disease shall be capable of propagation by the contact of the diseased with the healthy, it is not absolutely needful that every case shall show the same decided character or tendency to spread even when the material for its dissemination is within reach We are well aware, as already stated, that many cases and outbreaks of strangles are most satisfactorily accounted for apart from the question of contagion still we may not shut our eyes to many facts which point, as the only satisfactory explanation of its origin and propagation, to the inherent contagious character of the disease to the fact that there is given off from the actually suffering animal some organic material, whether active germinal matter capable of inducing active special changes

in the animal tissues with which it may come in contact, or living particulate organisms, either the carriers of the actual and potential contagium, or the contagium itself, but at all events capable of inducing in the previously healthy a similar train of phenomena to that which we observe in the diseased whence these organisms or potentialities come

VARIETIES, SYMPTOMS, AND COURSE OF THE DISEASE

In many instances the nature, development, and course of strangles are very complicated Instead of a few days of simple irritative fever, steadily maintained until the maturation of the submaxillary swelling, with regular but steady decline of symptoms, the discharge of the pus and the progress of the local healing process, we may encounter true 'hectic,' the fever of suppuration passing on to or terminating in the appearance of variously situated abscesses, more rarely *septicæmia*

In these cases, instead of simple and continued fever where the pyrexial symptoms are steady, with slight exacerbations from outset until the termination, or rather until defervescence, we have frequent remissions and accessions usually at periodic intervals, the paroxysms accompanied by local or patchy sweatings, and attended with emaciation and prostration

The pyæmic state, consisting of this hectic fever, with accompanying disseminated abscesses distributed over various parts of the body, but having a partiality for location in connection with lymphatic glands and vessels, generally succeeds the subsidence of the original or primary fever, and occasionally also the eruption of a primary abscess and discharge of pus It is characteristic of particular outbreaks of this fever of strangles, is a speciality of certain appearances of it as an epizootic, and sometimes seems much influenced as to the strength of its development by the character of the influences which surround the animals affected

With a view to give due consideration to these facts, observers, in speaking of this fever, have endeavoured to arrange it in forms and varieties These with advantage may justly and conveniently be all gathered or grouped under two divisions 1 Simple, benign, or regular strangles 2 Complicated, malignant, or irregular strangles The symptoms of both these forms of the disease result from the character of the fever and the phenomena attendant on the consecutive local lesions

1 **Regular or Benign Strangles**—This is a comparatively unimportant disorder, ushered in and accompanied by simple continued fever, which, however, is not invariably well marked, and which when pronounced reaches its acme with the abscess, defervescing with its decline and healing

There are ordinarily mild catarrhal symptoms The animal is rather dull, has a cough, with disinclination to eat, and when swallowing there is soreness of the throat. There may in some cases be a slight discharge of cellular matter from the nose, and frothy saliva from the mouth The head is poked forward, and shortly swelling may be observed in the submaxillary space, or at the base of the parotid gland.

The swelling or infiltration may occupy the whole of the space between the branches of the jaw on one or both sides of the inferior part of the larynx It may exist circumscribed at only one side of the space or throat; or it may be diffused.

The swelling steadily increases in size, becomes more painful to the touch, hard and defined, until the fluctuation indicates the presence of pus, which on evacuation is followed by subsidence of the swelling, amelioration of the general and local symptoms, and usually restoration to robust health

Cases may not unfrequently be met with where the general disturbance is less marked, and where the only abnormal feature attracting attention is the appearance of the swelling in the submaxillary space, which is subsequently developed into an abscess, with the formation and discharge of pus

In others, again, the constitutional disturbance, although not excessive, is much more protracted, the condition of ill-health continuing until the appearance and maturation of the characteristic abscess. Occasionally the local inflammation in connection with the structures in the vicinity of the larynx, the glands, and connective tissue, is more marked and earlier developed than the constitutional disturbance In such the symptoms are often alarming · the œdema of the glottis, and general infiltration of the submucous tissue of the larynx, with the implication of the connective and other structures around the upper portion of the air-tube, all tend to render respiration difficult of performance, giving rise to a loud and distressing sound, emitted during inspiration or expiration, according as the cartilages of the larynx have approached each other and so narrowed the tube, or as the tumefaction is more extensive in connection with the interior lining of the organ, generally, the sound is produced during both parts of the respiratory act, and may be trifling in its nature, passing off under a little judicious management, or the inflammatory condition may be so severe and so persistent as to endanger life by suffocation In such cases, also, there is a danger of the formation of an abscess, not superficially in the submaxillary space, but deep-seated in connection with the gland-structures contiguous to the pharynx and larynx, which may, even when progressing satisfactorily enough, endanger life, either by pressure upon the great air-tube, or by discharge of its contents into it.

In this regular form of strangles the abscess is generally single and well defined, and when matured and its contents discharged it does not return; occasionally there may be an eruption of one or more smaller pustules, or an appearance of a second and smaller growth on the subsidence of the primary one

2 **Malignant or Irregular Strangles**—Rarely is the irregular or complicated form associated with, or connected as a sequel to, the ordinary and regular, it generally appears and is developed *per se*, it is irregular and complicated from the first

By the term 'irregular' is meant that departure from the ordinary and recognised features of the disease both as to pyrexial symptoms and local manifestations The most frequent forms of irregularity and complication are those where the fever is still of the ordinary type, it may be more severe, but where the local inflammatory action and pus-production are removed from the submaxillary space, and attached to other gland-structures or their connective tissue, most frequently the intimate or contiguous structures of the parotid gland, the lymph-glands at the inferior part of the neck, under the levator humeri muscle, and less frequently the inguinal glands, or the glands of the mesentery or those in the chest

Although these irregular forms of the disease are as a rule irregular from the first, it is still not unfrequently seen that the local inflammatory action immediately antecedent to its establishment in the parotid region or other abnormal situations has made an appearance in the ordinary recognised situation, the submaxillary space, but only an appearance, proceeding a very short space and retrogressing. When the local diseased action seizes on these situations—such at least as are under our observation—the progress of the action in the formation of pus is as a rule tardy, and the systemic disturbance considerable; usually no well-formed abscess is the result, but the gland-structure may become permanently indurated and destroyed. At other times, particularly when affecting the lymph-glands at the point of the shoulder, the abscess is of great extent, and the pus well formed and laudable.

When the formation of the abscess occurs in connection with the gland-structures of the chest or abdomen, or with other internal organs, the symptoms of such disturbance vary in accordance with the organs and structures invaded. In all these conditions where there is a tendency to the formation of pus in connection with internal organs, we may expect a somewhat changed type of the fever; it will be subject to intermissions and regular paroxysms, these accessions accompanied with partial or local sweatings, accelerated breathing, and occasionally irregular cardiac action, marked wasting of tissue, exhaustion and prostration, together with local dropsies.

When the abscess is in connection with the mediastinum, there is usually embarrassed respiration or dyspnœa, with cough and anasarcous swelling at the inferior portion of the chest

When the mesenteric gland-structures are invaded, the probability is that the animal will exhibit fugitive abdominal or colicky pain, a depraved appetite, and an irregular condition of the bowels

In either of these situations the termination is apt to be fatal. In the thorax this is brought about either by suffocation resulting from the passage of pus into the bronchi and air-cells, or by the induction of inflammatory action in organs and structures of the chest. When occurring in the abdominal cavity, death is usually the result of peritonitis

Sequelæ of Strangles.—The most frequently occurring and damaging results or sequelæ of irregular strangles, and sometimes of the regular form, are those permanent structural changes which follow chiefly as a result of that form where the local diseased action is concentrated upon the larynx and structures associated with it. There is often left, as the result of an attack of this form, some textural change, either of the lining membrane and interior structures of the larynx, or of the surrounding and intrinsic muscles and their associated structures

Changes in either of these situations tend to the production of results precisely similar, viz , defective respiration. This disturbed functional activity is ordinarily recognised by some term taken from its audible manifestation, as *roaring*, *whistling*, etc.

By far the most serious sequelæ or results of strangles, however, are pyogenic fever, pyæmia, and general blood-poisoning, the result of absorption of certain decomposing or degraded materials, the product of local inflammatory action—most probably puriform constituents or certain liquid inflammatory products. We speak of this infective process as *pyæmia* when, in conjunction with the fever, there are numerous secondary disseminated abscesses in various organs ; and as blood-poisoning, or *septicæmia*, when, with the pyrexia, we have general and marked disturbance of vital functions, but not necessarily abscesses. There is, however, a great probability that no true pathological difference exists between the two named conditions. Both *pyæmia* and *septicæmia* result from the absorption of certain infective substances from some foci of local inflammation.

There is, however, a distinct difference between *pyæmia* and abscesses, the result of irregular forms of the disease.

Generally speaking, those large, well-formed abscesses or collections of pus seen in the lymphatic glands, in the region of the neck and limbs, ought rather to be regarded as belonging to the latter than to the former cases.

When *pyæmia* is encountered as associated with or rather resulting from strangles, it is following, not concomitant with, the occurrence of the primary abscesses ; or at least it rarely follows so closely in the wake of these as does the development of additional abscesses and purulent infiltrations characteristic of the ordinary irregular forms of the fever.

Usually one or more abscesses have either naturally or by assistance discharged their contents, and for a few days the animal seems convalescent, when suddenly the febrile symptoms start into greater prominence than at first, and are characterized by regular and recurring paroxysms, accompanied with partial and local sweatings, irregular action of the heart, and accelerated respiration

In some cases the temperature has continued steadily high ; more frequently the elevation is concomitant with the occurrence of the paroxysmal attacks; while between these periods of exacerbations it may be little, if at all, above normal standard.

Most of the cases exhibiting these symptoms of hectic are observed in animals unfavourably circumstanced either as to original constitutional stamina—that is, that they, previously to the attack of strangles, were not in a state of robust or vigorous health—or that at this particular time they are operated upon by depressing influences, hygienically and dietetically   They may be subjected to the pernicious influence of decomposing organic matter through the medium of the air or drinking-water, while the food supplied may be deficient in nutriment for an already exhausted system.

Immediately following those renewed indications of pyrexia, and certainly not previous to their establishment, there may appear on different parts of the body—chiefly the limbs—small, nodulated tumours, apparently situated in the subcutaneous connective tissue, placed along the course of the vessels on the inner surface of the limb, not unlike at this stage the first appearance of farcy-buds.   These shortly soften, and discharge a little pus.   More rarely the structures in the vicinity of the joints are specially invaded by similar small abscesses, the destructive effects of which may extend to and impair the integrity of the articulation with which they are connected.

The more fatal cases, however, are those where these multiple abscesses, developing from several centres of local inflammation, are situated in the more important internal organs—the lungs, the liver, or the heart. When these particular viscera are invaded, there are, in addition to the ordinary train of symptoms, others which specially indicate the visceral implications So long as the development of these multiple abscesses seems confined to the subcutaneous tissue of the limbs, the animal may continue to feed moderately well, and if they are restricted to these situations, it may ultimately recover When, however, pneumonic, cardiac, or enteric symptoms manifest themselves, consecutive to this condition of hectic, there is small chance of recovery Food is refused, a catarrhal and irritable state of the intestinal membrane may develop itself, the great serous cavities of the thorax and abdomen become charged with fluid, and rapid disintegration of lung-tissue ensue, with such conditions there is rarely sufficient stamina left to enable the animal to recover Fatal exhaustion may not be so rapid as we might anticipate; it is, however, certain.

Why these conditions of pyæmia and of septic contamination of the blood should not occur in every case, or at least in a greater number of cases of strangles than they really do, or why they occur in any instance, or what is the mode of their production, are questions which, although they have been much debated, may even yet be regarded as scarcely answered.

That it is due to the absorption into and admixture with the blood of some material or agent which thus acts in a deleterious manner, and by selective affinity is specially detained and operative at the particular centres of local inflammatory action, as also that this morbific factor or agent is in a certain manner related to the previously existing foci of inflammation and suppuration, is in these cases now under notice tolerably certain.

The idea that the passage into the blood of pus simply as pus, and which, either from the physical characters or size of its formed materials, and the operation physically or mechanically of such when located in the capillaries of an organ, or that its vital or chemical action on the blood in an ordinary and healthy condition, so to speak, is the true cause, explanation, or source of the multiple abscesses met with in cases of pyæmia following strangles, is at the present scarcely regarded as the correct explanation of this condition

It would seem rather that the facts and evidence with which we are acquainted point to the occurrence of a change, or further diseased condition, first occurring in connection with the puriform secretion and other inflammatory products, which, on being taken into the circulation, induce, under certain conditions, the phenomena recorded and spoken of under the terms pyæmia and septic poisoning of the blood Most probably the delay in removal of the inflammatory products, previous to pus-formation, renders these a fit soil for the development of bacterial forms, which, acting on these inflammatory products, render them infective and capable of producing secondary abscesses and blood-contamination, for it is an ascertained fact that bacteria are ever present in secondary or pyæmic lesions In this way we may so far account for the occurrence of this septic condition as a sequel of strangles in the horse in those cases where the animals, when suffering from the primary disease, are subjected to those unwholesome influences attendant upon defective sanitary and other conditions, or where, previous to the incursion of the fever, there existed a peculiar dyscrasia

Treatment — Simple or benign strangles rarely requires much medical treatment, properly so called Those various conditions and details which together constitute correct hygiene are the indications which require specially to be attended to When first affected, whether in the open air or located in the stable, if attainable, the animal is best placed in a good clean loose box or covered yard, where there is sufficient space for movement, a good supply of pure air and light, without being exposed to cold draughts Should the temperature be elevated from the normal standard, and other febrile symptoms pronounced, it is always advisable to allow in the drinking water, which ought always to be within reach of the animal, a moderate amount of such cooling salines as sulphate of soda, sulphate of magnesia, bicarbonate, nitrate or chlorate of potass By one friend of mine large quantities of solution of acetate of ammonia, with full doses of salicylic acid, are given from the commencement of the fever, and apparently with the effect of moderating its severity. These are taken in the drinking water Should angina be troublesome, attended with difficulty in deglutition, or in cases where the cough is distressing from the laryngeal irritation, good results generally follow the inhalation of simple or medicated hot-water vapour once or twice daily

7

In addition to this steaming of the upper air-passages, the exhibition of compound camphor electuary twice or thrice daily is much to be recommended. The external application of soap or ammonia liniment, or, what is probably better, of a mustard or mustard and linseed-meal poultice, or a smart cantharides liniment, is, in the majority of cases of troublesome angina and cough, productive of relief. When the swelling in the submaxillary space becomes evident, or tumefaction anywhere in the region of the throat, warm-water fomentations or warm poultices are probably the most successful means of hastening their development and the formation of pus. With some animals the application of poultices is a difficult matter; in such cases similar results will be obtained if a piece of fresh sheep, hare, or rabbit skin is placed with the raw surface to the swelling, and kept there for a few days, taking care during that time to remove it regularly, and keep the parts sweet and clean, either by washing or changing the membrane. Should the enlargement or tumour in the submaxillary space or elsewhere in this region fail to progress satisfactorily, seeming to remain stationary, good will result from the application of a little blister, or daily friction with common iodine ointment. Such treatment will generally confer fresh activity upon the local action, tending to development of the abscess; or it may, as sometimes observed, produce the opposite effects, and tend to induce absorption of the exudate.

When the abscess is fully matured, it will, either by softening and rupture of cutaneous tissues, discharge itself, or, if thought preferable, it may be opened.

It is certainly good in every case to allow the abscess to be fully matured ere it is opened. Some object strongly to open these in any case, advising that all be allowed to rupture without interference. The objection to this in every case is, that very many if left to themselves would rupture by such an extensive outlet as to cause unnecessary sloughing of skin and other tissue, and thus in healing leave an objectionably large cicatrix.

Again, on the other hand, there is no doubt that when opened too early, there is a disposition to re-form.

The abscess having discharged itself, nothing requires to be done save bathing with tepid or warm carbolized water as often as needful to keep it clean, and where the healing is rather tardy or seemingly not proceeding in a healthy manner, to touch the raw surfaces with a little nitrate of silver daily

During the entire course of the fever, and while the abscess is maturing, it will be very needful that we should give close attention to the dietary of the animal, so that should more serious results follow, the bowels in particular may not be found confined

With this end in view, allow scalded oats, with bran, twice or thrice daily, adding to this once daily from one to four ounces of good linseed oil, or double these quantities of treacle   Give the hay picked, good, and in small quantities Where green food, as grass or vetches, can be obtained, it is in moderation preferable to aught else, while where dry fodder is alone to be relied upon, it may be usefully supplemented with a few sliced roots

During recovery, even in the simple and mild cases, when we find that health and vigour are not returning so rapidly as we would desire, a trifling amount of exercise in the open air, and the administration of such tonics as preparations of iron, quinine, or arsenic, are always deserving of a trial

The more severe and dangerous cases of malignant or irregular strangles must be treated upon the same general principles   Avoid all depressing and debilitating influences ; ensure the animal s being benefited by good dieting and wholesome surrounding sanitary conditions   Where local inflammations and swellings indicate the probability of pus-formation, treat as advised in like conditions under the simple form, always remembering that heat and moisture favour the maturation of abscesses, and that as soon as such is complete, but not till then, give every facility for the escape of contained material   Where debility and exhaustion are marked constitutional features, which they almost invariably are in these forms, a certain amount of stimulation will be necessary so as to enable the creature to tide over the crisis of the disease

During the formation of the abscesses and continuance of the fever, although forcible administration of nutriment, whenever an animal refuses to take what we regard as a sufficiency of food, is not to be recommended, it will be found that here a large number imperatively demand it.

If ordinary food, in any form in which it may be offered, is persistently refused, a trial ought to be made of such as contain nutritive material more concentrated. Milk, when allowed, is sometimes drunk freely, and if so, may be mixed with good beef tea, or ale. And if absolutely needful to forcibly feed for a time, raw eggs whipped up and mixed with milk, brandy, wine, or good ale, are probably the most convenient and desirable form in which to administer the nourishment; and these are always better given in moderate quantities and often, than in larger quantities and at longer intervals.

When from the local inflammation and its effects on the organs and structures in the upper passages, particularly the larynx, the function of respiration is impeded, and there is a danger of suffocation, it may be needful to have recourse to surgical interference to obviate such untoward results

The operation of tracheotomy, although a purely surgical matter, may appropriately be glanced at in connection with the treatment of strangles

I am aware that some have condemned the operation as in reality of no ultimate use or benefit in this disease, even when asphyxia is imminent, asserting that the operation is likely to be productive of as unfavourable results as allowing the disease to take its course. Such, however, has not been my experience, as I am satisfied that in many instances the timely performance of the operation has saved the life of the animal, nor has the operation in these instances left any bad results.

The performance of the operation is not to be advised so long as there is a probability that it may be dispensed with. Hot-water applications, poultices, and steaming of the head ought to be persevered in for some hours continuously, and if the dyspnœa should increase, rendering it apparent that suffocation is impending, it will then become needful to give the relief so much needed by opening the windpipe. This opening of the great air-tube is of itself a simple operation, more judgment being required to determine when it ought to be done than skill needed in the actual performance. In addition to the simple opening of the tube, it is generally considered necessary to pass through the opening made in the trachea a variously formed metal tube by which communication with the outer air is rendered patent, this tube being retained in its position as long as needful

In performing the operation, it is rarely necessary to cast the animal, or even place him under restraint It is readily enough accomplished by simply elevating the head, which, being straightened upon the cervical articulation, so places the structures on the inferior surface of the neck in a state of tension The operator, selecting that portion of the trachea which is least covered with muscular or other tissue, which is about one-third of its length from the angle of the jaw, nearly where the subscapulo-hyoideus passes from beneath the diverging sterno-maxillaris muscles, makes an incision from one to two inches in length directly on the trachea, following the course of the tube, he may either pass the point of his scalpel straight through the wall of the tube, dividing transversely two or more of its rings, or he may pass a strong needle, armed with a stout ligature, through one of the rings, and with the knife excise a circular portion, probably of one whole ring and portions of other two, the one above and the other below, having the orifice a little smaller than the tube he intends to insert

Either of these methods will succeed; but if the first be adopted, the tube is grasped much tighter, a little care being exercised when it is passed to avoid carrying with it the edges of the trachea

The tube must be allowed to remain in its situation until the difficulty in breathing—the cause for its insertion—has been removed This is easily ascertained by at any time placing the hand over the orifice, with or without the removal of the inserted instrument On being finally removed, the wound may be left to close without further interference, or in some instances two or three sutures may be passed through the superficial edges

From the fact that during a few years of the earlier period of their lives a very large percentage of horses are sufferers from strangles, as also believing in the probability that animals once affected have conferred upon them an immunity from further attacks, many breeders and owners of horses show little disposition to adopt measures to prevent its occurrence or limit its dissemination However, as it does not appear that there is anything essentially characteristic in the constitution or temperament of the horse which renders it inevitably certain that all shall be affected with the disease, nor yet that it is necessary for his future development or vigorous health, added to which is the consideration of deterioration and loss attendant on an accession of strangles and the possibility of its propagation by contagion, it is assuredly a more rational procedure to put in force all preventive measures with a view to mitigate its severity or circumscribe its development   In addition to removing all causes extrinsic and intrinsic which may operate as predisposing influences, attention ought to be bestowed on the protection of the healthy from such agencies which, from their relation to, or association with, the diseased, may be considered capable of inducing it, as removal of the actually suffering from amongst the healthy, abstaining from using the same utensils in connection with both, and thoroughly cleansing and disinfecting stables and furnishings where the diseased have been located ere healthy animals are permanently or temporarily placed there.

CHAPTER IV.

GLANDERS AND FARCY —EQUINIA.

SYNONYMS.—Malleus, Equinæ Apostimatos, Malleus Humidus, Maliasmus, Farcinnia, Farcina equi, etc

Definition —*A specific contagious disease of a malignant type, the spontaneous origin of which has not been demonstrated. In the horse, the specific effects of the implanted virus are shown on the nasal mucous membrane, from which an aqueous, viscid or purulent fluid is discharged, and on which chancre-like sores are formed. The mucous membrane of the sinuses of the head, the larynx and trachea, as also the lung-tissue, are specifically affected. There may also be a general or local inflammation of the lymphatic vessels, lymphatic glands and skin, with a tendency to form small circumscribed tumours, known as farcy buds or buttons, which gradually*

develop into pustules, and ultimately suppurate and discharge
pus, which is charged with the specific virus of the disease

Historical Notice of Glanders and Farcy.—There is little
doubt that glanders and farcy, considering their wide geographical distribution, and their constant malignancy through
all time, must have been observed from a remote antiquity
The earliest notice of this disease—regarding glanders and
farcy as essentially one—is probably that by Apsyrtus, a
veterinary officer in the army of Constantine the Great, in the
fourth century   It is also, in the fifth century, described by
Vegitius.   Both of these, and others of the early writers on
the diseases of the horse, under the names of *Malleus, Morbus
humidus,* etc, have evidently grouped many dissimilar,
although dangerous, diseases of that animal.

Previous to the establishment of the fact that glanders could
be communicated to man, a wonderful amount of interest
attached to the disease, from its supposed relation to human
pathology, being regarded by some authorities as the source
from which the poison of syphilis had originated, both having
been reported to have appeared at the same time, at the siege
of Naples, at the end of the fifteenth century   These ideas
have, however, been overturned, experimentation showing
clearly that syphilis and glanders are distinct and not inter-
changeable diseases

The most notable points in the history of glanders, and
those which more than most others have furnished matter for
dispute, are its contagiousness and the modes of its development

As early as 1664, Sollysel recognised the contagiousness of
glanders , also Garsault, 1741 ; and both the Lafosses, 1754-
1772 ; while in 1797 Viborg, from accurately conducted experiments, demonstrated both its malignancy and inoculability
These experiments were confirmed at the beginning of the
present century by Gohier and Huzard   It is curious to observe
that, notwithstanding such experimental evidence, the supporters of the non-contagious theory, composed of able
and distinguished Frenchmen, should so long have held their
ground, and, through the dissemination of their ideas, entailed
so large a pecuniary loss upon their country

It was at the Alford Veterinary School, by Bourgelat and

Chabert, that the non-contagious nature of glanders was so strenuously upheld at the end of last century. While the school and teachers at Alford were mainly instrumental in upholding the non-contagious theory of the disease, the veterinary teaching at Lyons never ceased to be directed in the opposite direction.

The same diversity and opposition of opinion has been exhibited in the views entertained in respect of the nature of the disease.

Its relation, connection, or similarity to tuberculosis, or scrofula, have been entertained and written upon by Dupuy (1817), Dettrich (1851), Baron, Philippe, Roll, Falke, Spinola, Villemin, and others Not satisfied with this relationship, some of these veterinarians, with others equally industrious and learned, endeavoured to establish a connection and similarity between glanders and diphtheria, or pyæmia. Amongst the supporters of the former idea are to be ranked Dettrich, Kreutzer, Roll ; amongst the latter, Ercolani, Bassi, Brukmüller

From 1855-1863, by the investigations of Virchow and the researches of Leisering, much was done to improve our knowledge of the nature of glanders and to inculcate correct ideas regarding it.

The question of the birth or origin of glanders has, with that relating to its nature, been warmly debated, and opposing views regarding it have been registered. From the experimental investigations of Renault and Bouley (1840), it seemed tolerably well established that the disease might be developed autochthonously as well as by inoculation These and other investigators, both on the Continent and in our own country, claimed to have produced glanders in horses, not only by the injection into the circulation of puriform fluids, but also of various dissimilar noxious, irritant, organic and inorganic agents, in this way tending to invalidate the idea of the specific nature of the disease, and to establish that at most it was but a form of septic poisoning of the blood

Until a very recent period—indeed, until our own day—I am not aware of any veterinarian of note, here or on the Continent, with the exception of Gerlach, who has not accepted and adopted, it may be with some slight modification, the theory that glanders is capable of spontaneous development

Geographical Distribution — Glanders, and its variation, farcy, although very widely distributed, is apparently more extensively diffused where horses are treated in a highly artificial manner, and have operating on them such adverse influences as overwork, defective location, and insufficient dieting

It is said not to exist in our Australian colonies, and to be sparingly encountered in many parts of our Indian empire. It appears to prevail most extensively in temperate regions, and is of less frequent occurrence in very cold or very warm latitudes, although to this there are exceptions It is well known in Norway, and equally so in Java

Pathology *a Nature of Glanders* —The terms 'glanders' and 'farcy' are employed to designate merely phases or manifestations of the same diseased condition This condition is named 'glanders' when the specific or diagnostic symptoms and lesions are connected with the mucous membrane of the nose, upper air-passages, and the lungs, together with lymph vessels and glands adjacent thereto, and 'farcy,' when the morbific agent seems to locate itself, and is inducing specific changes in the skin and subcutaneous connective tissue, with the lymphatic vessels and lymph-glands belonging to these These two forms of the disease may be seen in the same animal at one time, or at varying intervals ; and the virus of the one may produce the other in its implantation from the diseased to the healthy Although in every case of well-pronounced glanders there is generally one particular organ or structure where the local lesions characteristic of the malady are more and better developed than in others, it seems, by experimentation, that on inoculation of a healthy animal with the matter from these dominant lesions of the diseased, the same distinctness and predominance of diagnostic lesions in organs and tissues similar to those from which the virus was taken does not hold good , that, in short, the results always, where successful, are diagnostic of glanders, but are not, as respects their dominant situations, to be determined from knowing the source from which the infecting material was taken Thus we may inoculate a healthy horse with the discharge from a glanderous

sore of the nasal septum, while, if the inoculation is successful, the specific lesions may be indifferently on the nasal
membrane, or in connection with the lymphatics of the extremities

When referring to the history of glanders, it was noticed
that different ideas had, at different times, been held by all
who had paid more than passing attention to the disease   By
many of our most able investigators in the field of comparative pathology, as Villemin, Roll, Falke, and some others, it has
been looked upon in all pertaining to its characters, causation,
symptoms, etc.—in truth, to its essential nature—as certainly
analogous to, if not identical with, tuberculosis or scrofula.
This relationship we cannot admit, as both its genesis and
entire clinical history clearly indicate that it possesses an
individuality and specificity entirely its own   By Virchow it
is placed amongst those diseases commonly described as
'granulomes,' or granulation tumours, it being regarded as a
diseased condition having a tendency to the formation of
granular cells and minute tissue disintegration, or local destructive processes   While the ultimate cause of these minute
or elemental changes is regarded as intimately associated with,
or probably resulting from, some alteration in the nutritive processes carried on in the tissues, the local capillary embolism
and phlebitis being in all these cases regarded as closely bound
up with this perverted nutrition tissue-decay, and death.

Again, it is particularly to be observed that in the acute
form glanders has a great resemblance to pyæmia or septicæmia; and by many has been regarded as the true repre-
sentation, in the horse, of these generally recognised morbid
states of the blood

Although certainly differing from these pathological conditions in which the degraded and infecting products of
inflammatory action are present in the circulation, there
is little doubt that the blood is in a diseased condition,
seeing we know by experimentation that it contains the actual
and active morbific agent of the disease, and thus we have
little difficulty to understand, so far, that healthy nutrition is
incapable of being carried on for any time, and that with impairment or arrest of healthy nutrition we have molecular or
systemic death

It seems abundantly clear, from experimentation by inoculation with secretions or animal fluids containing the active
virus of the disease, that the power of unicity of infection is
constantly maintained, and that in every case where persistent
disturbance is induced, the terminal processes and tissue-
changes are of an uniform character, that glanders will invariably produce glanders, and not tuberculosis or cancer.
Whether the obvious and accompanying elemental changes
are to be explained simply on chemico-physiological grounds,
without reference to individual life and life-processes in the
imported contagious elements, remains yet to be determined

b. Causation—Although peculiarly a disease of the equine
species, glanders is undoubtedly capable of transmission to
many other animals, and to none probably oftener than to
man. While the susceptibility of the human subject to
become infected with the poison of glanders is considerable, it
has rarely been brought forward—or, if instanced, has been
unsupported by proof sufficient to satisfy—as a disease which
in man is capable of development apart from inoculation or
infection   In the horse this is quite different, and, although
amongst the greater number of those who in our day are culti-
vating pathological inquiry through experimentation, the
autochthonous origin of this disease, as also of all contagious
specific maladies, is being received with less favour, there is
yet, I am satisfied, particularly amongst practical veterinarians
whose work is confined to the large centres of the horse
population, both in this country and on the Continent, a very
firm conviction in the frequency, or at least possibility, of a
direct and spontaneous origin of glanders in horses.

For my own part, reasoning from analogy, and the results of
a comparatively limited experience, I have ever regarded the
spontaneous origin of glanders in horses as very problematical

If capable of being originated *de novo*, it is unlike the particular class—the specific communicable diseases—to which it
belongs, a class feature of which is that they are only capable
of propagation by the reception in the healthy of the specific
virus manufactured or proceeding from the diseased   Every
case of glanders with which I have come in contact has been
most reasonably accounted for on the theory of infection or in-

oculation   in the majority they have been easily and directly
traceable to this source

As already stated, glanders and farcy are perfectly identical
affections, both owing their origin—whatever that may be—to
the same cause or causes, and differing only in their local
manifestations, farcy being simply the local and cutaneous
eruption incident to glanders, and although sometimes distinctly and separately spoken of, it is only as a matter of convenience, the distinction having no foundation in the nature of
the disease, nor yet in any recognised system of classification

The causes which are believed to operate in the direct and
spontaneous development of glanders are all such as tend to
debility and impairment of constitutional stamina, defective or
perverted nutrition, causes not at all dissimilar to those believed to be in ascendency in the production of typhus, tuberculosis, or phthisis in man

It is regularly induced, we are told by those who advocate this mode of development, where the laws which
regulate healthy animal existence, those connected with work,
location, food, and the apportioning of these to age and other
conditions of the organism, are persistently infringed   It is in
this way, it is asserted, and by the operation of causes such as
these, that glanders is so frequently seen in large studs of
horses, as tramway, omnibus, and colliery establishments, where
overwork, insufficient feeding, location in filthy, undrained,
badly ventilated, and ill-lighted stables extensively prevail.
Similar causes, it is imagined, account for it as a frequent
attendant on the transport of horses in ill-conditioned and
crowded vessels, and their congregation in camps and armies,
where the deteriorating influences resulting from noxious
emanations proceeding from decomposing animal excreta and
secretions have full play

Instances corroborative of the direct and spontaneous development of glanders under these differing conditions are
given by most writers on the subject past and present.   The
case of the celebrated Quiberon Expedition is pretty well
known to most who have taken any interest in this subject
Here horses said to have been embarked apparently healthy
were, after enforced confinement under the closed hatchways
of the transports during a storm, and thus subjected to a
deficiency of healthful respirable air, and the action of con-

fined secretions and decomposing excreta under a high temperature and much attendant excitement, found suffering from glanders, or farcy, or both. Mr. Fleming, in his 'Sanitary Veterinary Police,' mentions, as a necessary accompaniment or consequence of the collection of large numbers of horses, and the wasting and depressing influences operating on these when engaged in active campaigning during our more recent European wars, the sudden and extensive distribution of glanders amongst the cavalry horses composing the armies engaged in these operations. It is there particularly noted that 'the magnificent German cavalry that invaded France took the field after every care had been exercised that no glandered horses should be in the ranks, and yet at the end of the campaign every regiment, it is reported, was more or less infected, the necessities and hardships of war having as usual engendered it' I believe, however, that since this was written my learned friend has seen cause to change his views respecting the genesis of glanders. Very similar is the experience recorded by those connected with the British cavalry during our invasion of the Crimea

Many of those who have the professional charge of large studs of horses in civil life tell the same story.

It has also, it is stated, been found that locating horses in newly built, imperfectly dried, and untempered stables has been found to act prejudicially, by developing glanders

All these causes, essentially exhausting and depressing, favour the development of this or any other disease characterized by vitiated and depraved blood, and impaired, defective, or perverted nutrition, resulting in serious structural alterations and tissue-changes

They do this—(1) By the production of noxious miasm, deleterious agents resulting from the changes of surrounding organic compounds, and the entrance of these into the animal body. (2) By increasing the natural waste and tissue-change, and by further and pernicious alteration of these changed, as also of the imbibed materials (3) By preventing the natural elimination, through arrest of activities by which naturally the system rids itself not merely of the normally used-up materials, but of those which may have been unnaturally formed there, or introduced from without

Under such conditions as these, if glanders, either as glanders or as farcy, is not at once developed, the animals are so debilitated and predisposed, that even at some time subsequent, on being attacked by ordinary diseases of an enfeebling character, particularly in connection with the respiratory structures, they are more liable than others which have been differently circumstanced to develop glanders

Further, it is asserted that even apart from any apparently adverse and debilitating influences, recovery from certain exhausting diseases is not unfrequently arrested by the appearance of glanders. This has been particularly noticed in cases of *diabetes insipidus*, in malignant strangles, lingering cases of influenza, and in scabies.

The difficulties in the way of our acceptance of the theory of the spontaneous origin of the disease are certainly great, particularly the difficulty of obtaining in many cases sufficient evidence respecting the time and mode of infection, specially so when dealing with the insidious forms. The main support of the theory rests upon the results of a few experiments, which in the present state of our knowledge of pathological histology we are scarcely prepared unreservedly to accept.

The most significant of these experiments are those of Renault and Bouley, detailed in the 'Recueil de méd. Vétérin,' vol xvii p 257, 1840, in which there was injected into the veins of a horse, selected for the purpose of experiment, healthy pus, obtained from an issue that had been established in another sound animal Upon the sixth subsequent day there were developed upon the nose specific pustules, that were soon followed by ulcers. Death resulted at the expiration of eight days. The autopsy showed numerous nodules in the lungs, with tubercles and ulcers on the lining membrane of the nose. The retro-inoculation of another horse by means of the nasal discharge of this animal was followed by a positive result.

Laisné ('La clinique Vétérinaire,' t iv p 463, 1864) claimed to have implanted glanders by the introduction of healthy pus into the nasal cavity. Erdt ('Die Rotzdyskrasie,' etc., Leipzig, 1863), who regarded glanders as a form of scrofula, inoculated horses with scrofulous matter taken from the human subject, and asserts that he had in this manner produced glanders

Vines (*loc. cit*) went still further, alleging that he had seen glanders induced in mules and asses by the action of various irritating substances, for instance, by the injection of vitriol into the trachea, and by the introduction of the blood of a rabid dog (See Ziemssen—Bollinger, ' Glanders,' p 326)

When we know that in cases of pyæmia, the result of embolism, structural changes are often encountered, particularly in the lungs, much akin to what are observed in the same situations in glanders, we are not unwarranted in asking for further demonstration in confirmation of the genesis of glanders, apart from other causes than specific contagion; while, when we regard experiments which have been productive of negative or opposite results, this demand is further strengthened

In connection with and bearing upon this point may be mentioned the experiments of Leuret (' Archives générales de Méd,' t xi p 98, 1826), who injected putrid ichorus matter directly into the veins, and also into the subcutaneous cellular tissue of horses. In this manner he obtained the appearances produced by putrid infection, but he does not mention any alterations characteristic of glanders

Bilroth (' Allg Chir Pathologie und Therapie,' 5 Aufl p 97, 1871) refers to a similar experiment upon a horse, that was not followed by any symptoms of glanders.

Gamgee, quoting from Hering, reports a case of thrombosis of the vessels of the lungs, with abscesses of these organs, occurring in a horse after injection of pus into the jugular vein

Gunther, Spinola, and Lees injected pus into the veins of horses without producing glanders, while Waldenburgh, in conjunction with Köhne, inoculated several horses with tubercular, phthisical, and purulent substances without causing a single case of glanders The negative results as respects the production of glands from injection into the circulation of purulent fluid, I can corroborate from personal observation.

The conclusions to be drawn from experimental research as to the development of glanders from purulent injection are certainly not sufficiently convincing, while the clinical evidence is very often what may be regarded as too shallow and restrictive, and is drawn from a non-recognition of several important facts connected with the mode of the development of the disease in its more insidious forms.

We have been very apt to overlook the long period of incubation in certain developments of the disease, and also too much wedded to the idea that the early features or characteristic lesions of the disease are generally, if not always, to be encountered in the skin or mucous membrane of the nose ; whereas we know very well that in many cases, if not in the majority, the primary lesions are met with in the lungs, the trachea, or the larynx, the lesions of the nasal membrane being secondary or terminal, and in not a few no lesions may be discoverable.

It is a well-known fact that glanders may be propagated by horses which have not shown any unmistakable symptoms of the malady, and where, judging from what has been observed on examination after death, the lesions were confined to the lungs.

I have a distinct recollection of the propagation of glanders in a very malignant form by a pony in which no visible symptoms of the disease could be traced.

This animal had been bought at a distance, and when brought home by the purchaser it was placed in a stable along with a four-year-old well-bred colt, which had been bred and reared on the farm, and where no glanders had ever before been known to exist.

After being in company with the pony for about three weeks, I found the colt on examination to be exhibiting unmistakable symptoms of acute glanders. The left side of the nasal septum was possessed by several well-formed characteristic ulcers with eroded margins, and several small tubercles in the neighbourhood of these, with considerable swelling of the submaxillary gland of the same side, which was hard, nodulated, and closely adherent to the bone. The nasal discharges were also much tinged with blood, and the breathing was snuffling, indicative of the involvement of the membrane and structures higher up the nasal chambers.

The pony was examined repeatedly from this time until it was sent off the farm several weeks subsequently, but on no occasion could I detect aught characteristic of glanders, nor anything unnatural save a cough, a rather dry condition of the skin, and an open or staring coat. There was also to be observed on certain occasions a slight watery discharge from the nose, the membrane of which was always of a faint slate-colour, but certainly unabraded, untuberculated, and without erosion. Very similar details are given by Bollinger and by Bagge. The latter, indeed, gives as the result of the examination of one hundred and seven horses of a Dutch regiment, that were killed over a period of three years in consequence of being glandered or of showing symptoms of a suspicious character, that in the case of ten there were decided structural changes (ulcers in the nasal cavity), in thirteen the alterations were slight; in fifty-three there were merely nodules in the lungs and a few ulcers in the nasal passages (this number being to all appearance healthy during life), and in thirty-three no lesions whatever were found.

   c. *Modes of Propagation. Contagion, Infection.*—Although for a long time it was denied that glanders could be propagated in any other manner than by exogenous influences, and that consequently there was no specific poison connected with it, by general consent it is now regarded as a highly contagious malady.

   The certainty of the existence in the various fluids and secretions of the animal of a specific infecting virus has been abundantly demonstrated by experimental investigation.

   There certainly seem degrees of virulence amongst the varied discharges or fluid materials derived from the diseased animals, and with which inoculations have been made, or which have by accident become implanted in the living animal. And although its action does not entirely depend upon the channel through which an entrance is made into the system, it does seem that such has at least some influence either in modifying its potency or the extent of its absorption into the blood.

   The poison seems to exist in greatest potency in the nasal discharges, the discharge from the chancre-like sore, the various secretions, and the blood. Inoculation can be effected through the medium of the skin when this is abraded, the mucous membrane by employing friction or without it, and by injection into the connective tissue and the blood.

   Although at the present day it is almost universally ad-

8

mitted that glanders is a contagious malady, it is yet certain
that its propagation from the diseased to the healthy is to a
certain extent regulated by individual idiosyncrasy or susceptibility Neither from experimentation nor from clinical
observation or recorded history of special outbreaks can we
come to absolutely certain conclusions as to the exact mode
by which the virus finds an entrance into the system

The generally received opinion on this matter is that the
infecting material of glanders becomes attached to some
exposed or external surface of the body, where, by some breach
of tissue continuity already existing, or the production of
such through local irritation, it finds its way into the general
circulation   In this way it is sought to account for the production of the disease in cases where healthy animals are
brought into contact with the diseased, or where the former
have been placed in stables where diseased have previously
been located

That this is most probably the mode of infection in even
the greater number of cases, neither deductions arrived at
from a knowledge of the modes by which other infecting
poisons operate, nor yet the results of experimental research,
nor of clinical observation, would lead us to believe   If it
were true that the morbific material of glanders is, as a rule,
implanted in the animal system by direct contact, we should
expect to meet more frequently, as a primary diagnostic lesion,
the specific cutaneous and external changes so characteristic
of the disease

Now there is little doubt that these external structural
changes, whether in the true cutaneous tissues or in the nasal
membrane, are in many, probably in the great majority of
instances, not the primary, but the secondary or terminal
symptoms We know that when situated on the nasal mucous
membrane the tubercles and chancres are generally in the
upper part of these cavities, and in the larynx and trachea,
before they appear where they are capable of detection

If we discard the idea that the poison of glanders as a rule
enters the body through the external surface either of the skin
or the visible mucous membranes, it seems that we are driven
to admit the existence of a volatile infecting virus, and that,
as such, it must, where not actually implanted, find its way

into the body by means of the inspired air, or possibly by the food or drinking-water

By a volatile infecting poison, it is not meant that this must of necessity be gaseous; it need not be so · it may be an organized agent, vegetable or animal, of such a character as to be capable of being carried by the air to a certain distance from the focus of its production

By this vehicle it may be conveyed into the blood, first of all producing a poisoned condition of this fluid, resulting in the development of the peculiar and specific phenomena, the tuberculation, nodulation, and distinctive lesions in different situations in the lungs and air-passages, or it may at once produce the specific pulmonary lesions, to be followed as a sequel by general blood-poisoning

As so far confirmatory of the existence of a volatile infecting virus are the experiments of Viborg and of Gerlach, both of whom succeeded in producing glanders in healthy horses by inoculating them with the condensed exhalations and sweat of the diseased No doubt it is also true that other experiments, such as those conducted by Hertwig and Reynault, where the healthy and glandered horses were made to respire at the same time through a common bag or tube attached to the noses of both, were productive of negative results.

This is perfectly possible, for we know that certain animals possess a peculiar insusceptibility to the action of many noxious agents, and is very little, if any stronger evidence, against the idea that the virus is volatile, and does enter the system through the medium of the air, than many other experiments; than that of White's, for instance, recorded in his ' Compendium of the Veterinary Art,' in which he states having retained for a considerable time in the nasal chambers of a horse pieces of cloth saturated with pus from a diseased animal without producing this disease

The great probability of the infecting agent of glanders being volatile as well as fixed, and consequently its likelihood of being introduced into the economy through the medium of the inspired air, is] further strengthened by the fact that the disease is propagated from animals which have neither discharge from the nose nor external cutaneous lesions—nothing, in fact, diagnostic, save pulmonary nodules and infiltration,

8—2

as also from knowing that horses which have received the infecting material may for some time continue vigorous and to
all appearance healthy, and only after a considerable period
exhibit visible local specific lesions; while again the results
of experimental investigation may be cited as confirmatory,
for in cases where the poison has been introduced into the
system of horses and other animals susceptible of being contaminated, the selective affinity of the poison for the nose and
nasal membrane is distinctly manifest

These results I have observed in horses, and experiments
upon other animals corroborate them

When we regard the numerous direct experiments which
have been carried out by different observers in different
countries, there would appear to be no doubt that the virus
of glanders exists as a fixed infectious agent in the specific
local lesions of the diseased, as the ulcers of the nasal membrane, the tubercles from the lungs, and also in the blood and
blood plasma found as fluid in the softer organs and
tissues, also probably in most of the secretions and excretions
of the body, the sweat, the saliva, urine, tears, etc, although,
as respects some of these latter, we are well aware that
attempts to inoculate with them have occasionally proved
abortive (Viborg, Coleman, Hering, Chauveau)

Not only does it appear that the poison of glanders is communicated by immediate or direct contact of the diseased with
the healthy, it is in addition tolerably certain that it may be
propagated by mediate or indirect contact, that is, by some
intermediate bearer of the virus, which, being charged with the
infecting material, conveys it to the still healthy

The external media acting in this manner are the harness
and clothing of diseased horses, the woodwork, fittings, and
utensils of stables, as also the similar accessories of railway
and other carriages where diseased animals have been placed

It has also been stated that glanders has been propagated
by the acts of coitus and suckling, that in some instances also
it may be regarded as the result of hereditary transmission,
and that the poison may be conveyed into the system through
the medium of the food or drinking-water Certainly, if it is
(which there is little reason to doubt) capable of propagation
in this latter manner, the power of communication is

infinitely less certain than through other channels, and probably in some animals is not in this manner capable of entering the economy at all

Seeing that the possibility of developing the disease through means of the introduction into the intestinal canal of matter containing the specific discharges is a question of great sanitary importance, and has large practical bearing, and knowing that many even now have grave doubts of this possibility, I will quote somewhat in detail one of several experiments carried through under the direction of my predecessor, Professor Simonds

'May 10th—Gave a donkey at 4 pm a quantity of glanderous matter mixed with water. The matter was two days old, and had been obtained from a horse killed while affected with glanders. May 12th—Animal apparently well, temperature 100° F., 13th, temperature 103° F., 14th, temperature 104 3° F.; 15th, temperature 103 2° F., 16th, temperature 103° F. At this latter date the animal is reported as not feeding so well it is also often heard coughing, and frequently observed lifting the right hind leg. May 17th—Temperature 105 2 F, appetite very fastidious, pulse 64 per minute, animal dispirited. May 18th—Temperature 101° F.; 19th, temperature 98° F., scarcely takes any food, very dispirited, frequent lifting of hind legs. May 20th, temperature 104° F., depression great, no appetite, lymphatic glands under the jaw on the left side tender and slightly swollen, lifting and abducting both hind limbs now present, 21st, temperature 104 2° F, general symptoms the same, 22nd, temperature 103° F, nasal discharge, mucous and white, 23rd, nasal discharge, copious from both nostrils, sinking from choking produced by nasal obstruction, temperature 100° F. 24th, autopsy. tuberculous deposit extensively distributed throughout nasal passages, producing great thickening of membranes, which were highly injected. The specific deposit extended into the fauces and commencement of the pharynx, ulceration existed at several distinct spots of the membrane, covering the deposit, but no indication of this change on other parts of the structure epiglottis and surrounding parts inflamed no inflammation of great air tube; lungs a mass of tuberculous deposit, lymph vessels and glands in different situations indurated and enlarged'

d Nature of the Virus.—Although we are perfectly assured
that in every case of the disease there is present in the
economy, and exhibiting itself with varying power or intensity
in not merely the specific lesions or local manifestations of the
disease, but also in the greater number or the whole of the
secretions, excretions, and fluid tissues of the body, a peculiar
specific morbific agent, which, when introduced into the
tissues of a healthy horse, possesses the power of inducing a
similar diseased condition, we are nevertheless not yet in a
position to say what this infecting virus is   Whether it is
detached, wandering, plasmic, or bioplasmic material proceeding from the diseased, or spores of specific organisms,
remains yet to be determined   The tendency of our present
knowledge certainly points in the direction of living particulate organisms as the active inducing factors in the production
of glanders as of many other infectious diseases.

For some time it has been well known that observers have
occasionally detected a parasitic growth in the nasal discharges
of glandered horses, this parasitic growth, known as puccinia,
is, however, found in the nasal discharges from almost every
horse, and is probably not specific as to its association with
glanders, but is rather to be regarded as proceeding from the
fodder.

More recently, bacterial forms have been met with, it is said,
in both the blood and other fluids of animals—horses as well
as men—also in the pus from the specific sores, and their
existence has been regarded by Hallier, Zurn, Rindfleisch, and
others, as intimately associated with the materies morbi of the
disease   Bollinger, who says he has most carefully examined
both the blood and other fluids of animals affected with
glanders, has failed to verify the statements of these investigators.   He has, however, satisfied himself that the virus of
glanders, like that of some other specific infectious diseases,
possesses the property (pointed out by Schonbein) of exciting
a decomposing or catalytic action upon certain substances with
which it is brought in contact.

The poisonous agent in the disease may safely be regarded
as fixed and volatile

The fixed virus is attached to, or associated with, the specific
local manifestations of the disease, the ulcers, tubercles, and

pus from these, with the blood the secretions, probably the excretions, and all the animal tissues which are permeated by blood or lymph The volatile infecting agents seem closely connected with the sweat and exhalations of the diseased

Chauveau, in his investigations, gives it as his opinion that the active infecting agent, the materies morbi of glanders, is contained, not in the truly fluid or serous portion of the infecting material, but in the formed or corpuscular elements

Virchow, however, seems rather inclined to regard the most active disease-inducing factors or elements of the discharges to be, not their anatomical, but their chemical characters, regarding these as chiefly disturbing from their acridity and power of inducing irritation

The power of life, or the period during which, after separation from its source of origin, the virus of glanders will retain its activity, is considerable, but varies in accordance with the nature of those conditions to which it may be subjected It is destroyed when mixed with water at a temperature of $133°$ F. Similar results follow when brought in contact with such chemicals as carbolic acid, chlorine, sulphuric acid, etc It is said also to lose its virulence through putrefactive decomposition (Gerlach) We know, however, that the vehicle in which the infecting virus is contained may be desiccated, and in this condition maintain its vitality and power for weeks or months

I am acquainted with one case where the dried nasal discharges of an animal suffering from chronic glanders conveyed the disease to a healthy horse in the form of acute glanders and farcy, when placed in the stable previously occupied by the diseased, two months after the removal of the latter

Renault and Bouley state having produced acute farcy after inoculating with dried mucus taken from a glandered horse six weeks before

It would also appear from experimental inquiry that the poison of glanders is not to any perceptible extent reduced in virulence either by propagation directly through other horses or by its passage through other animals, as man, it is also equally active when propagated by retro-inoculation It is said to lose its power in the digestive canal of man, dogs, swine, and fowls, and to be less active when introduced into the horse in this way   Although it may thus be propagated both mediately and immediately, directly or by a secondary agent or carrier, the virus itself is only capable of multiplication within, not without, the animal body   In this latter situation it is distributed by the blood and serous canals, and partly by the inspired air

b Anatomical Characters.—The anatomical features peculiar to glanders, which a naked eye examination takes cognisance of, are mainly embraced in the existence of certain neoplastic growths, nodules or tubercles, in certain situations and tissues for which they have a special affinity, or of diffuse infiltrations in certain organs and textures   These growths occur chiefly in the mucous membrane of the air-passages, as the membrane lining the nasal chambers, the sinuses of the head, the larynx and the trachea, and in the lungs and pleura They are likewise encountered in the skin and subcutaneous connective tissue, the muscles, and in certain internal organs, as the liver, the spleen, kidneys, etc   The lymphatic vessels and glands are similarly affected

When the tubercular form of glanders occurs on the mucous membrane of the air-passages—the situation most obviously invaded—the form is that of raised or slightly elevated nodules on an inflamed and indurated base, surrounded by a ring or zone of similarly indurated and vascular character, they are of a tolerably firm consistence, light in colour, and in their centre prone to disintegration and the formation of ulcers The surface of these sores is glistening, covered with a sticky puriform fluid mingled with blood   These ulcers have a tendency to extend, occasionally involving the underlying tissues, whether cartilage or bone.

In the lungs these tubercles present an appearance somewhat like the miliary tubercle of man, but in less masses   To the naked eye they appear as small circumscribed spots of congested tissue, or as firmer indurated nodules, with an encircling hyperæmic zone and a soft yellowish centre   In substance they are chiefly composed of proliferating nucleated cells of varying size, apparently depending upon their age and period of growth   After a certain time, these cell elements are prone to undergo change, they lose their distinctive characters, soften, and suffer fatty and calcareous metamorphoses, this alteration proceeding from the centre to the circumference of the growth These nodules seem to possess an irritating action on the surrounding textures amongst which they are situated, for they are generally accompanied with inflammation and infiltration of a gelatinous or hyaline character, while occasionally they are practically encircled by a fibrous capsule, which, however, is not perfectly distinct from the nodule itself In some instances this inflammatory and exudative process from its extent is spoken of as the 'pneumonia of glanders.' It is of the lobular character These nodules are scattered throughout the entire substance of the lungs

In cutaneous glanders or farcy, the nodules or growths are found in the cutis and subcutaneous connective tissue They are not sharply defined, are of different sizes, and in their manner of growth and intimate structure resemble those situated in the lungs and mucous membranes. They also take on disintegration and form ulcerous sores

The lymphatic vessels are enlarged as the result of inflammatory action, they contain a yellowish purulent liquid, and are knotted, or possess numerous bulgings throughout their course. The glands with which these vessels are connected may not be much enlarged; they are, however, indurated and distinctly nodulated

In the infiltrated forms of its development there may be few tubercles, but instead, we observe swelling and infiltration of the mucous membrane, with death and removal of its epithelium in granular masses This is to be looked for chiefly in the membrane of the nasal passages, the infiltration, however, occurs also in the lungs. In very few cases of glanders will the lungs be found perfectly healthy or free from the lesions of existing nodules or specific infiltration Bollinger mentions that in fifty-two carefully examined cases the lungs were perfectly sound in only four. When other organs, as the liver, spleen, or kidneys, as well as the voluntary muscles, become the seats of the specific growths of glanders, and wherever these are found, the same general and special characters are associated with them, and the same tendency to elemental disintegrative changes

Incubation, Symptoms, etc *Incubation* — Like all other

specific infectious diseases, there exists in glanders a period of
quiescence, so to speak, between the reception of the poison
and the development of the characteristic symptoms There
is, however, in this disease in the horse a most wonderful disparity, if we are to depend on the correctness of statements
made, in the duration of the incubative period—a disparity
utterly irreconcilable, considering the natural history of specific
infectious diseases—if no regard were had to defective or imperfect observation, which, in the circumstances of such cases,
cannot be remedied

When resulting from direct inoculation, it is usually from
four to seven days, or even more When following the
normal mode of propagation, that of infection, mediate or
immediate, it is somewhat longer ere the diagnostic symptoms are developed In these cases an interval of several
weeks, or even months, is said occasionally to elapse between
the reception of the morbific agent and the appearance of
characteristic symptoms.

In all probability such lengthened periods of incubation do
not actually occur, but may be accounted for very simply, if
we are to regard it as certain, or at all probable, that the
reception of the glander virus as a volatile agent acts primarily
on the blood and internal viscera, and that this contamination and induction of specific organic changes in the lungs,
trachea, and upper air-passages, does not for long interfere
with the enjoyment of apparent good health and activity, and
that the symptoms which at last diagnose the disease are of
secondary importance , or if local lesions have, at the period
of the reception of the virus, been produced, they have shortly
afterwards healed, the contamination of the system moving
slowly but steadily on, until subsequently the local lesions by
which the disease is recognised are established.

During the latent period of the disease, certain conditions,
if brought to bear on the animal so circumstanced, seem to
have a power of hastening the development of the diagnostic
symptoms Long-continued, or rapidly performed work, and
other adverse conditions such as placing animals in unhealthy
stables, exposure to cold and damp, with insufficient food,
have all been noted as operating in this manner Indeed, so
well has it been understood that any sudden change, sanitary

or dietetic, is likely to operate thus unfavourably, that, in suspected cases, the common practice has been, by bleeding or purging, to convert suspected into confirmed cases, and so lessen the risk of cohabitation

There are to be found, in some of the German veterinary journals, most remarkable cases of extension of the period of latency in chronic glanders   Many of these carry with them the impress of correct reporting and authentic statement of fact   (See Fleming's 'Sanitary Police,' article 'Glanders') Still, I am rather inclined to view them as cases which in all probability were, for a long period prior to the exhibition of specific symptoms, suffering from structural changes of an occult character, situated in connection with internal organs and structures, and where the constitutional symptoms were not pronounced enough to indicate any serious disease   In all such cases, where the lesions are confined to the lungs, trachea, larynx, or any situation where the true morbid deposits or changes are hidden from view, the disease—merely from evidence derived from observation on the animal itself— cannot be diagnosed

In speaking of the symptoms of glanders and farcy, it is probably better to separate the so-called forms of the disease, and to note the different appearances or signs which each form exhibits ; also, seeing that both are known to us in the somewhat different aspects of acute or rapidly developed, and chronic or indolent, to observe in what respects the differing phases of this one disease resemble or disagree with each other.

1 **Symptoms of Acute Glanders.**—Acute glanders may be developed primarily by inoculation or infection, or it may, and indeed often does, follow as a sequel to the chronic form   This latter mode of its development is denied by some, as Reynal , still, even in my comparatively limited experience of the disease, I have encountered several.

Wherever occurring, the symptoms may be regarded as constitutional and local   The general or constitutional symptoms are very pronounced ; they appear first, and are shortly followed by the diagnostic or local, on the accession of which there may be a slight mitigation of the former

The earliest symptoms are those indicative of great febrile disturbance   rigors or shivering-fits, often persistent, with a dry, staring, and unthrifty condition of the coat; the pulse is increased in frequency, quick, soft, and of little volume; the respirations become frequent, and the temperature rapidly rises and remains high, often standing for several days at 107° F.

The animal is much distressed by enforced movement, the breathing becoming rapid and spasmodic, disturbed or snuffling, indicative of infiltration in the submucous tissues of the upper air-passages   The secretion of urine is often—not always, and generally when the constitutional symptoms have somewhat abated—augmented, clear and watery-looking, containing an extra amount of albumen or albuminoids.

There is much exhaustion and great emaciation   The visible mucous membranes are much congested, the membrane of the nose of a swollen hyperæmic condition, at first of a yellowish or straw colour, shortly becoming darker   In the course of a few days, from three to five, there is generally a defervescence of the pyrexial symptoms, which, however, return at a variable interval; with this remission of the fever, there is the development of the specific local lesions

Over the surface of the pituitary membrane, most frequently over that in the nasal septum, and at the alæ of the nose, we see small nodules or tubercles, either in groups, or scattered less thickly; or in some instances there is a diffuse elevated condition of patches on the membrane of a yellowish colour, as if the epithelial covering was raised by subjacent infiltration.

The nodules or tubercles, varying in size from a large pin's head to that of a hemp-seed, appear as projections on an elevated and injected base or background, and are rendered visible by the white or yellowish-white centre   This centre is surrounded by a greyish transparent zone, which again is encircled by a red areola

In a few days from their first appearing, these papules soften and disintegrate on their centres, the larger diffuse infiltrated patches also undergoing a similar change.

The removal of the epithelial covering results in the production of the characteristic chancrous sore or ulcer; this sore is marked by the possession of irregular excavated edges, which, as well as the floor of the pit or ulcer, are inclined to nodulate and become covered with prominent and very vascular granulations

These ulcers or sores are not disposed to heal, but extend, and by the removal of the septa or sound tissue existing between several small sores, one large rodent ulcer is produced, and should the animal survive long enough, we may have necrosis and penetration of the septum nasi

When these lesions have existed on the nasal membrane for even a short time, or probably contemporaneously with their appearance, the larynx and membrane of the sinuses of the head become similarly affected

The nasal discharge, which at the beginning of the fever may have only slightly differed from that of a common catarrh by being of a yellowish colour and slightly viscid, becomes, on the development of the papules into ulcers, thick and mingled with puriform matter, and as erosions advance and capillaries are ruptured is sanguineous, more copious, and sometimes flaky The neighbouring lymphatics and lymphatic glands become swollen, specially those in the intermaxillary space, sometimes only on one side, occasionally on both, depending upon the fact whether both or only one nasal cavity is involved At first the gland-structures and surrounding textures feel soft and slightly painful, as if they might suppurate, which they rarely do shortly this enlarged condition becomes better defined, harder, and less painful

Generally, in this condition of ulcerated nasal membrane and tumified lymphatic glands, there is the accompaniment of swollen or corded lymph vessels, those passing between the nose and mouth to the glands in the maxillary space becoming distinctly marked out, corded, nodulated, and ulcerated

The scalp, face, and particularly the structures around the nose and mouth, become œdematous, while the farcied and inflamed state of lymph vessels is not confined to the head and face, but extends to the extremities, on which, in the course of the swollen lymphatics, tubercles or nodules develop themselves, which after a time soften, disintegrate, and discharge purulent matter

The breathing, if not snuffling and hoarse from the outset, very shortly becomes so, partly owing to the œdema of the nose and nasal structures, but chiefly from the extension of the destructive and ulcerative action to the larynx and laryngeal structures, this diseased process being invariably marked by extensive infiltration and thickening of membranes and tissues In these instances there is usually frequent and painful cough, and tenderness on manipulation of the laryngeal region

The pneumonia and bronchitis attendant on acute glanders are often overlooked ; they may, however, be made out to satisfaction by careful physical examination of the chest These conditions, when existing, appear to be intimately connected with the formation of the glanderous nodules in the pulmonary tissue, and the circumferential infiltration attendant on this condition   When the lung-tissue becomes involved, exhaustion is rapidly progressive   the appetite, which may for some days have only been capricious, is now gone; dyspnœa from pulmonic changes and blood-poisoning becomes distressing, while œdema of the inferior parts of the body and specific cutaneous infiltration ensue   Life is rarely prolonged beyond twenty or thirty days

2 **Symptoms of Chronic Glanders**—Glanders in a chronic, or at least not in an acute form, is the manifestation of the disease we most frequently encounter in this country   In this form it may continue for many months without making marked inroads on the animal's constitutional health and vigour, or by very obvious symptoms proclaiming the establishment of the fatal disease

As in the acute form, we may regard the symptoms as partaking of the same double character, constitutional and local. In chronic glanders, the local phenomena are certainly the more important, from being the specific , they are also the more numerous   The constitutional, besides being more trivial, are also not invariable, and are dependent for their existence or character on varying surrounding conditions Unlike the acute form, the chronic is more apt to develop constitutional symptoms, at the latter, rather than the early, stages of the malady

The diagnostic features in chronic glanders are the local, and are connected with · (a) changes in the nasal chambers ; (b) with alterations or changes in the lymphatic vessels and lymphatic glands

a Changes in the Nasal Chambers —The very earliest indications of aught being amiss with a horse affected with
chronic glanders may be the altered condition of the discharge from the nose, or even previous to this, attention may
be drawn to the case, and an examination instituted because
the animal is not in such good condition, or looking so bloom-
ing or so well as he ought to be ; that for a few days his appetite has been capricious, or he has had slight rigors, or he has
perspired excessively under moderate exertion   In exceptional
cases there may be no discharge. In all, however, where
nodules or ulcers exist in the cavity, there will be a discharge
great or less in amount, and of a character varying in accordance with the development of the lesions   In the early stages,
the material flowing from the nasal passages is not very dissimilar to what is observed in common catarrh, only it may be
discharged from one nostril, the left, when from both it is
evidence that changes are progressing in both ; gradually it
becomes thicker, viscid, and mingled with purulent matter,
rather green in colour, and inclined to adhere round the margin of the external nasal openings, or it is expelled from the
nose by snorting in small pasty masses

The peculiar character of the nasal flexu, although it has
always attracted attention, and has by all writers and teachers
been much spoken of and regarded as a prominent characteristic symptom of the disease, must never of itself be
depended upon as furnishing from merely physical characters
undoubted evidence of the existence of glanders, its physiological character being alone diagnostic.

With such a discharge, a little careful examination will in
all probability disclose the existence of nodes, or of nodes and
chancres   When these conditions exist only in the superior
or posterior parts of the chambers—they are usually not
largely distributed in the chronic form, and most frequently
only on one side—their discovery is not always attended with
success   The head being held in a favourable position as to
light, the exploration will be materially aided by using a
reflector, or the finger may be passed up the cavity along the
septum nasi, when the nodules or ulcers may be detected by
the sense of touch. When situated on the lower portion of
the septum, or at the alæ of the nostrils, the appearance of the

nodules is in all essentials similar to what was described in
the acute form

Their further development from the stage of nodulation,
and their destruction of tissue by ulcerative invasion, proceed and are accomplished by processes analogous, but only
less active, to those exhibited in acute glanders The larger
eroded cavities, which result from extension by circumferential invasion of tissue or by coalescence of original sores,
whatever may be their shape—and it is often very irregular
—always possess the same generic features of the smaller and
original chancres, the eroded base and slightly swollen or
everted edges

Both upon the edges of these larger excavations and upon
their base or floor, new nodules or tubercles similar to the
original arise, which by the carrying out of the disintegrative
changes and removal of destroyed tissue rapidly extend the
area of the sore As these sores extend, the amount of
secretion naturally increases the discharge, seemingly excessive, when the extent of the suppurating surface is
regarded The puriform secretion is generally spread over
the surface of these tumified and vascular-looking ulcers, as if
for a protection, forming a loosely adhering yellowish-coloured
crust, tinged with blood

In addition to this disintegration of tissue and formation of
chancrous sores, another form of lesion is occasionally
observed in connection with the membrane of the nasal
septum It consists, not in papules or erosions of the texture,
but appears to the eye as mere abrasion or denudation of the
parts affected of the entire epithelial covering, this denudation
extending no deeper than the superficial covering of the
membrane, but occupying a considerable space. The place
of the removed epithelium is apparently supplied by soft
granular material, which is readily removed by passing the
finger over the part

The removal of epithelium is not, however, the earliest appearance of this condition ; it is rather a sequel. The first is of
an opposite character, in which the membrane seems to suffer
from an ordinary inflammatory action, is slightly exuberant,
and swollen from infiltration by a pale gelatinous fluid amongst
the interstices of the connective tissue The result of this

infiltration of fluid and varied forms of cell-growth is the displacement of the entire epithelium, which previous to removal is elevated and heaped together, giving that soft granular character to the structure which has been noticed as evident when touched with the finger

This process, and the peculiar results of it as regards the infiltration of low cell-growths and accompanying products prone to change and removal, bear a considerable resemblance to the ordinary diphtheritic inflammation of mucous membranes   This erosion of superficial structures may not be seen in every case, but it has for long been observed in many which have existed for a lengthened period   It has in this form been spoken of as 'Inflammatory glanders,' 'Infiltrated glanders,' and 'Diffuse glanders' (Bollinger and Röll)

Certainly this is not the same condition of the membrane which is seen after extension and development of the primary sores resulting from the rupture and softening of the nasal papule or tubercle   These may be seen at the side or around this abraded space, which, however, does not owe its existence to the removal of the superficial tissue in the way indicated in the case of these nodular changes and softenings, but to the process of infiltration by products seemingly the result of specific inflammatory action, or possibly having a close connection with the condition of thrombosis of both venous capillaries and minute lymph-vessels, which in such cases is found pretty well established in these situations

Neither the large irregular-shaped rodent ulcers, the smaller and shallower chancre sores, nor yet the diffuse superficial erosions of which we have last spoken, are in ordinary cases disposed to heal, rather are they disposed to progress, the ulcerative and destructive process not resting with the mucous membrane or its subjacent tissues, but in course of time invading the harder structures, the cartilage and bone   Occasionally it may be observed, however, that some of these ulcerative or abraded surfaces, by a changed, more active, and reparative process, lessen in depth and superficial extent, gradually healing over in an unique manner by the development in the vacuities of cicatricial or fibrous tissue   The cicatrix thus formed, when perfect, is sometimes slightly depressed where the depth of the erosion previously existed, of

9

a clear white colour, with well-marked fibrous bands either branching off from one main band where the cavity has been extensive, or crossing each other stellate fashion, where the ulcers or sores have been less extensive

Sometimes, when thus healing, a glanderous sore of a little more penetrating character may still be left open, yet to undergo the healing process, while the remainder is covered with fibroid cicatricial tissue.

These specific cicatrices and callosities of fibroid tissue represent, therefore, ulcers or erosions that have actually healed

These, Bollinger remarks, 'occur exclusively in the chronic form of glanders'—the only cases I have seen were in such— and he states that they were first accurately described by Leisering, whose views on this point were corroborated in the main by Virchow, the latter differing from Leisering in this respect only, that he admitted the possibility of genuine specific cicatrices being formed from ulcers, whereas Leisering maintained that the cicatrices produced by the infiltration and development of fibrous tissue were not to be regarded as evidence of the healing of specific lesions, but merely as a specific form of neoplastic growth concomitant to the disease From all, however, which I have observed myself, and from what I am able to glean from those whose experience on this point is considerable, I am disposed to regard this production of cicatricial tissue, whether found in connection with specific ulcers, the result of softened nodules, or of infiltration, as the evidence of a healthy healing and reparative process in connection with these specific sores

Although I freely allow thus much, I would at the same time caution all who may observe this action in connection with the glanderous sore, and who are intimately associated with such cases of the disease, not to be misled with the idea that the appearance of cicatrization of the ulcers is evidence or indication of restoration of systemic or general healthy functional activity

It ought ever to be remembered that these ulcers or sores on the nasal membrane may most certainly heal or cicatrize in the way indicated, and still the specific dyscrasia remain ; that it is highly probable that even with this local healing process there may exist in the lungs, as previously, the specific nodules and tubercles characteristic of the disease of which these local nasal sores now healed are but partial manifestations and exhibitions of the peculiar general diseased condition, and that it is almost certain, should the animal survive long enough, that these local sores will again appear

The certainty also that in such cases, even with the cicatrization of the chancres, the power of infection is not lost, that from such an animal an acute case of glanders may be propagated, must ever be kept before our minds, so as to regulate our conduct and the advice given

b Changes connected with the Lymphatic Glands and Lymphatic Vessels —Concomitant with the phenomena taking place in the nasal chambers are the changes encountered in connection with the lymph-glands situated in the inter-maxillary space. In the swelling and induration of these structures there is a distinct symmetrical accordance with the situation of the lesions of the nasal cavities. When the nodules or ulcers exist in both chambers, the gland-structures of both sides are affected. When only one cavity—usually the left—is the seat of the lesion, the glands of that side only are involved

When participating in the morbid processes going on in the course of the development of the disease, these structures first become full and enlarged, partly from infiltration in the true gland-structures, but chiefly from the same condition occurring to the surrounding connective tissue amongst which they are placed. When both glands are affected the swelling is at first most distinctive in the middle of the sub or inter-maxillary space; and whether one or both are the seat of the morbid action, the feeling is at first of a soft and doughy character, attended with a trifling amount of pain. Gradually this soft swelling is replaced by a condition of greater firmness and less sensibility, while with the disappearance of the doughy feeling we have the establishment of the distinct nodulated condition, which is persistently maintained The swelling, whether of one or of both glands, is more marked as increasing the bulk of the gland antero-posteriorly than across the space

With the acquirement of the nodulated condition we also

9—2

notice that the ability to be moved from place to place by pressure with the fingers is much impaired, gradually to be lost altogether, the gland becoming fixed both to the super-adjacent connective tissue and to the jaw

Although these phenomena or conditions which have been detailed—the albumino-muco-purulent, or slightly sanguineous nasal discharge, with nodules, tubercles, ulcers, or superficial abrasions on the nasal membrane, together with indurated and adherent maxillary lymphatic glands, and occasionally cuta-neous specific changes, with little constitutional disturbance, or febrile symptoms—are what may usually be regarded as diagnostic of chronic glanders of the horse, the form with which in this country we are probably most conversant, it is yet certain that many cases occur where some of these, or it may be all of them, are absent, and yet we know from many sources that such are undoubtedly deeply infected with the specific poison

3 **Symptoms of Acute Farcy**—Farcy, in its two forms of acute and chronic farcy, being but a manifestation or peculiar development of the general empoisoned condition known by the generic term 'glanders,' we can understand that the same factors operate in its production which are charged with the appearance of that other development known specially by the inclusive or general term 'glanders'

It may be induced or owe its origin to artificial inoculation with the specific discharges of the sores of glanders or farcy: or it may appear in animals from intimate cohabitation or infection, or, if we allow that it is possible, under certain conditions unfavourable to animal health, to originate glanders, so named, we are also necessitated to believe that under similar degrading and debilitating influences it is possible to originate acute farcy

Why the reception in both classes of cases of the same infecting virus should in the one specially exhibit its specific action in connection with the mucous membranes and struc-tures of the upper air-passages, or with internal organs, and in the other select the cutaneous or cutaneous and connective tissues and superficial lymphatics, is rather difficult to deter-mine, probably the causes which thus operate are largely and intimately associated with the soil in which the seed is implanted   The symptoms indicative of the existence of acute farcy may, as in acute glanders, be regarded as general or constitutional, and local or diagnostic

The general or systemic symptoms are in their nature essentially febrile   elevation of temperature, sometimes to an extent as great as indicated in the pyrexial condition attendant upon or preceding an attack of acute glanders—as a general rule, however, it is rarely so elevated—rigors with a staring coat and unthrifty state of the skin, thirst, loss of appetite, and general impairment of healthy functional activity

The local infiltrations and swellings, although not always, are generally confined to the extremities   When the limbs are thus affected the œdema may appear—1. As a very diffuse and general swelling, invading a very considerable extent of cutaneous and underlying tissue, the local heat and pain, together with lameness, being very marked.   This condition of superficial and extensive swelling may not be persistent from its first appearance, but it may exhibit distinct accessions and declines each recurrence or increase of the swelling, being more distinctly marked with diffuse, irregular, and indurated patches of tissue   At length, when the infiltration and general œdema have permanently subsided, the specific nodules, or circumscribed swellings, known as ‘farcy-buds,’ together with the enlarged and tense condition of the vessels, veins, and lymphatics, recognised as ‘cords,’ become more distinctly visible   2 The infiltration and œdema, instead of partaking of the general character now spoken of, are essentially local and circumscribed, the specific nodes or buds arising at once from these infiltrations, between which and the nearest lymphatic glands, or between each nodule, the enlarged and corded condition of the lymph vessels is seen.

The immediate appearance of these farcy-buds is generally sudden—that is to say, the infiltrated, swollen, and painful condition of the limb may have existed for a day or two without showing distinctly where these nodules are to appear, when rather unexpectedly they may be projected beyond the general surface, and so attract attention

These specific tubercles, so characteristic of farcy in either its acute or chronic form, are situated in the cutis, or the subcutaneous connective tissue, or they may penetrate deeper, affecting the muscles   Individually they vary in size from a pea to a hazel-nut. they are not sharply circumscribed, particularly in the acute form, their base shading off and extending into the more diffuse infiltration already noticed, which, however, closely surrounding the nodule is more indurated than elsewhere.

In a few days central softening, and disintegration, with rupture of skin, take place in these individually. The openings or sores thus formed, now known as farcy ulcers, are deep, angry looking, with rounded ragged edges, they are disposed to extend and discharge a foul, greyish-white creamy liquid tinged with blood   These buds, or nodules, are often developed in groups clustered over a limited space, and the ulcerative process proceeding with much rapidity from each centre, shortly converts two or more of the original chancres into one large, many-pitted, irregular-margined ulcer

The extensive rodent sores, when regarded minutely, give evidence of varying degrees of activity, as of colour, in the destructive process   both in the floor of the sore, and on its sides or edges, we observe the rounded forms noticed in the specific sores of the nasal septum, resembling actively developing granulation tissue.   These are very tender, and when touched are disposed to bleed.

The discharge from these sores is very abundant, and, although mostly distributed over the adjacent surface, does in some cases, and to a limited extent, collect and harden in brownish crusts around the openings of the sores

In addition to the existence of these buds, or ulcerating sores, we have also a characteristic prominent, projecting, or corded condition of the lymphatics   The inflammation of these vessels may take place coincident with the appearance of the nodes, and previous to their suppuration, or it may not be obvious until the open suppurating sore has been established   These vessels, when thus affected, seem and feel full and hard, as well as being painful to the touch—in these respects resembling the nodules and infiltrations   Shortly following these appearances there are developed, in the course of the distended vessel, distinct nodules, or swellings, which ultimately soften, and discharge a yellowish purulent fluid akin to that poured forth from the ulcers, these nodules, or buttons, like the larger buds between which the lymphatics stretch, have a tendency to coalesce and form larger ulcerous sores opening into the lymph canal, now charged with a tenacious, blood-stained, purulent fluid.

The adjacent lymph-glands are also largely involved in the diseased action they become swollen from hyperplastic infiltration, are nodulated and painful on manipulation. It is generally stated, that although thus enlarged, tense, and painful, the formation of abscesses in these is like suppuration in the tumefied glands of glanders—a very rare occurrence

During the continuance of these phenomena, the formation and development of the buds, or nodules, their softening, and the progressive ulcerative changes and continued suppuration, the fever never entirely disappears It can scarcely, however, be regarded as continued, or as a good specimen of continued fever; it is more truly remittent or hectic, and its exacerbations are very often clearly marked by rigors and patchy perspiration , while in all cases, even when the horse is allowed to live and feeding tolerably well, the emaciation and prostration are rapidly progressive

Not unfrequently the terminating scene in a case of acute farcy is the development of glanders in an acute form, with all the characteristic lesions in the nasal chambers, glands, and air-passages

4 **Chronic Farcy.**—This, while an exceedingly common form of the manifestation of equina, is probably also the only one, or at least that which more frequently than any other seems susceptible of being successfully combated by medical treatment Less distinctly indicated by general or systemic disturbance, our chief means of recognition—its diagnostic features—are eminently local When accompanied with fever this is even more distinctly remittent than in the acute form. Ordinarily the general functional derangement is neither distinctive nor yet attractive ; occasionally cases will come under observation where a prolonged or lingering malaise, or want of vigour, out of all proportion to other existing and extrinsic conditions, distinctly precedes or ushers in an attack of chronic farcy.

The special local manifestations of this condition are the occurrence of circumscribed inflammatory swellings, tumours,

nodules, or buds, in connection with the skin and subjacent
tissues, which after a time soften and ulcerate, leaving an unhealthy open sore discharging a puriform liquid, and not disposed to heal

The situations in which these tumours are encountered are
various, a preference being shown for those localities where
the skin is thin and vascular, as over the facial, the maxillary,
and laryngeal regions, along the sides of the neck, inferior
parts of the chest, inside the fore-arms, along the belly, over
the flanks, and inside the thighs

These tumours vary in size, like the same growths in acute
farcy, and like them also, they vary in a similar manner as to
the exact seat of their development.

The smaller are usually situated in the cutis, are more
numerous, more generally distributed over the body, and in
any particular locality where they occur they are more given
to coalesce after ulceration and suppurative action have been
established. The larger are chiefly confined to the subcutaneous connective tissue, and frequently only involve the
skin when undergoing the softening and ulcerative process.
They are also less numerous, not so disposed to be closely
grouped together over circumscribed surfaces, and consequently less apt to become confluent. In chronic farcy we
may sometimes see certain of the nodules or swellings which
seem distinct enough, and likely to proceed to perfect development, retrogress, or at least remain perfectly indolent for a considerable time, and finally disappear

The course of their appearance and development varies much
They may appear in an isolated order over different parts of
the body at the same, or nearly same, time, or a few may first
make their appearance, remain for a few days isolated, to be then
joined by a fresh eruption of papules over some particular
part, or even distributed over the greater portion of the body
In this latter case they are most probably of small size. The
greater number of the nodules in chronic farcy are not much
elevated above the surface of the surrounding skin, they are,
however, as a rule, more sharply defined than the similar
growths in the acute form, the accompanying infiltration of
the meshes of the connective tissue being less extensive, and
shading off at the base of the tumour less gradually than in

that, the defining or separation of the diseased from the comparatively healthy surrounding textures is better marked as the nodules approach maturation, the infiltration becoming less diffused, the node acquiring a characteristic form and indurated base.

The natural changes which occur in these fully formed tumours are similar to what has been noted as taking place in the same growths in the acute form; these are central softening, disintegration and ulceration of the skin, with the discharge of a thin pale yellow-coloured pus

The period occupied in the perfecting of these changes, from the appearance of the tumours until the formation of the sores, varies according as these growths are only situated in the skin or in the underlying tissues. When in the former situation the changes may be gone through in a week; when in the latter, several weeks may be required to accomplish the processes of softening and ulceration. Once formed, these ulcers, like similar sores in all the forms of glanders or farcy, have little or no disposition to heal, but extend in superficial area and in their invasion of subjacent tissues by extension of the ulcerative process. When these nodes are numerous and closely set over a limited surface of skin the ulcerative process steadily removes the portion of tissue intervening between the several chancres, forming at length one or more large, irregular-margined, foul-looking ulcers.

In all their forms the farcy sores, whether of the character of widely distributed, comparatively superficial erosions, or isolated deeply-seated rodent ulcers, we find maintained the same generic and distinguishing characters: the pus at the first eruption tolerably laudable in appearance, shortly becoming thin, viscid, and of a pale yellowish colour, the margins or walls of the sore full or vascular-looking, slightly everted, ragged in outline, excoriated, and surrounded by a zone of indurated tissue; the bottom of the sore not smooth, but nodulated and indented, and resting on a base of similar texture and character to the circumferential zone of the superficial opening

The inflamed, swollen, and corded condition of the lymphatic vessels, which both in this and the acute form is so distinctive, is here more likely to follow than precede or appear contemporaneously with the nodular swellings   Sometimes these inflamed vessels are so much enlarged from infiltration, the result of the morbid action, as to stand boldly out in relief from the surrounding surface, at others they may of themselves be equally enlarged and swollen, and yet from adjacent cellular infiltration give no evidence to the eye of their existence   Their true state, however, in such circumstances, may always be discovered by steadily passing the fingers over the tract where they are likely to be situated

The physical appearances and characters of these 'cords,' or inflamed lymph-vessels, are not always precisely similar Generally of the thickness of a goose-quill, they are rarely, either in their bulk or the uniform resistance or tension of the swelling, continuously alike   At irregular points along their course, usually at the situations of the so-called valves, there are dilatations or small circumscribed spots of induration and elevation of tissue, which have not inappropriately been likened to a string of beads or pearls   When these small indurated swellings are fairly developed they do not often disappear, but, like the primary farcy-bud, gradually take on ulterior changes, terminating in central softening and discharge of puriform material.   These smaller buds further comport themselves in a precisely similar manner to the larger ones, by widening through ulceration, and ultimately coalescing, thereby forming not merely an ulcerous sore, but an ulcerous sinuous tract or cavity , those unhealthy secreting sinuosities have generally been known as ' farcy-pipes.'

In some mild and decidedly chronic cases, although the lymphatic vessels are distinctly corded and projecting from the cutaneous surface, the nodulation generally observed on their course may not be reached, but the lymphatic distension and immediately surrounding infiltrated connective tissue may remain in an inactive and indolent condition for a lengthened period , while should the general health be restored, and the primary farcy sore take on a healthy healing action, the corded and accompanying infiltrated state of lymphatic vessels may disappear

Following as a sequel of the development of these specific nodules or tumours, and of the diseased condition of the lymphatic vessels, is the swelling and induration of the adja-

cent lymphatic glands. This condition is much similar to
what has been mentioned as existing in acute farcy, only the
surrounding and interconnective cellular tissue of the glands
is here less swollen as the infiltration seems less; the induration and nodulation, or superficial irregularity, is, however,
equally well marked, but the tenderness on manipulation is
not so attractive.   Generally at the commencement of the
swelling the infiltration of the surrounding and interlacing
tissue is most distinctive, gradually decreasing to a certain
point, and in this way allowing the indurated and nodulated
condition of the gland to be observed and felt.   Although
this enlargement and induration may continue for a lengthened
period, softening and suppuration are here even more rare than
in either glanders proper or the acute form of farcy.

Additional Lesions and Textural Changes —These peculiar
conditions of irregularly developed neoplastic formations,
their growth and further disintegrative changes, together
with the specific inflammation of the lymphatic vessels
and lymphatic glands, although constituting the great diagnostic features of chronic farcy, are, like the similar manifestations of the specific poison in nearly all the other forms
of equina, occasionally and in particular cases added to by the
occurrence of phenomena which, if not specially diagnostic,
are at least peculiar in their association with the different
developments of this general infective process in the horse

These phenomena and manifestations of morbid activity are
the occurrence in different parts of the body of (*a*) *circumscribed tumours or abscesses*, and (*b*) *of diffuse infiltrations*

a. Circumscribed Tumours or Abscesses —These are perfectly distinct from the tumours or nodules diagnostic of the
disease, and must not be confounded with them   They are,
when occurring, generally situated on the more exposed parts
of the body, the scapular region, the sides, and haunches
They are evidently inflammatory in character, of much larger
size than the ordinarily encountered adventitious growths of
farcy; they are tolerably well defined, and, unlike the true
farcy tumours, are not disposed to take on the ulcerative process. Neither at their base nor around their border is there
the characteristic infiltration and induration of the nodules
In all their characters, with the exception, probably, of the

contained fluid, which is very similar to what we find in the common and true glanderous growths, and in their disposition again to fill when evacuated, and the slowness of the healing process, these tumours or abscesses bear a greater resemblance to ordinary cysts or abscesses than to the specific farcino-glanderous sores

b Diffuse Infiltrations—The infiltrations or diffuse swellings are the usual accompaniments of the pseudo-rheumatic symptoms, and are chiefly located on the limbs in the vicinity of joints

Unlike those already noted, they are not circumscribed or defined so as to give a distinct and definite form to the enlargement, but the infiltration is largely diffused, and gradually shades off until it meets or terminates in the normally conditioned connective tissue

They differ also from those adventitious abscesses in their want of permanence or stability, for one of their distinguishing features is their metatastic character, in this simulating the onset of rheumatic inflammations

They neither resemble the abscesses nor the true farcy tumours, in as far as they rarely soften or suppurate, and that when they do not remove by rapid change of situation, to appear in connection with some other articulation, or are apparently accessory to an outbreak of acute glanders, they steadily become less by induration and removal of the more fluid parts of the infiltration

Occasionally these conditions of specific infiltration have been mistaken for and spoken of as farcinous invasion of the constituent textures of the joint affected   Such in some cases may be true, still in the entire number of those which I have encountered there has been involvement chiefly of the connective and fibrous tissues external and extraneous to the joint proper.

The pain and lameness on the first appearance of these infiltration swellings are well marked, the former gradually disappearing as the infiltration reaches its height, the latter continuing not exactly as lameness which it showed at first, but as a peculiar stiffness seemingly from the mechanical impediment offered to the movements of the joint from the exuded and infiltrated material.

Neither of these phenomena, the 'abscesses' nor the local 'infiltration swellings,' can be regarded as essentially characteristic or diagnostic of farcy, acute or chronic; they are certainly not always, nor even very often, met with. They are not unfrequently regarded as the result of injuries received, the special character and development of the swellings being accepted as the result of a local injury sustained while the economy is pervaded by a specific and malignant virus. That such causes never tend to or assist in the development of these changes we would not venture to maintain; they are certainly very often situated on those parts most liable to suffer from blows or external violence, still there seems evidence enough to satisfy that external violence is not always, or in every instance, the determining agent in their production.

Between the two extremes of so-called acute glanders and chronic farcy there are many varieties of the diseased action presenting many features and phenomena of an intermediate character; these variations in the form, and the apparent divergence of the phenomena exhibited during the developments of this malignant disease, render it exceedingly difficult always to form an exact and perfectly correct classification of it and in dealing with it in daily practice are apt to mislead the most experienced and careful.

Diagnosis—Correctly to diagnose the existence of equina in any of its varied manifestations, or as a general diseased specific condition, is for us, as experts and scientifically equipped sanitary officers, of infinite importance.

It may seem to the uninitiated a rather strange matter that in a disease so generally accepted as undoubtedly malignant there should be room for any doubt, particularly amongst skilled witnesses, as to its existence in any particular case. Undoubtedly very many, probably the greater number, of the cases of farcy-glanders exhibit features and indications sufficiently diagnostic to keep even the least skilled and most careless or reckless observer from being mistaken; still it must not be forgotten that not a few developments of the disease are so insidious and undemonstrative in the exhibition of their specific features as to mislead, or cause the most competent and careful investigator to hesitate, while it is well

known that those cases where the symptoms are occult are
usually the most dangerous in a sanitary point of view

As experts called upon to give an opinion, or as sanitary
inspectors charged with the preservation of the health and life
of an important section of the animal population, which, in
their intrinsic worth and labour-executing power, represent a
vast amount of money—not to enter upon the importance of
the subject from the possibility of the disease being propagated
to man—it behoves us to have regard to the extreme difficulty,
or even impossibility in some cases, at once to give a positive
and well-grounded opinion as to the existence of glanders
This is particularly true when the case is one of those known
by the terms of ' occult,' or ' pulmonary glanders '

In forming an opinion as to the existence of glanders, regard
must be had to the presence or absence of the local diagnostic
symptoms of the disease.   These, as we have already stated,
are the character of the nasal discharge, the condition of the
nasal membrane, whether or not the true specific nodules,
tubercles, ulcers, or abrasions, exist, together with the condition and form of the submaxillary gland   Certainly the
most important of these indications is the existence of the
specific growths or sores of the nasal membrane, seeing that it
is possible that both an unnatural nasal discharge and a tumefied condition of the lymphatic glands may exist apart from
the specific glanderous contamination

In all doubtful cases, when one or more of the indications
upon which we must rely for forming our opinion are absent,
much care in examination is needful, and the animal must be
kept under observation sufficiently long to admit of the
development of those which are defective or wanting   Sometimes the administration of a dose of aloes will hasten the
appearance of what is desired.

With the occurrence of the peculiar nasal discharge, and
when the nodules, or chancre-like sores, together with the
induration and fixing of the intermaxillary glands, are present
in any horse, which may or may not exhibit constitutional
disturbance or indications of ill-health, there is little difficulty
in satisfying ourselves that the diseased condition is specific,
and distinct from every other.

With acute glanders there is, as a rule, little difficulty in arriving at a determination, as the symptoms and indications connected with this development are generally sufficiently pronounced. It is the chronic form which presents the difficulty, and which may be confounded with several diseased conditions chiefly of a local and restricted nature. Chronic catarrh of the mucous membrane of the nose—'nasal gleet,' disease of the bones connected with the nasal chambers, and coincident inflammation of the mucous membrane—ozæna; disease of the fangs of the molar teeth, with or without accumulation of matter in the sinuses of the bones; post-pharyngeal abscesses, collections of pus in the Eustachian pouches, and irregular cases of strangles, with protracted formation of pus, have all been considered as likely to mislead the incautious or unskilful. None of these affections, however, with the exercise of sufficient care, ought to present much difficulty to the qualified veterinarian.

In all cases where the diagnostic lesions of the disease are absent, but where we have reason to suspect that the system is contaminated with the poison, too much care cannot be exercised in regulating the contact and intercourse of the suspected animals with the undoubtedly healthy. The many records relating to the propagation and spread of glanders, both in this country and on the Continent, and the serious losses arising from the spread of the disease, undoubtedly originating from an unsuspected case of the occult form, are sufficient to warrant us in adopting any reasonable means to secure safety from the poison and to circumscribe its ravages; still although in the exercise of our professional duties, and as sanitary officers, we are bound to take every warrantable precaution to prevent glanders from being distributed, we must at the same time be equally certain that the disease exists before condemning any animal, or at least before positively asserting that it is suffering from glanders. In no instance, probably, are we warranted in giving an opinion in the affirmative in this matter until the specific growths or sores are exhibited on the nasal membrane, or, in cases where the diagnostic lesions are not visible, until by inoculation with the secretions or organized fluids of the suspected animal, or enforced cohabitation with it, we have certainly produced the disease in others previously healthy.

As a means of assisting our diagnosis in these doubtful
cases, the opening of the sinuses of the head or face has been
suggested with the object of detecting the existence of the
characteristic growths or sores on the membrane lining these
cavities, which by some is said in every case to be invaded by
them Now, although in every examination of ordinary
glanders which I have made, and where the specific changes
existed on the visible mucous membrane of the nose, the same
were detected on the membrane of the sinuses, examinations
conducted by other competent observers seem to throw doubt
on the constancy of this phenomenon

Farcy, both acute and chronic, must be diagnosed by watching for and recognising the specific local lesions A remembrance of the characters of these, and a careful examination to
see that they really exist, will save us from much vexatious
annoyance, and is, in truth, the only means generally available
by which we are able to arrive at a positive conclusion. In
acute farcy, as in acute glanders, there is always greater probability of our being able to speedily determine the question of
the specific character of the lesions which may be presented to
our view. The diseases which specially simulate farcy, and
which, in certain stages of their development and under
certain conditions, may be mistaken for it, are chiefly those
which invade the extremities, or which in their progress exhibit special symptoms in local changes connected with these.
'Lymphangitis,' idiopathic and traumatic, both acute and
chronic; 'variola equina,' horse-pox, either of itself or complicated with the former, and simple local 'œdema,' are the
chief affections with which farcino-glanders may be confounded.

The usual form in which 'idiopathic lymphangitis'—weed
—makes its appearance, or the suddenness of its attack, the
marked febrile symptoms, pain of the limb and lameness, with
the swollen, inflamed, and corded condition of the large lymph-
vessels on the inner surface of the limb, together with the
infiltration of the subcutaneous connective tissue and consequent swelling of the whole limb, together with swelling and
pain of the lymphatic glands of the inguinal region, is not
unlike the early stages of acute farcy In some subjects, in
certain situations, and with certain surroundings, we are
necessitated to wait for a few days ere being sufficiently satisfied

that the case is not one of acute farcy, for we know well enough that in some developments of farcy the only abnormal features for a few days are not diagnostic, being merely such as we have noted as existing in lymphangitis—viz pain, swelling of the limb from infiltration, and it may be indurated and swollen glands   Very shortly, however, if the case is one of farcy the diagnostic lesions will become manifest. farcy-buds will appear and steadily pass through their different changes, terminating in ulceration with its specific characters. Should the general tumefaction and inflamed state of the lymph vessels and glands be only that of the commonly occurring and benign affection, they will, in something like the same time, gradually subside, together with the accompanying fever and pain, and certainly without the formation of farcy-buds, or tumours, or the existence of chancrous ill-conditioned sores

This subsidence of the symptoms of illness and a return to health will be expedited by a course of treatment which, if the œdema and pain were the concomitants or precursors of farcy, would in all likelihood hasten the production of the specific and diagnostic lesions, the growths and ulcers   When 'lymphangitis is due to wounds of the limb, which may exist either in the superior but more frequently in the inferior part, of the member, the general symptoms and indications of irritation, with the swelling from infiltration, the result of the inflammatory action, and the corded full, and sharply defined condition of the lymphatics, together with the fact that a wound exists, which may probably, at the period of inspection, not be of a remarkably healthy character, all tend to give a certain feasibility to the suspicion that the case is one of farcy The absence, however, of specific growths on the course of the lymphatics, which are not bulged or knotted as in farcy with probably the history of the wound, and the fact that only one exists, as also its character and the obvious effect which a moderate amount of soothing treatment will produce on its condition, in a very few days afford substantial evidence that no farcy exists

In the chronic manifestation of lymphangitis, or rather, it should be said, in that peculiar diseased condition of the sub-cutaneous connective-tissue consequent on repeated attacks of ordinary lymphangitis, and known as elephantiasis, when,

10

from the character of the morbid changes proceeding in connection with the connective-tissue of the limb, there exists a
disposition to a steadily progressive increase in its bulk,
there seems less danger of placing the animal in the
dangerous position of being considered affected with farcy
Although there is here much swelling, it is not of the character
of that associated with farcy, the infiltration has here gradually,
and in stages, become indurated , there is, however, no active
hyperæmia, little pain, and no glandular induration, with the
absence of corded lymphatics, nodules, or ulcers.

With equine variola, a comparatively rare disease in Great
Britain, farcy may possibly be confounded, and particularly so
if local œdema, or partial organization of previous inflammatory
products, be existing at the time of the eruptive fever   With
a moderate amount of care, however, there ought to be little
difficulty in diagnosticating the two diseases   In variolous
fever the course is rapid and determinate, having a tendency,
after passing through its regular stages, to terminate in
restored healthy functional activity ; while the local lesions,
when fully developed, do not result in chancre-like sores, but
possess a natural tendency to heal by healthy cicatrization
With farcy its course is prolonged and irregular ; the nodules,
when ripe, result in unhealthy sores, which have no tendency
to healthy reparative action, but are disposed to pass on
to progressively destructive changes, and ultimately to destroy
life

No doubt many of those affections which have been regarded
as simulating farcy, and likely to be confounded with it, are
much more annoying when occurring in animals where, from
age, previous debility, and other vicious and depressing
influences, the probabilities of suspicious symptoms, culminating in what is regarded as confirmed farcy, are considerable   We must not, however, in our desire to arrive at a
decisive opinion, rest satisfied, when giving that opinion in
the affirmative as to the existence of farcy, with evidence
less satisfactory, or less strong, than that which rests on the
presence of the specific growths or buds, the true ulcerous
character of the sores, the nature of the discharge from these,
and the condition of the lymphatic vessels and glands   In
addition to an available knowledge of those diseased conditions,

which may be mistaken for any exhibition of this special affection, we must never forget that in assisting us in determining as to the existence of glanders in any of its forms or developments, and in guarding us so as not rashly to pronounce an opinion as to the freedom of animals suspected from contamination with the infecting virus, we will ever find careful interrogation of attendants and owners, and the collection of as much information relating to the history of the antecedents and associations, certain and possible, of the horse, of much benefit; often more to be relied upon for guidance than the conclusions arrived at from the observance of existing physical signs.

Dissemination—Amongst those who are best informed, and most capable of judging, it is a generally admitted fact that glanders in any of its forms is of less frequent occurrence and less widely distributed in our country at the present day than in periods which have preceded. The opinion formerly dominant both here and in other countries of Europe, that it was not capable of being propagated by contagion or infection, was certainly productive of incalculable mischief; while the adoption of the idea of its infectious character, and the moulding of our actions and of our management of horses in accordance with this idea, have probably had more to do with lessening the numbers diseased than all other measures taken together. While there seems every reason to believe that in proportion as the idea that it is more frequently caught than generated, or that it never originates autochthonously, gains ground and takes possession of the minds of those intimately connected with the management of horses, in like proportion will our losses decrease, and the rapidity and frequency which mark its extension from centres of infection be curtailed and circumscribed.

Although many of our veterinarians still strenuously hold to the belief that farcy-glanders may arise spontaneously, even they now more willingly allow that it is largely distributed by the direct contact of the diseased with the healthy, or indirectly by the medium of contaminated agents or carriers. So long, however, as we entertain the opinion that glanders is largely capable of spontaneous development, or that its genesis is brought about by the operation of adverse influences, and in-

10—2

dependently of a prior existence of the specific virus; so long as
we regard the specific infecting medium or contagion as only
fixed and not also volatile, so long will our endeavours for
the extinction of this disease want definiteness of purpose and
unity and strength of action, without which they must ever be
vacillating, weak, and inadequate to accomplish the ends con-
templated. By those who favour the idea of its spontaneous
development we are pointed to those recurring outbreaks, after
its apparent disappearance, in stables where large numbers of
horses are located, when these have been suddenly subjected to
vitiating and depressing agencies, such as overwork, defective
food, and bad sanitary arrangements. This coincidence and
the determining influence of these adverse factors are most
willingly allowed, but they may at the same time be susceptible of an entirely different interpretation; for aught we
know to the contrary, these are only the agents in the production of a visible and local development of symptoms proceeding
from a previously existing and long-established though occult
disease. Like every other specific contagious disease, its
existence is always favoured by the care with which it is kept
alive in individual cases and in centres of origin by medical
treatment of the affected, by disregard or imperfectly carrying
out of properly digested measures for the prevention and
eradication of the disease.

All who are connected professionally with horses congre-
gated in large numbers, particularly in our centres of trade
and population, know how difficult it is when glanders once
obtains a location among hard-working horses to arrest its progress and secure its disappearance. In all such cases there is
little doubt that unhealthy and crowded stables, overworking,
and underfeeding aged and otherwise debilitated animals, tend
much to furnish at least a suitable soil for the development of
the specific infecting material when placed there.

It is probably more through timidity, and a desire to save
both life and money by retaining in the establishment animals
which may be designated only suspicious, and which at the
particular time of examination could not conscientiously be
condemned as undoubtedly glandered, than by the simple and
uncomplicated influence of vitiating agents, that the continuous though intermitting appearance of the disease is main-

tained, and that stables and particular collections of horses
have occasionally obtained an unenviable notoriety.

Treatment—Although in some cases of chronic farcy recoveries may appear to result from the judicious employment
of therapeutic and sanitary measures, it is probably better,
considering the risks incurred, particularly when we remember
that all forms of the disease are capable of resulting from
inoculation or infection with the virus or infecting material of
even the chronic manifestations of it, and also its universally
acknowledged malignancy, that all should be classed together,
also, when evidence of its existence is sufficient, that all should
be prevented from doing further damage as the centres of
infection by ensuring their destruction

There seems pretty strong ground for believing that with
respect to glanders, the Act of 1878, and orders founded
thereon, have not had either a full or fair trial Until the
inspection of localities and stables is thoroughly well carried
out, and the isolation and slaughter of all diseased horses
faithfully executed, with proper attention to the carrying out
of the general instructions connected with disinfection, we
need not hope for much lessening of the mortality from this
contagious malady

**Sanitary Measures necessary to adopt in connection with the
Prevention and Eradication of Glanders**—When we consider
the fatal nature of this disease, and its acknowledged contagiousness in every form of its development, the great pecuniary loss entailed upon the community by its existence and
distribution, not to mention the more serious danger to human
life, the importance of well-considered and energetically carried out preventive and suppressive measures becomes obvious
to all but the most thoughtless and ignorant.   Until, however,
veterinary medicine is duly recognised and takes its proper
place in that considerable section of 'social science,' public
health, we can scarcely expect that executive measures sufficiently comprehensive to satisfy even our present knowledge
will be adopted and carried out

'The Contagious Diseases (Animals) Act of 1878,' and the
several orders founded thereon, are, so far, a step in the proper
direction, and although I doubt that in their operation these
have been as fruitful of beneficial results in the case of glanders

as in that of contagious pleuro-pneumonia and epizootic aphtha, it yet behoves all veterinarians to acquaint themselves with the provisions of these, that when called upon to carry out the duties of sanitary inspectors, they may be able to do so truthfully, and in accordance with the spirit and in the entirety of these enactments

However, whether acting as inspecting officers under this State order, or otherwise, it is needful that, as professional men, charged not merely with the cure of disease, but also with advising as to its prevention, we should be able to give directions and instructions to owners of animals, as well as the attendants upon these, which, if carried out faithfully, are calculated to give as large a measure of protection as our present knowledge will admit of

From what has already been said in speaking of the spontaneous development of glanders, it will be obvious, whether we regard it possible in this way to induce the disease, or only view the subjection of horses to the depressing influences indicated as more likely to facilitate its propagation by direct or indirect infection, that the first and most irreproachable recommendations as preventive measures are such as operate in maintaining animals in the full enjoyment of health and vigour, that general indications be given as to what ought to be considered suspicious signs of the disease, the dangers attendant on contact or close cohabitation of suspected animals with others as yet obviously healthy; and the necessity in all suspicious cases of obtaining at once the opinion of a professional man. While when so engaged we ought ever to be careful if any suspicions symptoms exhibit themselves, to at once isolate the suspected and steadily keep such under observation and treatment, strictly enforcing the separation from the healthy until sufficiently satisfied that no danger is likely to occur from again returning to company with others

When glanders is known to exist in any particular district, much circumspection is needful both in taking healthy horses into stables of unknown character, and in allowing strange horses to be placed in uncontaminated ones; while, should it be absolutely impossible to carry out this latter advice, a useful precaution before placing healthy animals in the stalls or boxes tenanted by strangers is that these be first thoroughly cleansed and disinfected

When once established in any particular locality, thoroughly effective suppressive and eradicative measures can only be carried out under the authoritative sanction of Government To detail what ought to be considered as effective and satisfactory is not our province here or at this time Such measures as in this country presently concern us are contained and dealt with in the State Act and orders already mentioned, in which form only can suppressive measures be carried out

There is one item, however, in compulsory eradicative measures generally insisted upon in such enactments—viz, disinfection—of the necessity of which it is not difficult to convince the greater number of sufferers in cases of outbreaks of the disease, and the details of which it is consequently advisable that we should be familiar with.

Into the consideration of the various theories of disinfection, the methods by which those agents termed disinfectants are supposed to act, it is not intended to enter, suffice it to say that by the term employed we mean the use or action of such means or agents as facilitate the destruction or removal, or both, of the supposed contagia or infecting material, or of the vehicle which may contain and convey this, thereby removing the probability of the contamination of the healthy when brought into situations where animals previously suffering from communicable diseases have been located Prior to and during the employment of either mechanical or chemical means of disinfection, all horses, manure, and litter must be removed, the latter—manure and litter—ought to be burned or buried, and air and sunlight admitted freely into the interior of the building The walls, from floor to ceiling, ought to be well scraped, by which all loose lime, plaster, or other superficial covering may be removed the same to be done to the floors, and if these are not composed of a close, compact material, as concrete or pavement, the separate stones or bricks forming the floors must have the sand or earth contained in the interstices removed by picking, which can be replaced with fresh material when the disinfection is complete All fittings of wood, iron, or other material to be well scraped, then thoroughly washed with hot water and an alkali, as soda or

potash Immediately succeeding this mechanical cleansing the
chemical and other appliances are brought into application.

First, the fumigation with sulphurous acid evolved from
burning sulphur is to be recommended, from its thorough
penetrating and diffusive character. To be successfully done
the stable must be rendered tolerably close, so as to prevent
the egress of the vapour, which is readily obtained from burning sulphur in separate iron or earthenware vessels distributed
throughout the building The doors ought to be kept close
until the vapour has been well distributed and had a sufficiently long contact with the walls Chlorine gas, generated
from treating the black oxide of manganese with hydro-
chloric acid, is also an efficient disinfectant of the gaseous form
And seeing that in all processes of disinfection thoroughness
and certainty in the destruction of the virus or infecting
agent are most surely obtained by varying the disinfecting
agents employed rather than by employing an extra amount
of any one, it will, after the fumigation, be a wise plan to wash
the walls, the floors, the whole of the woodwork and iron
fittings with a mixture of carbolic acid and water, in the proportion of six or ten ounces of the acid to the gallon of water
This mixture may also be further used in slacking the caustic
lime with which the walls ought to be finally washed it also
ought to be repeated over the permanent fittings which are
not removed   Having done all this, the stable ought not to
be occupied until exposed for some time to the action of the
air by allowing the doors and windows to remain open

At this time also attention must be directed to the drains
of the stable see that no foul material is allowed to obtain a
lodgment there, and flush them first with water, followed by a
mixture of carbolic acid in water, or a solution of chloride of
lime or sulphuric acid

All stable utensils which are not capable of being thoroughly
disinfected with hot water, chemical mixtures, or by passing
through the fire, or which are of little value, ought to be
destroyed by fire   Horse-clothing, harness, and other articles
which have been in contact with diseased or suspected animals,
must, if retained for further use, be well steeped and washed in
hot water and soda, disinfected by fumigation, and exposed to
the air for some days ere being used   Stables of wood of a

temporary character, and all internal fittings of wood when much worn or of little value, are much better destroyed by burning than retained to be washed and disinfected

CHAPTER V.

VARIOLA EQUINA—HORSE POX—CONSTITUTIONAL GREASE

Definition—*A specific, mild, continued, or intermittent fever, having in addition an eruption appearing on the skin and mucous surfaces, the result of the entrance into the system of a specific and palpable animal poison, which after a period of latency passes through the distinct and definite stages of fever, papular, vesicular, and pustular eruption, to be followed by decline*

Nature.—Variola or variolous fever, as occurring in the very different species of animals which we know are sufferers from it, from man downwards, although marked by much similarity or even many points of identity, is yet characterized in its development, its characters, and propagation in these several species by many features which seem to stamp it as in its essential nature specifically distinct in each

In none of our patients, save the sheep, has the appearance of variola, even in an epizootic form, given us much cause for alarm While with respect to the relations which variola of one animal bears to that of another, there seems even now in our day, after much experimentation and the extensive record of facts which exist, no very general agreement

By some the existence of a distinct variolous fever in the horse has been denied, and this is scarcely to be wondered at when we consider that, unless in the most distinctly marked and pronounced form in which it is seen in that animal, the eruptive affection, which is known by the name and classed as equine variola, is in the horse, in the majority of cases, either passed over without attracting observation, or is confounded with an aphthous eruption, or with the irregularly recurring skin affection, commonly recognised by the term 'grease' In this way, probably, has the fever, which really seems to

have a distinct claim to be regarded as variolous, been held
to be a comparatively rare disease, even in the country where
its existence was first indicated more than half a century
ago

Believed originally by Jenner and his contemporaries to be
the source of vaccinia in the cow, it seems by experimentation
to be capable of transmitting that, both to the bovine species
and to man, either directly or indirectly; and when so transmitted, to be capable of protecting these from their variola, as
well as the human subject from vaccinia; while vaccination
protects the horse from its own variola

That the disease which by our German *confrères* has been
designated *stomatitis pustulosa contagiosa*, and by French
veterinarians *stomatitis aphtheuse*, or *herpes phlyctenoide*, and
by some of our English authorities regarded as true equine
variola—that this disease is frequently met with I am thoroughly
satisfied; that it exhibits some of the characters of variolous
fever I am free to admit, while additional resemblances to
variola, which have not been proved by me in actual practice,
seem powerfully supported by those upon whose ability and
judgment we may depend   Still there does not seem sufficient
evidence to compel us to regard it as true equine variola

The theory generally accepted regarding the accession of
variolous fever is, that a specific poison, proceeding from previously existing variola, is received into and affects the
economy; that after a certain period of latency this originates
the primary fever, which lasts a few days, to be followed by
the secondary and diagnostic symptoms, the local disturbances
and lesions, the eruption on the skin and mucous membranes
This eruption passes through certain stages of papule, vesicle,
and pustule.   In the horse these local changes are chiefly
observed in the cutaneous surface of the inferior parts of the
extremities, particularly the hind ones, and on the mucous
membrane of the mouth, and skin immediately connected with
this membrane   When occurring on the extremities, the
eruption—partly from friction, and partly from soaking of the
epidermic scabs with the secretion—is extremely prone to
become confluent, and the abundant discharge of purulent
material from an extensive surface has often caused this affection to be confounded with the skin disease known as 'grease.'

Symptoms—The general symptoms or disturbances constituting the primary fever in horse-pox are usually very slight
—so slight that they rarely attract observation The period
of incubation is somewhat variable, when resulting from inoculation, it rarely extends beyond eight days

For two or three days previous to the appearance of the
local phenomena, general disturbance, as indicated by slight
rigors and staring coat, may be attractive ; in the greater
number, however, even these premonitory symptoms of illness
are unnoticed · and it is not until the animal refuses his food,
and appears either disinclined or unable to eat, that any fear
of illness is felt. At this time the pyrexia is distinct, and
seems to vary in accordance with the seat of the local eruption

It is said that the constitutional disturbance is most marked
when the eruption is situated on the extremities, and least so
when this is developed in connection with the skin and mucous
membranes of the head   When the skin of the limbs becomes
the seat of the eruption, there is an increase in its vascularity,
if colourless, the first indication of disturbance is the appearance of red patches, which shortly become slightly elevated, and
feel hard or firm when pressed between the fingers   As it advances in growth this elevation becomes depressed in the
centre, elevated at the edges, with an encircling zone or
areola

This umbilicated appearance of the eruption, and its being
surrounded by an areola, is usually characteristic of the
variolous papule in most animals   In three or four days
after the appearance of the pimple, the contained fluid or
serous material becomes more opaque, the epidermis dry and
crust-like, but movable, and if abraded, easily detached from
the soft or fluid state of the tissue beneath

When abraded and detached by friction, the removal of the
crust or epidermic thickening is followed by a discharge for
some days of a limpid, straw-coloured fluid, which gradually
subsides, the small circular cavity or depression filling by
granulation. When not detached by force, the natural process of cicatrization generally detaches this crust, with little or
no suppuration, in from twelve to twenty days

When from the situation of the pustules in the flexures of

the joints, or from any untoward circumstances, these do not heal by the natural cicatrization, the purulent discharge is very apt to become excessive, and the healing is delayed being accomplished by granulation beneath a scab formed by the desiccated discharge. During the continuance of the eruption, and even after perfect desiccation, there is usually considerable swelling of the limbs, and even of the inferior surface of the body—this swelling remaining persistent for weeks after the animal is otherwise perfectly restored to health.

When the eruption of equine variola is situated in the membrané of the mouth, it is somewhat different from that which is situated on the cutaneous surface of the body. Tenderness and pain are indicated by the difficulty or inability to masticate and swallow, and by the ejection of fluids from the nostrils. Ropy saliva is abundant in, and dribbling from, the mouth.

On examination the mouth exhibits vesicles of somewhat varying character and stage of development, scattered singly or collected in groups over the buccal membrane, covering the cheeks and along the sides of the tongue. When occurring on the membrane of the mouth and lips, as also over the margin of the nasal openings, these vesicles are smaller than such as are encountered on the limbs; they, however, pass through similar regular stages of development, and usually heal more kindly.

The entire course of equine variola may be regarded as rather rapid, and not prolonged, but perfectly benign. The entire period of its duration, from the reception of the infecting material to the occurrence of the desquamative process, is rarely over three weeks: of this period the most important is that occupied by the eruptive stage, or the time during which the diagnostic lesions are most readily distinguished—this may be said to be eight days: the period taken up by the fever prior to the appearance of the eruption is only a few days. Although the last stage, or that of desquamation, is generally completed in twenty days from the appearance of the invasion fever, the complete restoration to health is often retarded by the appearance of a secondary eruption, or by complications connected with the results of the localization of the virus in the skin and subcutaneous tissues. The pustules, from being confluent, may produce, by infiltration and other inflammatory results, death of considerable portions of the cutis and subjacent tissues, with accompanying or consequent ulceration and a tardy healing process, extensive local œdema continuing as a troublesome sequel for some time   Unless irritated by bits or halter-ropes being placed in the mouth during the period of the eruption, the pustules, after discharging their contents, very quickly scab over, or where an open sore exists, it is rapidly filled by healthy granulations, and in a very short time is so perfectly cicatrized that no scars or indentations are left.

Contagium and Mode of Transmission—It is said by the majority of observers that equine variola is only propagated from horse to horse, or from the horse to other animals, by direct contact; others, however, particularly our American brethren—who, from the accounts which they have published, seem to see more of it than we do—believe that the virus is not only fixed, but also volatile, that the disease may be transmitted by cohabitation as well as inoculation or direct contact This is certainly what we should expect, and is in accordance with what we know occurs in connection with variola in the other animals which come under our care.

What may be the exact nature of the *materies morbi*, whether organic germs, granules, molecules, or living particulate forms, we do not know, this, however, we are satisfied of, that while some of the animal secretions seem capable of transmitting the disease when implanted in the body of the healthy, the most active and fruitful is the fluid from a well-formed vesicle before the contained material has become lactescent   How long, or under what conditions, the infecting virus of horse-pox may be preserved and still retain its powers of propagation when tested by inoculation, there appear no reliable data upon which to form an opinion   Most probably the vehicle, the vesicular fluid, when dried, may retain its activity for a lengthened period, only needing favourable circumstances to bring its infecting powers into life   It is equally probable that it may be rendered inert by such chemical agents as sulphurous acid vapour, chlorine gas, carbolic acid, and by its subjection to a high temperature.   If we are only to regard the contagium of horse-pox as a fixed and not volatile or

diffusible infecting agent, its transmission, mode of access to
the system, and its extension amongst a number of animals, or
over a considerable district of country, can only be accounted
for by the contact, mediate or immediate, of the actually
diseased with the healthy. No doubt many of the outbreaks
of the disease which have been chronicled, being exceedingly
difficult, or it may be at the time of their investigation impossible to trace to their source, have been regarded as of
spontaneous origin This, however, judging from analogy, is
improbable, and would, to be received, require very convincing evidence

In the transmission of the virus of this disease, where the
specific lesions are situated on the head and extremities—parts
of the animal most constantly in contact with fodder or litter
—we may comprehend how readily a healthy animal, when
placed where the diseased have previously been located, will
become contaminated. Placed in direct contact, either during
work, in the stable, or at pasture, there is little difficulty in
the transmission of the disease The infecting material, most
probably the saliva, having mingled with it, the lymph from the
vesicles or the secretion from the sores on the limbs may be
brought in contact with and placed upon the mucous membranes, or on some abraded cutaneous surface frequently existing on the parts most susceptible of receiving the inoculation,
the heels and fetlocks

That equine variola may be transmitted to the horse and
other animals by artificial inoculation, experimental investigation abundantly proves. It also proves that the susceptibility
to the action of the virus of variola when inoculated varies in the
different species, being greatest in the horse and less in cattle
and sheep, it also indicates that the individual susceptibility
of different animals of the same species varies considerably.
Further, we seem to be taught from experimentation that the
virus loses its power after passing through the systems of
several animals Whether the passing through one attack of
the disease exempts the horse from a successful reinoculation,
does not from experimentation or observation amongst the
diseased appear to be determined.

Diagnosis.—When considering the subject of glanders and
farcy, attention was directed to this disease as one likely to be

confounded with it. Now, although it may be true that mistakes have been made in the diagnosis of these diseases, I am rather inclined to believe that this equine variola when encountered has more frequently been mistaken for glanders or farcy, not been recognised or regarded as of a varioloid character, but accepted as simply stomatitis or aphtha when the eruption has been prominently developed on the membrane of the mouth and of the cutaneous surfaces contiguous, and as the recurrent skin disease known by the name of 'grease' when the pustules were largely present on the skin of the extremities. That it should in its early stages and when examined cursorily be mistaken for glanders is easy enough understood. It has so long been regarded as settled that erosions on the membrane of the nasal cavities and in the vicinity of the nose and mouth, accompanied with swelling of the adjacent gland-structures, are to be regarded as diagnostic of glanders without further considering the nature of these erosions and swellings, that the existence in horse-pox of the pustules, either singly or in groups, might readily enough be regarded as symptomatic of the more malignant disease. And this is even more likely to be the case when similar sores exist on the external cutaneous surface of the limbs, which through abrasion, to which they are very liable from their situation, may induce a corded state of the lymphatic vessels; while to any observer who has not previously encountered this affection the alarm will be greater, and the suspicion of glanders more likely to be confirmed, when the disease is found to spread, and apparently by contagion

It is only, however, in the earlier stages, and when examined hurriedly, and when there may, from other circumstances, be an apprehension of glanders, that the danger of this mistake is at all great. The resemblance disappears when the eruption is more closely looked at, or when the disease in its different features is watched in its general development; the longer equine variola exists, the older the eruption, the more unlike is it to that of glanders.

The differentiation of the eruption in the various modifications of glanders and of horse-pox having already, in describing the former, been sufficiently entered into, it will be unnecessary to recapitulate the distinguishing features here.

From 'grease,' 'steatorrhœa,' and 'eczema impetiginodes '—
with which in their severer forms horse-pox has much in
common—it may be distinguished by carefully observing,
first, the nature of its attack, second, the character of its
pustulation; and third, its course and termination In its
attack horse-pox is sudden, usually accompanied with a certain
amount of fever, and the local inflammation and phenomena
are subsequent to, or coincident with, the pyrexia   In grease
the attack is gradual   we are probably not aware of its existence until it has made so much progress that the local
lesions are evidently acting in the production of systemic disturbance, which thus as a rule follows, and does not precede,
the local changes

When the pustules of variola are discrete on the skin of the
heels and lower parts of the extremities, they are not difficult
to diagnose, and when they have become confluent, and the
scabs are matted together, and remain partially floated, as it
were, over a considerable raw surface, on their removal by
washing with soap and water, the same characteristic features
of the sore will be revealed which mark the isolated pustules
It is circular, comparatively shallow, with occasionally numerous hairs projecting from it, indicating the non-destruction of
the deeper layers, or where suppuration has been longer continued and more severe, loops or projections of granulation-
tissue will be prominently displayed

Most frequently at the full development of the eruption all
the affected surface is covered with a firm brown crust, partially
adherent, chiefly by means of the hairs which project through
it this crust, or at least a crust so distinct and of this
character, does not exist in specific grease   The character of
the course of the eruption, which in reality is the essential of
the disease in equine variola, is benign, proceeding through a
short and ascertained course to perfect restoration to health,
in grease the local lesions are not disposed to heal, and they
do not pass through definite and understood phases, and are
sometimes difficult to control

Treatment —Belonging to the class of eruptive fevers which
naturally tend to restoration to health, after passing through
an ascertained and definite course, interference with this is
likely to be productive of undesirable results   Our object

must always in these be directed to the guiding of the patient safely through the natural development of the disease, interfering as little as possible with its regular phases, and only when complications occur, or when the animal activities seem to need support. In this, as in most fevers, excessive febrile action may be moderated by the exhibition of such salines as sulphate or hyposulphite of soda, allowed *ad libitum* in the drinking-water, or four drachms of chlorate, with two of nitrate of potass given twice daily in a similar manner.

When the sores on the membranes of the mouth are troublesome, and mastication and deglutition are performed with difficulty, we may harden the tender parts, and thus confer more liberty in both chewing and swallowing, through the use, for a few days, of an astringent gargle of sulphurous acid and water, or a mild solution of sulphate of zinc, to which a little glycerine has been added.

The food allowed ought to be of a character permitting of its easy mastication, and such as will tend to maintain the bowels in a healthy state. The horse will also, in the majority of cases, require a little exercise or the use of a good loose box.

CHAPTER VI

ERYSIPELAS

Definition.—*A specific, febrile disorder, attended with peculiar local complications in connection with the skin, and frequently also the immediately underlying tissues. The local inflammatory action occurring in the skin and other tissues is diffuse and spreading, accompanied with an eruption, much pain, and swelling.*

Pathology. *a General Characters and Varieties.*—This peculiar local inflammation of the skin and subcutaneous tissue shows itself in somewhat varying forms and modes of development and in accordance with these modifications of its exhibition has received somewhat different names; these names indicating some accepted idea of its origin, some distinctive phenomena exhibited during its course, or the invasion by the diseased process of a particular organ or class of tissues.

11

For us, however, all the varied developments of the disease may be grouped under the three different forms of—1 *Simple cutaneous erysipelas*, in which there is diffuse inflammation of the skin alone, the underlying textures being little, if at all, involved   2 *Cellulo-cutaneous or phlegmonous erysipelas*, in which both the skin and subcutaneous connective-tissue are affected. 3. *Cellular erysipelas*, in this the inflammation is confined to the underlying cutaneous connective-tissue, the skin itself being little involved.   This last form I have rarely found in the horse

Erysipelas has also, having a regard to what are considered as causes, been spoken of as *idiopathic* when appearing spontaneously, and *traumatic* when associated with an appreciable injury.

In some of its forms of development it is encountered amongst all our domestic animals ; while the horse, with which we are more particularly concerned, is probably the greatest sufferer   In him we meet with it, both as an independent or idiopathic affection, and associated with, or resulting from, an obvious injury The latter form, as being more properly included in the province of surgery, will not at this time engage our attention.

b Nature and Causation.—Both in the essential nature of the local morbid process which characterizes erysipelas, and in the entire ætiology, much difference of opinion has been ex pressed   By some it has been regarded as a common inflammatory action, arising from general or local disturbances, and owing any feature of individuality which it may possess to some condition of temperament or extrinsic agency.   On the other hand, it is probably more generally accepted as the visible manifestation of the operation of some specific poison, animate or otherwise, which has found an entrance into the animal body   Although in the horse not appearing to be capable of propagation by contagion, it does in all its features and results seem more than a common inflammation

I have observed that it is more apt to occur in animals in a debilitated and exhausted condition, and when these are exposed to the operation of influences which undoubtedly are potent factors in the production of disease generally   Also it is deserving of note that in many other animals it seems directly related—in some as cause, in others as effect—to other infective conditions which are surely propagated by contagion

In many of its principal features, which seem associated with or owe their existence to a vitiated condition of the blood, the result of the entrance into it of a specific morbific material, this disease bears much resemblance to some other conditions resulting from blood-changes or contaminations, as *scarlatina* or *purpura hæmorrhagica* As in these, there is a marked disposition to seize upon and exhibit peculiar blood-changes in connection with mucous membranes, while when they terminate fatally, they all appear to reach that result by processes not much dissimilar

In its mildest form, as simple cutaneous erysipelas, existing as a diffuse spreading inflammatory action ot a benign character confined to the skin, it is not often met with , more frequently we encounter it in the form known as the *phlegmonous* or *cellulo-cutaneous erysipelas* of rather a malignant type, and in which there is involved, to a greater or less extent, the subcutaneous connective and other tissues

When appearing in the horse in the idiopathic form, one of the hind extremities seems almost invariably selected as the situation for the manifestation of the local phenomena, the most characteristic of which in connection with the local inflammation is the peculiar serous exudation, which may either occur uniformly distributed over a considerable surface of the skin in the form of a copious perspiration, in which form it is commonly found around the upper part of the hoof and in the hollow of the fetlock, situations largely supplied with sebaceous follicles, or projected on its surface in the form of considerable vesicles or bullæ, which in the severer forms contain a bloody serous fluid and are chiefly observed situated over the inner surface of the thigh and hock, situations where, in the horse, the skin is remarkable for its great tenuity

Along with this external cutaneous exudation there is invariably, to a greater or less extent, effusion amongst the subcutaneous connective-tissue of serum or liquor sanguinis Coincident with these changes, and with the infiltration of the subcutaneous connective-tissue with inflammatory products, a change of a somewhat similar nature is going on in the submucous layer of several of the mucous membranes

11—2

The connection between the two changes and structural alterations, the one proceeding in the underlying layer of the connective-tissue of the skin, the other in the same layer of the mucous membranes, is evidently close and intimate, if not precisely similar in character.

c. Anatomical Characters—The pathological changes which occur during the progress of the disease vary with its nature and intensity In the milder forms there is simply furfuraceous shedding of the scarf-skin from desiccation of the serous exudation, or rupture of the vesicles with discharge of the contained fluid, followed by the healthy reproduction of tissue beneath In the more common and severe cases, where the vesicles are larger or more numerous, and filled with a darker-coloured fluid with accompanying infiltration on the inferior surface of the skin and amongst the subdermal connective-tissue, circumscribed patches of skin gradually lose their vitality, and are ultimately removed by sloughing, leaving an open and not rapidly healing sore with rough edges inclined at first to extend from the disintegration of the effused material occupying the subcutaneous connective-tissue, and discharging a fœtid sanious fluid mingled with shreds of lymph and areolar tissue; this death and removal of tissue may extend to sloughing and laying bare of tendons, ligaments, and joints In other instances again, where the inflammation seems to have more rapidly reached its height in the subjacent structures, and where the effusion has been extensive and the tension great, collections of pus are apt to form, and to be met with both circumscribed and diffuse

It is in such cases of gangrene of the skin, and extensive destruction of the cellular and other tissues, that we may look for changes of an analogous nature to occur in connection with the membrane of the mouth and nose Previous, however, to the erosion or actually ulcerated condition of these membranes, marked changes occur at the parts, which ultimately suffer destruction , these changes are represented by irregularly formed but circumscribed spots, varying in colour from dirty yellow to dark purple These markings, as far as can be distinguished, are in every respect analogous to those which occur in scarlatina, and seem, as in that disease, to bear a direct relationship to the period and severity of the fever.

It is to be observed that the suppurative process in the more severe forms of phlegmonous erysipelas is accompanied by well-marked serous effusion, and that the pus of a thin and sanious character is more frequently infiltrated amongst the areolæ of the tissues than circumscribed and bounded by adhesive inflammation so as to form a well-defined abscess.

Necroscopic examination discloses alterations chiefly in connection with the local manifestations of the disease, some peculiar changes in the composition of the blood, and certain adventitious appearances in the organs of respiration and digestion The character of the exudate permeating the meshes of the connective-tissue and vascular layer of the cutis varies from a structureless hyaline material to one of considerable density and distinctly fibrilated. When the inflammatory process and attendant disintegrative action extend to other and deeper-seated organs and structures, the changes observed by the naked eye are those consequent on the peculiar morbid action ; specially we encounter infiltration of tissues with the products of this action, and general and minute structural changes, disintegration, death, and removal not merely of the normal structures, but also of the new products themselves.

The question of the presence, both in the local lesions and in the blood itself, of certain low forms of organization, probably constituting the animate contagia of the disease, requires further proof ere it is received without certain modifications.

Symptoms—These are of two kinds, the constitutional or general, and the local ; they are of very differing degrees of intensity

The constitutional fever, which as a rule precedes, or at least is coincident with, the appearance of the local symptoms, is in young subjects, and those of a full habit of body, generally of the acute or sthenic type, in older animals, or those previously debilitated or suffering from the depressing influences of adverse local sanitary or dietetic conditions, the low or asthenic form is likely to prevail. Whatever may be the form of the fever at the outset of the disease, it will in all but the very mildest cases become truly hectic, most probably passing on to a low, prostrating form, and when having a fatal issue terminating by collapse.

When closely watched, the first symptoms of indisposition will be the ordinary shivering-fit of simple fever, with staring coat, exalted body-temperature, and evidence of muscular pain. The digestive organs appear to have suddenly become deranged, the mouth is hot and clammy, the tongue furred, while the breath has a disagreeable acrid smell, the bowels disposed to be confined, and the fæces coated with tenacious mucus.

Like other severe febrile disorders, there is, during its progress, obvious wasting of the muscular system indicative of tissue-change, and, as it advances, much prostration, the irritation and excitement being always greatest at the outset. All these constitutional symptoms, the character of the fever, the condition of the digestive, circulatory, and other organs, vary with the stage of the disease, its intensity, the existing susceptibility of the system, and the depressing and vitiating influences of adverse atmospheric and sanitary conditions.

Of the local symptoms, the earliest seldom manifest themselves more than twelve hours prior to the commencement of the constitutional disturbance. When the inflammation is simply located in the skin it is not, considering the covering and pigmentation, easy to observe the first indications of disturbance, consisting of simple redness, which disappears on pressure, to return immediately the pressure is removed; however, the roughness and perceptible elevation above the surrounding surface is easily enough detected, as also the oozing of serum, or the existence of vesicles filled with serous or sero-purulent fluid. Even when the skin is chiefly or entirely the seat of the inflammation, if it be supported on an abundance of connective-tissue there will be œdema from serous infiltration, although the connective-tissue itself is not involved.

In the *cellulo-cutaneous* variety, which is probably the most commonly met with in the horse—indeed there is some doubt whether in him the skin is ever, in a pure and uncomplicated form, the seat of this morbid action, but is not in every form complicated with the invasion more or less of the subjacent cellular tissue—the effusion into the subdermal connective structure is at first purely serous, and consequently the swelling resulting from this infiltration pits easily on pressure, the indentation being as rapidly filled up again when the pressure is removed. As the disease advances, however, the effusion is more strictly inflammatory, the pain is greater, the skin feels resisting, tension being increased, the material extravasated is less susceptible of indentation when pressed upon, and the parts acquire a firm, brawny feeling

The presence of numerous well-defined phlyctenæ or vesicles, although a characteristic symptom of the disease, is nevertheless not met with in every case, and the serous exudation found preceding as well as accompanying them occurs at intervals over considerable areas of the skin The tendency of the epidermis to become detached is well shown by pressing on the vesicles, when the contained fluid is readily distributed over a large surface , while the character of this fluid may be taken as a fair criterion of the severity or malignancy of the seizure, it is more truly serous in the milder forms, and bloody and albuminous in the less benignant

When the inflammation in the subcutaneous tissue has terminated in the process of suppuration, or when patches of skin are losing their vitality, ultimately to be removed by sloughing, the hair falls off or is easily removed, and the skin appears of a leaden hue and of a moist feeling

Pus, whether in circumscribed cavities or diffused through the areolar tissue, is detected beneath the skin by the sense of fluctuation imparted to the finger, this more distinctly in the former than in the latter case When this is evacuated, either by natural processes in the course of the disease or through incision, it will rarely be found of a laudable well-developed character , it is more frequently watery, mixed with blood, shreds of imperfectly organized lymph, and the debris of broken-down tissues The wounds thus formed are uncovered by any plastic exudation, while the areolar tissue becomes infiltrated, the skin undermined, and both take on ulceration and sloughing In very severe cases the inflammatory and subsequent disintegrative action does not rest with the invasion and destruction of the textures primarily involved, the skin and subjacent areolar tissues, but may, either in virtue of the character and severity of the action, or as the result of maltreatment, extend to the structures deeper seated, or to those contiguous to them The muscular and intermuscular

structures, the ligamentous appendages of joints, or the periosteum, may all inflame and suppurate, while the presence
and extension of purulent matter beneath these fibrous
structures, in addition to excessive pain, may cause inflammation and death of bone-tissue, or by finding its way into joints,
destroy their integrity by inducing anchylosis or general
disturbance sufficient to terminate in death. It is at this
period, subsequent to the first stage of the constitutional
fever, that changes somewhat analogous to those occurring in
the skin of the affected limb are met with in connection with
the visible mucous membranes particularly of the mouth and
nose

Course and Termination —The milder forms of erysipelas
generally run their course in from ten to fourteen days, the
inflammation and fever increasing for the first week, when
defervescence takes place, the local heat and swelling diminish,
and the superficial layer of the epidermis is shed in bran-like
scales. With this decline of general and local disturbance pain
disappears, and the limb is again used freely, this is the most
favourable termination, and is spoken of as the termination by
'resolution.' Rarely, however, in the horse do we recognise
erysipelas in this simple and benign form. Usually the
inflammatory action, involving both dermal and subdermal
connective-tissues, proceeds to the effusion of serous and
other products of established inflammatory action; vesicles, or
bullæ, are thrown out from or projected above the external
surface, the effused material in subjacent structures giving the
parts a more or less tense and firm feeling. Should the
morbid action not be excessive or proceed to the suppurative
formation, the subcutaneous effusion is arrested and gradually
becomes absorbed, the vesicles speedily desiccate, form into
scabs, and after a time scale off

Occasionally the bullæ in parting with their serous contents
do not desiccate, but on rupturing are succeeded by small circumscribed sores or abscesses, which for a time discharge
purulent matter, and may, previous to fairly taking on a healthy
reparative action, penetrate the underlying textures; this
tendency to infiltration and impairment of cutaneous nutrition
at these particular points, with the tension exercised by the
confined inflammatory products, rarely fail to produce destruc-

tion of the superimposed tissue and the formation of an irregular, ill-conditioned sore

When the constitutional fever, having reached its height, does not steadily although slowly defervesce, but seems rather to experience a fresh exacerbation, resulting in the development of truly hectic symptoms terminating in extreme exhaustion and prostration, when the local sores, upon which the constitutional disturbance seems now to depend, continue to extend by destructive infiltration and steady disintegration of tissue, a fatal termination is alone to be looked for

Diagnosis.—The recognition of erysipelas, although ordinarily not a difficult matter, may in particular instances be confounded with some of those disturbances in which hæmal contamination is a prominent feature, as scarlatina or purpura, with acute farcy, or with lymphangitis. With the exercise of a little care, however, it is easily enough differentiated from all of these From scarlatina it is distinguished by its non-association with a previously diseased condition, and by, in the severer cases, the more sthenic character of the pyrexial and inflammatory symptoms In erysipelas the tumefaction of the limb is uniform and firm, not in patches as in scarlatina; although both have oozing of serous fluid from the skin, the manner of oozing is different. In erysipelas pain on manipulation is more marked, while in scarlatina there are no circumscribed or diffused ruptures of the cutaneous tissue, infiltration and swelling of gland-textures are characteristic of scarlatina, not so of erysipelas From purpura it differs by the more sthenic character of the entire morbid process, by the local tumefaction being uniform and confined to one particular part of the body, usually the limbs, and most frequently a hind limb, while in purpura the swellings are irregularly distributed, sharply defined, and the head is early and markedly affected by these The swellings in purpura are also comparatively painless, not, as in erysipelas, acutely sensitive

From the local swelling of acute farcy it differs in that here we have no corded lymphatics nor any of the peculiar growths, farcy-buds or nodules; for although there may be sores in both cases, the character of these sores is dissimilar, they have no hard base and circumference of indurated tissue as in farcy, while the exquisitely sensitive condition of the entire dermal surface, so marked in erysipelas, is not so prominent in farcy.

With lymphangitis it has certain resemblances, particularly in the early stages of both affections, as the diseases progress, however, there is little danger of their being confounded, while all through their respective courses there are certain distinguishing features In lymphangitis the swelling, heat, and tenderness appear first in the inguinal region, and after a time extend downwards, in erysipelas the same local conditions almost invariably originate in the vicinity of the hock, or between that joint and the fetlock, and extend in both directions There is rarely any exudation from the skin in ordinary lymphangitis, and never any of the vesication, local gangrene and sloughing sores so characteristic of erysipelas; nor is there any liability to structural changes in the membrane of the mouth and upper air-passages

Treatment —Acting upon the understood and admitted inflammatory and febrile character of erysipelas, the whole of those remedial agents known as antiphlogistics, the principal of which are blood-letting and purging, have been employed and carried to their fullest extent, without, however, I believe, such success as will warrant their recommendation ; by some they are even yet advocated as superior to aught else. Now although it may be true—notwithstanding the doubts as to the universality of its truth—that these are the legitimate means whereby inflammatory action, whenever occurring, may be successfully combated, it is even now certain that their indiscriminate employment, even moderately, in every case of erysipelas is attended with anything but desirable results.

In actual practice it is found that the exhibition of purgatives, and especially the abstraction of blood, is borne with impunity only in young or strong subjects, and when the fever is of the sthenic or active type, and at its very outset. In other circumstances, i e where the animals suffering are old, or previously debilitated, or subjected to depressing influences, or where the fever is in its second stage, or is from its outset of a rather asthenic type, their employment is productive of decidedly dangerous results In robust cases at the commencement of the fever, bilious symptoms, indicative of derangement of the digestive organs, being almost invariably present, a small dose of aloes, from three to four drachms, combined with thirty grains of calomel, sufficient to induce an action of the bowels, and repeated after an interval of two or three days, will be found of greater benefit than active purgation Bleeding, unless in the cases indicated, is not to be recommended, and even in these is of doubtful efficacy.

Having obtained an action of the bowels, should the horse be inclined to feed moderately, care must be exercised that only such food is given as will tend to maintain a natural or rather moist condition of the canal. Not being disposed for movement from the pain of the limb, a loose box is not so absolutely needful in any stage of erysipelas as in many other affections

As we cannot expect to cut short the development of constitutional symptoms, the more rational system of treatment seems to be that of directing all our energies and appliances to moderate the course of these—preventing complications, supporting the system, and maintaining unobstructed those natural channels of the body through which poisonous and effete material is thrown off From its general soothing and mild diuretic action, a mixture of sweet spirits of nitre with camphor and solution of acetate of ammonia, given in moderate doses three times daily, will be found to serve these purposes well , or, as in the case of other febrile disturbances, both specific and common, and particularly when the internal temperature is high, the continuous use of salicylic acid in full dose twice or thrice daily is deserving of being fairly tried As the disease advances and stimulants become more necessary, the liquor ammonia acetatis may be supplanted by an ounce of the solution of ammonia carbonate, two ounces of aromatic spirits of ammonia, or the same quantity of brandy or whisky When the thirst is great, such salines as sulphate or hyposulphite of soda, or chlorate of potass, are readily taken with the drinking-water, and appear productive of benefit, more particularly during the height of the fever

With some practitioners—even from the earliest stages of erysipelas in all animals—treatment by tonics, particularly preparations of iron, is spoken of favourably , still I have always looked upon these agents as likely to yield, and fancy that in practice they have yielded, better results when given on the subsidence of the fever as aids to convalescence   At this period tonics, and especially iron, either alone in the form of the tincture or solution of the perchloride, or combined as the sulphate, or the sulphate of iron and quinine with sulphuric acid, or in bolus with vegetable tonics, and alternated with the stimulant draught aheady mentioned, is productive of good

Of local applications the best is warm water : cold I have tried in various ways and extensively, but with indifferent results   To obtain the full benefit from the warm-water applications, they ought to be employed as soon as the swellings commence—not for a few minutes two or three times daily, but for an hour or two continuously ; and when the pain is severe, a little tincture of opium may with advantage be added to the water.

When exudation has taken place in the subdermal tissues, free scarifications are of much benefit, both in relieving the tension and in permitting the effused serum to drain off. these may probably require to be performed daily, and are best done immediately previous to the fomentation, by which the discharge is favoured during the after-application of the warm water   In both these methods of treatment, with or without the employment of scarifications, a certain amount of protection and relief from pain appears to be afforded by dusting the limb with wheaten flour, having previously smeared it with carbolized oil   Whenever it is certain that pus has collected beneath the skin, a free incision ought to be made so as to allow of its escape.

Patches from which the skin has been removed by sloughing, unhealthy sores resulting from abrasions or incisions which are discharging fœtid sames, should be kept clean and dressed twice daily, so as to promote healthy action and destroy the fœtor, with carbolized oil, a solution of permanganate of potass, or chloride of zinc   The application over the skin, at the union of the healthy with the diseased parts, of tincture of iodine or solution of nitrate of silver, with a view to arrest the progress of the local inflammation, does not in our patients appear to be productive of much or any effect.   Even free scarification and cauterization, carried out on the boundary of the healthy tissue, seem equally impotent for the attainment of a like result.

When, however, convalescence has been established, and a certain amount of swelling of the limb still remains, resulting from partial organization of the material effused, I have seen good result from daily application, by smart friction over the swollen limb, of common iodine ointment.

However, even when seen early, and with all the attention it is possible to give them, amongst the severer forms of erysipelas there is always a large proportion of fatal cases

---

CHAPTER VII

CEREBRO-SPINAL FEVER—EPIZOÖTIC CEREBRO-SPINAL MENINGITIS

Definition—*A general diseased condition, sudden in appearance, partaking of the character of an acute specific disease, often appearing as an enzooty or epizooty, characterized by variable pyrexial symptoms, disturbed innervation, particularly impairment of voluntary movement and clonic spasms of the muscles of the cervical region, when terminating fatally, exhibiting hyperæmia and structural changes in different parts of the cerebro-spinal nerve-centre.*

Pathology   *a. Nature and Causation.*—This diseased condition, which, notwithstanding all that has been said to the contrary, ought probably to be regarded as a true specific fever of the horse, has for a very lengthened period been observed in different countries and under different conditions   It has frequently been considered as simply a sporadic local inflammation of those structures, the great nerve-centres, in connection with which the diagnostic lesions are chiefly encountered   This is hardly to be believed when the extensive involvement of the entire nervous system is had regard to, its occasionally wide distribution, its extreme fatality, and the absence of relation between the severity of symptoms exhibited and the extent of textural change observable after death.

From its not unfrequent association with the well-known disease *specific catarrhal fever, distemper,* or *influenza* of the horse, it has by many been regarded as merely a sequel or

complication of that fever, this view I for long entertained
Still evidence is not wanting to show that, although such
phenomena as are characteristic of this fever may be observed
in certain manifestations of *distemper*, there are still many invasions of 'cerebro spinal disease' more easily explicable on
the supposition that the disturbance is an abnormal condition
per se, and that whatever may be the immediate inducing
factor, it is specific and distinct.

The febrile symptoms, when existing in this disease, seem to
be directly related to the local lesions as a result or sequence,
and are not developed as the effect of the blood-contamination
direct, the inducing agent operating primarily on the nerve-
centres.

The cause or causes of this disease, which comports itself
in most respects like other manifestations of that entire class
which owe their existence to the entrance into the animal
body of a specific poison, are not understood

The predisposing conditions do not, as in many other
diseased states, seem intimately connected with indifferent
sanitation or defective food-supply, probably with overwork
and climatic disturbances, although these are not at all
definite

In America, where it is more generally distributed and more
frequently encountered, dietetic errors have by many been
credited with its production, particularly under certain conditions, as the excessive use of Indian corn

b Anatomical Characters.—The most obvious and extensive of the structural changes are connected with the membranes of the brain and spinal cord, and are indicative of
inflammatory action.

These changes are not always in direct relation to the
length of the disease or its severity In all there is hyperæmia
of the pia mater, with often a congested state of the entire
vessels of the cranium and spinal canal, and the presence of
an extra amount of fluid of a turbid character in the sub-
arachnoid space occasionally there are hæmorrhagic spots
on the dura mater, and a gelatiniform and feebly organized
material between the arachnoid and pia mater This latter
material may exist over the posterior and superior convolu-
tions of the cerebrum and cerebellum, but is oftener encoun-

tered at the base of the brain and in the sacro-lumbar region of the cord.

Even when the hyperæmia and blood-stasis are not conspicuous in the vessels of the meninges, the muddy colour of the existing spinal fluid and dull opaque character of the former structures are distinctive

In addition to the membranes, the proper substance of the brain and cord are excessively vascular, and may also be somewhat softened

When pneumonic symptoms have been conspicuous during life, the lung-tissue is found congested or inflamed, the solidified structure undergoing in some instances further distinctive changes.

Symptoms and Course.—In its onset this disease is very often sudden, there being no premonitory indications of illness, the characteristic symptoms at once attracting attention Impairment of motor-power is often so complete and so rapidly developed that the horse falls to the ground in a most unaccountable manner, or this complete disturbance of muscular power may have been shortly preceded by vertigo or staggering, particularly noticeable on moving the animal around, when a disposition is exhibited to twist the hind-feet one over the other, through inability to control the movements

When laid on the ground there are ordinarily much struggling, and perspiration of a patchy character, pulse and respirations quickened—these disturbances of a very irregular character as respects the relation of the one to the other In many instances there is marked hyperæsthesia, particularly of the anterior parts of the body, with clonic and convulsive contraction of the superior cervical and dorsal muscles, in some instances passing on to opisthotonos. In the majority, although from the wild appearance of the eyes and injected conjunctiva, with restless tossing of the head, it is evident that the internal cerebral parts are invaded, consciousness is not extensively impaired, and the creature seems acutely sensitive to every impression

When the cerebral centres are more affected there are proportionate coma, contracted pupils, slower pulse, and stertorous breathing

Very early in the affection, and all through the disease,

unless when the brain-lesions are great, pain is evidenced on pressure being exercised with the fingers along the spine. The bowels are usually confined, and the urine is not discharged with regularity, often not until from its amount it is forced in a continuous small stream or repeated small discharges from the urinary conduits.

On the point of internal temperature, as indicated by ther-mometric observation, there is a strange discrepancy of opinion; some observers emphatically declaring that no elevation is ex-hibited in any stage, others giving high readings as habitual. My own experience is that this state is rather variable and uncertain, the greater number indicating considerable elevation, while a few continue normal, with an occasional instance of depression. The condition seems one to which from its un-certainty it is not possible to give any typical range; an elevated temperature has, with my observations, been more frequent than the opposite.

There are also to be observed not unfrequently during the entire course of the disease well-marked cases of intermittency in the pyrexial symptoms, these, I have noticed to occur in instances where recovery has apparently taken place, and I have been inclined to associate this return or exacerbation of dis-turbance with the advent of reabsorption of exuded material, or with the development of complications which are apt to appear in severe and protracted cases.

In the milder attacks of the fever, which may be encountered at any time, but are oftener seen at the termination of an epi-zooty, the development of symptoms is not so hurried, the advance of the severe and diagnostic being heralded by dul-ness, want of vigour, impaired appetite, slight rigors, and a peculiar sluggishness. In these, when complete paraplegia or more extensive paralysis with affections of the cerebral centres does not show itself during the first three or four days, with careful attention a fair proportion will recover. When, however, the loss of control of the posterior extremities is very early in the seizure and very complete, with well-marked and persistent muscular contractions and convulsions, together with impairment of consciousness, or exalted sensibility, the probabilities of an early and fatal issue are great. The chief complications which are apt to occur during the course of such cases as are protracted or fatal are pulmonary With the appearance of these congestions and inflammatory advances the chances of recovery are materially lessened

Prognosis —Any attempt to forecast the course and termination of this disease in the early stages of the fever is most uncertain ; it ought always to be remembered that it is both an erratic and a fatal malady In every outbreak with which I am acquainted the percentage of fatal cases has been large, but rather irregular, ranging from ten to eighty , while in many it has been shown that the death-rate has usually been highest at the commencement of the epizooty

In some of the American States, where it has on several occasions been extensively distributed, the fatality has not been so large

Although, when terminating fatally, the larger number succumb during the first week of the attack, we yet find that relapses and complications are liable to augment the death-roll after this time, and that the common results and complications so largely operative in determining, if not in inducing, death do not develop until some time has elapsed

Treatment —It is to be feared that until a more definite knowledge is obtained of the active inducing agent, no real advance will be made in attempts to give certainty to our efforts in controlling the spread or movements of the fever. A consideration of the morbid anatomy of the malady would lead us to believe that endeavours directed to the controlling of the supply of blood to the great nerve-centres, and lessening its tendency to retardation and effusion, as also, failing the securing of these results, the employment of such agents as are likely to expedite the reabsorption of exuded material, were those from which most benefit might be expected Practically, the former of these ends is sometimes attained by the application to the region of the spine of ice-bags, or heat with or without moisture, and by inducing a free movement of the bowels by the administration of aloes combined with, or followed by, saline purgatives

Following this, and subsidence of the more active symptoms should the animal survive such, recovery of tone and removal of exudation is favoured by the employment of tonics, as iron with sulphuric acid, and stimulants with mild diuretics In

12

more protracted cases good has resulted from the use of compounds of iodine and of strychnine   When prostration is a
marked feature at an early stage of the fever, neither purgation
nor local applications of cold or heat seem to do so well as
general and local stimulation.   This may be carried out by the
exhibition of small and repeated doses of alcohol with quinine,
or ammonia compounds, and by daily friction to the spine
through the use of ammonia or soap liniment.   When pain,
muscular convulsions, and tetanic spasms are severe, the
administration of opium affords more relief than aught else;
this may be exhibited in the usual manner by the mouth, but
is probably more effectually and economically dealt with when
employed hypodermically   Belladonna, given internally, and
applied by liniment or plaster to the spine, has been highly
spoken of by some, and the use of ergotina by others

The employment of this latter drug has not in my experience
been attended with the favourable results anticipated   In all
save the more active cases, and in those in their convalescent
stage, I have imagined that the greatest benefits have followed
local stimulation, the steady exhibition, in not too large doses,
of tonics and stimulants, particularly preparations of iron,
iodine, strychnia and ammonia.   Considerable objections are
entertained by some to placing the suffering in slings; this
must be regulated by the stage of the fever, the temperament
of the animal, and accessory advantages we may possess. From
experience, I should advise the use of this mechanical support
in all cases where the animal was not utterly powerless, and
when the restraint did not seem to cause aggravation of symptoms.   Complications which arise during the course of the
disease must be treated as they occur, and in accordance with
their character

In the matter of food, nothing special probably is demanded,
save to see that it is good, easily assimilated, and such as will
not tend to constipate, where little food is taken, nutriment
should be combined with the medicine

CHAPTER VIII

ANTHRAX—SPLENIC FEVER—CHARBON—CARBUNCULAR FEVER—
GLOSSANTHRAX—BLAIN, ETC

History —Regarding the relative position allotted by comparative pathologists to this disease in the equine species, and in accordance with our previously expressed intention of avoiding to trespass on the domains of general pathology, we must but cursorily glance at the history of anthrax, though probably we are in possession of more which relates to it historically than to any other general animal disease. Referred to in Exodus, chap. ix., it is presumed, as the 'boil which came forth as blains upon man and upon beast throughout all Egypt,' in response to the casting forth of 'ashes from the furnace' by Moses, the modern names of Charbon, Anthrax, and Carbuncle, all signifying 'burning ashes,' would seem somewhat remarkable. Greek and Latin writers on diseases of the domesticated animals evidently describe it under the head of Οἴδημα, Sacra ignis, Gutta rosea, etc, etc, while applied to man the former termed it Anthrax, and the latter Carbunculus, and in Arabian manuscripts of the middle ages it is found mentioned as Atshac-al-Humrah, or Persian fire—each of these several terms evidently intended to convey some idea of the lesion. It is worthy of notice that though anthrax is in our day a comparatively rare disease among horses, from records we have of animal scourges in the past it seems certain that as a malignant epizooty it frequently ravaged both the Continent and the Islands of Europe. Mr Fleming, in his 'History of Animal Plagues,' refers to several graphically described outbreaks in Great Britain and central and western Europe of what is perfectly evident were visits of both anthrax proper and glossanthrax. The last of these, an epizooty of glossanthrax related by Scheuchzer, occurring in 1731-32, appears to have committed great ravages amongst all domestic animals in the states of central and south-western Europe

The literature of the subject assumed no approach to a definite form till, in 1780, Chabert grouped many separately described diseases under the one head, considering them

12—2

several manifestations of the same. About this time Fournier, Bertin, Montfils, and others, sought to demonstrate its power of propagation by contagion, though soon Kansch disputed this, and enunciated a theory which attributed the disease to paralysis of the pneumogastric nerve. In the *rôle* of observers we can scarcely forbear mention, as prominent among a large field, of Larry (1811), Remer (1814), Greve (1818), Hoffmann (1830), and Delafond (1843)—whose experiments, principally with sheep, induced him to deny its contagious nature, and to attribute it to condition of locality, soil, and dietetic errors; Gerlach (1845)—who, by direct experiment, proved its contagious nature, and concluded it was a form of septicæmia. In 1850 Heusinger, as the result of his investigations, wrote of it as a malarial neurosis of the ganglionic system, in which the nerves of the spleen were first paralyzed, then followed by death of the tissue, hence the name, Milzbrand, inflammatory death of the spleen. After this there are circumscribed extravasations due to local paralysis in different organs, and death of tissue in patches. Further, that in the disease a poison was developed which had the power of conveying its specific effects to men and animals, concluding that the different manifestations in these are essentially those of the same malady. He asserted that the disease is primarily developed in herbivorous mammals. Virchow, writing in 1855, confirms these views regarding the cause as some 'specific ferment.'

In 1855 Pollender started a fresh epoch in the history of medical science, for, in connection with anthrax, he actually demonstrated countless masses of rod-like bodies, to the class of which is now relegated so important a part in the ætiology of diseases of this order. From their micro-chemical behaviour he placed them in the vegetable kingdom.

In 1857 Brauell, experimenting with the blood of sheep, arrived at similar results, and regarded the existence of the rods which he found during life as diagnostic; though from the fact of his producing the disease with blood in which these bodies did not exist, he concluded that these were neither the cause nor the carriers of the cause of the malady. He also found that they appeared in the blood only a few hours, or less, before death. He was of course unaware of the spore-bearing nature of the organism.

At this period of the history of anthrax the nature of these bodies absorbed a large share of attention from many biologists and pathologists, being variously considered living organisms, shreds of fibrine, blood-crystals, etc

In 1863 Davaine, who studied the subject with much pains and precision, first named them *Bacteridia* to distinguish them from bacteria of putrefaction, whose presence he demonstrated were destructive to the rod-like bodies of anthrax, which he maintained were the true contagia of the disease

Since this date many foreign and British investigators have pursued, with notable success, investigations into the life-history and pathological significance of this organism, now generally regarded as a vegetable and a schizomycete

Geographical Distribution—Among the diseases of animals the geographical distribution of anthrax is unique, for in one or other of its varied forms it is encountered wherever animals are found The regions of the northern or southern latitudes are no more exempt from its ravages than are the temperate or equatorial zones It appears as an epizooty among the herds of the Laplander—as such the Russian too well knows the deadly *Jaswa*—and as an epidemic and epizooty among men and animals over the vast plains of Siberia, where it is spoken of as 'Siberian Plague' Neither do the great upland deserts of central Asia escape its visits, and as Loodiana Disease it is well enough known amongst horses over central Hindostan The great Australian stock-owner dreads the havoc of the scourging 'Cumberland Disease,' while it is not unknown on the wide pampas of the South American Republics, nor on the rolling prairies of the great Western State of the northern continent While, from the descriptions of the ailments to which animals are subject, it seems to be as well known, if not so frequently recognised, in the fertile valleys and plateaux of southern and central Africa, where our acquaintance with it as 'Cape Horse Sickness' is intimate, as it is over the central plains and river-basins of middle and western Europe

Although certain conditions, geographical, thermal, meteorological, and those dependent on the character and quality of soil and subsoil, may to some extent influence the development and spread of anthrax, even in virtue of these it cannot be said to be confined to any particular district or territory; though these are, however, sufficient to render the causes of production distinctly abiding and extremely virulent when brought into action

We shall again draw attention to these when treating of the ætiology of the disease.

GENERAL CHARACTERS AND NATURE.

Definition.—*As a short definition or description of anthrax we may with propriety say it is an acute infective disease, generally enzoötic, characterized by the rapidity of its development, generally fatal termination, and by the visible alterations in the blood, which is viscid, dark-coloured, and indisposed to coagulate, and which in many cases before death is crowded with minute organisms known as bacteria, believed to be of vegetable origin, and capable of inducing a similarly diseased condition when introduced into the blood of many other creatures.*

The universality of its distribution geographically, and its disposition to attack all animals, are among its most prominent features. All animals which domestication has placed under our care seem liable to its influence, though of these probably the larger ruminants are most susceptible, while solipeds manifest the tendency in a much less marked degree. Out of the pale of domestication the same species exhibit similar predisposition, while in anthrax districts the smaller feral creatures, with birds and fishes, are said to be not unfrequently affected. Inoculation with material from any one species of animal under the other requisite conditions will produce the disease in another, and in its treatment we must consider these matters of grave importance; indeed, anthrax cannot be studied out of the region of comparative pathology.

Though, as we have remarked, anthrax is not confined to any particular soil or climate, it stands beyond dispute, as the result of observation and experiment, that certain conditions connected with these have a great influence in its development and spread. Great manurial or organic richness, moisture, and an elevated temperature are in the highest degree favourable.

Most frequently occurring as an enzootic, or epizootic, it may, however, though more rarely, be met with in isolated instances as a sporadic disease

That it is contagious in the ordinary sense of the term has been variously admitted and denied by different writers, whose opinions are highly esteemed in such matters, but deductions derived from experiment, and the behaviour of the bacillus anthracis in relation to artificially produced disease, compel us to subscribe to the theory of its being communicable by the alimentary tract, the air-passages, or by cutaneous inoculation, and, though generally fixed, the virus may be more rarely volatile That it is transmissible is now beyond dispute, and may, either fresh from the source of the poison or after a long period of preservation, be conveyed by mediate objects to fresh habitats and means of development

To the condition of receptivity of the species and individual we are inclined to attach the utmost importance, and from our observation we are led to look to this for much explanation as to the apparently erratic behaviour of the anthrax virus

We have before said the manifestations of this disease are not invariably one and the same, either in species or individual But we feel justified, for purposes of description, in dividing them into two groups, viz .

1 *Anthrax proper as a general blood disorder, without external and readily appreciable local manifestations, and known to be connected with hæmal parasitism*

2 *Anthrax as a blood disease, with external and readily appreciable manifestations, included with which is one form in which the hæmal parasitism has not yet been so clearly demonstrated, and probably, until more definite information respecting its pathology, especially ætiology, is obtained, should be classed as ' Anthracoid '*

When occurring in the first form its course is usually shorter and its fatality greater than in the latter

It is deserving of notice, in having regard to the varied manifestations of anthrax, and the peculiarities which mark its development as to the respective liability of different animals to any or all of its forms, that although in Great Britain our horses are comparatively exempt from attacks of anthrax, as compared

184 ANTHRAX.

with our cattle and sheep, we must remember that this exemption is not enjoyed by equidæ over every quarter of the world, or even through our own empire. It is also worth knowing that liability or susceptibility of particular districts to special forms of anthrax have been known to change. And, although I cannot endorse what Mr Fleming says, quoting from Reynal, who, in speaking of the malady as it manifests itself in France, remarks, that ' splenic apoplexy, after prevailing in a malignant form for a certain time in a locality, becomes comparatively benignant,' I am yet satisfied that this acute form of anthrax, splenic fever, after having existed for years in some districts, has gradually given place to another form of anthrax, most frequently the erysipelatous, and that where anthrax fever existed in cattle, this succeeding anthrax erysipelas appeared in sheep. This has been the result of my experience in more than one district where anthrax, as an abiding disease, has been known for two or three generations, and where splenic fever was prevalent some twenty years since.

Although investigations have been carried on both in this country and on the Continent, with much energy and acumen, to determine the nature of the poison of anthrax, modern science has not yet been able to furnish us with irrefragable evidence and facts capable of affording thoroughly satisfactory answers to all our questionings. As to the general features of the disease and the manifest blood and tissue changes, there is little divergence of opinion ; but the rationale of the process by which these are brought about continues a moot-point. These alterations, formerly regarded as natural sequelæ of simply disturbed and perverted digestion and assimilation, are now more generally allowed to be the result of, or intimately connected with, the presence in the blood of certain minute specific organisms, which of themselves are either the actual cause, the agents which produce the actual cause, or the mere carriers of it. The reception of this theory, feasible in most points as it is, leaves much scope for further investigation ; and when calling to our memory many instances of sporadic nature in our own experience of anthrax, we confess they are not in all particulars explained by it, though we would not withhold our conviction that the weight of evidence is undoubtedly in its favour, and we confidently accept it as hæmal parasitism.

In every appearance of the naturally produced disease, it is argued, the state of animal habit is inclined to partake of the plethoric rather than the anæmic, that the nutriment supplied to the animal, whatever be its form, is never below the requirements of the organism, generally in excess; that the greater number of seizures are among animals the digestive and assimilatory organs of which have not attained the maximum of vigour, and are consequently not so fitted to resist any strain thrown suddenly on them—they are young, or at least have not reached maturity. The offspring of animals attacked with anthrax, which were *in utero* at the time of the attack, seem to enjoy an immunity from the disease throughout their course of life; while the preservation of their life in the uterus has been attributed to the filtering action of the fœtal membranes

Although interchangeably transmissible among the various susceptible species, inoculation with anthrax material from one animal or species may produce different manifestations of the disease from those noticed in the case from which the virus was taken We notice also, that in the transference of the *materies morbi* through different species a certain attenuation occurs, or, at least, the ultimate is not usually as severe as the original attack. In some interesting cases reported in the *Veterinarian* for December, 1873, the outbreak was originally noticed among sheep; the victims of the disease formed the food of certain dogs which usually took their meals in a field, from a pool in which the horses of the farm received their supply of drinking-water. While pasturing in this field one horse and then another died, and then carcases, which showed proof of anthrax, were so disposed as to be above the source of potable water used in the stable Within a month five more of these horses fell victims to anthrax; probably the poison had been conveyed by soakage from the carcases to the water, and thus to the healthy animals

Ætiology and Pathology—Though in connection with no department of medicine has more real work been done and positive results arrived at during the past decade than in the study of anthrax, we find ourselves now encountering many difficulties in attempting to explain all the phenomena in its causation That the study of the life-history of the

vegetable organism 'bacillus anthracis' is inseparable from
the study of anthrax proper, is now a matter beyond question,
and though, as we before stated, this disease in Great Britain
at least does not claim a very important part in hippopathology,
we shall further on give some little consideration to the more
essential points connected with the bacillus

In the *rôle* of inducing causes undoubtedly conditions
telluric, atmospheric and meteorological play a very important
part, though we must allow that these are subservient to the
growth and development of the bacterial organism, apart from
the effect they may have in rendering the subject of attack
suitable soil for these   In matters agricultural and horti-
cultural the consideration of the adaptability of the soil to
habits of the plant is certainly a matter of no secondary importance, and we think we should err if we lost sight of the
fact that a certain condition of animal constitution is essential
to the taking root and flourishing of our vegetable   And in
the study of no disease has this been more clearly shown than
was done in the experiments of Pasteur with anthrax-inoculation
in fowls   These creatures were long credited with possessing,
by virtue of their high temperature, an immunity from anthrax,
as they resisted the ordinary inoculation.   To prove the dependence of this on the thermometric state, the illustrious pathologist immersed a fowl, into which some anthrax virus had
been introduced, in cold water to lower the temperature, in a
short time it had died, and its blood, spleen, liver, lungs, etc,
were found swarming with bacilli   Other fowls uninoculated
were kept in the water with the former, with in them negative
results, while a counter-experiment substantiated the former
Colin also found that young buds, whose temperature is
normally lower than adults, were susceptible

Rats fed entirely on an animal diet resisted inoculation,
while some fed on bread readily contracted the disease   Again,
certain individuals prove refractory to all inoculation and even
intravenous injection; and this is apparently substantiated by
the well-known experiments of M Chauveau with Algerian
sheep, in which, though the instances were numerous and
carefully followed out, the disease could not be induced by the
ordinary artificial means of inoculation : in these cases virus
taken from the same vessel, and at the same time, proved their

immunity by producing the disease in other sheep at the first operation

With two conditions of system favourable to the development of anthrax we are from long experience familiar. These are, that there be no other disease present, and, as we also mentioned when speaking of its general characters, that the animal be in what is commonly known as a 'thriving condition,' and it appears to us that where the elaboration and assimilation processes are put to their utmost tension we have the most genial soil or the highest state of receptivity In the same light we may view the reason of youth being the most frequent period of attack. To induce this plethoric habit of the animal it is essential that its food shall not only be abundant but highly charged with nutritious matter. That food of this character is grown more especially in low-lying moist lands in warm weather is well enough known to most people, as is the fact that manurial richness is most conducive to its production

Here then we have three conditions which seem to be most favourable to the growth of highly stimulating fodder—moisture, heat, and manurial richness. As we proceed to look more closely into the life-history of bacillus anthracis, we shall find that the same conditions are probably the most congenial to its growth and development

Though there has been much variety of opinion as to some parts of the pathology of anthrax, there has been a general agreement that it is much more prevalent in low-lying lands and swamps—thus it has been attributed to malaria, etc.; while as to the beneficial results of removing water from the surface of lands by draining, etc, we have abundant proof That heat is essential to render conditions favourable to activity of bacillus anthracis is sufficiently evident to us, not only from experiment in the artificial cultivation, but also from actual observation of the disease as naturally occurring The same may be said when referring to the effect of vegetable infusions, as we may, we think, appropriately term the stagnant moisture we meet with under certain circumstances on swamps, morasses, etc. Having regard to these facts, it is scarcely to be wondered at that, at a time not far distant, anthrax was held to be the result of malaria and miasmata

Again, that soils of certain characters have been credited
with the production of the poison is not extraordinary when
we think of the capability of some of retaining moisture, and
of the organic richness, etc, of others. Results succeeding
the removal of these conditions, under a more rational and
improved system of agriculture and the employment of other
means calculated to lessen what were termed malarial emanations, seem to confirm this view by showing a most marked
decline of the disease, which in the same districts, under the
former conditions, was very prevalent. Thus Buhl reports
that a form of anthrax, which raged for a long time in the
Neuhof stud, at Donansworth, ceased entirely after some
stagnating water, to which the animals had recourse, was
drawn off. According to Wald, in many of the districts around
Potsdam, anthrax, which at one time had been common there,
gradually disappeared after the swampy land had been dried
by extensive improvements and drainage, and a suitable
outlet had been furnished for the stagnating water. We need
not, however, go to Germany or any part of the Continent
to seek for well-attested facts bearing on this point. In our
own country, probably easier than elsewhere, may facts of a
similar nature be gathered. I am acquainted with several
districts in the low-lying land of the Merse—the level plain of
Berwickshire, where the soil is clay and retentive—where half
a century since anthrax was one of the most common diseases
to which stock were liable, but now, by adoption of a system
of thorough drainage, and by the clearing and deepening of the
larger watercourses, together with a generally improved system
of agriculture, the disease is comparatively rare. To a superficial observer the decrease of anthrax in this and other
countries, by the adoption of means which are calculated to
remove malarial emanations, would seem to point to a certain
power in the soil itself of originating and developing the
specific and inducing factor of disease ; but for the production
of anthrax proper, at least, we think we have sufficient
grounds for saying the presence of bacillus anthracis or its
germs is a *sine quâ non*, as we should find it very difficult to
reconcile our minds to the fact that these living organisms,
which we can examine and cultivate, can come from any other
than living organisms, themselves having an independent

existence, and we imagine the recent advances in the study of the ætiology of specific diseases must have dealt severe blows to the 'spontaneous generation theory,' which has always been supported by negative rather than positive evidence

Though we wish to confine our attention specially to the diseases of the horse, the character of that now under our consideration demands that it be studied in connection with other animals on account of the common susceptibility to the effects of the poison producing the malady, and in no section is this comparative study more to be insisted on than in the present For, having regard to its highly contagious nature, we cannot place too much significance on the part which the bodies of animals dying from anthrax have in its causation To the improper disposal of cadavers, etc., many of the outbreaks may be traced, and if we accept the germ theory, all may be attributed The abiding enzootic character which anthrax manifests must be due to the same cause. There seems much to satisfy me that the bad name which many of our Highland and mountain sheep-walks have acquired as thoroughly unsound grazing-grounds, from the notorious prevalence of anthrax, is unquestionably to be traced to the extremely careless and reckless manner in which the carcases of animals dying from the disease are disposed of.

In many instances no attempt is made to bury these; they are simply thrown into some more obscure corner of the hill, behind a rock, or into some gulley, where their bones may be found whitening the ground months afterwards.

When we consider the period which the spores of the anthrax bacilli have been known to retain their vitality and capability of producing the disease after being buried in the soil, it is certainly somewhat startling to us, being cognizant of the extreme indifference with which these matters have been treated, that anthrax is not more prevalent in Great Britain It will now be seen that any medium by which the contagion of anthrax may be conveyed from diseased to healthy animals must be looked on as a factor in its causation

Pasteur credits the earthworm with doing much mischief, by raising with its upheavals the spores of the bacillus, for he found the soil above the graves of animals which had died of

anthrax, and been buried ten or twelve months before, literally
teeming with spores. And, as we have noticed before, dogs,
crows, and other carnivorous creatures become distributors of
the disease by bringing parts of affected carcases and deposit-
ing them in previously healthy situations.

Though it would seem, from the history of the disease, that
the most fruitful mode of contagion is inoculation at the
particular place where animals have died, been slaughtered, or
buried, it is yet sufficiently well established that the poison
generated in the diseased may by healthy men and animals be
carried and implanted in others which may become mortally
affected. Gerlach reports the transmission of anthrax by dogs
as inoculators. When shepherds' dogs are called away from de-
vouring anthrax carcases and are used in working the healthy
sheep, some are bitten, and perish of anthrax very quickly.

Davaine was early in pointing out that flies which had been
feeding on blood of animals which died of charbon possessed
in their proboscides material which on inoculation gave positive results. Bollinger in 1873, in the viscera of flies removed
from the carcase of a charbonous ox, demonstrated the presence of the characteristic bacilli, and by introducing them
into the system of rabbits produced well-marked anthrax.

We are conversant with several cases where shepherds who
have removed the skins from animals dead of anthrax have a
week afterwards conveyed the disease to other healthy animals;
and to show the extreme care and inquisitiveness which is
required in investigating the processes involved in the disease,
I may be excused for mentioning a case among sheep which
occurred within my own practice.

In two instances the original cases were acute charbon in
sheep, with local swellings in the region of the throat and
tongue. After having removed the skins from the dead
animals the carcases were buried, and nothing further thought
of the matter. Some eight or ten days elapsed, and the individual who skinned the sheep took his part in the annual
shearing, which lasted some days. Daily serious losses
occurred among the shorn sheep, and we were called in professionally, to find the carcases and the dying presenting positive
indications of anthrax. Knowing that in most labour executed by the hand there is some individual peculiarity attach-

ing to each person's work, we made use of this in endeavouring to discover the cause of death, and had the gratification of
having each carcase identified both by owner and shearer
himself as bearing the handiwork of the latter, who had
skinned the first-mentioned diseased sheep. It may be worthy
of remark here that in none of the cases, though there were
several small wounds in the skin, could we discover any special
lesion at any of these points

In woolsorter's disease, internal anthrax, or malignant
pustule of man, we have remarkable evidence of the manner
in which anthrax may be propagated. This form of the
disease is frequently seen among the *employés* in our woollen
factories, and has been specially and carefully studied by Dr.
Bell, of Bradford, who elicited that the disease is contracted
by the workers in wool and hair brought from certain districts
where anthrax is known to be common, and by these only
when the wool is undergoing a certain process (sorting)

The materials, working on which is associated with a certain
amount of danger, are alpaca, mohair, and camels' hair. The
maintenance of vitality of the organism, and the power of
transmissibility, are here proved to extend over great changes
of temperature and considerable periods of time. That knowledge of this to us, as veterinarians, is highly important, a
report in the *Veterinarian* for August, 1880, clearly shows.
As evidence of the close relation between the diseases of man
and the lower animals, this is well worthy of perusal. We
will only say here that in this instance some cattle and sheep
died of anthrax, lower down the course of a stream than
Keighley, where there are some woollen manufactories. It
appeared, from information gathered by some gentlemen who
investigated the matter, that these animals were supplied with
drink from a source contaminated with the 'sud-water' from
certain mills where van and Cape mohair are largely worked,
and where handling these several persons had suffered from
anthrax.

In a serious outbreak of splenic fever on a farm, a donkey
and a pony were employed at different times for conveying
the skins of the diseased; these beasts of burden died of acute
anthrax, probably inoculated through small wounds which
existed on the withers.

And we are acquainted with another instance in which a bone from an animal which had died of anthrax, by abraiding the tongue of an ox which had taken it into its mouth with food, appeared to be the cause of malignant glossanthrax

Other bearers of the contagion are of course very numerous, and such articles as harness worn by the diseased animals, or, indeed, anything connected with their management in or out of the stable, which by contact with secretions, etc, of the diseased have become contaminated. Fodder of every description may be the medium by which the poison is conveyed to its host, as may be water also   The former, particularly when grown upon lands where anthrax carcases or offal have been deposited, can scarcely fail to be a common form of conveyance   At the present time there are several attempts to introduce into this country as bedding for our animals moss from Germany, and we shall look with some curiosity to the effect of this material on health, since, considering the situations in which moss is usually found, we think there is just a possibility of this proving a source of anthrax-production, a quality which has by some been attributed to artificial manures

That water must afford many facilities for the distribution of the contagious principle we are quite convinced   Percolating through the soil, it carries with it the disease-germs and distributes them in various manners—both by drinking-water and by deposition in situations with which actual anthrax material had not before come into contact   Nearly twenty years since, on a small farm in the low-lying lands of Berwickshire, where only eight horses were kept, I witnessed the death of six in two years, all from that form of anthrax known as carbuncular fever   Believing the disease had a direct and intimate connection with the existence of a stagnant pool of water close to and a little more elevated than the stables where the horses stood and where they all died, I obtained, after persuasion, the removal of the pool, since which I have seen no disease amongst the stock of this farm having any resemblance to anthrax

That the atmosphere may transfer the minute spores, or even bacilli, from the diseased to the healthy, and that they may gain the circulation through the air-passages, there seems every probability, though to our knowledge this has not been so undeniably settled by experiment as some of the foregoing However, though not specially referring to anthrax, some observations, made by M P Migale to the Academy of Sciences in Paris, as the result of experiment with organized bodies found suspended in the atmosphere, are quite compatible with this mode of distribution and the pathology of anthrax He says · ' 1 The prevalence of organized corpuscles, which exceed $\frac{1}{1000}$ millimetre in size, in the air, is low in winter, increases rapidly in spring, remains almost stationary in summer, and diminishes in autumn 2 Rain arouses the organisms into activity.'

As we have before remarked, when speaking of the general characters of anthrax, that all animals, though liable to be affected by the disease, did not in every species and individual show the same susceptibility ; so, in estimating the power of the contaminating agent, we must not lose sight of the fact of varying receptivity shown under various conditions by different species and individuals

Instruments used at post-mortems, and in removing the skins of animals improperly cleansed, are proved to have been the means by which the disease has been conveyed to healthy men and animals

To summarize what we have said respecting the causation of anthrax 1 We feel bound to give in our adhesion to the theory which accepts the disease proper as the result of the action and influence of certain living and particulate organisms upon the different elements and tissues of the body, and thus it may be classed as hæmal parasitism 2 That this organism is a vegetable—a bacterium—the bacillus anthracis 3 That the bacillus may enter the animal body, either by cutaneous inoculation, by the digestive tract, or the air-passages It is not distinctly proved that an abraded surface is necessary, though in two at least of the foregoing media it would seem probable 4 That a certain condition of animal system is necessary to form a suitable pabulum for the operation of the poison, and that circumstances favourable to the production of this condition are also favourable to the existence and activity of bacillus anthracis. 5 That though under certain circumstances this organism may lose its vitality—as in the presence of *bacterium termo*, the germ of putrefaction—it resists extremes of low

13

tempeiatures, regaining its activity after iemaining at $-40°$ C.
for long periods, on being placed in conditions suitable

Life History of Bacillus Anthracis.—That we may more
readily comprehend the recent and generally received view of
the pathology of anthrax we will here briefly glance at a few
of the piincipal facts in the life-history of bacillus anthiacis,
and its artificial cultivation in relation to protective inoculation, and some arguments in favour of the adoption of the
theory that this bacterium and anthrax stand in relation to
each other as cause to effect—indeed, that the organism is a
true "pathophyte'

After much debate as to whether vegetable or animal kingdom should rightly claim among its orders the little living
particle under consideiation, I believe it is now unanimously
allotted a place in the former, botanists putting it among
the 'schizomycetes' (literally, fungi which split up), with
which the term 'bacteria' is used interchangeably Biologists
have variously arranged these 'protean organisms,' but this
part of the subject is not within our province, so we content
ourselves with saying bacillus anthracis, the bacteridium of
Davaine, is a rodlike body of the bacteria class It consists of
elongated cylindrical iods, homogeneous or almost granular
in appearance, which multiply by transverse fission Sometimes
forming long chains by union of these rods, at the junction of
which there are no constrictions, they curve in various directions, and the mass may assume different forms These bodies
have periods of rest and motion Spore-pioduction goes on in
these filaments, which are seen as round or oval bodies, highly
refractile, on the sides or ends of the rods, enclosed within a
soft membrane which ruptures and allows their escape, which
may take place singly or in masses or swarms ; or the sheath of
the filament may persist, enclosing a number of spores The
spores may again undergo division, geneially into fours They
do not always form into rods The rods developed from the
spores are said to increase their length 120 times in twenty-
four houis, and in forty-eight hours to present a dotted appearance—spore-production This process is most active at
from $24°$ C to $28°$ C. An idea of the rapidity of development
of the bacillus anthracis can best be conveyed by narrating
the following experiment The $\frac{1}{1000}$th of a cubic millimetre

of fluid, taken from the peritoneum of a guinea-pig which died of anthrax, and on examination found free from rods, was inoculated into the tail of a mouse In twenty-four hours the mouse died with symptoms of anthrax Immediately after death, the blood and spleen were found to be literally swarming with rods Ewart says the spores are motionless Temperatures of 40° C and above, and − 40° C and under, check the development of both rods and spores. Free oxygen is necessary to the activity of the bacillus, and Pasteur terms this characteristic 'aerobic' Carbonic anhydride destroys it Thus putrefaction, in which this gas is generated, is not compatible with anthrax After death the rods putrefy, and the spores remain intact High pressure of oxygen destroys the filaments and not the spores, though Ewart asserts they are inactive Desiccation kills the filaments, and a temperature less than 100° F Spores retain their vitality for extremely long periods in the dried state.

I have myself partaken daily for some days of roasted beef from an ox killed because affected with splenic fever, without unpleasant results Boiling for two minutes entirely destroys rods and spores in all conditions, fresh or old, dry or moist Both rods and spores retain their vitality if hermetically sealed and kept at a low temperature—near freezing-point They exhibit all the phenomena of their existence in various fluids, and may be cultivated in many vegetable and animal infusions, as that of cucumber, hay, malt, or fowl-broth ; also in neutral or alkaline solution, as the urine of some herbivora

When the bacilli or spores are introduced into the susceptible animal system, certain conditions are produced which are specific ; and though manifesting themselves in various ways, these conditions are recognised under the general term 'anthrax.'

The manner in which the bacterium gains the circulation is still somewhat obscure Cohn—from the fact that the glands in the course of infection are tumefied, and contain bacteria—concludes that the symptoms are due to some poison, the product of bacteria, and that these remain in the glands in large numbers ; and are first taken up by the lymphatics, pass through them to the glands, and thus to the blood-stream Toussaint contradicts this, showing the symptoms to be com-

13—2

cident with their entrance into the blood-stream. Pasteur
and Joubert believe they pierce the capillaries, and thus gain
the blood-stream, and this latter would be the most satisfactory way to account for their presence there, as they have been
seen under the field of the microscope passing through the
walls of capillary vessels

In artificial and natural cases the general blood-stream may
contain but a small number of the rods   In speaking of
splenic fever, Siedamgrotsky says, 'Germs in the blood of
animals affected with anthrax adhere to the white corpuscles,'
and he believes that the filter-work of the spleen retains the
white corpuscles hence the lesion there, and scarcity of
bacilli in the general blood-stream

The presence of bacilli in blood renders that fluid less
coagulable, acting either mechanically or chemically.

When introduced into the blood of living animals, by their
rapid growth and multiplication they become so numerous
that they are found blocking up capillaries, and it is believed
by thus affecting the essential organs death of the bearer is
produced   Toussaint attributes the occurrence to asphyxia,
from blocking up of minute vessels of the lungs, asserting that
an atmosphere of oxygen will not keep a patient alive

M. Pasteur believes the fatal phenomena arise from the
bacillus robbing the red discs of oxygen, and producing carbonic anhydride   With these have to be taken into consideration the accumulation of effete material, by plugging
of vessels of kidneys, mechanical impediment to the heart's
action, etc

From some experiments of Toussaint and others, there
would appear to be some definite relation between the number
of bacilli introduced into the system, or at least the blood-
stream, and the time at which their fatal effect occurs
Toussaint finds that, when calculating the number inoculated
at 15,000,000,000, death occurred in seven hours, at 75,000,000
in twelve hours, and at 1,500 in thirty-six hours

Protective inoculation by artificially cultivated bacteria, or
as preferably but erroneously termed 'vaccination' by Pasteur,
has by this distinguished scientist been made a most successful
subject   The attention which it has drawn from every scientific
and specially interested circle has scarcely been surpassed

since the gigantic discoveries of Harvey or Jenner began to be appreciated.

After much diligent research, M Pasteur has arrived at knowledge from which he asserts that the disease-producing germ of anthrax may be so modified by artificial cultivation that healthy animals, inoculated with the attenuated virus, receive a certain immunity from the fatal effects of the disease whether naturally or artificially encountered.

The following is the method adopted to obtain the inoculation-fluid, or, as Pasteur calls it, 'vaccine' A drop of blood, taken from an animal about to die of anthrax, on a glass rod is, under antiseptic precautions, placed in a small vessel containing some fowl-broth (bouillon de poule), or other suitable pabulum, perfectly clear, and rendered sterile by being previously raised to a temperature of 115° C If this little vessel be now kept in pure air at 42° to 43° C., a cloudiness is seen, and cultivation goes on, though no spores are said to be produced (at 45° C. cultivation ceases) In this crop there is a certain amount of attenuation acquired Now one drop of this crop is introduced into another vessel containing fowl-broth, and placed under the same conditions as the first ; and so the process is repeated until the required number of generations is produced It is highly essential that the above temperature be maintained in the cultivation, as the vital point, the object of the process, attenuation, rests upon it, namely, that under this circumstance no spores are produced. It is equally important that certain definite periods should elapse between each impregnation, and according to the length of these periods, and the number of sowings, will be the virulence of the different cultures The longer the interval, the less potent will the next cultivation be, and the process will be continued till, by experiment, the required strength is ascertained

This inoculation-fluid, introduced into the susceptible animal system, is said to produce there such a change as to render it in the majority of cases incapable of contracting anthrax, or, as it were, a certain *vis medicatrix* is given to the constitution to encounter and resist its effects The vaccine is generally injected into the subcutaneous tissue, and there may be more or less swelling at the seat of puncture , by some the amount of this is said to bear a relation to the protection afforded

It will be seen that the greatest care is required in obtaining the proper stage of attenuation of the virus, and that in unskilful hands it may become a source of grievous loss and annoyance, while in the hands of the skilled the benefits we may expect from it, having regard to report of results from abroad, are almost incalculable. In the hands of Pasteur and others, knowledge of these facts—the attenuation of the virus, and the effect of the inoculation of this modified poison—has been found of great practical use, and has been applied by the former to vast numbers of animals, especially sheep, among which anthrax is more prevalent in France and Germany than among other species

From the foregoing facts the following deductions suggest themselves to us as having a more practical bearing 1st That spores are a phase of the life-history of the bacillus; 2nd. That these spores are in a high degree capable of producing the disease; 3rd. That these spores resist extremes of temperature, desiccation, and other circumstances which are fatal to the rods, 4th That much of the doubt which arose respecting the part played by bacteria in the earlier study of the disease was due to the fact that spores were not then recognised in their development—and as filaments could not be detected in the blood at all times, the organism was not deemed essential, 5th That the boiling-point is fatal to the spores and rods, 6th That inoculation with cultivated virus is said to afford a certain amount of protection from the naturally or artificially produced disease

SYMPTOMS OF ANTHRAX

Generic Symptoms—Although anthrax, both in the different species of animals in which we meet with it, and the several manifestations of the disease in the same species, has in these several manifestations, both in origin and development, much that distinguishes the one from the other, there are yet certain generic or class features characteristic of the disease which stamp these several forms as merely forms, and not separate or distinctive diseases. The disease itself differs less in the symptoms which are exhibited in the different animals than in its different forms in the same animal

Anthrax proper, in both horses and cattle, is more uniform, and possesses greater similarity in symptoms than we find existing between anthrax proper and glossanthrax of either animal, and at the present stage of pathological research we have some hesitancy in placing them both under the common heading, more especially after having, when speaking generally of the disease, endeavoured to show the close connection between certain organisms and the pathology of anthrax. However, with some reservations which we think future investigation may remove, we propose describing them in the same chapter, though in our present knowledge it were perhaps preferable to class them separately as anthrax proper and anthracoid diseases We shall follow the course before suggested, and recognise—

1 *Anthrax proper as a general blood disorder, without external and readily appreciable local manifestations, and known to be connected with hæmal parasitism.* 2 *Anthrax as a blood disease, with external and readily discernible manifestations, which probably, until we possess more definite information respecting its pathology, and especially atiology, should be classed as 'anthracoid'*

Of the features which may safely be regarded as common to anthrax in all animals, and in every form of its manifestation, the chief are obvious—physical and chemical changes in connection with the blood, which in character is viscid, in colour darker than natural The relation of the blood and its conduits is also much deranged, so that the latter cannot perform their function, and there is leakage All signs in our patients which will convey a knowledge of these facts must therefore be taken as generic symptoms

1 **Symptoms of Anthrax Proper, Anthrax Fever, Acute Anthrax in the Horse, Apoplectic Anthrax, etc**—The period which may elapse after the reception of the infecting agent or virus, according to most observers, is rarely uniform, even when this may be calculated in inoculated cases Probably it may be set down in the horse and larger animals at from a few hours to three or four days

Of the very acute or truly apoplectic form the occurrence in the horse is not common, certainly in Great Britain a rare form of the disease. From those records we possess of the symptoms indicative of acute anthrax in the horse, it would

appear that these are in all their essential features analogous
to what we observe in cattle with which, in this country, we
are most conversant, though, from the rapid progress of the
malady, few opportunities are afforded to medical practitioners
for observing these

The animal seized, perhaps more generally while at work,
has given no premonitory indications of any dyscrasia or impending illness Violent muscular tremors, sudden general
or partial perspiration, wild tossing of the head, paroxysmal
breathing with dyspnœa, reeling in the gait, complete loss of
control of the muscles of the limbs, are the first and only inti-
mation of illness After a short period of unconsciousness and
convulsive movements while on the ground, the animal succumbs to the attack

In other cases, where the course of the symptoms is less
rapid, there may be cessation of the more distressing features
of nervous complication, and time is given to take further
notice of the disease In these subacute cases of anthrax
proper, which, when terminating fatally, generally continue
over two or three days, the onset of the illness may be
ushered in by an acute seizure, similar to that just described,
which suffering subsidence may shortly proceed in a somewhat
milder form, or the symptoms from the first may be less
sudden and violent. In either case there is a certain amount
of coma and lethargy, disinclination to move, or, when compelled to do so, a certain want of power in the muscles of
locomotion, giving the idea that the animal is weak in its loins;
there are partial sweating-fits, with spasmodic twitchings or
tremblings of the muscles of certain regions of the body; in
the interval the skin is unnaturally cold and wants pliability

The respiration is sometimes at the outset not much altered;
at others it is hurried or protracted and laboured The pulse,
increased in frequency, is feeble and small, this condition becoming marked as the disease advances. Temperature is much
elevated, and, as a rule, continues so until shortly before death,
directly before which it most frequently shows a decline The
heart's action is usually marked and somewhat tumultuous.
A symptom which has been remarked by several observers is
the swelling of some of the superficial lymphatic glands, which
in one situation or another is very common.

It has been stated that these symptoms, which we may term
the early or premonitory, in some cases disappear, and are
replaced by a critical eruption (see Fleming's 'Sanitary
Science' and Williams's 'Veterinary Medicine') This I have
never found They may remain stationary for twenty-four
hours, but are oftener characterized by a steady increase in
severity, or by an addition of others of a more acute nature.
The pulse becomes weaker, the respirations more hurried and
'catching,' and in some dyspnœa is marked. The nostrils
are distended, and the visible mucous membrane presents a
cyanotic appearance ; or it may have a dirty yellow colour,
and be marked with blood-spots, or in place of petechiæ we
may have considerable patches of dark colour from blood-
extravasation in the submucous tissue, particularly on the
nasal septum There is a straw-coloured discharge from the
nostrils, sometimes mingled with blood, the mouth seems full
of pasty mucus and frothy saliva, having a peculiar fœtid
odour.

Often the termination of an attack of this subacute anthrax
in the horse, succeeding the febrile symptoms we have described,
is in the form of an attack of colic, with delirium, or at least
unconsciousness, in which wandering around the box, or restlessly thrusting the head against some resisting object, is a
prominent symptom The signs of abdominal pain are generally developed rather suddenly, and accompanied with
paroxysmal sweatings and shivering-fits, or rather more properly localized muscular tremors or clonic spasms, and an
irritable state of the bowels, in which more rarely the discharges are mingled with blood When the urine has been
observed it has been of a dark or port-wine colour, and limited
in amount. The temperature, high at first, declines when
coma and other signs of cerebral involvement continue,
although some cases exhibit, even at the last, very slight
decrease of animal heat as indicated by the thermometer

When delirium or unconsciousness, with dilated pupils,
haggard expression of countenance, and increased dyspnœa,
or where enteric disturbance of a sudden and severe character succeeds the febrile symptoms and muscular twitchings,
the horse rarely survives long, control of movement is
gradually lost, and falling suddenly to the ground he is rarely

able to rise again, and after struggling convulsively for a short time quietly succumbs.

The course of this form of anthrax in the horse has in my experience been uniformly progressive. There has been no well-defined remission of symptoms, but in all, even if at some time during their rather short course they have given any evidence of improvement, it has only been that of the symptoms remaining stationary, and after a very short time they have again shown fresh activity, or have to the original ones of special pyrexia added those indicative of the disturbances of other organs and functions. In no case which I can recollect have I been favoured with a recovery.

2. **Symptoms of Anthrax as a Blood Disorder** in which certain external manifestations are a prominent feature, but which from want of more positive knowledge as to its ætiology, and taking anthrax to be essentially hæmal parasitism, it would probably be orthodox to regard as simply 'anthracoid;' still from its having been described by most writers on the subject under this head, and its not having been proved not to be anthrax, we follow the same order.

Amongst our patients, others than members of the family 'equidæ,' we are aware that anthrax with local complications is a very common form of the disease; with the horse, at least in this country, it is, we are inclined to believe, not at all common.

A diseased condition, spoken of by German writers under the term 'anthrax typhus,' and named by English pathologists purpura hæmorrhagica, we do not consider has yet been satisfactorily determined to be a form of anthrax, so we have preferred to consider and speak of it separately.

The only forms of anthrax with local complications with which I am conversant as occurring in the horse in this country are those known as *glossanthrax*, or *malignant glossitis*, and *anthracoid angina*—malignant sore throat.

Neither of these conditions are common; the first I have seldom seen in the horse unassociated with the latter, while this latter independent of the former is even of rarer occurrence.

Whether *glossanthrax* be due or owe its origin to a general infected condition, a primary charging of the system with some infectious virus, or to contamination and poisoning by inoculation, it is tolerably certain that the local symptoms from which the diseased condition derives its name are coincident with, or probably slightly precede, the constitutional and general disturbance

The local manifestations, the characteristic swelling of the tongue and appearance of vesicles or phlyctenæ over the dorsum of the organ, the sides, and more rarely the frænum, are rapidly developed symptoms

The animal, though occasionally disposed to eat, is unable to do so This is generally the first attractive sign of indisposition On more careful examination the tongue is found swollen, tense, and firm, with, very early in the disease, the existence of several larger or smaller vesicles along its dorsum and sides The mouth is filled with ropy saliva, if the tongue be examined on its venter surface, vesicles may or may not be found, and according to the amount of swelling is the protrusion of the organ from the mouth. The sublingual glands and adjacent tissues will be seen swollen and infiltrated with a straw-coloured fluid At first the vesicles are small, and the contained material may be of a pale colour

Very rapidly, however, they increase in size, and become darker from the apparently bloody matter which they contain The swelling of the tongue itself is also rapid, and in a few hours it will be protruding from the mouth, livid-looking, indented or lacerated from contact with the teeth The saliva which drops and hangs from the mouth will now be rusty coloured from being tinged with blood, either from the torn tongue or ruptured vesicles, which also in some cases are found on the lips and buccal membrane At this time the ability to swallow even fluids is gone, and constitutional disturbance, hitherto not a marked feature, becomes gradually more severe

The vesicles which may have ruptured show an unhealthy, angry looking surface, particularly around their edges, which often have a gangrenous appearance They rapidly become coated with a yellowish aplastic exudate, which as rapidly becomes removed, exposing a further eroded and corroding sore, partly from the pain of which, and partly also from the impossibility of having the thirst quenched and the impeded respiration, the horse becomes restless, moves uneasily from place to place, looking anxiously around him for relief, and if water be within his reach, plunges his head into the containing vessel.

As we have already said, this condition of the tongue is very often complicated with specific inflammation and swelling of the throat and structures of and around the throat—anthracoid angina When swelling becomes obvious externally, we may, as a rule, consider that a condition much similar is taking place in deeper-seated parts. This swelling from infiltration of connective-tissue and glandular structures, when commenced, progresses with great rapidity Very shortly, from pharyngeal œdema and œdema of the glottis, the respiration becomes embarrassed and the dyspnœa distressing, while from the swelling extending from the lips and buccal membrane, the head puts on a very unsightly and unnatural appearance

The swelling around the throat and larynx, when occurring, is hard, hot, and painful Accompanying this we have generally a rusty or blood-tinged discharge from the nostrils, from its effects on the surface over which it passes, apparently of an irritating character. In some cases the swelling has been noticed to extend along the course of the trachea even to the sternum

When local complications confined to the tongue and structures of the laryngeal and pharyngeal membranes are imminent, the course of the disease is exceedingly rapid, a few hours sufficing to produce such alterations of the throat and upper air-passages, that unless relief is afforded by tracheotomy the animal will fall asphyxiated. The performance of this operation, however, is rarely effectual except in very temporarily relieving the symptoms

Diagnosis—At the first glance the diagnosis may appear easy enough Still we must not shut our eyes to the fact that mistakes have been made even by the experienced in this as in other matters.

Anthrax in the horse being a disease that we have hitherto not been taught to regard as at all common, I have not unfrequently imagined that it is oftener met with than recognised; and indeed I am far from being satisfied that a great number of apparent ordinary bowel affections of rapid course and fatal termination, usually described as enteritis, are not truly anthracoid   How often do we encounter cases where a young, vigorous, rather plethoric subject, apparently well and in the fullest enjoyment of health, is suddenly seized with what in many of its features is akin to a severe attack of colic, after the exhibition of only moderate abdominal pain, becomes unaccountably prostrate, and in a few hours succumbs, falsifying a rather favourable prognosis given only a few hours previously ! When examined after death, the usually obvious changes are excessive sero-hæmorrhagic effusions in connection with the subserous and submucous tissues of the bowels, this exudation often exceedingly well marked between the layers of the mesentery close to the margin of the bowel, and of a characteristic yellow colour, mingled with streaks of blood, while the submucous exudate is always extensive, of a dark colour, and evidently hæmorrhagic   Collections of similarly constituted exudate are often encountered in the areolar tissue of the pelvic cavity, and occasionally the character of the blood in the large venous channels approaches that of the more determined and recognised attacks of anthrax.   We regret that up to this period we have been unable to so thoroughly investigate the ætiology of this condition as to allow us to speak positively on the subject, but hope opportunity may shortly occur for more careful attention to the matter.

    In determining the nature of suspicious cases, when there is some probability that anthrax is the disease with which we are dealing, due attention must be given to the existence of certain influences and surrounding circumstances, as well as to the symptoms and ætiology; whether the case is an individual and isolated one, or an indication of some generally disturbing element at work and attacking a number of animals , whether anthrax exist in the district among other species of animals, and if the affected have been in any way exposed to the virus of the diseased if cases have occurred   It is also advantageous to know the history of disease in the neighbourhood, and that if anthrax has, at some previous time, been known in the locality, a great source of infection may at any time, for a lengthened period, be started by the disturbance of soil where dead animals or their offal have been interred, while we must remember that what is capable of carrying the bacterium is also capable of conveying the disease. Of course a careful examination of the blood, with the object of detecting the specific bacterial forms, is a point to be always insisted upon. When these are capable of demonstration the diagnosis is satisfactorily settled, but we must never lose sight of the fact that anthrax may exist without the detection of these organisms in the general circulation being possible. This fact should also always be among our considerations when we think of adopting those means we are disposed to consider most crucial and satisfactory—the inoculation of some small animal; for it is found that when anthrax blood, in which bacilli could not be detected, is inoculated into these creatures they die of well-marked anthrax, and *their* blood actually swarms with the organisms.

Morbid Anatomy.

General Features—Although the discussion of the morbid anatomy is not our particular province here, we must of necessity give so much attention to this point as will render us capable of detecting the necroscopic appearances usually presented to our observation. Though a point upon which we would expect there could be little or no difference of opinion—the tendency in cases of death from anthrax to a rapid decomposition of the body—we find that regarding this, at the very threshold of our examination, much difference of opinion meets us: some observers, both foreign and English, giving it as the result of their experience that no unusual tendency to destructive tissue-change is, as a rule, to be met with in the cadavers of the victims of anthrax; others again as distinctly stating that early and rapid decomposition is always a marked feature. Amongst the latter we must undoubtedly place ourselves, as we have observed that immediately life is extinct decomposition is particularly rapid, especially if the weather be hot. In truth, the crepitant swellings characteristic of one form of the disease, and their emphysematous nature, are, as respects their size, in large measure due to change occurring in the effused blood during life; this may be readily enough demonstrated in cattle, where these are, as a rule, most extensive.

In many animals shortly after death, besides an ill-established rigor mortis, there exists the usual feature of general distortion from uniform distension of the submucous and interconnecting connective-tissue with gases, this, to a casual observer, is the most obvious abnormal condition. In addition to this generally swollen condition we will, in many cases, observe a collection of frothy rusty-coloured mucus around, and issuing from the natural openings, with a red, swollen, and everted anus and vagina. When the skin is cut, or an incision freely made into the subjacent tissues, we have an exit of gas with a hissing or bubbling noise, foetid smell, and black fluid blood.

When the skin is removed the subcutaneous connective-tissue will be found more or less infiltrated with a pale straw-coloured serosity; while in patches, where the local swellings or tumours, when found, have existed, the infiltrating and effused material is rather more consistent and of a much darker colour from the blood mingled with the jelly-like exudate. The skin itself, over the tumours, is deeply stained and impregnated with a bloody serosity, the cutaneous tissue being swollen, soft, and apparently undergoing a destructive change. Amongst the connective-tissue existing between and amongst the muscles and muscular tissue the infiltration exists, the muscular tissue being soft and dark coloured; and in connection with the local swellings this softening has, as with the skin, gone so far that the cohesion of texture is largely destroyed.

The abdominal cavity, on being opened, emits a quantity of foul-smelling gas, and contains a varying amount of sero-hæmorrhagic fluid. The parietal and visceral peritoneum present varying ecchymoses. The intestines in submucous as well as subserous tissue show patches of extravasation of gelatinous, more or less coloured exudate; this is most extensive in their borders connected with the mesentery, and extending between the folds of this membrane. There are also patches of dark-coloured markings from distinct blood-extravasation, both beneath their external covering and in their submucous texture.

The glands of the mesentery are swollen and infiltrated, both in their intimate structure and beneath their peritoneal covering, with the characteristic exudate so largely distributed, and they are very friable The mesentery itself is in patches, or throughout its whole surface dark in colour, its vessels being very prominent The large veins of the abdomen and body generally are filled with a dark viscid tarry-looking blood indisposed to coagulate, and staining not merely the lining membrane of the vessels, but every tissue with which it has contact.

On opening the thoracic cavity we find the parietal and visceral pleura presenting the same ecchymosed or generally stained appearance as the serous membranes of the abdomen The cavity usually contains, in varying quantities, coloured fluid of different shades, according to the absence or amount of hæmorrhage The heart is soft and flabby in texture, the cavities containing a moderate quantity of dark viscid blood, and both pericardium and endocardium marked with large dark patches of hæmorrhagic effusion beneath the serous membranes, which, in the interior of the cavities, in addition to these blood-markings extending into the muscular tissue, are uniformly stained with the altered blood This same dark hæmorrhagic marking and uniform staining exist in the lining membrane of the bloodvessels proceeding from the heart In the pericardial sac is also to be found a varying amount of bloody coloured serous fluid, while in the connective and adipose tissue around the root of the lungs, and where the heart is attached through the medium of the large vessels, there is much effusion and infiltration of the characteristic exudate, mingled with spots of a darker colour from blood-extravasation. The lungs are uniformly, or in patches, congested with dark blood, and on being cut into, this, mingled with more or less of a rusty coloured fluid, exudes The mucous membrane of both large and small air-tubes is infiltrated in like manner, and their lumen is occupied by frothy mucus

The large abdominal glands, the spleen and liver, and the kidneys somewhat less so, give the most constantly occurring and specific lesions in all animals, when the spleen is most extensively altered the liver is less so, and *vice versâ* The obvious changes in the spleen are enormous enlargement, deepening of its colour, and excessive friability In weight it may become equal to three or four healthy spleens, its colour, darker than natural externally, is on being cut into perfectly black, and in many cases the parenchyma so much softened that the entire organ resembles nothing more than a quantity of tar enclosed in a membrane. Over the surface, in particular cases, nodulation, or moderate elevations, may exist, over which the investing membrane has in some cases been found ruptured

The condition of the liver and kidneys is very similar to that of the spleen—in neither, however, do we ever see the retained blood so dark and tarry-looking; and although the friability of the liver is often very marked, it is rarely of that perfectly diffluent character we so often encounter in the splenic pulp. The membrane in the pelvis of the kidney may be ecchymosed, as also that lining the bladder, which often contains a moderate amount of bloody coloured urine

The lesions of the brain partake much of the same character as those of the parts described. thus we may have congestion of cerebral and meningeal vessels, and effusion of the peculiar material into the cavities and substance. The pia mater, velum interpositum, and choroid plexus especially present this turgescence with dark-coloured blood. The spinal cord and the theca vertebralis present similar conditions. The nasal cavities, the pituitary membrane, the structures about the eyes, the mammary gland, the scrotum, indeed every region and organ, may be the seat of its attack

Besides these obvious physical and chemical changes which the blood has undergone in anthrax, and the important part it plays in the existence of the characteristic exudations and extravasations, together with its tendency, and all connected with it, to rapidly undergo further changes, there are, when we examine it more closely, marked alterations which have occurred to it; and although all these may not be special to the disease, there exists, at least, a close relation between them and the production of the phenomena we have been describing. In addition to the alteration in colour so obvious, we find, on examination, the blood has somewhat increased in density from loss of its more fluid portions; there is also a marked decrease in its fibrine-producing elements, which in a large measure accounts for the want of power shown by anthrax blood to coagulate.

In the formed materials of the blood we also notice a

14

difference   there is an increase in the white corpuscles, while
the coloured show a variety of changes, some being shrivelled,
shrunk, or crenated, and having a disposition to crowd together,
not in strings or rouleaux as in health, but into a jelly-like
mass   The latter conditions seem to be due to withdrawal of
the more liquid portions from the blood, seeing they are reversed if to blood devoid of fluid, or to anthrax blood, a moderate
amount of water be added   Besides these changes of a disintegrative or minus character, we have the frequent presence
of those organisms to which we gave a considerable share of
attention when treating of the ætiology—bacteria, bacilli, or
their spores.

We have already noticed these forms as present in the blood
in anthrax proper, and stated what was known, or believed to
be known, to be their action on the blood, and in the living
organism where found.   There is still among pathologists some
difference of opinion respecting their effect

In order to observe the bacilli, a small quantity of the
blood containing the organisms should, with great care as to
the exclusion of bacterium termo, be placed on a slide, covered,
and put under the field of the microscope   When fresh and
viewed with a 500-power, there are seen cylindrical rods of inappreciable breadth, and about ·007 to ·012 mm. in length.
These elongate rapidly, and may assume a variety of forms, as
single and straight filaments, zooglea masses, intricate coils,
loops, bundles of parallel rods, etc.   On the addition of water
their sides may present a beaded appearance, on account of
spores becoming more prominent.   Short straight cylinders
may have spores, as it were, protruding from either or both
ends   At a temperature between 30° C. and 35° C., by carefully
watching, they will be noticed to have certain periods of rest
and motion   a rod will move in an oscillatory manner for a
short time, then perhaps wriggle across the field to the other
side   Cossar-Ewart says he has 'noticed under the No X
Hartnach filaments moving about appearing from one third to
half an inch long.' The rods may occasionally be noticed rapidly
elongating into filaments of various lengths ; and, if particular
attention be paid to them, transverse striæ will soon be
apparent at the point where scission (their mode of multiplication, hence the appellation schizomycetes) is about to take

place. In from eighteen to twenty-four hours at this same temperature spores will be noticed. If the temperature be lower the development of spores will be retarded, and if above 47° C to 40° C, all apparent developmental changes are said to cease. On the advent of putrefaction in the tissue, the bacilli are noticed to be motionless, disappear and the blood becomes inert in the production of anthrax. Deprived of air, they soon become inactive and their development is said to depend on the presence of oxygen, while bacterium termo under the same conditions loses its activity.

We are certainly as yet not satisfactorily informed respecting the behaviour of these bacterial forms when in the body, or their exact relation to many abnormal conditions during the progress of which we find these organisms in the blood. However, whether these be the direct cause or only the carriers of the specific virus of the disease, or merely indicative of certain peculiar altered conditions of the circulatory fluid, their presence in the blood is undoubtedly intimately associated in some way with the lesions and perverted functions observed, and as such constitutes an important feature in their development.

In pursuing our investigations in this disease, we must not lose sight of the knowledge that there are other bacteria which are morphologically identical with bacillus anthracis, and thus can be distinguished from it only by their effects on living animals. It is on record that one, bacterium subtilis—the hay-infusion bacterium, quite harmless in this state—may by cultivation in the animal body acquire the property of being capable of producing anthrax; while we must notice that in bacillus, attenuated for protective inoculation purposes, recrudescence may be effected by repeated cultivation in a series of animals of a species susceptible to anthrax.

Special Necroscopic Appearance in the Horse.—In the non-localized forms of anthrax of the horse, the special lesions and changes observable after death are in no way different from the appearances we have now attempted to sketch. In addition to the marked changes and characteristic alterations of the great glandular structures and organs of the abdomen and thorax, we observe there is probably a more evenly distributed condition of infiltration of the connective-tissue of the body,

14—2

external and internal, with the citron-coloured, jelly like exudate so common to anthrax.

When the symptoms have been marked with much severity, rapidity of development, and with a fatal termination, I have not been able to observe structural changes so marked as in cases where the animal lived longer, and the severity of the symptoms was less obvious. This would seem to obtain in more general diseases than anthrax. The animal seems cut down by the poison before time has been given for structural alterations.

In the foregoing observations we have glanced at the principal changes which may be expected in anthrax generally. It will be evident that we shall not frequently meet with the whole of them in one individual case, though such may occasionally happen; but that the different symptoms will lead us to look to the various localizations of the lesion.

Thus when delirium, or other disturbance connected with the nervous system, predominates, we shall expect to find the most marked structural changes in the nerves or nerve-centres. When enteric pain is specially manifested—in the bowels, and so on—and as there is most frequently a complication of symptoms, so on post-mortem examination do we find more than one organ or set of organs affected.

Of that condition of the intestines associated with carbuncular elevations, sloughing, and formation of deep yellow-coloured ulcerated cavities, indisposed to heal—spoken of and described by some German authors—I have had no experience.

When occurring as glossanthrax, the additional characteristic tissue-changes are associated with the tongue, larynx, pharynx, and structures connected with and contiguous to these.

The infiltration, with the peculiar exudate, is usually very extensive on the retro-pharyngeal and laryngeal tissue; while the glands, both lymphatic and salivary, are much enlarged, chiefly with the exudate, mixed with dark-coloured blood. Along the buccal membrane, as also on the tongue, we may sometimes see an angry looking sore, which has resulted from the rupture of a vesicle, and the after-irritation of the exposed surface, the entire submucous structure being either generally or in patches swollen and infiltrated. The membrane over the dorsum of the tongue may be elevated in patches from the phlyctenæ present. They are, however, often absent   The muscular tissue of the organ is swollen and dark-coloured, and its cohesion and integrity much interfered with   It is soft, and may be easily lacerated   Along the under surface of the tongue, by the sides of the frænum, there is often a considerable elevation or cord-like projection, resulting from the infiltration of glandular structures and connective-tissue.   Over the lining membrane of the pharynx there are petechiæ, or larger blood-markings, with a general cyanotic condition of the entire membrane, which looks swollen and pulpy from the infiltrated submucous tissue   The lining membrane of the larynx exhibits conditions very similar, œdema of the glottis being often present

Around the course of the trachea, and in the jugular groove —extending in various cases to considerable distances into the cervical region, in some instances even to the mediastinum— there is a varying quantity of the effusion peculiar to the disease   All the structures of the cervical region—vessels, nerves, muscles, etc.—are occasionally involved

We have elsewhere spoken of the forms of anthrax prevailing among horses in India and South Africa—Loodianah disease and Cape horse-sickness   The appearances on autopsy present precisely the same typical characters as those described. From information at our disposal, we are inclined to think the lesions are more generally distributed than in this country The presence of the bacillus is also, we believe, even more frequently detected   The rapid decomposition of the cadavers has been remarked by all who have given us the benefit of their observations

In inoculated cases, bacilli or their spores are usually found at or around the seat of inoculation, though they may be absent from the general blood-stream.

Treatment —Anthrax, in every form and in all animals, is a disease which, as regards the employment of curative measures, yields very unsatisfactory results.   In its acute form in the horse as anthrax proper, its development is so rapid that it usually results in death before the majority of remedial measures employed have time to produce any effect on the system.   Even when there are early signs of illness which culminate in a manifestation of the symptoms of anthrax, unless in an outbreak in which animals have been previously attacked, we have little to lead us to suspect this special disease. However, when we are aware of the fact that we have to deal with an outbreak of anthrax, our attention should most assuredly be directed to both curative measures for those which are attacked, and prophylactic for those which appear to have been in dangerous relations with the diseased, or with the cause of the disease.

In its acute form, when opportunity occurs, it matters little what be the class or character of the symptoms, as soon as our suspicions of its being anthrax are aroused, we should at once proceed to administer those agents which rapidly taken into the circulation seem immediately to act on the bacterial organisms, so as to render them inactive, and to produce such a condition throughout the system that the pabulum it provides should be in no way suitable for their development; at the same time, if possible, attention should be directed to those symptoms which show that the effects of the poison predominate in certain regions or organs. Thus, when the indications are those of cerebral congestion, with a slow oppressed pulse and stertorous breathing, partial coma, and a disposition to remain stationary, with head depressed, or resting on or forced against the manger, blood-letting is by some said to be indicated. This will usually at once relieve the urgency of the symptoms, and the patient may appear benefited. The relief is, however, of brief duration, for, although the coma may not again seem so marked, other nervous symptoms become prominent, and cardiac disturbance intensified. When bleeding has been deemed needful because of the head-symptoms, the application of cold water or ice-bags to the poll would appear indicated. Quickly following this, unless enteric symptoms are prominent, a dose of laxative medicine should be administered; the most useful, we believe, is from two to four drachms of aloes given as bolus. By exciting the bowels to action we secure a chance for the excretion of effete material from the blood, which is so rapidly altered in the disease.

To produce through the vital fluid that condition of system inimical to the life and increase of the bacillus anthracis and its germs, to which we just now referred, we certainly advise the administration of some agent with what are known as antiseptic properties Of these we prefer carbolic acid, and some very recent experiments by three French veterinarians, MM Arloing, Cornevin, and Thomas, quite confirm this choice, which, some time previous to these results being made known, had been used by us and publicly advised by members of the profession generally In these experiments the 'fresh' and 'dried' virus of anthrax were severally operated on It was found that those agents which destroyed the dried, also destroyed the fresh, but that the converse was not the case Thus the following destroyed the activity of the fresh, but had no effect on the dried a saturated solution of oxalic acid, 5 per cent solution of permanganate of potash, 20 per cent solution of soda, chlorine gas, and sulphurous acid vapour The following rendered inactive the 'dried' virus a 2 per cent aqueous solution of carbolic acid, a solution of salicylic acid, 1 in 1,000, nitrate of silver, 1 in 1,000; perchloride of mercury, 1 in 5,000; bromine vapour, strong solution of boracic acid or sulphate of copper while many agents usually credited with considerable antiseptic properties had no effect on the dried

Thus, as a fundamental point, we should start in all cases of anthrax by the administration of one of the above an aqueous solution of carbolic acid, ʒss. of the acid in a pint of water three or four times daily, is a very convenient mode of administration, and the agent is generally to be obtained everywhere with little trouble We should, at the same time, be inclined to use inhalation of chlorine gas, generated in the ordinary manner, thus endeavouring to impregnate the system with materials directed to subduing the action of the poison This, as we before said, is to be followed by some stimulant to the emunctories to rid the constitution of the effete matters with which it must now be charged To combat the disintegrative process, which is such a marked feature of the disease, we would suggest the exhibition of nutritive materials; and an abundance of these in the liquid form is probably best adapted to the circumstances, being most readily assimilable and also supplying a great deficiency in the fluids of the body, which the heightened temperature and drainage from the vascular system must necessarily have rendered deficient in quantity

as well as quality. Of course these may also be used as
vehicles for the medicinal agents, and such salines as chlorate
and nitrate of potash may be readily conveyed in them without
interfering with their being voluntarily taken, should the disposition and power to do so be shown. In the event of difficulties arising from interference with the ability of swallowing,
or otherwise, the foregoing may be administered as enemata.
In cases where abdominal pain has been evident, we have
applied to the abdomen woollen rugs wrung from hot water,
and given every two or three hours subcutaneous injections of
℥xxx. of the solution of morphia, ℥ii of carbolic acid, ℥xxx.
of water, and have noticed that apparent relief has been
obtained

Somewhat more hopeful, however, than the treatment of
anthrax proper is that of the disease with localizations in the
mouth and throat. We say hopeful, not that we consider this
a promising affection to treat, because we have seen a few, a
very few, recover from glossanthrax, while from the former we
have never seen one. In attempting to treat a case of glossanthrax we do not deem it a good practice to bleed indiscriminately, even when the subject is young and plethoric; such
treatment is recommended, we are aware, by both our own and
continental veterinarians; from this we should certainly abstain
unless there were distinct symptoms of cerebral involvement,
when probably we are warranted in abstracting blood. When
vesicles appear upon or under the tongue, it is better to
open them, and to treat the parts with a strong solution of
carbolic acid, we prefer this to one less powerful, as it seems
to produce less pain than cauterizing, and having a numbing
or soothing influence on the nerves, and likely to destroy any
disease-germs which may exist in connection with the localization of the poison

When the tongue or buccal membrane is much swollen from
infiltration, we do not hesitate to scarify deeply, and afterwards
gargle with a 3 per cent solution of carbolic acid. These scarifications and after-treatment may with advantage be repeated
if tumefaction does not subside. We have, in severely swelling
cases, removed the tip of the tongue, which had become gangrenous; and have not observed after subsidence excessive
disposition to slough at these incisions. We have here also

applied warm water to the swollen parts, which, we before said, reached sometimes down the neck as far as the fore-limbs. Hot-water vapour inhaled has been thought to afford relief, and of course this may be medicated in any manner which suggests itself to the practitioner

In cases where the swelling of the internal or external structures is likely to produce suffocation, recourse must be had to tracheotomy.

In other forms of localization, though with such in this country we are not familiar, the same principles must evidently be adopted

In anthrax, as in every other disease under our treatment, symptoms must be assiduously watched; the condition which they indicate must be combated as the circumstances require. The cauterization of local tumours we strongly advise, as also the administration of carbolic acid in small and repeated doses The injection of the same agent hypodermically for effect on the entire system, and into the tumour, is certainly worthy of trial During convalescence, a course of tonics and food of a highly nutritious character should be given

In the same tone as we commenced to speak about treatment, so we must conclude we cannot, with our present knowledge, give much encouragement as to the likelihood of benefit from curative measures in a large majority of cases, but that is no reason why perseverance in further investigation into the matter should not be stimulated; and we would by no means muffle any attempts even in this direction, as in every sense the study of the disease is of the highest importance, both to the profession and the community at large

However we may find ourselves paralyzed in endeavouring to bring about the healthy process in the diseased, we have no inconsiderable command of means at our disposal for its prevention; and under present circumstances we feel we can do very much in arresting its progress and averting its consequences A knowledge of the true pathology of anthrax in all its bearings, and a due regard for its several phenomena, especially those involved in its aetiology, are necessary before consistent prophylactic measures can be suggested or carried out. Though, when studying this part of our subject, we admitted there was yet more to learn as to the causation of

anthrax, we know sufficient of the influences which predominate as factors in the production of the condition to
entitle us to make an attempt in this direction with reasonable
hope of success   And from a somewhat extensive experience,
though more particularly with cattle and sheep, we are satisfied
that if we cannot cure we can largely prevent   The several
methods of propagation have been discussed, and in considering its prevention not one of these should be overlooked   Our
first efforts will of course be directed to the separation of the
healthy from the diseased   Then the medical treatment of
these, and, in case of death, the proper disposal of the cadaver-
ous offal, and everything which may have become contaminated,
demand our attention. The most satisfactory manner in which
to get rid of all these is to burn them, or, where this is not
practicable, to submit them to boiling   All excreta, straw,
water, food, to which the diseased have had access, etc., should
be placed under the destructive process   The stable and surroundings, when the patients have been suffering indoors,
should be scrupulously cleaned and disinfected   Every effort
of the medical adviser must immediately be directed to discover the source and nature of the food and water supply, and
all other animals which have in any way come under the
same conditions as the affected should be removed from these
conditions, and kept isolated from them until the cause of
the outbreak is elucidated, and removed when this is possible.
Of course this is not always an easy matter, and often defies
the most careful investigation ; and it is only in these cases,
after all possible sanitary precautions have been attended to,
that the animals may be returned to cohabitation. Coincident
with the separation of healthy and diseased should be the administration, to the former as well as the latter, of some antiseptic, as already advised for the affected, in the form of carbolic
acid, hyposulphite of soda, etc   These remarks apply equally
to animals stabled or grazing   Further, our memories, and
those of others possessed of local knowledge, should be taxed
to ascertain if a previous outbreak had occurred in the same
locality, and more especially the spot at which the animals
had been affected, or, more important still, where the carcases
had been deposited   It will then be our duty to see if these
spots have been disturbed, or if anything has occurred to

bring the germs into positions accessible to the animals through pasturing, or indirectly by food or water brought to the stable The water-supply should be traced to its source, and our attention given to ascertain if there were chance of its being contaminated in its course by any means All pools and ditches should be thoroughly cleaned out, and the greatest care given to the proper disposal of the 'clearings;' while the animals should have no access to the situations where the disease was supposed to have been until every one of these has been put under the most favourable conditions in our power All tools used in operating on the living body, or at the autopsy, should be scrupulously cleaned and disinfected, as should everything which could have been contaminated. When we consider the extreme facility of transmission of the virus in some cases, such for instance as we have noted in woolsorters' disease, it certainly seems extraordinary, considering the carelessness shown by the class, how knackers' men, butchers, and others having to do with the affection and the corpse, should escape so frequently as it would seem they do

Most of the foregoing directions are in their entirety only applicable to rural districts; we do not often meet with the disease in the large towns, but when such does occur we must advise that all these measures which are in any way practicable be stringently carried out. Also when the disease has to be combated in India, South Africa, or elsewhere, all measures having for their object the prevention of anthrax must be based on the same general principles as here laid down; the details will of course be as various as the several outbreaks.

In a former chapter we drew some attention to the method of 'protective inoculation,' and although in Great Britain the disease does not assume proportions sufficiently important for us to advocate its use generally here, in the two countries we have just mentioned, as well as for the Cumberland disease in our Australasian colonies, we do recommend it as worthy of every consideration. The date of the birth of its practice is not as yet sufficiently remote for us to quote our practical experience of it, or to draw from any source information which will warrant our advising its adoption as a simple operation, successful in most men's hands, and one whose success has been undoubtedly proved Nevertheless, those who have had most experience in this matter certainly express unbounded confidence in its ultimate success

The effect of oxygen in the attenuation of the bacillus should also not be lost sight of, and should prove an incentive to improved ventilation.

Added to the treatment of our patients, it will be our function to advise our client as to the communicability of the disease to the human being, and to impress on him the facility with which anthrax may prove a source of fatality among his family or dependents, as well as among his other than equine stock.

Loodianah Disease and Cape Horse-sickness

If in the British Isles in our day anthrax, as appearing in horses, is a rather rare disease, in two of our colonies—India and South Africa—it is of common occurrence. In the former known as Loodianah Disease, and in the latter as Horse-sickness, it is frequent and fatal, both in epizootic, enzoötic, and sporadic forms.

Loodianah Disease—now clearly demonstrated to be a form of anthrax, and connected with the presence of bacillus anthracis in the blood—took its name from the fact of a memorable outbreak occurring among the horses of a battery of Horse Artillery at Loodianah, in 1841 Known under that name since, it has been a source of great annoyance to owners of horses in India Behaving as we described to be characteristic of anthrax, and generally known throughout the empire, it is much more commonly met with in low-lying, damp situations, though cases have been reported at an altitude of 7,000 feet Showing a preference for attacking the plethoric, it at times spares animals in no appreciably special state of system. Outbreaks have been ordinarily noticed a short time after rain, when the surface-water has been evaporated or absorbed

Grass—considering the source from which it is usually derived, and the manner in which it is offered as food to the horses (having a good deal of earth attached)—is by some, who have had practical experience with the disease, thought to be a frequent bearer of the contagium ; while drinking-water can be scarcely less important in this point of view Indeed, what we have said respecting its ætiology, when speaking of anthrax generally, obtains here, though possibly the relative importance of each factor may be somewhat different. There are some instances of outbreaks which have apparently been traced to alluvial soil underneath the floor of stables, on removal of which, and adoption of other sanitary measures, the disease has disappeared: and it seems probable this influence of the soil was due to the presence in it of the spores of bacilli.

As far as we can gather from the literature of the subject, Loodianah disease differs in no essential manner from anthrax, as we have described it occurring in Great Britain, however, in the form characterized by external manifestations, we may notice the tongue is not so specially involved as in gloss-anthrax   The swellings, frequently commencing about the head, rapidly extend backwards, even to the extremities of the fore-limbs. The rise in internal temperature is very marked, there being records of the thermometer reaching 108° and 109° F.

The course of the disease, generally rapid, varies from six hours after the earliest symptoms to six days   There is a very small percentage of recoveries   Imported—especially Australian—horses are supposed 'to yield a little more readily to the fatal effects of the disease than native-bred animals.

Owing probably to extrinsic favourable conditions, putrefaction takes places rapidly after death, rendering post-mortem examination a most offensive task

The most successful remedial and prophylactic measures are precisely those we have mentioned in that category elsewhere

Horse-sickness, Cape Horse-sickness, Paard-zietke, Dikkop-zietke—as anthrax is termed among equidæ in South Africa—appears to an alarming extent throughout the length and breadth of the colony: showing itself in epizootic, enzootic, and sporadic forms; committing devastation among studs, civil and military. The losses recorded during the Zulu campaign were of a most serious character   Though here its geographical distribution is general, it also shows a preference for the lowlands ; and the Dutch settler knows too well the effects of placing his horses and cattle in the ' bush veld,' and the relative freedom from Paard-zietke enjoyed by the ' high veld.'

Although to be met with in every season of the year, those dry months following the wet are quoted as 'the horse-sickness season.' And great importance is attached to the fact that animals grazing while the dew is on the ground are much more liable to contract the disease than those turned out after the dew has dispersed

In connection with the disease in South Africa, another matter is worthy of attention—the immunity enjoyed by 'salted' or 'gezout' horses, which are very much sought after by intending purchasers These animals are said never to contract the disease, or, if they do so, to have only a mild attack, which is rarely fatal. This condition—and there seems every reason to think it does exist—suggests to our minds the possibility of these horses having been naturally inoculated with attenuated virus, having had a mild attack, recovered, and acquired this freedom from susceptibility Indeed, as we hinted before, we think there is in this colony a fair field for a thorough testing of protective inoculation

Anthrax among the domesticated animals would appear to be comparatively most fatal to horses in South Africa Thus we have on record, out of many other instances, one in which a stock-owner on the same pastures lost on his cattle 30 per cent, on his goats and horses 100 per cent, and gained 45 per cent by his sheep in eight years

As far as the morbid processes of the disease are concerned, horse-sickness is so clearly allied to what we have described as anthrax proper that we will forbear from further mention of these.

CHAPTER IX

PYÆMIA—SEPTICÆMIA

ALTHOUGH these conditions may more correctly be regarded as subjects pertaining specially to surgery, it is probably advisable that a short notice be taken of the chief facts connected with them, as they occasionally demand our attention in the province of medicine

Definition.—*Both pyæmia and septicæmia may be regarded*

*as febrile conditions, with general disturbance, closely allied
to the ordinary specific fevers, consisting in contaminated
states of the blood, the result of infection from without, or of
changes occurring in the animal tissues within, resulting—in
true pyæmia—in the formation of abscesses and particular
lesions in internal visceral organs and other particular parts
This state is often subsequent to an infective inflammatory
condition of wounds and suppurations in certain structures,
particularly bone; while, when abscesses occur, the pus they
contain is largely charged with bacterial forms*

Pathology *a Nature of these Conditions*—Both these
manifestations, pyæmia and septic contamination of the
blood, which are probably in their essential nature one, although long and extensively known, particularly in their
manifestations and results, and although we possess a mass of
facts and information bearing upon their different relationships, still afford material for differences of opinion as to the
interpretation which ought to be given to these facts, as well
as give rise to many questions which yet remain unanswered

The meaning originally attached to the term 'pyæmia,' viz
that the phenomena of the diseased condition were to be
accounted for by the existence of pus in the circulating blood,
has for some time been abandoned , and although the name
indicating this assumed condition is retained it has now
very different significations attached to it Experiment and
investigation lately carried out clearly point to differences,
more or less important, existing between conditions often
spoken of under terms understood by many to be convertible,
as pyogenic fever, pyæmia, and septicæmia, etc The results
of these experiments point to the fact that pyæmia and septicæmia, like other infective diseases, are produced by animal
fluids in particular states of change or decomposition, and that
in some way bacterial forms are intimately associated with
their production , that these organisms are either the direct
contagia, the carriers, or the manufacturers of it from fluids in
which they are found

In its nature pyæmia has often been regarded as but the
natural result of embolism and thrombosis, and dependent for
its peculiar manifestations on the softening, breaking up, and
distribution through the mass of the circulating blood of the

material of which the thrombus is composed, the material thus distributed causing blocking of the capillaries, with the production of secondary abscesses This, however, is not absolutely nor fully correct, for although capillary thrombosis may be a feature of pyæmia, it may also, we know, exist without the specific changes attending this process, while the distribution of the broken-down clot may be prevented by secondary plugging from entering the blood-current The existence of micrococci on wounds, and otherwise gaining entrance into the tissues of the animal body, where they find a suitable soil and conditions favourable for their assuming certain activities and potentialities, seem better able to explain the phenomena of pyæmia added to which, we know that certain fluids in which bacteria exist are decidedly septic—these same fluids on abstraction of the organisms being innocuous That they may not always be detected where expected to be found, is explainable on different hypotheses—they may be destroyed by advanced processes occurring during the diseased action, or they may be so altered that our ordinary means of recognition fail; while that they should be present, and not produce pyæmia, may be accounted for because of the absence of material suitable for their growth and operative activities They are usually found where the blood-current is slowest and by their presence produce irritation and vascular changes, the results of which seem favourable for the operation of their powers of septic production It is not in the blood itself that the powers of septic infection reside most powerfully—rather in serum and serous fluid, the result of local irritation, consequently, in the cases of ordinary wounds, the serous material in the adjacent tissues, the result of inflammatory action not yet taken possession of by the suppurative process, is the most powerful agent of infective influence This conveyed artificially, or naturally, to distant parts is more certain than other fluids to induce abscesses and septic changes

Instead of restricting our ideas of this morbid state to particular local changes, whatever these may be, it seems certain that we ought to regard it as contamination of the whole blood, which is altered by the entrance of some poisonous material, that in this way the relation of the circulating blood to the tissues is altered, so disposing to coagulation and obstruction of vessels, these changes being accompanied with fever and specific lesions in internal visceral organs   Independent of this origin of pyæmia or septicæmia, by introduction of an infective agent from without, it seems that similar results may follow from peculiar inflammatory changes in the tissues of animals themselves.   We know that micrococci and bacterial forms are usually to be found in the tissues of even healthy animals.

b Causation—The immediate cause of pyæmia is to be looked for in the existence of some diseased part or tissue which so operates and influences the blood passing through it, either by addition to it of some active and distinct entity, or through an alteration of its already existing elements, that it is prone to induce disturbance, change, and suppuration in distant situations to which it may travel   These situations are usually in the capillaries of the lungs, the liver, the kidneys, and also in other parts of the body more superficial   In those cases which follow suddenly after the occurrence of extensive wounds or operative interference, chiefly in situations where there is difficulty of obtaining a free exit to purulent matter, or where, from other conditions, such is unduly retained, there are few or no local lesions, and death is brought about by excessive blood-contamination

In those instances which occupy longer time in the perfecting of the process, and where the poison, after its introduction, is augmented by self-multiplication, and where distant local suppurative changes are conspicuous—true pyæmia—we will usually find that such is sequent to suppurative action in some part, often to necrosis of bone-tissue   Another point of which we are tolerably certain is, that inflammatory action and pus-formation, in their capacities to induce pyæmia, are not always alike, but are modified by the type of the action, the tissues affected and the conditions with which the animals are surrounded

To understand pyæmia completely Dr Sanderson, in dealing with experiments relating to it, states, we ought to consider its origin, its symptoms, and its anatomical characters   In defining it he says

' 1 Pyæmia originates by the introduction into the blood of a poison which is itself the result of the inflammatory action

15

'2 This poison shows itself by alterations of the blood and disturbance of function   The former of these is shown by the presence of bacterial and other physical changes of the blood ; the latter in fever and, in severe forms, collapse, terminating in death

'3. That more remotely the condition shows itself in the production of secondary or metastatic abscesses in varying situations, and that the pus of these abscesses contains numerous bacteria.'

All, however, are not agreed that the active principle of the diseased blood and other fluids is directly dependent on these bacterial forms, or that they are the essential condition of infectiveness ; some look to a chemical change of the fluids, others to the condition of phlebitis, or inflammation of the animal's own tissues.

c. *Anatomical Characters* —1. Certain changes in appearance and character of the blood. It is of a darker colour than natural, not disposed to coagulate, while the red corpuscles appear to have lost their colouring material, and are shrunk and altered in form   There is also the existence in it of varying forms of bacteria, with an acquired power of inducing irritation when introduced into the circulation of another animal, tending to the production of a condition similar to that which affected the animal from which it was taken. 2. General congestions or inflammations of various organs and structures throughout the body   3 Hæmorrhages and blood-extravasations, extensively distributed, and appearing in different forms in different structures   as petechiæ and blood-markings on the skin, serous and mucous membranes ; as effusions in serous cavities ; as blood-clots in the parenchyma of internal organs —these clots prone to softening and breaking up, with capillary and venous thrombosis, or more extensive embolism   4 Disseminated abscesses in internal organs and subcutaneous tissues, with inflammation of surrounding structures   These abscesses possess certain specific characters, appearing at first as minute spots of congestion, to be followed by the presence of effused material like inflammatory exudate, ultimately possessing pus-like elements, variable in size ; they are in the internal visceral organs, surrounded by a boundary wall of condensed tissue, beyond which they are encircled by a hyperæmic zone. Their contents are of a modified puriform character, true pus-cells are in limited amount, the chief bulk being various cell-growths, much changed, mingled in a grumous liquid with many bacterial forms When occurring in the subcutaneous or muscular structures these collections of pus are disposed to become infiltrated, passing amongst the meshes of the connective-tissue and the interstices of the muscles 5 Extensive changes in connection with the fibrous investing and synovial membranes of joints, pus-formations, and textural alterations of the component parts

From these variations in anatomical characters and symptoms we observe that pyæmia and septic contamination of the blood may exhibit in their development somewhat varied phases; we may, in some instances, be able to detect nothing abnormal save changed characters of the blood with much enlargement and congestion of the great glands of the abdomen, in others we notice particular hæmorrhages and blood-markings on serous and mucous membranes, as the peritoneum, the membranes of the joints, or the respiratory and digestive tract and skin, in a third, the changes take the form of numerous scattered abscesses with embolism and thrombosis, chiefly in internal visceral organs

Symptoms —Although pyæmia may develop itself insidiously and gradually, giving few or no indications of its existence until the system is seriously invaded, its usual form is entered upon suddenly

In the horse, as with other animals, its occurrence is chiefly in connection with injuries and wounds, particularly when suppurative action is progressing in bone, and where small venous conduits are numerous

It is from knowing these facts that we so much dread suppurating wounds of the feet, particularly when the structure of the pedal-bone is involved Here we observe that the blood in the vascular canals is exceedingly apt to be contaminated from the permanent dilatation of these, because of their peculiar lodgment in bony channels.

The more attractive symptoms are rigors, with patchy perspiration; an anxious expression of countenance, indicative of suffering rapidly proceeding to exhaustion; sudden elevation of internal temperature to a point generally in excess of

15—2

most febrile states, this high temperature being markedly un-
steady, and, although always high, it is subject to much variation : the entire symptoms partake of a rather remittent
character, the changes being of a very erratic type. In some
instances where numerous abscesses form in internal organs,
there are special indications of such in accordance with the
situations where these are encountered. From their frequency
in lung-tissue, pneumonia is a rather frequent accompaniment.
The digestive organs are much disturbed, while the mucous
membranes, and even the skin, may exhibit petechial markings
or a distinctly icteric condition. When following injuries or
wounds inflicted in operative interference, there is usually
at the outset of the pyæmic state, from three to five days
subsequent to the infliction of the injury, certain marked
local changes around the wound itself. the tissues seem
infiltrated, the wound being of an angry character, this
infiltration steadily but rapidly passing on to œdema and gangrene of the connective-tissue, with a discharge of ichorous
material and the development of gases in the subcutaneous
structures. Embolism may or may not occur, but the condition is probably more serious with obstructed vessels than
apart from such. When accompanying such diseased states
as the specific fevers, the symptoms of its accession are usually
delayed until the fever has passed its height, a fresh development of physical symptoms marking its inroad. Cases of
pyæmia or septicæmia when fully established, whether associated with external wounds or appearing during the course of
any disease, are extremely dangerous, and in the majority of
instances prove fatal.

Treatment.—When occurring as an accompaniment or sequel
of some general disease, the line of treatment which promises
most favourable results is that of affording direct support to
the suffering by the use of good, easily assimilated food while
the animal still continues to feed ; or ordinary food may be
supplemented with such articles as milk, raw eggs, good beef-
tea, and the administration of alcoholic stimulants, with such
tonics as quinine, iron, or arsenic. In some cases benefit has
seemed to follow the addition to these of regular and moderate doses of carbolic acid. In the case of wounds, in addition to the constitutional treatment indicated, every atten-

tion must be given to remove all influences likely to favour putrefaction, disintegration, and change of blood-clots or tissue-elements undergoing removal This may be attained by careful manipulatory dressing, and by the free use of anti-septics These latter may be applied directly to the wound, also sprinkled over the stall or box The injection into the swollen lymphatic glands of dilute pure carbolic acid, from trials which have been made, deserves a more extended em-ployment, as likely to destroy the infective nature of materials passed through these structures In all cases it is worthy of remembrance that a full and free supply of fresh air in cur-rents seems to be beneficial to animals suffering from these conditions

---

CHAPTER X

RABIES—MADNESS

Definition—*An acute or subacute infective disease of a febrile character occurring in the horse, as the result of inocu-lation with the saliva, through a bite, of a rabid dog, or pos-sibly also some other rabid animal It is characterized by distinct disturbance of several functions connected with inner-vation, notably by much excitement and irritability, a dispo-sition to bite, and with clonic contraction or convulsive move-ments of certain muscles*

Pathology *a Nature and Causation*—Although it has been stated that in certain animals of the canine or feline species rabies may arise spontaneously—a condition we much doubt—it has not, that I am aware of, been regarded as appearing in our larger mammals save as the result of direct inoculation

It is possible to conceive of the occurrence of a collection of symptoms analogous or similar to those we speak of under the term 'rabies,' providing certain conditions are fulfilled with respect to particular parts of the nerve-centres Pro-bably, however, this condition is only known to us in our patients as the direct result of inoculation Usually the virus is conveyed into the system by the dog at the moment of the infliction of the bite, which to secure successful inoculation need not be extensive, the slighter abrasions being equally dangerous with the deeper or more extensive wound. It has been supposed that following the implantation of the virus, an augmentation and change occurs to it, first at the point of inception and afterwards throughout the body; that the blood thus contaminated acts prejudicially on all parts nourished by it, particularly on those of the nervous centre situated in the medulla and anterior portions of the cord

This idea has so far support when we know that for some time, until the development of the characteristic symptoms, nothing abnormal may be observed at the seat of the wound, and that at the period of the manifestation of the constitutional symptoms there are evidently changes either of an irritative or other character, as the attention paid to this part by the animal itself clearly indicates.

Occasionally the horse may be bitten while removed from the observation of its owner or attendants, the wound inflicted being of so trivial a character that no indications of its infliction may be detected, thus rendering the future development of symptoms rather mysterious. That this disease may be produced in the horse from the bite of one of its own species under the influence of the specific poison is, from certain somewhat analogous cases, highly probable, the actual occurrence of it in this manner I am not aware of, the rabid dog having in all instances been the offending individual

Although the period which we are certain has intervened between the infliction of the bite and the first symptoms of illness is in our patient subject to considerable variation, we have no authentic account of such lengthened periods of incubation as are claimed for the disease in man, from twenty to forty days being the usual periods in the horse.

b Anatomical Characters — Although in many instances structural changes and unnatural conditions of many and various organs and structures are obvious enough, none of them are so constantly present nor so uniformly marked in their intensity or ascendency over all others as to enable us to regard them as diagnostic. In some the lesions in connection with the nervous system are more distinctive than changes observed elsewhere; with other cases the digestive and circu-

latory organs seem to have borne the force of the diseased
action So that alone the simple morbid anatomy is not
enough to enable us to decide whether or not rabies has been
the cause of death In the majority of cases we may observe
general congestions and inflammations in connection with
nearly every organ and structure

In the abdominal cavity ecchymoses and spots of blood-
extravasation are scattered over the different viscera, appearing in different forms in the serous membrane of each. The
gland-structures, particularly the liver and spleen, have been
noted as giving evidence of many textural changes One or
other, more rarely both of these, are said to be engorged,
swollen, and friable from hyperæmia and other blood-changes
The lungs are usually congested, and the smaller air-tubes
filled with slightly coloured mucus The heart, while exhibiting sub-endocardial blood-patches and superficial blood-stain-
ing, contains imperfectly formed coagula, often fibrinous clots
The visible character of the blood is variable, being sometimes
darker than natural, and giving evidence of its ability to stain
membranes and tissues from an altered condition of its
coloured corpuscles Throughout the alimentary canal, from
fauces to rectum, we may observe a variable amount of congestion or blood-extravasation rather than of inflammatory
action In the nervous centres and around certain nerve-
trunks we may notice a distinctly hyperæmic condition, with,
in rarer instances, effusion of a peculiar material It seems,
however, rather doubtful whether these conditions ought to
be regarded as consequences of the disturbed activities, or as
inducing factors of them

Various careful examinations of the tissue-elements of the
different parts of the nerve-centres likely to afford evidence of
disease have at different times been made, and much believed to
be abnormal has been stated to have been detected. How much
of these elemental changes is adventitious and how much is
specific does not seem possible to determine On several occasions microscopic examination of nerve-centres from other
animals than the horse has shown considerable and rather
varied changes in connection with the minute vascular conduits, these changes are chiefly capillary thrombosis, much
invasion of the perivascular sheath of the veins, with a pecu-

liar small-celled growth which, not confined to the sheaths of
the bloodvessels, is apt to extend into the adjacent tissue.
These peculiar and minute cell-elements seem to partake of
the character of the ordinary wandering leucocytes And all
these altered conditions are chiefly located, or rather confined,
to that portion of the medulla known as the respiratory centre
where the nerve-nuclei reside which are regarded as presiding
over or controlling the respiratory act.

Symptoms.—As with other animals successfully inoculated,
there is not during the period of incubation any indications
which are likely to draw our attention to the horse until the
disturbances indicative of the systemic poisoning declare
themselves These are increased activity of the general sen-
sorial functions, excitation from the operation of what may be
regarded as inadequate causes ; or in some instances the
earliest indications of the disturbance have been impairment of
control over certain voluntary muscles, particularly those of
the posterior extremities, or a certain amount of rigidity or
tonic spasm of others, as of those of the neck or back, not unlike a mild attack of tetanus Very shortly the state of simple
excitability or of impairment of motor activity is followed by
symptoms of unmistakable madness and ungovernable fury.

At the outset of these symptoms the temperature is raised
two or three degrees, the pulse rather full and hard, with
increase in the frequency of the respirations The appetite, if
at the first capricious, is now gone, and the creature is more
disposed to be vicious and destructive with everyone and
upon all with which it is in contact Trifling disturbances in
the stable cause it to start, and often with flashing eye and
open mouth, from which abundant saliva is discharged, the
horse will make a dash and grasp with his teeth anything
which he can lay hold upon or destroy.

These paroxysms are largely subordinate to impressions
apparently conveyed to the animal by actions carried on
around him To everything taking place the sufferer seems
acutely sensitive, and rarely is anyone able to carry out anything like a careful examination

During the development of these symptoms it has been
noticed that the part of the body which sustained the bite
receives much attention, at first gently rubbing it with the

muzzle, or against any resisting object, to be shortly followed by increase of this friction, or a furious gnawing at it
with the teeth to the extent of inducing laceration of the
parts

As the disease advances the intervals between the fits of
excitement become less and the fury more confirmed, until
the state of exasperation or madness is permanent. Often in the
last stages somnolence and stupor, with paralysis, are developed previous to death

Diagnosis —The only diseased conditions with which rabies
in the horse may be confounded are tetanus, and certain inflammatory conditions of the cerebral structures. From the
former, with which it is only likely to be confounded in the
early stages, and where excitation is not a prominent feature,
but rather spasm of muscular tissue, it is easily differentiated
by the spastic state of the muscles of mastication, the restricted
movement or closure of the jaws in tetanus, and the absence
of these features in rabies. With varying forms of cerebral
inflammation there may be more difficulty, and unless a
history indicative of rabies is attached, we may be compelled
to wait a little ere diagnostic symptoms are developed.
Although both excitation and depression of nerve-power may
be exhibited in certain manifestations of brain disease, there
is not accompanying these any purposely directed attempts of
a violent or destructive character, nor have we wilful self-
infliction of injury

Treatment —Considering the experience which has been
accumulating for ages, and the nearly invariable and universal
fatality of rabies in all animals, it would seem that with the
horse, as with other of our patients, the most expedient as well
as humane course, when satisfied of the nature of the disease,
is the destruction of the sufferer. In the face, however, of this
certainly fatal termination, we are justified in adopting any
measures which the advancing knowledge of healthy or
diseased processes would seem to hold out of hopes of a
favourable termination

In cases where we are aware that the horse has been bitten
by a dog, regarding which suspicions may be excited, every
attention ought to be given to preventive treatment. The
wound, if seen early, should be well irrigated with water, so

that all infecting material which may be adhering to the parts
is removed   If the situation will admit of it, the entire tissues
forming the boundaries of the wound had better be cut away
with the knife ; while, if this is not practicable, or only imperfectly accomplished, cauterization with an iron adapted so as
to reach the entire surface and depth of the wound is to be
carried out , or, failing this, attempted destruction of the
parts may be sought through the use of nitrate of silver or
caustic potash in the solid or liquid form, or liquid nitrate of
mercury, or pure carbolic acid

CHAPTER XI.

SURRA

VERY recently, through the untiring exertions of some members of the profession, whose duties lie in our Indian Empire,
we have been put in possession of information of a most interesting character concerning a condition well and widely
known there as Surra, a brief *résumé* of which we propose
giving here, with the object of furnishing a certain preparation
to those who may yet meet this disease   The literal signification
of the term *surra* is ʻrotten,ʼ and we presume this name has
been applied to indicate the most appreciable effect of the
disease, as, without to the casual observer any marked external
manifestation, the animal attacked would seem to be the
subject of a decaying, or what we term a ʻpining awayʼ process, which sooner or later terminates fatally

Recognised to a greater or lesser extent throughout the
empire, we have it recorded by Mr Griffith Evans, A V.D , that
it is more frequently met with west of the Indus   To this
gentleman's exhaustive efforts, especially in the Dera Ismail
Khan, the profession is deeply indebted for much that is
highly interesting and instructive on the subject.   The information gained could only result from patient investigation
under adverse circumstances, and should future work confirm
the apparent outcome of the related experiments, a fresh page
will have been added to veterinary pathology, and an original
revelation in biology must be acknowledged

Surra may be conveniently defined as a specific blood disease of the horse, enzoötic, marked by general tissue-waste, elevated temperature, extravasations on visible mucous membranes, dropsical swellings; by possessing the capability of being propagated by subcutaneous or intravenous injection and introduction into the stomach of blood containing a parasite, and by the presence of this parasite in the blood during the attack.

The symptoms of the affection are somewhat varied in character, though some of the more prominent are pretty constant, fever is present, a yellowish discharge is noticed at the nasal orifices, the submaxillary glands may in some cases be enlarged, and even discharging. In mares there are frequently anasarcous swellings between the fore-legs, in horses in the sheath. The visible mucous membranes are of a sickly yellow colour, and scattered over them are seen petechiæ; these are said to be most marked at the inner canthus of the eye, and in the female at the vagina. These structural alterations in the mucous membranes are generally continuous, even during defervescence of other symptoms. Occasionally appetite may be wanting or deficient, but it is usually retained throughout the disease. Thirst is evinced, the urine is high-coloured, and on examination found to contain albumen. Marasmus is marked, and there would seem to be little relation between this and the amount of food consumed; for when ample food has been partaken of even until the later stages, the patient almost invariably becomes much emaciated before death. In the earlier stages there is in some cases evidence of loss of power, manifested by stumblings and ineffectual attempts to move the limbs.

The progress of the disease is of an undulatory character it usually continues from about seven to ten weeks, when the animal may drop down and expire suddenly, he may become delirious, and death ensue after a short period; or the patient may linger on in the lying position for several days, continuing to partake of food, and then to succumb without apparent pain. The pathognomic symptom is of course the presence of the parasite in the blood.

The revelations of the post-mortem examination are quite in accordance with the manifestations during life. The intestinal mucous membrane is of a yellowish colour, and marked with small blood-spots. The peritoneal and pericardial cavities have been found to contain layers of lymph. The other internal organs are generally free from macroscopic alteration, except that occasionally a *sodden* appearance of tissue is met with—the result of effusion into connective structures. It is in the microscopic examination of the blood of animals suffering from surra that our attention is drawn to the presence of certain organisms which give speciality to the condition. When a small quantity of fresh blood is placed on a slide, and viewed with the aid of a six-inch power, the parasite—which may be present singly or in groups—is observed to possess a somewhat rounded body, inclining to a neck, surmounted by a spheroidal head, and a tail tapering to a long flagellum. In both cervical and caudal regions there is a papilla-like eminence. In length it is about three or four times the diameter of a white corpuscle. In colour it appears to be white. Closely watched, interesting movements are noticed. The filariæ seem to have a special affinity for the red corpuscles: one, two, or even more, after wriggling about the field of the microscope, become attached to a red corpuscle, and appear to be tugging at it until disintegration takes place. This disposition towards white corpuscles is never noticed; but these are in the disease supposed to increase in number.

In order to observe these phenomena, it is essential that fresh blood be used.

From the tabulated records of Mr Evans, there would appear to be some relation between the febrile symptoms of the disease and the appearance of the parasites in the blood-stream; and that when these are most numerous, the temperature is in proportion much elevated.

In the blood of animals which had six days previously been inoculated with blood from surra patients, there were to be seen swarms of the parasites; while the same result followed the examination of blood of horses which had drunk surra blood seven and a half days previously. Blood which has been drawn from the affected living animal, twenty-four hours before the experiment, has proved incapable of producing the disease by introduction into the body by any of the foregoing means.

Inoculation of blood containing the parasite into the dog was successful in one instance.

The manner in which the disease is spread is not yet ex-plained; but a more intimate study of the life-history of the parasite will doubtless be fraught with significant results in this aspect of the subject. While reasoning from analogy in the history of animal forms of the lower classes, it will be ad-visable that due regard be had to the nature of the drinking-water, which, if possible—and we appreciate the difficulties encountered in tropical countries—should not be procured from unprotected stagnant storage. Much protection would probably be afforded if the boiling of such, where no other is attainable, could be carried out.

As to the success of medicinal treatment little has been made known. The insidious nature of the attack would appear to admit of much constitutional damage being done before treatment is adopted; thus prophylactic measures are espe-cially called for, while, on the principle of deleteriously affect-ing the parasite, the administration of such agents as carbolic and salicylic acid, in frequently repeated doses, would be worthy of trial.

B. CONSTITUTIONAL DISEASES

CHAPTER XII.

OF THE NATURE OF THE GENERAL DISEASES INCLUDED IN CLASS B.

THOSE diseases—some of which, as more particularly affecting the horse, have been so far considered, and regarding which it was agreed to consider under the terms of 'general' or 'systemic' diseases—comprehended in Class A, represented by, and in-cluding the specific febrile diseases and some allied affections, may all be looked upon as largely, if not entirely, resulting from, or developed in, the animal body through the direct in-fluence of agencies acting from without.

In contradistinction to these, it is now intended to consider in a similar manner certain other diseases, 'general' or 'sys-temic,' in the sense that their manifestations of deviations from normal or healthy condition are not confined to any particular organ; but differing, however, from the already noted general

or systemic diseases included in Class A, in that the influences which seem to operate in their production are not
found extensively, if at all, gendered without the animal itself,
but are the result of changes or influences originating or operating from within

From the circumstance that this class of the general
diseases has been chiefly regarded as of endogenous growth,
and inseparably connected with specialities and individualities
of form and temperaments, they have come to be spoken of as
constitutional diseases

These diseases differ from others with which they are grouped,
as general or systemic affections, by such features as the
tendency which they possess to appear in continuous succession, or at uncertain intervals, in individuals of the same
family, by the fact that the local lesions, however pronounced
they may be, are only understood when regarded as the
circumscribed manifestation of an indwelling disposition or
bad habit of body, usually spoken of as a *dyscrasia*; and that
this disposition we find acts as a modifying influence on the
development and course of many processes, healthy as well as
abnormal. Also that the diagnostic, anatomical features of
these affections are chiefly those of the local lesions, which are
usually specific for the several diseases.

CHAPTER XIII.

RHEUMATISMUS — RHEUMATISM — ACUTE RHEUMATISM — CHRONIC RHEUMATISM

UNDER the term of Rheumatism are included several rather
different diseases, some of which seem more properly regarded
as local affections, but which for various reasons it is proposed
to consider together

I ACUTE RHEUMATISM

Definition.—*A specific febrile disturbance, most probably
owing its origin to a morbid, inbred, or constitutional state
of the system, and characterized by the manifestation of much
pain, and a special tendency to the involvement of certain*

structures or textures, as the coverings of muscles and
tendons, and certain structures entering into the formation of
joints; these local manifestations showing a disposition to
shift their situations to other textures or organs of a similar
nature but remote situation

General Characters and Intimate Nature of the Disease.—That
rheumatism is more correctly considered as a general rather than
a local disease, seems tolerably evident when we recollect such
prevailing features as—1 The regularity with which systemic
disturbance accompanies its appearance 2 The considerable
tissue-changes, as alteration in the composition of the blood,
and occasionally in the urine, previous to the development of
the local phenomena. 3. The fact that certain animals are,
from a peculiar inherent diathesis, liable to develop the disease,
apart from any apparent cause.

Although a wonderfully common disease amongst men, its
existence in our patients has often been doubted, and even
now is denied by some There appears to be, however, sufficient evidence to convince any but such as are determined
not to be satisfied with any proof, that all our domestic animals
are subject, with varying susceptibility, to rheumatic disease

The inbred morbific agent in the development of rheumatism
is, in the exhibition of the local inflammations and phenomena,
not confined to any one organ or texture, although markedly
disposed to invade the white fibrous tissues—those chiefly met
with as investing and covering membranes of the muscles,
the component parts of tendons, ligaments, their sheaths, and
the fibro-serous visceral membranes. It is one of those diseases
which are considerably influenced in their appearance, extent
of distribution, and severity of attack, by meteorological and
telluric agencies; in this way may we account for its existence
or prevalence in certain districts and not in others.

Very various and rather contradictory statements have from
time to time been made, both by observers of the phenomena
of the disease and by those who have attempted to study its
pathology by experimental investigation; so that even at the
present the true nature and modes of action of that which we
have good reason to believe exists as the main factor in its
production, viz. a specific inbred morbific agent, are points upon
which pathologists are not agreed At one time, and by many,

regarded as being the result or external manifestation of the
action of some miasmatic influences, it seems now very generally
accepted as originating from intrinsic causes that although
there has not yet been detected any peculiar or hurtful material
circulating in the blood, it is yet highly probable that the
general and local diseased manifestations owe their origin to
some constitutional and inbred morbific agent, the result of
some imperfectly executed chemical or vital process connected
with the exercise of animal function; or at least, that for its
existence this inducing agent, or specific factor, is not dependent on anything, or is itself received into the body, from without It has been spoken of by some as a blood disease, and
evidence of the poisoned state of the blood has been pointed
out as exhibited in the coincident occurrence of fever and
certain regularly appearing local phenomena and internal
structural changes, by the symmetrical development of local
symptoms, and the often exhibited metastatic character of
these However, the only abnormal condition as yet well
established, and proved to have a constant existence in the
blood in rheumatism, is the large increase in the fibrinogenous
materials, and the relative disproportion which exists between
these and the saline ingredients as compared with the usual
proportionate relations in health Probably from the knowledge that certain secretions and excretions of the body, in
acute rheumatism, are distinctly acrid and acid, the idea may
have originated that the true rheumatic poison was some
special and distinctive organic acid produced in excess during
the exercise of natural function, or if not manufactured in
excess, at least unnaturally retained in the system from some
defect in convertive or eliminative function The idea first
suggested by Dr. Prout, that all the phenomena, systemic and
local, exhibited in rheumatism might be referred to the retention in the system of an extra amount of lactic acid, has been
extensively adopted, enforced, and expounded by many succeeding pathologists The source of this lactic acid is believed to
be the ordinary one of the transformation of the starch of the
food into this agent, which, in the further steps in the heat-
production, is converted at the lungs by combining with
oxygen into carbonic acid and water; and that the extra
amount of the acid is to be accounted for by the occurrence of

any disturbance in the various steps of these chemical and elemental changes

The constancy of the occurrence of structural lesions of the endocardium on the left side of the heart, is by those who hold the theory of the lactic acid origin of rheumatism explained by regarding the final perfecting or development of the morbid agent to occur only in the pulmonic circuit of the circulation The theory of this origin of rheumatism has received some confirmation from certain experiments in which the injection of various watery solutions of lactic acid into the peritoneal cavity of animals was attended, not with peritonitis, but with certain cardiac changes, as inflammation of the lining membrane of the left side, with valvular alterations and fibrinous deposits, and with metastatic affections of the joints   The universal acid condition of the blood and other animal fluids has, however, not been accepted by every observer or experimenter, some declaring that the opposite condition has in very many instances been found to exist

Although we may not be able to state precisely what is the nature of the *materies morbi* in the rheumatic inflammation, nor yet to explain the mode of its action or development, it is yet tolerably certain that some specific poison, or morbid agent, exists in the economy, most probably as the result of some faulty or deranged activity, and that to the action of this inbred agent, so erratic in the exhibition of phenomena, the product of a constitutional diathesis, the various general and local symptoms owe their origin

In the local inflammatory action occurring in acute rheumatism, it is deserving of notice that although the action may be severe, and the exudation abundant and largely infiltrated amongst the connective-tissue, in the situation invaded, it is rare that the process advances to suppuration, at least, it is seldom as compared with common inflammation of like severity and extent   Whether the phenomenon of the persistent invasion of one class of tissues, the fibro-serous, by the rheumatic poison is always to be accepted as an ultimate fact, the explanation of which we may not reach, or whether we are yet, through the investigation of those chemical actions which occur in the animal economy, particularly the relations which subsist between the results of the secondary digestive process,

16

the character of used animal tissues, and the process of nutrition, to arrive at a more satisfactory understanding of cause and effect, remains to be seen

Causation.—The causes which seem to operate in the production of rheumatism are generally spoken of and regarded under two groups

1 *The Indwelling, or Predisposing,* which are also often hereditary. We may not as yet be able to lay the finger upon the specific indwelling factor of the disease, and say of this something definite and tangible that its existence in the animal body, and it alone, is the predisposing cause in producing this diseased condition Still reasoning from analogy, and from comparing the phenomena occurring with other strange appearances, the causes of which we are tolerably well aware of, we are forcibly drawn to the admission that in all cases of rheumatism it is highly probable that a peculiar something, whether it be formation of solids, composition of fluids, or peculiar modes of manifestation of nervous or other power, which we have named a diathesis, or constitutional tendency to develop this special manifestation of symptoms which we find characteristic of rheumatism, exists in certain animals This constitutional tendency is in some so marked, and constitutes so striking a peculiarity, that the outcome and appearance of the disease are often, to our observation, called into existence without any inducing agency whatever While whatever adverse influences are brought to bear on animals so constituted, which in others tend to the production of very different and opposite diseases, in them, as a rule, terminate in rheumatism

That this constitutional predisposition is hereditary, or capable of transmission as an inheritance from parent to progeny, can be satisfactorily established by evidence collected by many and competent observers, although this point has not, in my experience, been so well established and so prominently brought forward, as respects the horse, as it has in cattle, I am still aware of facts sufficient to satisfy me of its truth

2 *Exciting or Directly Operating.*—These include all influences, sanitary and dietetic, which result in a lowering of the vital energies, or disturbance of the process of nutrition, as undue confinement, want of cleanliness, imperfect ventilation,

fatigue with exposure, without sufficient attention to sudden alternations of temperature, particularly when accompanied with excess of moisture in the atmosphere, and probably also age We are aware that when examined carefully these inducing agencies are found to operate with singular irregularity, are often disappointing and always erratic: it is, however, abundantly certain that, with animals possessing the constitutional predisposition, their exposure to such extrinsic influences as indicated is more likely to be followed by the exhibition of symptoms of rheumatism than others where this inherited constitutional tendency is unmarked.

Of the directly operating agencies some appear more powerful or more constantly in operation than others, such as age—the young being more liable than the matured—and what are spoken of as atmospheric That young animals should suffer more from coincident depressing influences is not to be wondered at, in them all those functions subservient to the development of the body are in the most vigorous operation, this very functional activity rendering them more susceptible to the action of adverse agencies The small amount of exercise to which they are often compelled to submit is injurious from the enforced inactivity to which the joints are subjected; while it not unfrequently happens that they are turned in great haste, without preparation, from too warm paddocks and close confinement into the open air and perfect liberty—the transition is too great, both as to temperature and exercise

When referring the immediately developing causes of rheumatism to atmospheric influence, location, and disturbed nutrition, there is little doubt that we are speaking of agencies the exact mode of whose operation we may be unable satisfactorily to explain 'Atmospheric influence' is a term of much ambiguity, and is often employed to veil our ignorance There are, however, certain conditions of the atmosphere, as its temperature, its moisture or dryness, etc, the actions of which we can with tolerable certainty predict Even when very young, animals can with impunity endure a comparatively low temperature if unaccompanied with moisture; when, however, a damp lair is added to a dry cold wind, a very actively exciting cause of rheumatic inflammation of the joints exists; the animals are disposed to lie, the circulation becomes flagging, and if there

16—2

exists the slightest constitutional tendency to this unhealthy condition the system rapidly succumbs   A deficiency of shelter and of food, with a naturally damp condition of soil, will further ensure an earlier and more confirmed form of the malady, while the opposite conditions and influences, when existing, may delay or prevent the development of the constitutional taint

Anatomical Characters—In the great majority of deaths from acute rheumatism—chronic rheumatism cannot be said to be fatal—the result is reached through the extent or the severity of the cardiac complications, consequently the appreciable structural changes are as a rule most distinctive in connection with the heart and the structures immediately associated with it. These cardiac lesions vary in accordance with the stage or period of development of the symptoms at which death occurs.

In all cases, even where the heart and investing or lining membranes are the seat particularly of the diseased action, it does not necessarily follow that these symptoms are at once and speedily fatal. The acute stage of the inflammatory process may entirely pass away, the animal may survive for a lengthened period, ultimately to succumb to conditions following as sequelæ of the structural changes developed as the result of inflammation of the heart or associated structures

When the animal has yielded to the active stages of the cardiac inflammation the changes are generally very well marked, and probably connected with the pericardium or endocardium rather than with the muscular tissue of the heart itself The pericardium is thickened mainly from organization of the inflammatory exudate on its inner surface   This exudation of organizable lymph is not laid on in a uniformly smooth manner, but is characterized by being disposed in an irregularly papillated or reticulated form, while occasionally adhesions connect the visceral and parietal membrane. The sac of the pericardium contains a greater or less amount of fluid of a reddish colour, with occasionally small shreds of lymph floating in it

When the endocardium is involved the changes are more frequently and distinctly seen as affecting the valves guarding the orifices, chiefly those of the left side. These are found thickened both in their structure proper and also the cords stretching from them to the papillary eminences of the cardiac wall. When the morbid action in connection with the heart has existed for a somewhat longer period prior to death, there will be less fluid probably in the pericardial sac, the extravasated inflammatory products will possess a greater consistence and more distinct reticulation, while on the cardiac valves the depositions will have acquired a more perfectly fibrinous character, and are better distinguished from the valves upon which they are situated

The joints and other situations of the limbs which have been the seats of local inflammatory action are swollen from the infiltration of the integral textures of the different structures invaded, and the capsules of joints and sheaths of tendons are distended with simply an extra amount of the natural fluid, or with a mixture of this and sero-cellular matter

As it is generally in the earlier stages of the disease that a fatal termination occurs, it is the softer tissues which most distinctly show the results of the diseased action, the harder textures, as cartilage and bone, are not at this stage much changed. The entire structures surrounding the joints, the ligaments and tendons, are frequently adherent to the connective and subcutaneous tissues by the extension to these of the specific diseased action, and the intimate union of all by the diffusion of the products of the inflammatory process In the more advanced cases ulcerative changes occur, and sinuous communications extend from the capsule to the surface, while peculiar and extensive alterations, as loss of substance, of cartilage, expansion of bone-tissue with deposition of lime, salts, and subsequent eburnation of the altered articular surface, are likely to follow should the animal live long enough

Symptoms—In many well-marked cases of acute rheumatism, particularly in young animals, I have noticed that there has preceded the development of the more characteristic symptoms a deranged condition of the intestinal canal, with a particular acridity of the evacuations, also, in the majority of such cases, either showing themselves antecedently or synchronously with certain local changes, there are the usual febrile symptoms—elevation of internal and external temperature, as indicated by the thermometer, being particularly well marked, with a rather frequent, full, and unyielding pulse

In all, at this stage, the bowels are rather confined ; there is thirst, while the secretion from the kidneys is of the true febrile type, small in amount, and of high specific gravity.

Besides these features of general disturbance common to many febrile affections, there is to be noticed the special cardiac disturbance. When the involvement of the heart is trifling, the inconvenience may be so slight and the symptoms so little attractive that this complication may escape observation. There seems good ground for believing that all cases of acute rheumatism show specific inflammation of some part of the structures of the heart ; but from the fact that the serous fluid effused is rapidly taken up, and any fibrinous adhesions are very early effected, the disturbance of function has not been sufficient to attract attention

When, however, there is much effusion in the heart-sac, pressing upon and confining its movements, complicated with inflammation of the muscular tissue, the inner lining membrane or valvular structures, both general and local symptoms become distressing and distinctive.

Pain is exhibited on exercising percussion over the region of the heart, intensified by pressure in the intercostal spaces of the left side. There is some restlessness, anxious expression of countenance, slight cough, difficulty in breathing, and palpitation when rapidly moved or sharply turned round. These conditions may attract us to make a more careful examination by auscultation, which will reveal a somewhat altered condition of the natural sounds of the organ. Very often all that we can be certain of is that there is some irregular contraction about the orifices, or that the natural impulse of its movements is deadened by the presence of fluid in the pericardial sac

Of the local symptoms lameness is the most attractive ; it is severe as well as sudden. The animal, when last seen, may have had perfect freedom of locomotion ; it may now be totally incapable of movement, or only able to accomplish this with the greatest difficulty. Manipulation of the affected limb or limbs—for lameness is often symmetrical—will at once satisfy us of the nature of the affection ; one or more joints will be found excessively painful, they may or may not be tense and swollen.

The articulations most liable to be thus affected in the horse are the stifle and fetlock, the hock and knee less so. When the pain in the joints is severe the horse is dejected, and at times restless. The swellings, when occurring, show themselves at those parts of the joints which are least bound with ligament, and by their peculiar fluctuation are at once indicative of capsular distension. The advent of the swelling does not seem to relieve the pain, which is augmented by the least handling or movement of the joint, the latter when enforced causing copious perspiration. All these symptoms may be most marked, and for several hours the condition of the limb or limbs remains much as indicated, when, in a most unaccountable manner, the pain and swelling become alleviated or entirely disappear, only to be reproduced in one or more of the as yet unaffected extremities, this shifting, with relief and exacerbation of symptoms, being distinctly characteristic of rheumatism.

At this, the earlier stage, there is merely increased vascular action, with an evident increase of the natural fluid of the joint. Very shortly, however, should the symptom not abate, certain structural changes set in, the synovial membrane becomes thickened, soft, and not so clear-looking; while flakes of plastic material show themselves in the more fluid contents of the capsule, to the walls of which, as also to the loose synovial membrane, they become attached. In exceptional cases the process does not stop here; the fibrinous exudations do not seem very capable of taking on healthy organizations so as to finish the adhesive process, but the morbid action proceeds to the production of a puriform material. With these changes in conditions are developed a change or new train of symptoms, both constitutional and local.

The general febrile symptoms, which may have become somewhat lessened, exhibit exacerbation; the local pain and swelling increase, while the peculiar fluctuation conveys to the touch the tolerable certainty that something more than simple serum or synovia is now contained within. Following the evacuation of this material there will generally be relief from pain—not, however, of long continuance, as the inflammatory process will shortly renew its supremacy, and proceed with fresh vigour until the articulation is completely altered.

Although aged horses do suffer from this acute articular rheumatism, it seems more prevalent amongst animals before they reach maturity, when occurring in the aged it is often as an accompaniment or a sequel of the specific fever 'Distemper,' and in such the tendons and their fibrous sheaths are as apt to be involved as the joints themselves.

Course and Complications—We cannot from observation of the earlier symptoms of rheumatism predict the probability as to time of recovery, it is not like some continued fevers where the crisis is reached in a determinate number of days, which as a rule is closely adhered to. In acute rheumatism the fever may reach its height, and defervescence be established, at the end of the first week; the greater number of cases, however, are prolonged considerably beyond this period.

With the subsidence of the fever the local inflammations may seem much relieved. they generally, however, continue stationary in the exhibition of their varied symptoms for a considerable time after the general symptoms of illness have disappeared.

There is in the development of the different symptoms, the constitutional and local, some considerable difference as to time and sequence of individual appearance. While, in whatever way these two classes of symptoms show themselves, there does not, from the relative precedence as to time in their occurrence, seem to be any rule established either as to their subsidence, disappearance or probability of a severe or slight attack, or yet of the chance of ultimate recovery or of a fatal issue.

In the instances of metastasis of the local symptoms there cannot be said to be any indications or warnings given by which we may become aware that any change is to occur, while when the change is being accomplished there is no certainty that the local phenomena will continue to develop and remain in the situation to which the action has been removed.

The cardiac complications, which are neither offshoots nor developments, so to speak, of the systemic disorder, nor of the local inflammatory processes, and are only related to these probably in so far as they are the development or results of one and the same morbific agent or specific poison, in their appearance seem to be regulated by no fixed law which we can discover as to the time of their occurrence.

It seems highly probable that they are more frequently seen and developed during the course of the fever than delayed until defervescence of pyrexia and amelioration of local phenomena. When not proving fatal from their severity or extent, they are apt by structural changes to ensure confirmed ill-health and inability to perform ordinary work

Treatment.—In the treatment of rheumatism, especially of the acute form, blood-letting has almost invariably been resorted to. This has been thought to be indicated by the urgent febrile symptoms, the character of the pulse, together with the extra fibrinogenous condition of the blood, a condition which we know is in health rather increased than diminished by blood-letting.

Now, although I have noticed its employment result in the immediate abatement of certain prominent symptoms, there are yet objections to it, founded on its ultimate results, which militate against its employment in any save young animals in vigorous health and full habit of body, and even then only sparingly The early and free abstraction of blood has by some been spoken against because of its tendency to favour the development of cardiac symptoms, which all dread so much For my own part, I have not observed this tendency, but have noticed that although immediate relief has followed its employment, this relief has been only temporary, and was generally followed by an increased severity of symptoms coincident with the reaction In all cases good will result from getting the bowels early under the action of a mild saline purge, and being afterwards kept moist by the diet or some appropriate medicine Considering the nature of the alterations in the blood, alkalies and neutral salts would appear indicated, and practically they are of the greatest benefit They are best administered as the bicarbonate or nitrate of potass, and when the thirst is considerable are readily enough taken dissolved in the drinking-water For the production of their desired action they ought at first to be given in full doses, and frequently

For foals, from one to three drachms of each salt, according

to strength and age, will be found sufficient when given every
third or fourth hour largely diluted with water. For adult
animals three times this quantity will be necessary.

This treatment must be persevered with for some days, or
until obvious benefit is derived from its administration. This
is generally shown by abatement of febrile symptoms, as lowering of temperature, an increased secretion of urine, and
relief from pain

Should the more active symptoms not seem relieved by this
treatment in a few days, there had better be given, alternately
with the alkaline solution, a little colchicum wine, with acetated
liquor ammonia or instead of the bicarbonate and nitrate of
potass, the iodide of potassium may be substituted and alternated with the colchicum and the acetate of ammonia The
treatment of acute rheumatism by salicylic acid and its compounds, while in many cases evidently attended with good
results, has not, in my experience with the horse, yielded such
continuous and general benefit as the use of those agents
mentioned Both here and with the more truly chronic
manifestations of the disease, particularly when pyrexia has
disappeared, benefit has sometimes seemed to follow the use
for some time of moderate doses of arsenic and quinine, or of
ounce doses twice daily of Donovan's solution

Locally all stimulating agents—the usually resorted-to remedies—ought at the earlier stages to be carefully avoided
Instead, apply continuously some cooling or evaporating lotion,
or swathe the part, where this is possible, in woollen bandages
kept damp with a saturated solution of bicarbonate and nitrate
of potass; or, where the pain is excessive, warm poultices are
more likely to afford relief, or woollen bandages kept warm and
moist by means of hot water, medicated with tincture of
opium and a small quantity of tincture of aconite, the animal
being at the same time kept perfectly quiet Should the characteristic local symptoms of pain and difficulty in locomotion
not become ameliorated during the first week, or even in all
cases of a less acute nature, which have nevertheless continued
persistent as to their localization and severity, a somewhat
different mode of treatment may be necessary and productive
of good results Local stimulating applications may now be
had recourse to, varying in strength from ordinary soap to

cantharides liniment.   In many instances where the local
action is settled in connection with individual joints, smart
vesication with some cantharidine application I have almost
invariably found followed by relief from pain, a great point to
be gained even while freedom of movement is still much
impeded

II CHRONIC RHEUMATISM

Although this form may follow as a sequel of acute rheumatism, it is also met with as an independent and idiopathic
affection   In either case the symptoms of its existence may
be regarded as merely modifications of the more pronounced
form, minus the pyrexial features   Chronic rheumatism is
also less liable to exhibit metastatic features, less disposed to
seize upon the cardiac structures, and probably also less inclined to yield to curative measures.

The only recognisable symptoms consist in inflammation of
the aponeurotic expansions over the articulations, which
gradually extends to the periosteum and the component
elements of the joints, resulting in such textural changes as
alteration of synovial membrane and cartilage, while a porcelain-
like material takes the place of the latter, which, although
admitting of movement, does so only in a modified manner,
and together with the general thickening of ligament and
other structures, tends to stiffen and impede the natural freedom of the joint   In many cases, although pain and lameness
exist, and are largely influenced by atmospheric and other
extrinsic conditions, swelling is not always a constant feature

Treatment —In the manifestations of rheumatism the sequel
of the acute type, and where the articular structures are
evidently undergoing change, the preferable treatment is the
application of the actual cautery   When, however, the disease
is decidedly of a chronic type from the first, where the constitutional fever is little if at all marked, or of a truly intermittent
character, such severe means are rarely called for

Regarding the local manifestations, which are certainly the
most prominent feature, as merely the development, or at least
owing their existence to the specific constitutional diathesis, it
is found that much mitigation of pain and restoration of function may be obtained through the use of constitutional

remedies   Horses which have become the subjects of well-developed and confirmed chronic rheumatism are not as a rule very hopeful patients, still so much benefit may sometimes be obtained from careful attention to the dietary, and by the administration of an occasional laxative, with the steady employment in the food of a moderate quantity of bicarbonate of potass or soda, that a fair amount of slow work may be done without distress to the animals   Half-ounce doses of oil of turpentine, or two-drachm doses of iodide of potassium twice daily, or the addition to the alkali given in the food of a few grains of arsenic, are, considering the chances of their benefiting as tonics, severally deserving of a trial

Locally, in such forms, we are often puzzled what to do, as nothing which we employ seems to result in much good, in practice I have found more benefit from the employment, where this was possible, of woollen bandages soaked with hot oil, or warm alkaline solution applied to the parts for an hour or two at a time, and when removed, smart friction with a liniment composed of equal quantities of soap liniment and tincture of opium   I have found this better than strong blistering agents, which in old animals do not seem productive of much good, while in their use they necessitate a great loss of time from the enforced rest

The treatment by hot fomentations or bandages, and afterwards friction with anodyne liniment, does not necessitate rest, in truth, it seems to do better when the animal is steadily but not too severely working

III   MUSCULAR AND TENDINOUS RHEUMATISM

It is generally allowed that the muscles and their fibrous investing membrane and continuations are subject to a peculiar painful affection aggravated by movement or manipulation, and believed to be of a rheumatic or rheumatoid character It is usually of a subacute nature; occasionally it appears suddenly and unexpectedly, and, once established, is rather liable to recur.

This disturbed condition seems to owe its origin, wherever the pre-existing disposition exists, to the operation of causes much similar to those which we recognise as inducing factors

in the other manifestations of rheumatism   Here it is to be
noted that fatigue, general improper treatment, and exposure
to vicissitudes of weather are regarded as specially obnoxious
It may affect any of the voluntary muscles, but is chiefly
known to us in the horse as seizing upon the great muscles of
the lumbar and gluteal regions, those of the neck and shoulder,
and probably also of the chest

Although not ordinarily exhibiting systemic disturbance or
constitutional symptoms, we do find that when this form of
rheumatism is referable to the great mass of muscle situated
on the loins and haunch, which we often enough observe in
agricultural horses, or those engaged in draught in towns, that
there is also well-marked symptoms of general illness or discomfort, usually a certain amount of fever, with more of
derangement of the digestive system   The pulse is somewhat
increased in frequency, and harder than natural, with suffused
or injected conjunctival membranes, the tongue coated, mouth
pasty and smelling sour, the bowels confined, urine scanty and
turbid   The pain in the muscles and fascia covering these
causes the animal to exhibit a cramped or drawn-together
form, with back slightly elevated, and not at all disposed to
move; on causing him to turn or execute a backward movement, the gait is very ungainly and straddling, the horse
occasionally giving audible expression to its suffering   That
the pain is really in the region mentioned may be further
demonstrated by drawing the fingers with steady pressure
along both sides of the spine

When invading other regions a train of symptoms somewhat
similar, and called into exhibition or intensified by special
movement or manipulation, is well enough made out

Treatment—The management of muscular rheumatism,
particularly when acute or sudden in its appearance, is always
most successful when carried out both constitutionally and
locally; in the decidedly chronic manifestations our chief
reliance is on measures more strictly topical   All those
remedies and systems of dietary which seem to be productive
of good in other developments of the disease are deserving of
trial in this, while probably such as partake of more strictly
tonic properties may be expected in the lingering cases to
yield the more favourable results   Of local treatment rest,

with heat and moisture, and the daily use of moderately stimulant and anodyne liniments, such as contain opium, belladonna, aconite, turpentine, or camphor, seem from experience to yield the most satisfactory results.

Generally, in all cases and every form of chronic rheumatism our success in treatment is of a doubtful character, rarely is it abiding; while the occasional fact of a recovery after a prolonged attack will always give hope when amidst our endeavours we see little to encourage or satisfy.

CHAPTER XIV.

SCROFULA—TUBERCULOSIS

Definition—*A constitutional disease evidencing itself in a specific deposition or infiltration in connection with various tissues—known as tubercle, and in mass as scrofulous or tuberculous matter—or in specific inflammations, ulcerations, or disturbances of developmental or nutritive processes.*

Considering that this is a disease to which the horse is less liable than any of our patients, as also that numerous questions connected with its nature, causation, and modes of development are yet in a transition stage, and liable to undergo change as respects our opinions regarding them, it is unnecessary to do more here than very briefly note some of the generally accepted ideas and facts connected with it.

Meaning of Terms—By the term *scrofula* is understood the indwelling constitutional predisposition, or diathesis, to exhibit under favourable conditions the local changes which in their development are spoken of as *tuberculosis.* *Tubercle* is the minute local product existing in the state of tuberculosis, the larger masses recognisable by the naked eye being spoken of as *tuberculous* or *scrofulous* matter.

Pathology *a Nature of Scrofula*—The proper understanding of the entire subject of scrofula and tubercle, besides being darkened and rendered intricate through the misapplication of terms or their varied interpretation has often been further confused where a separate value has been placed upon each

through the divergence of opinion as to the identity of variations of the diseases spoken of as scrofulous and tuberculous,
some regarding them as identical, others as separate and
distinct. A very common cause of confusion, it will be found,
is that of using the term *tubercle* to express the meaning now
understood to be conveyed by that of *scrofula*—the indwelling
disposition to the production of the lesion

Scrofula may in our present nomenclature be taken to
express the indwelling predisposition which precedes the
development of tubercle, that this latter is but the local
expression of the constitutional taint known as scrofula. This
bad habit of body, it is probable, is intimately related to faulty
conditions of the assimilatory process in either or both the
primary and secondary digestion

b. Nature of Tubercle—At one time tubercle was believed to
be an exudation from the blood which, at first fluid, ultimately
developed cellular characters, this is now proved to be incorrect,
although it is yet, in a somewhat modified form—in which
certain of its cell-elements are regarded as wandering leucocytes—the view held by a few Others regard this adventitious
material as the result of degenerative changes of normal or
morbid elements, in which specific activities carry out definite
changes, succeeded by retrogression and death Some—the
more modern investigators—maintain that the masses are
merely hyperplasia of normal lymphoid or adenoid tissue, a
structure extensively distributed in animal bodies, and particularly abundant in those situations where tubercle is chiefly
found. Changes in the minute lymph-vessels themselves,
particularly their endothelium and tissue-elements surrounding
these, have also been stated as being the true source of
tubercle, while quite recently attention has been directed to
its parasitic or bacterial origin

c Causation. 1. *Scrofula*—In whatever way explained,
there is nearly a general consensus of opinion in regarding
heredity as the first great factor in the production of the
scrofulous diathesis—transmission of a something, either
textural peculiarity or dynamic or formative power from parent
to progeny, whereby in certain conditions this tendency or
scrofulous condition may develop in tuberculosis or specific inflammatory action. By some, common inflammation is regarded

as capable of resulting in the production of a material identical with tubercle ; this is, however, doubtful, unless the scrofulous diathesis exists. Caseation is something different from tubercle. It seems, from comparison of facts and data, that tuberculosis may be propagated under favourable conditions from the actually diseased to the healthy. These conditions are close and intimate cohabitation, partaking of milk from tuberculous animals, and the using of their flesh as food. The latter probably require further confirmation. All influences which tend to depress and lower the general vital activities in animals seem to render them more liable to develop tuberculous diseases. Under this group we must rank indifferent food, bad sanitary conditions—particularly defective ventilation —over-work in contaminated atmospheres, previous disease, prolonged lactation, etc. These influences are all more powerful when operating on animals in confinement.

2. *Tubercle*.—As respects the direct or immediate causation of the tubercle, several operating agencies have been accredited with the power of production : (1) Tubercle has been regarded as merely the local expression of that constitutional cachexia or diathesis known as the scrofulous. (2) That it arises from local irritation of that particular tissue, the adenoid, in which it is largely found, apart from any constitutional tendency. (3) That it always arises as the product of an infective action proceeding from some previously existing centre of inflammation, poisoning the lymph and blood-streams, and developing a specific inflammation. This is the view largely supported by experimentation, but it seems to need modification.

Anatomical Characters *a General Features*—The typical tubercle, grey granulation or miliary tubercle, may be regarded as a non-vascular, round or roundish microscopic body, well-defined, of variable consistence and greyish colour. These are either discrete or aggregated in masses of variable size, or they may be infiltrated throughout the structures where situated.

Yellow tubercle, so-called, is probably degenerate common inflammatory product, or changing tubercular matter, which may have become mingled in the caseous mass. This adventitious material is found on the free surface of mucous

membranes generally, and in the tissues of the alimentary canal,
in the pleura, peritoneum, and arachnoid, in the structure of the
lymphatic glands, particularly the mesenteric and the cervical,
also in the lungs, spleen, liver, etc   It is characteristic of this
disease that it attacks many organs, and that in cases of acute
tuberculosis miliary tubercle is encountered in nearly every
organ of the body.

b. Minute Structure—Although the minute anatomy of
tubercle has been most patiently wrought at for years, perfect
agreement on this point, as also the parts which the several
histological elements play, has not, in our day, been arrived
at   The chief elements of tubercle may be stated as:
1 Lymphoid elements—small round bodies, slightly granular,
and containing a single nucleus, 2 Epithelial cells, rather
large and delicate, 3 A giant cell, consisting of a granular
mass of protoplasm with many nuclei, and processes stretching
in different directions—this, together with other fibres, forming
a hyaline structure or meshes, 4. Intercellular matter of
varying character, 5 Free nuclei   Opinion differs as to the
relative proportion and relation of these several elements
Probably age of the product, as also situation, may have some
influence in both these directions

Although possessed of neither vessels nor lymphatics of its
own, tubercle is liable to undergo retrogressive changes
(*a*) It may be softened and absorbed, (*b*) it may calcify,
(*c*) it may undergo fibroid change.

Occurrence in the Horse.—That this constitutional condition
of scrofula may in our patients exhibit itself in the form of
acute tuberculosis is not impossible   The probabilities, however, in adult life are largely in favour of its appearance as
localized tubercle, although even in this development I am
rather doubtful if I have ever encountered it   When exhibiting itself in this latter form, the situations are chiefly the
lungs and pleura, with the gland-structures of the abdomen
In all such developments its diagnosis is rather difficult, seeing
that such changes simulate and may be mistaken for those the
result of common inflammation, or other textural alterations
connected with special diseased processes   The nearest
approach to true miliary tubercle in the organs of the horse is
probably the diffuse granulation masses found in the lungs

17

and other parts of the pulmonary tissues in glanders. All other collections of adventitious material in these organs or elsewhere which have come under my notice, whether distributed in minute particles of a friable character, or as larger pus-like or caseous masses, seem rather to have resulted from ordinary changes occurring in the ordinary products of common inflammatory action affecting the structures where they have been found

In all such instances, in addition to the history of the cases, which may or not be suggestive, the general symptoms of fever and wasting, either continuous or of an intermittent character, have been supplemented by others pointing to local disturbance of function or textural change, very similar to what may be expected in localized tubercle

Relation of Specific Arthritis to Scrofula—Although not claiming for every case and form of development of arthritic disease in young horses the character of tubercular, I am yet rather disposed to regard many of the well-pronounced and malignant cases in their nature scrofulous. Regarded in no other light do we find such rational explanation of the numerous phenomena which are connected with and surround this disease

Apart from this manifestation, I regard scrofula, with or without the development of tubercle, as a rare disease in the horse. In this phasis, as specific arthritis of a tuberculous character, it is common, and probably within the last quarter of a century has been on the increase.

Causation.—This specific inflammation, which affects the joints of young horses, possesses, in the matter of causation, the strongest resemblance to local inflammatory and other changes, the result of a scrofulous disposition. It seems (1) Dependent on an inbred or constitutional peculiarity, being more prevalent in some families than others, and is modified in all pertaining to heredity, as other congenital affections are. (2) Like every other constitutional and inbred disease, there is little doubt that its appearance is largely favoured by external influences, which are much within our power of control. These are chiefly of a character bearing upon our manipulatory interference with the breeding, locating, and feeding of these animals, with a view to the perfecting of their forms and general improvement in many directions   It is peculiarly a disease of our finer breeds, and is more apt to show itself when those conditions unfavourable to animal life are in operation   So well marked is the influence of external agencies in the development of this disease, as of many manifestations of undoubted scrofula, that, like the constitutional cachexia, many have come to regard it as capable of propagation apart from an inherited disposition, which is doubtful.

It is certainly capable of mitigation by attention to the breeding of animals, and to correct hygienic and dietetic conditions   Not only is the advent of this tubercular arthritis in the young animal heralded by dyspepsia and disturbed digestion, but a condition of mal-assimilation and perverted formative power in either or both parents seems largely to determine its appearance

Although the ordinary form of the appearance of this scrofulous tendency is as specific arthritis with disseminated tubercle or changing products of a specific inflammatory action, it may yet exhibit itself in a fatal form apart from collections of the specific adventitious material

The production of this constitutional cachexia, which shows itself by the peculiar local tissue-changes, will, when a large and comprehensive view is taken of the subject, appear intimately related to disturbed assimilation and perverted tissue-formative power   To the time and manner of performance of the various acts or steps in the complex process of nutrition we must look for the explanation of the production of the unhealthy condition.

General Anatomical Characters — Regarded from an anatomical point of view, the obvious textural changes here are precisely those of inflammatory action operating under the determining influence of the scrofulous diathesis   These changes are general or local   The former is exhibited—1 In wide-spread want of perfectly developed and carried out formative action, or the beginning of degenerative changes, seen in the unclosed urachus, with its lining membrane studded with a puriform varying-coloured aplastic material, the great blood-conduits and connective-tissue in which all are enclosed being texturally altered, with numerous circumscribed

17—2

abscesses and collections of soft cheesy-looking material , 2 In
retrogressive changes in the great gland-structures of the
abdomen and in the pulmonary substance, particularly its vascular part   The local structural changes, those confined to
the joints, are not restricted to one tissue, but are met with in
all. Not merely is the enveloping membrane thickened and
changed, and the capsule distended with fluid, but the cartilage
of encrustation, the bone epiphyses, and the cartilage of development are undergoing retrogressive changes   In the one case
there is rarefaction of the bone-tubes, and filling of them with
caseous material , in the other, the matrix of the cartilage
softens, and the cell-elements increase   And these do not
occur as results of the local inflammatory action, as merely a
further development and extension of the process, but are
seen in many instances at the very outset of the disease

Symptoms and Management of this Condition —The evidences
of this local development of a constitutional state of ill-health,
both of a systemic and local character, are sufficiently distinct
and attractive to enable us to distinguish it from every other
disease to which these young animals are liable

It is probably only when occurring as an enzooty or epizooty
that we are somewhat staggered to connect this general extension of the affection with an unhealthy condition of individual constitution   And even here we may be much assisted
by recollecting that this systemic deterioration has generally
been culminating for generations, and that a general eruption
is only determined by peculiar surrounding conditions   If we
are correct, or even nearly so, in attributing the general disturbance and extensively distributed change of tissue-elements,
as well as the local phenomena or alterations more intimately
related to the articulations, chiefly to the existence of an
indwelling disposition, an agency of evil operating from
within, and probably received as an inheritance from progeni-
tors, only culminating in extensive and serious manifestations
when adverse influences are brought to bear from without, it
will be easily understood how unsatisfactory all measures of
a curative character must be   The correct indications for the
control of all such disorders must move backwards long anterior to birth, and obtain in the parents such a condition of
vigorous health and freedom of taint from inherited disease, as

will ensure to the progeny a fair prospect, under favourable conditions, of ability to execute the ordinary functional activities necessary to ensure development of body and fitness for the purposes for which they are bred.

CHAPTER XV

LYMPHANGITIS—INFLAMMATORY ŒDEMA—WEED.

Definition—*A constitutional disturbance of variable extent in the process of assimilation, intimately associated with inflammatory action and œdema of one of the extremities ; this inflammatory action first showing itself in connection with the lymphatic glands of the limb, and during the continuance of the disease most distinctly manifest in these glands and in the course of the absorbents and bloodvessels.*

Pathology *a Character and Distribution*—Although its most diagnostic features are local, so much so that everywhere these have determined its ordinary name, modified, of course, by the amount of intelligence possessed by those who have observed it, there yet appear sufficient reasons from its history, distribution and modes of manifestation to warrant us in attributing it primarily to general disturbance of function, particularly in connection with the process of digestion and assimilation

Although this disease is widely distributed, not only in our own country but wherever horses are utilized, it is yet particular as to the subjects of its attack. Amongst well-bred horses, or those of the lighter draught variety, it is not common, the more highly susceptible are to be found amongst the heavier draught animals of dull, sluggish, or lymphatic temperaments, having an abundant growth of hair on their legs, and a large development of cellular tissue, while it is to be noted that even horses of this type possess a greater predisposition to suffer when reared on certain varieties of soil and under certain conditions In particular districts, at certain seasons and amongst certain classes of agricultural horses, this affection is extremely common, being only exceeded in frequency of manifestation by disorders of the

bowels and air-passages   In animals so predisposed very
slight disturbance of that natural equilibrium which ought to
subsist amongst the different steps of the assimilatory process
most surely tends to the appearance of this disorder

 b Nature.—Peculiarly a disease of hard work and exalted
functional activity, it is occasionally met with under opposite
conditions, and is intimately connected with the infringement
of certain dietetic and sanitary laws   Non-contagious and
generally susceptible of amelioration by treatment, it is still a
matter of much importance from its liability to recur, and the
certainty that after one or two seizures the structural alterations in connection with the absorbents of the limb, the
glandular structures, and surrounding tissue are such that
permanent thickening, unsightliness, weakness, and consequent
unsoundness are the result   It seems highly probable that
the first step in the act of derangement is in connection with
the passage into the blood of material appropriated during
intestinal digestion ; whether this is the result of simple
redundancy of material, or some abnormal action, chemical or
vital, it is rapidly extended to, and is first and most clearly
visible in that other process connected with the elaboration of
material for nutrition, in which the lymphatic glands and
vessels act so prominent a part   It is in this manner that
sudden alterations as to quantity or quality of nutriment
and enforced rest during seasons of good feeding and hard
work are found to act so powerfully as exciting causes , the
former of these we meet with in the case of horses being
rapidly made up in condition for sale or show, and the latter
in hard-worked and well-fed animals on being confined to the
stable on Sundays, or in consequence of weather or other unfavourable circumstances preventing their being employed as
usual

 In all the milder forms of the disease where fever and
general derangement are slight, there is evidently a disproportion between the nutritive material thrown into the system
and the powers of assimilation and excretion   This redundancy of nutritive pabulum is very early shown in the altered
condition of the blood   When abstracted in these cases the
alteration is shown by the increased tendency exhibited by
the formed and coloured constituents to separate from the

others, and to sink to the bottom of the vessel in which the blood may be received. Although it is rather difficult to form any correct estimate of either the character or the composition of blood from merely observing the mode of its solidification, the character of the clot, or the relative amount of this as compared with the fluid portion, seeing these are largely modified by various trifling circumstances, it is yet evident to any careful observer that something of an abnormal character exists, although he be not able to pronounce what the abnormality is Here there is little doubt that we have a more marked tendency than in health for the several elements, the formed or corpuscular and the liquid, to separate from each other, also that there is an appearance of want of stability in the red globules themselves, and a great inclination to aggregate in masses, that in the liquid portion there seems an increase in such nutritive materials as are represented by the fibrinogenous or fibrine-forming elements, and of albumen

Seldom, however, save in the most simple cases, is the local disorder confined to merely functional derangement, in a number, in addition to marked febrile disturbance, we have in the affected limb true congestive or inflammatory action. These morbid processes are the primary and active agents in the production of structural changes in the locality invaded; the material naturally resulting from inflammation of lymphatic glands and vessels is extravasated into the connective-tissue adjacent to these, it is rarely ever perfectly removed either by natural absorption or degenerative processes, but remaining in the situations where effused, becomes more or less perfectly organized. Like all other structures which have been the seat of such unhealthy actions, those connected with the limb where the local manifestations of this disease have occurred have conferred upon them not merely permanent functional incapacity but also structural weakness One feature connected with the manifestation of lymphangitis is deserving of notice, although it is difficult of explanation—we mean the preference which is shown for development of the local symptoms in the left hind-limb over all the others The fore-limbs, although liable to be invaded by the local diseased action, are much less so than the hind ones

c. *Causation* —Of the rather numerous causes operating in

the production of this disturbance, all may be grouped as—
1. *Intrinsic*, or those more properly belonging to the animal
itself, comprehending such as are spoken of as remote or predisposing, connected with speciality of individual temperament,
form, and organization—generally inherited 2 *Extrinsic*, those
more truly operating from without, comprehending (*a*) the
reception by the system of nutritive material in excess of the
natural waste or requirements and powers of disposal,
(*b*) disturbance of the balance which ought at all times to
exist amongst the different phenomena of the living body,
particularly those of food-assimilation, secretion and excretion,
whether this disturbance is brought about by the infringement
of hygienic laws, or by the action of adverse operating agencies
over which we may have little or no control

1. *Intrinsic Causes*—The hereditary or inherent tendency
of certain horses, under very trifling or even no apparent cause,
to contract this disease is a fact tolerably well known to all
who have paid any attention to the subject ; while there is
little doubt that it is simply because this and other cognate
matters associated with the physiology of breeding have not
been known, or if known, systematically ignored as to the
practical inferences to be drawn from the knowledge, that we
find distributed over the country so many constitutionally
faulty and unsound animals   Amongst the agricultural and
heavier breeds of horses, which are the great sufferers from
lymphangitis, there are various modifications of type   Some
there are with large, it may be, but compact and well-knit
muscular bodies, supported upon limbs well-placed in relation to
their bodies , and although their legs, below the knee and
hock, may be well clothed with hair, it is found that this hair
is rather long and soft than remarkable for thickness, that
these limbs in the metacarpal and metatarsal regions feel, on
being handled, clean and hard, the flexor tendons and great
suspensory ligament distinctly prominent, there being no filling
up of the spaces between bone and ligament, and ligament and
tendon, with soft, pulpy connective-tissue, the entire leg in this
region below the knee and hock having the appearance of
great breadth

Others, again, seem the opposite of all this : their bodies may
be bulky or of small size ; they invariably, however, give to the

observer the idea of defect in form and muscular tonicity
They seem soft, sluggish, and lacking energy, their limbs,
frequently badly placed in relation to the body, are apparently
of extra size, not, however, so much from increase of muscular development as from abundance of connective-tissue, which in the
inferior part of the limb confers upon it a full rounded appearance,
and imparts to the hand a sensation of general filling up or
padding between bone and ligament, and ligament and tendon,
the entire limb taking the character of rotundity and puffiness,
not, as in the others, of flatness and firmness of texture, the
hair is generally inclined to be thick and abundant rather
than long and silky It is amongst horses of this latter
character, of lymphatic temperament, bulky, badly-formed,
sluggish, and having full, rounded legs covered with a profu-
sion of coarse, thick-set hair, and showing a great amount of
connective-tissue distributed throughout the body, that we find
the greatest predisposition to weed

2 *Extrinsic Causes* —Of the factors operating from without
in the production of this disturbance of function and subsequent structural changes, the most potent—in connection with
congenital disposition—is probably the importation into the
system of nutritive material above the normal demands or
wants of the animal, and which may not be utilized by converting it into a source of reserve   It is perfectly possible, we
know, to throw into the animal economy a greater amount of
nutritive material than is required to replace the usual waste
and to allow for increase of growth, and yet this excess of
nutriment to do no positive injury, it being set aside as a
source of reserve   Here, however, whether the material provided in excess is too rapidly supplied, or whether it is
generally of the variety not most readily converted into fat,
the formation of a source of reserve nutrition is less likely
to be the result of a rapidly increased supply of nutritive
material than the production of a disordered state of assimilation

The powers of those vessels connected with nutrition,
suddenly called upon to bear a great strain, are over-taxed,
and gradually or at once they become incapable of exercising
their natural functions   Over-taxed and over-loaded, the
change from disturbed function to alteration of structure, the

result of inflammatory action in connection with both lymph
glands and vessels, is natural and easy

The same engorgement, arrest of functional activity, and
irritation is as apt to follow any great and sudden change in
the habits and work of horses as they are in the case of the
supply in excess of nutritive material This is particularly
evident with horses which have for some time been doing
good regular work, and receiving a full supply of even wholesome food on a sudden cessation or lessening of the work
done The absorbent and lymph vessels, in such cases
regularly and for a lengthened period kept in tone and full
activity by the steady muscular contraction and movement of
the limbs, and by the regularity with which their contents
are disposed of in the regular exercise of animal activity, at
once and suddenly receiving a check, engorgement and irritation follow, not because an extra amount of nutritious
material may be poured into the system through the primary
digestion, but because the activity in the secondary is suddenly brought to a stand by the non-demand for its products,
owing to arrested animal functions It is in this way that we
account for the occurrence of weed amongst our hard-worked
full-fed city and town dray and heavy draught horses on
Monday mornings

Rarely in country districts is this disease encountered
where we cannot trace it to an over-supply of food or to
enforced idleness on account of vicissitudes of weather, or to
both combined

Sudden and prolonged exposure of horses to depressing
atmospheric influences, as cold and moisture, after smart exertion, even when previously in the enjoyment of the fullest
amount of health and vigour, will often in certain animals
develop an attack of weed by suddenly disturbing or arresting
normal functional activities connected with digestion and food-
assimilation

Although most frequently encountered and chiefly interesting to us as a systemic or constitutional disturbance terminating in local structural changes, lymphangitis is sometimes seen as simply local inflammation of the absorbent
vessels of the limb or other parts of the body, the result of
injuries In the limbs the most fruitful cause of this form of

lymphangitis and lymphadenitis is that of wounds to the feet from foreign bodies, as nails picked from the ground, or carelessly driven in the act of shoeing

In all these cases, however, the character of the inflammatory action in both vessels and glands is considerably different from what occurs in the constitutional affection Although the lymph-glands may be early involved in the morbid action, they are rarely the part from which we observe the action to originate, this is generally in the course of the vessels themselves and in the inferior portion of the limb, not as in the systemic disturbance, where the inflammation and consequent pain and swelling obviously spring from the inguinal or brachial glands, and steadily proceed in a downwarddirection.

d. Anatomical Characters.—It is rarely that uncomplicated lymphangitis results in death, the great majority of cases making recoveries more or less perfect, and under many forms of management and medical treatment. When a fatal result is attributable to an attack of weed, death is usually the immediate sequel of irritation The structural lesions are nearly always confined to the situation of the local inflammation, where, to the unaided eye, they are plainly marked. The general swelling of the whole limb is the most distinctive feature, the greater amount of œdema existing at the superior surface in the inguinal region. When the skin is removed from the limb the subcutaneous tissue and the fascia are found loaded with a yellowish-coloured imperfectly organized lymph, which in cases of long continuance, or where several attacks have previously occurred, on being cut into disclose the fact that the natural fibrous stroma or framework of the connective-tissue is increased in amount or hypertrophied, that it is toughened, and more distinctly fibrillated or indurated than in health. The interconnective tissue existing amongst the muscular and other structures is changed and infiltrated in a similar manner; to this tissue the vessels, particularly the lymphatics, seem intimately united, so much so that these latter are rather difficult to demonstrate. The gland-structures in the inguinal region are swollen, their intimate connective-tissue hypertrophied and infiltrated with a similar fluid; while if decidedly chronic the true gland-texture, in addition to in-

creased volume, feels firm and indurated ; in recent cases, parts
of this structure may have become softened and broken down,
forming small circumscribed abscesses.

Occasionally the glands of the mesentery and of the abdomen are found enlarged and infiltrated with a hyaline or gelatinous straw-coloured exudate, and the abdominal cavity contains a considerable amount of a similarly coloured fluid

In the very well-marked cases of elephantiasis, the skin
itself is much thickened, the hypertrophy seemingly occurring
in the fibro-vascular structures of the dermis ; in this situation
the organization of the material effused has been more perfect
than in the meshes of the subcutaneous and intermuscular
tissue The corrugation or doubling of the skin in this condition does not seem, on more careful examination, to be folding
of the whole structures, but rather to spring from its vascular
or papillary layer, as if a hypertrophy merely of this particular
portion, which, however, carries the more superficial structures
along with it The lymph-glands in these very chronic cases
are sometimes found infiltrated with calcareous material,
giving a feeling of grittiness when divided with a knife

Symptoms—The symptoms of weed are very obviously
separable into two classes : (1) Local, which are the truly
diagnostic ; (2) Constitutional or general, common to this and
many other affections

1 *Local*—The horse is found lame in the morning, most
probably no suspicion having been excited on being left on the
previous evening Although there are cases which at first
rather puzzle us as to the cause of lameness, in the majority
there is little difficulty, while in all a careful examination
will direct us to its origin. In making these examinations,
a short history of the case will materially assist us, always
remembering that enforced rest in the midst of hard work,
and liberal feeding, are exceedingly likely to induce this disease , also the breed and character of the animal under
observation.

Swelling and tenderness are first shown in connection with
the lymphatic glands in the inguinal or brachial region. The
swelling, which at first may not be large, is tolerably firm,
although truly œdematous, slightly irregular, from the nodulated character of the gland-structure, and is more extensive

in an antero-posterior direction, it feels hot, is very painful when manipulated, and sometimes bedewed with perspiration

Gradually the swelling extends downwards, first as a narrow line in the course of the vessels, steadily extending in breadth until it covers the greater part of the inner surface of the limb to which it is confined until the hock or knee is reached, from which point to the foot both sides of the limb are involved, and, with the pain and lameness, increases in severity until the crisis is reached, when all are stationary for a day or two. In severe cases, where the distension of tissue is great, a slight serous exudation is seen and felt over the inner surface of the limb in the course of the vessels, particularly at the flexures of the joints, the hocks, and fetlocks

From the first appearance of these local symptoms until they reach their full development, the pain and lameness are persistent, if not of gradual increase.

2. *General.*—Immediately succeeding, or synchronous with, the appearance of these local symptoms, is the manifestation of the constitutional fever. It is, however, highly probable, were particular attention bestowed on each individual case, that the constitutional disturbance would be found in every instance to precede the local changes

Between these two classes of symptoms, the constitutional and local, there is exhibited, as regards their severity, a direct relation to and mutual dependence on each other, a high development of the one never occurring while the others are in abeyance

Like the local symptoms of œdema, pain, and lameness, this fever or constitutional disturbance is sthenic in its nature, and moves rapidly through its different stages of development. It is occasionally ushered in by the shivering-fit so common to most febrile disorders; the pulse is early indicative of much systemic disturbance, from its normal standard of forty-five to fifty beats in the minute it is increased to seventy-five or ninety-five, the artery feeling tense and cord-like under the finger; the respirations unaffected in mild cases, become hurried, short, and catching in the more severe. The internal temperature is elevated two or three degrees, the mouth feels clammy, the bowels inclined to be confined, while the urine, not at first increased in amount, is of higher specific gravity than natural

In addition to these, which we may consider the more truly diagnostic symptoms, there is greater or less impairment of appetite, an increased desire for fluids, slight restlessness, sometimes amounting to colicky pains, and an anxious expression of countenance, with repeated turning of the head and pointing with the muzzle backwards

Course and Termination—Although the local manifestations both of functional disturbance and of tissue-change connected with lymphangitis may continue for a lengthened period ere they are completely removed, in their acute characters they are of comparatively short duration. Both general and local symptoms continue to increase in severity for twenty-four or forty-eight hours, when, having attained their height, they remain stationary for at least a similar period before any distinct sign of defervescence is obvious Rarely do we encounter any serious complications during the development of the constitutional disturbance, while, when such do occur, they are usually pneumonic or enteric ; the latter are the more serious In the ordinary and uncomplicated cases of lymphangitis, the general symptoms, as a rule, defervesce before any change except the abatement of pain takes place in the extent or severity of the local. The absorption and removal of the exudate characteristic of the disease is in no case so rapidly accomplished as its extravasation, while where the vessels and connective-tissue of the limb have been weakened and lost their tonicity through previous disturbance and invasions of a similar nature, or where the material thrown out as the result of the inflammatory action has been largely composed of fibrine-producing agents, the removal of the adventitious material is always more tedious, and never perfectly completed.

In all recurring attacks there is at each fresh invasion less chance of a good recovery ; the whole vascular and inter-connective tissues of the offending member are steadily and in an ever-increasing ratio weakened, the material effused on each succeeding disturbance is added to the organized remains of the extravasate of the formerly existing disease, to be itself in all probability organized, and thus adding so much to the existing abnormality and weakened condition   These repeated attacks, even in a mild form of lymphangitis, resulting in hypertrophy and induration of the interconnective-tissue of the limb, ultimately terminate in permanent organization of the products which, from the appearance conferred upon the skin, and the truly fibroid condition of the cellular connective-tissue, the result of the often-recurring diseased action and steadily progressive change of the exudate, has received the name of 'Elephantiasis,' or 'Elephantiasis fibroma' These cases of chronic lymphangitis are always the result of several attacks, rarely of one, of the disease, and very often these are not of the most severe character, but follow closely upon each other. while I have remarked further that such as terminate in this chronic induration and hypertrophy of the inter-connective-tissue of the limb, are more frequently attacks upon the absorbents themselves than of the glands, or of the glands and absorbents combined

When fairly established this condition is very marked, the entire bulk of the limb is much augmented, the hair is removed in patches, while the skin is rough and coriaceous-looking, sometimes projecting in ridges or folds, generally dry and scaly, more rarely moist and exhalent

In the course of the diseased action which has invaded the subcutaneous tissue, the skin has become involved, for it is also in its fibro-vascular structure, its papillary and connective-tissue layers, become hypertrophied and indurated. Not all cases, even after repeated attacks, terminate in this condition, but only particular instances, while, even when observing cases of the disease, it is not possible to indicate the ones which shall terminate in this manner.

Occasionally, as the result of a first or second severe attack, we have the formation chiefly on the inner aspect of the limb of disseminated abscesses The occurrence of these is some time subsequent to the disappearance of the systemic fever, when the infiltration of the limb not showing signs of lessening, we may, on examination, discover some circumscribed portions of tissue where it is evident, from the increased heat and pain, that inflammatory action is in active progress; it may never have subsided, or a fresh exacerbation may have been established. The detached portions of tissue become distended, slightly elevated, gradually soften on the top, and bursting, dis-

charge more or less of a not very well-conditioned pus, leaving
an angry-looking sore, which, after a little, is disposed to heal
The abscesses are generally situated in and confined to the
subcutaneous connective-tissue, and only implicate the skin in
the process of pus-formation by the pressure of contained fluid
They are usually found in the vicinity of joints, with which
I have never seen them communicate; the sheaths of certain
tendons, however, are sometimes involved.

Diagnosis—The diseased conditions with which lymphangitis
may be confounded are those where we find local swellings or
infiltrations, accompanied with constitutional fever, as the
diagnostic features   Both of these conditions, the general and
local, are seen in ' Purpura hæmorrhagica,' ' Erysipelas,' ' Scarlatina,' in ' Farcy glanders,' and some other affections.   From
all these, however, it is sufficiently distinguished by variations
in the local symptoms chiefly, which ought to prevent any
careful observer from mistaking it for any of them.

From purpura it is to be distinguished by the absence of
swellings about the head and throat, which are so common in
that disease, while the tumefaction of the limbs in purpura,
when these occur, are totally different   In lymphangitis the
swellings extend over the whole limb, beginning in the inguinal
region, and moving downwards ; in purpura they may start into
existence on any part of the surface in the form of circumscribed
patches   In this disease there are no blood-markings or
petechiæ on mucous membranes, and no effusion of blood as in
purpura.   With erysipelas it is more likely to be confounded,
still the character of the local swelling is different.   In that
disease the swellings, equally painful as in lymphangitis, start
into existence, not at the glands in the superior part of the
limb, but usually in the median portion, these are also more
disposed to form open sores by sloughing of the skin, while
petechiæ and blood-markings on exposed membranes are not
uncommon   From scarlatina it differs by the absence of
angina, the want of the blood-markings on the visible mucous
membranes, and from the fact that the local changes of the
skin are, in scarlatina, quite superficial, and do not seem to
affect—certainly not by inflammatory action—those tissues
subjacent to the skin.

With farcy it has, in common, an inflamed and swollen con-

dition of the lymphatic vessels and glands ; the swelling, however, is different. In lymphangitis the swelling originates in
the superior gland-structures of the limbs, and extends to the
absorbents, producing uniform and general infiltration of the
connective-tissue In farcy, the swelling more often originates
by the production of papules, around which infiltration takes
place, and from which it extends and spreads in different directions The sores, too, when such exist, differ in position and
character

Treatment—The course of treatment all but universally
adopted in the management of this disease is the antiphlogistic
Generally regarded as one of those disturbances which are most
successfully combated by the early employment of free blood-
letting in conjunction with active purgation, the same system
has been advocated and carried out in all stages, and under
somewhat opposing conditions Although I have pursued this
treatment largely, and observed its action carefully, I am
satisfied that it does not in every case yield the results we
desire, and that in its general employment much discrimination
is needed In cases where the attack of lymphangitis may be
associated with, or follow as a sequel of, some debilitating
disease, blood-letting is counter-indicated Local bleeding,
either from the greater saphena vein, or the circumflex of the
foot, formerly much extolled, does not possess anything to
recommend it in preference to the now more commonly adopted
practice of taking blood from the jugular ; while, beside other
disadvantages, it is open to the objection of inflicting a wound,
which, from the diseased action in the limb, is likely to prove
troublesome in the further local treatment of the case

Of the beneficial results to be obtained from the general
employment of mild purgatives in lymphangitis there are
fewer doubts, although, like every other curative means, they
are capable of being abused , excessive purgation being here
apt to result in enteric complications, or congestion of the
lungs or feet In the early stages of the disease, and where
the febrile symptoms are marked and persistent, it will always
be advantageous to administer every three or four hours a little
of the ordinary saline febrifuge mixture—composed of nitrate,
or chlorate of potash, or both, with solution of acetate of
ammonia, and sweet spirits of nitre—to which from four to six

18

minims of Fleming's tincture of aconite have been added; or, taking advantage of the thirst usually present, sulphate of soda or magnesia may be given liberally in the drinking-water. Following the action of the purgative, it is good to administer daily, or every alternate day, a mild diuretic, to which, in some cases, may be added with advantage twenty to thirty grains of calomel. When the disturbance is in any way connected with a previous state of debility the calomel should be withheld, and a similar quantity of sulphate of iron substituted

As respects local treatment, the best is fomentation with simple warm water; this relieves the tension of the vessels, favours effusion, lessens pain, and so reduces the fever and systemic disturbance. It is most readily applied through the medium of woollen bandages, or loosely twisted hay or straw bands wound from the foot upwards, and as high as it is possible. When the pain is distressing, and in very sensitive animals, relief is obtained by the addition of a little laudanum to the warm water employed in the fomentations; this is most economically done by adding it to a limited quantity of water at the termination of each act of fomentation

As soon as the animal is able to take a little exercise, the fomentations may be discontinued, and moderate friction with the hand and a little oil substituted; while where there exists disinclination to move, enforced exercise is generally beneficial, and the application, when in the stable, of dry woollen bandages

Throughout the course of the disease a careful regulation of the dieting must be attended to. The indication at first is by lessening the supply of nutritive material, and by presenting such as may be deemed needful in the least stimulating or irritating form, to give the organs connected with food-assimilation as much rest as possible, an increase of stimulating nutriment to be given when the needs of the system demand it, or the organs are capable of appropriating it, but not until then In cases where the limb has suffered from more than one attack, and where there is much thickening from organization of diseased products, but following the subsidence of the acute symptoms of the fever, the employment of iodine both internally and externally is often of benefit. Internally, it ought to be given twice daily in a soluble form as the compound solution, which in some cases is taken in the drinking-water, but if not, it must be exhibited in draught

A very good preparation in many of these conditions is Donovan's solution, given in moderate but repeated doses for some time

Externally, the most useful form is the compound iodine ointment, applied with gentle friction all round, but chiefly on the inner surface of the limb, once daily   This last treatment may be persevered with even while the horse is doing moderate work, which, if it is possible for it to engage in, is rather an advantage than otherwise.   Issues, in the forms known as rowels or setons, smart blistering, or even the actual cautery, applied over different parts of the limb, have been, and are even yet, employed, with a view to reduce the unsightly swelling, and thereby restore the natural freedom of movement, none of these, however, seem to yield results superior or even equal to the more easily applied and more humane treatment which has already been indicated.

CHAPTER XVI

PURPURA HÆMORRHAGICA

Definition —*A general or systemic disease intimately connected with or having its origin in extensive changes of the blood and capillary bloodvessels, characterized by the presence of petechiæ or blood-spots on the mucous membranes, and by the existence of elevations of the cutaneous tissue. From the mucous membranes there is hæmorrhage, and from the cutaneous swellings an oozing of bloody coloured serum. There is also a disposition to blood-extravasations in internal organs*

Pathology. *a Nature*—Although the diseased condition of the horse recognised by the term Purpura hæmorrhagica is now pretty well known, and is rarely confounded with any other, there is yet little agreement as respects its pathology, which, besides being disputed, is but imperfectly understood   We are not agreed as to the interpretation of, or the value which ought to be placed on, the several symptoms which mark the

18—2

development of the disease. By some it has been regarded
and spoken of as essentially a local affection, as a disease of
the cutaneous tissue; this is clearly not correct, seeing that
during its progress we have evident and severe constitutional
disturbance manifested by disorder of nearly all the functions
of the animal body, while we find that with marvellously
trifling cutaneous manifestations there are not unfrequently
serious constitutional phenomena; that the local changes bear
no adequate relation to the severity of the systemic disturbance. It is also, we are aware, most successfully combated not
by local remedies, but by the employment of constitutional
means, and is most liable to terminate fatally when the constitutional character of the affection is overlooked or ignored.
By others it has been classed with the charbonous diseases,
and spoken of as a form of anthrax; this at the present, and
with the knowledge we possess, seems also a wrong estimate of
its nature.

Unlike anthrax in its varied forms, it does not appear
capable of propagation by infection or inoculation, nor has
there yet been demonstrated to exist in the blood of animals
suffering from this disease the specific organisms of pure
anthrax. The local swellings, too, both as to character, mode
of development, and their relation to the termination of the
disease, are totally different in purpura from those of
anthrax.

Peculiarly a disease of the horse rather than of our other
patients, it is chiefly but not exclusively met with as a sequel
of such exhausting febrile disorders as influenza, strangles, or
even common catarrh. Largely a disease of debility, it appears
to consist in a morbid condition of the blood and capillary
bloodvessels, from which there results a marked disposition to
effusion or extravasation of blood in connection with the skin
and mucous membranes. Although there may be doubts as to
the exact nature of the changes which occur in the earlier
stages of purpura, the most rational explanation of the phenomena seems that which refers these to alterations in the conditions, vital and chemical, of the blood, and to certain
structural changes of the capillary bloodvessels.

We speak of it as referable to a morbid state of the blood
and bloodvessels; still we are inclined to believe that these

morbid conditions of tissue-elements are not invariably of one and the same character, and that these differences of abnormality originate from different causes, manifest themselves in somewhat different ways, and in their management demand somewhat different treatment.

In one form we have certainly an altered condition of the blood itself as the most prominent feature of the disturbance, but even this alteration may not be invariably of the same character. There is evidence that it presents itself for our consideration in at least two forms: 1 In what we may term the aqueous condition, where an excess of water is present and a deficiency of albumen and fibrine factors. 2 A condition in which the colloids of the blood, the albumen and fibrine-producing materials, are in undue solution, and probably also the formed materials, the blood-globules. While in many, if not in all, there is another, a third, abnormal condition which must be taken into consideration—viz, the changes which the capillaries have undergone, most probably textural degeneration, by which the blood-elements are allowed to transude and permeate the surrounding tissues.

It is deserving of remark that, troublesome and serious-looking as the cutaneous patchy elevations resulting from the capillary extravasation are, they cannot be taken as true or good indices of the amount of danger attendant on the attack; the greatest danger in connection with which is the chance of blood-extravasation into the intimate texture of, or in connection with, organs and structures essential to life.

Although the accompanying fever as a rule is not great, weakness and prostration are marked features. The weakness we can understand, as well as the marasmus, when we observe the imperfectly carried on assimilatory functions and great tissue-waste; these indicated by the altered state of the nutritive fluid, the blood, and the excreted fluid, the urine. The former of these is to a considerable extent rendered unfit for healthy nutrition from both physical and chemical changes; the latter becomes increased in density from excess of tissue-elements, the result of increased tissue-change.

b *Causation*—Although it may seem a perfectly rational way of accounting for the phenomena characteristic of purpura hæmorrhagica, and in no way doing violence to our ideas of the fitness of things and the relation of sequence and cause, to attribute the occurrence of the disease to the natural effects of such exhausting diseases as prolonged catarrh or influenza, effects specially showing themselves in a deteriorated condition of the fluid tissue, the blood, there are still cases where we encounter this disease in which it would appear, at least as far as we can discover, that such deteriorating influences are not and have not been in operation. Carefully and impartially giving all supposed causes their due consideration, and placing them in connection with ascertained facts relating to the disease, it would seem that all which minister to the production of this peculiar condition are capable of being grouped as causes indigenous and causes exogenous, the former probably predominating

Seeing that purpura is to a great extent a disease of the blood and capillary bloodvessels, we must look for the chief cause of its production to those influences which operate in disturbing or preventing the healthy formation of blood And as we are aware that the fluid tissue, blood, is the result of the action of formative processes in connection with these combinations of phenomena we call primary and secondary digestion, any impairment or disturbance in the details of these will operate injuriously in the formation of this tissue, which depends for its support and correct maintenance on the regular and healthy action of these activities. It is only by placing its causes first of all on such broad bases as these that we can in some degree comprehend how, if it be true—of which none entertain any doubt—that purpura, largely encountered as a sequel of certain exhausting diseases, and peculiarly a disease of debility, should also be met with under conditions apparently the opposite. It is seen to follow exhaustive catarrhal diseases where animal force and tissue-formative power in every structure are largely impaired and at the minimum, and when every organ and function are depressed by the presence in the system of materials which, having served their purpose, are now changed and effete, and ought to be eliminated, but which from some functional disturbance are still retained, and by their further disintegration and change render the blood impure. It is also, although not so frequently, seen where the animals are seemingly in perfect health, and their

condition, instead of showing exhaustion, indicates plethora
When observed in these latter conditions, however, it will be
found on examination that the animals, although to appearance plethoric, are not in full and vigorous health, that the
fulness of body is the result of defective, unnatural and unhealthy dietetic conditions, that the material upon which they
have been fed has not been calculated to produce healthy and
well-elaborated blood-tissue

Animals in either of these conditions when exposed to such
direct adverse influences as proceed from improper location,
and particularly such as result from imperfect ventilation,
defective drainage, effluvia arising from decomposing animal
or vegetable matter, are extremely liable to experience a rapid
and full development of those tissue-changes which have
already been faintly traced out and rendered possible

Thus, although undoubtedly true that the causes acting
in determining the production of purpura may often seem
rather obscure or apparently conflicting, not operating with
what we may regard as uniformity, we may, nevertheless, see
through all cases traces of certain general laws which regulate
its appearance, and thus be able to follow in detail the inducing
agencies of many individual developments of the phenomena
characteristic of the disease

c *Anatomical Characters*—The earliest and most extensively affected tissue, the blood, is altered in general appearance
and intimate characters; it is darker than natural, possessing
greater tenuity, or a disposition for the watery portion to
separate itself from the other constituents, it is not disposed to
coagulate either in or without the vessels   Examined more
minutely, there is often a preponderance of watery constituents
and an alteration of the red globules, these have in part
become destroyed, they are shrivelled in appearance, as if their
contained material had become lessened, and they occasionally
become heaped together in mass; the amount of colourless
corpuscles is increased

The cutaneous swellings, which were so diagnostic during
life, show on removal of the skin a condition of infiltration
with more or less blood-stained imperfectly coagulated gelatinous material, the infiltration extending throughout the subcutaneous connective-tissue, and the colouring matter, apart from

the jelly-like exudate, marking the underlying muscular tissue This exudate does not, in the depositions of longest duration, show any disposition to fibrillate or become organized   In some instances these local cutaneous swellings, in addition to the peculiar colloid or jelly-like and coloured exudate, have true extravasation of blood as blood, and this, when so met with, possesses the characters already spoken of, excessive tenuity, altered state of the red corpuscles, and indisposition to form coagula.

In the greater number of cases of the ordinary type, next to the obvious changes in the blood and general connective-tissue, the most striking are those pertaining to the great serous cavities and structures   Petechiæ, vibices, and larger blood-markings are observed on the peritoneum, sometimes on the pleuræ, more often on the peri- and endo-cardium, and occasionally on the membranes of the cerebro-spinal centres. In the cavities with which these several membranes are related we have also not unfrequently a considerable quantity of a more or less highly coloured fluid, the quantity varying with the obvious extent of the tissue-changes which the structures have undergone, particularly with the extent of the blood-markings or extravasations into the subserous struc-tures

In some instances there is, in addition to the blood-markings on the visceral layer of these membranes, a collection of the characteristic coloured gelatiniform exudate found so largely in other situations   This is oftenest seen connected with the kidneys and heart

The mucous tract of the elementary canal, particularly in the intestinal portion, may show scattered ecchymoses or larger blood-stainings, and more rarely in the ordinary cases turgescence of the mucous membrane, from infiltration into the submucous connective-tissue. When during life we have had much abdominal pain, either with or without blood being mingled with the natural discharges, free blood will be found in the canal, or the fæcal matter and ingesta extensively coloured, from admixture with blood or blood-products.

The glands of the mesentery, as might be supposed from their connection with the process of assimilation, are visibly altered in character; they are enlarged, somewhat changed in colour, and of greater friability than in health. Most probably all these changes are the direct result of structural alteration, closely related to effusion of fluid material into the intimate texture of both cortical and medullary portions; the lymph-spaces, or alveoli, are certainly distended, and the trabeculæ stretched and less resistant

Both the liver and spleen are somewhat texturally altered. This alteration, however, is not of a constant or uniform character, either in the organs themselves and individually, nor as to the relative extent to which they are severally affected

Sometimes the liver is simply congested; at others there is obvious want of colour and great friability. When this organ is comparatively little involved the spleen will most probably show greater changes; these are chiefly in connection with the composition and character of the blood which it contains, and the relative amount as compared with its normal condition. The lungs, besides the petechial markings which may exist on their pleural surfaces, are congested and engorged with blood, presenting the same general characters as are exhibited by it in other situations and tissues of the body, while there is often, in the smaller bronchi, a quantity of rusty coloured spume.

It is certainly not always the case that the whole of these morbid appearances are presented equally well developed in all fatal cases of purpura. The ordinary forms are those where the lesions and peculiar vascular changes are more distinctly marked and of a dominant character in one organ or region of the body, being much less distinctive elsewhere. It is perfectly possible that a fatal result may occur with little or no extravasation apart from the petechial markings on certain mucous and serous membranes

Symptoms—Although purpura hæmorrhagica in the horse does show itself as an idiopathic affection unassociated with other diseased conditions, it is yet most frequently encountered, as we have already said, as the result or sequel of some other affection, particularly of the air-passages and organs of respiration

When associated with such diseases as catarrh, strangles, or influenza, it is not found developing during the height of the febrile symptoms, nor even at the period of defervescence; it is usually when the condition of convalescence has been so far entered upon that good hopes are entertained of a speedy restoration to health   Nor from the previous history of the character, course, or severity of the primary fever can we with certainty predict what cases are likely to be followed by this troublesome affection ; the mildest as well as the most severe attacks of these fevers are alike liable to have this condition attendant on their dispersion

Usually the earliest symptom which awakens our suspicion, or which yields indications of the onset of purpura, is the appearance of the local swellings   These swellings are diagnostic ; they are sudden in their appearance, occurring in different parts of the body, generally the limbs, the abdomen, or the head, particularly the inferior portion of the face and around the nostrils and mouth   They are sometimes limited or in patches, often uniform when in connection with the limbs, always elevated above the level of the surrounding skin, and terminating abruptly, not gradually by shading off into the level of surrounding parts   They are tense, pitting slightly on pressure, but neither very hot nor very painful. They owe their existence to the transudation of blood or degraded blood-constituents into the subcutaneous connective-tissue.

In a number of cases, after a variable period, bullæ, or vesicles, appear, and rupturing, discharge a reddish-coloured serosity, or a uniform oozing of a similar material may occur instead   The fluid thus discharged is disposed to irritate the parts with which it comes in contact, and further to induce discomfort by hardening in cakes, ultimately cracking and disposing to fissures in the skin   When occurring in the region of the head these swellings are more disposed to coalesce than elsewhere, presenting a somewhat uniform appearance, most severe over and around the nostrils and the angles of the mouth, seldom extending above the eyes

A feature quite characteristic of these, particularly in the early stages of the disease, is the disposition which they exhibit to suddenly disappear and again return, probably in a more severe form either at the original situation or at a part as yet uninvaded, and that with their return there is an increase or exacerbation of the other existing untoward symptoms   This disappearance of local swellings and subsidence of symptoms may occur oftener than once during the course of the disease.

In some special instances, where these elevations are particularly well developed over the floor of the abdomen, the skin loses its vitality, and becomes removed by sloughing, leaving an ulcerous, ill-conditioned sore, not much disposed to heal.

Very early in the course of the disease, or it may be delayed for some time, is the altered condition of the lining membrane of the nasal cavities. It is at first merely heightened in colour, and studded with petechiæ, which gradually extend, chiefly by coalescing, until they cover the greater portion of the septum which is visible, and steadily assume a darker colour or they may be observed to alter in colour, as also in extent, with the changes and remissions of the other symptoms When these blood-spots and submucous blood-extravasations are fairly established in connection with the nasal structures, we observe that a sero-sanguineous fluid, or blood, of a darker colour than natural, and not disposed to coagulate, trickles from the nostrils. This condition of vascular disturbance, when observed in connection with the nasal membranes, is probably very extensively distributed throughout the body in connection with the cutaneous structures and mucous membranes, and is only not a regularly observed symptom because of the pigmented and largely developed epidermic portion of the one and the hidden character of the other

From the infiltration of the subcutaneous tissue of the external, and the submucous of the upper and internal air-passages, and consequent swelling, the breathing becomes embarrassed or accompanied with a troublesome cough

Fever, although rarely absent, is seldom a very prominent feature The pulse is more frequent than in health, soft, or thready and weak, the respirations accelerated, and the internal temperature increased by 3° or 4° F

There is usually impaired appetite all through the course of the disease, sometimes refusal to take anything for days, digestion invariably weak, bowels rather inclined to be confined

Occasionally very early in the development of the affection, usually after the diagnostic symptoms have been fully matured, and in severe cases on the occasion of a remission of symptoms and their renewed appearance, local blood-extravasations, either extensive or more restricted, occur in connection with internal structures and organs essential to life , such internal extravasations are very serious, and are characterized by sudden and fatal collapse, or by the development of symptoms indicative of disturbance or change of those organs in connection with which the blood-extravasation has occurred

Course and Termination —When purpura hæmorrhagica is fully established, and the diagnostic symptoms indicative of the peculiar blood-changes have declared themselves, if the diseased condition does not rapidly terminate in a fatal issue its course is generally protracted

During the continuance of the disease we cannot say that any definite, well ascertained, and clearly marked out course belongs to it. The character of the symptoms, taken in entirety, may be regarded as decidedly intermittent This very character is often the cause of much disappointment, the animal being, on the subsidence of the more severe and diagnostic symptoms, apparently on the way to convalescence, but when seen again, all have reappeared with greater severity, and without any cause for this accession, as far as we are able to discover The existence of unhealthy sores, resulting from death and removal of the skin over certain cutaneous swellings, seem to exercise an evil influence and to retard convalescence , or probably we ought rather to say that the existence of these unhealthy sores is more surely indicative of a greater deterioration of animal health and vigour than regard them individually as capable of retarding recovery.

When purpura hæmorrhagica does not kill by blood-effusion and tissue-change of organs essential to life, the subjects affected usually recover and ultimately regain their previous condition , there are, however, exceptions where, although not fatal, the lesions occurring as sequelæ of the disease permanently invalid and debilitate the animal, and some, such as those of a cardiac nature, may prove fatal years after the disappearance of the causes from which these changes have originated. The ordinary form which the disease assumes, or rather, we should say, the conditions in which it terminates when convalescence is not established, are those of the formation of abscesses in various glands, and the infiltration of connective-tissue and parenchymatous organs, with pus and purulent matter, not unfrequently resulting in extensive tissue-change, gangrene, and pyæmia. These undesirable and fatal terminations may not with any certainty be predicted at the outset of the disease, seeing that cases which may at the first appearance of symptoms promise to terminate favourably, are found at last to develop the most intractable results, while others which begin unfavourably occasionally prove more responsive to treatment.

Diagnosis—Although distinctive enough in the great features of its development, purpura may yet be confounded with such diseases as scarlatina or erysipelas. From scarlatina it is distinguished—1 By the character of the cutaneous swellings; 2 By the nature of the blood-markings on the mucous membranes; 3 By the existence or not of angina.

In purpura the swellings, whether circumscribed or extensively distributed as over a whole limb, are always marked by the considerable elevation of these above the surrounding skin, and by the suddenness and the abrupt manner of their termination, they stop as if checked by a ligature.

In scarlatina there is little or no elevation, only a raising of the hair with a slight oozing and hardening from coagulation of the exuded fluid, and these conditions merge gradually into the surrounding tissues. In purpura the petechiæ or blood-spots on the mucous membranes, if not at the first much larger than in scarlatina, rapidly become so by coalescing, they are of a darker colour, and from the membrane on which they are situated a sero-sanguineous fluid, more bloody than in scarlatina, is found trickling, while it is not at all uncommon to find that in purpura these petechiæ take on disintegrative changes, the superficial membrane becoming removed and an ulcerous discharging sore remaining. This condition of circumscribed molecular death and ulcer-formation does not as a rule take place in cases of scarlatina.

Again, angina is usually a characteristic symptom of scarlatina, and is accompanied with swollen cervical glands and cough. Sore throat and cough, although met with in individual cases of purpura, are not regular, far less diagnostic, symptoms.

With erysipelas it may not be confounded because (1) of the difference in their systemic developments or symptoms. In erysipelas, fever is a most characteristic and constantly abiding phenomenon; in purpura it is less sthenic and not diagnostic. (2) From the variations in the character of their local features. In erysipelas the local phenomena are those of inflammatory action invading the skin and subcutaneous tissue. We have swelling, but not the swelling of purpura, it is steady, gradual, and continued, not remittent in character, acutely sensitive and painful. Its physical characters are also different in erysipelas from purpura; in the former it does not appear in patches and extend by coalescing; it is not, when occurring in any situation, sharply marked off and bounded as by a line. When destructive changes take place in the skin in erysipelas, they do so as the natural results of the active inflammatory process; when occurring in purpura, they are the outcome of another action entirely—death of intimate tissue-element is in it independent of the morbid action of inflammation. Although petechiæ may occur in erysipelas, they are less pronounced than in purpura, and rarely have we the sero-sanguineous or blood-discharge from the visible mucous membranes so characteristic of the latter affection. The subcutaneous infiltrations and swellings of the head and facial region, so marked in purpura, are rarely seen in erysipelas.

Treatment.—Although it is no uncommon circumstance to find that both the functional and structural changes associated with purpura are of so serious a character, developed so rapidly, and following closely on an already weakened system, that little hope can be entertained of aught save a fatal issue, there are yet many cases not marked by such malignant and rapidly fatal conditions, and where by judicious management much may be accomplished in the direction of arresting this termination.

Acting upon the conviction that serious results are usually immediately connected with changes in the vascular system, the blood, and minute bloodvessels, our efforts ought to be directed to the restoring of the lost equilibrium which naturally subsists between the several elements of the blood, and to

the maintenance of the blood-conduits in a healthy and
tonic condition, thereby lessening the tendency to effusion,
the characteristic local feature of the disease. There are,
it may be, many cases where the earliest efforts must be
directed to remove certain evil results which have attended
early symptoms, as blood extravasations and effusions in connection with certain internal organs and structures, which, if
not relieved, would still farther complicate and render more
serious existing conditions. When, however, these are
relieved, the first object of attention must be the cause or
source from which these have proceeded: the morbid state of
the blood and vascular system. This in every case is not
readily accomplished or attended with equal certainty, the
adverse conditions being most refractory in cases where
previous disease has lowered the vital force, disturbed assimilation in some of its many steps, and where exhaustion exists as
an established condition. When speaking of the pathology of
the disease we noticed the fact that it is extremely probable
that all forms of purpura may not be dependent on precisely
the same conditions or combinations, and that there seems good
reason to regard these as susceptible of amelioration by somewhat different modes of treatment. This may to a certain extent
explain the varying opinions given by different practitioners
with regard to the employment of the same agents and modes
of management, for in this respect there is much divergence
of opinion, which, concerning what might otherwise be regarded as simple matters of fact, is otherwise inexplicable.
In undertaking the treatment of any cases of purpura, it is
desirable for the success of our therapeutic treatment that
good sanitary conditions be enforced; for apart from any
consideration as to the power of indifferent sanitation
under certain states of inducing this disease, there is the
established evidence of fact and observation, that there is
probably no abnormal state of the horse in which the animal
is more susceptible of being acted upon unfavourably than in
purpura.

A number of cases evidently closely connected with the
fibrinogenous and other colloid elements being in a peculiar
and excessive state of solution, together with an excess of
water in the blood, seem most successfully treated by the

exhibition of certain salines, some acids, and terebinthinates
Of salines, the preparations of potash, particularly the chlorate,
are most largely employed, this latter for the first few days
may be given alone in three or four drachms two or three
times daily, and is readily enough taken in the food and
drinking-water, after this period we have generally preferred
to allow it in smaller doses—two drachms—combined with
one of the nitrate, and continued for some days longer. The
salts of iron usually employed are the sulphate or solution
of the perchloride—the former is to be preferred, combined
with diluted sulphuric acid—thirty grains of the sulphate
with half a fluid drachm of the acid in cold water twice or
thrice daily. This may either be given alternately from the
commencement of the treatment with the chlorate of potash, or
its administration may be deferred for some days, and then employed in this alternate manner   When benefit does not seem
to follow the use of the iron salt in conjunction with the
potash compound, when the local swellings do not give
evidence of subsidence, the substitution of the oil of turpentine
for the former is advisable, the quantities to be administered
being from six to ten fluid drachms in combination with
linseed oil, good gruel, raw eggs, or a combination of the last two

In those cases where exhaustion and depression are great,
and where sufficient food is not being taken into the system, a
steady but moderate stimulation is indicated, this may be
accomplished while the administration of the medicines already
mentioned is being carried out, and alcoholic are to be preferred to the ammoniacal stimulants.

As an agent capable of acting on the capillary bloodvessels
through the vaso-motor nerves, maintaining their tonicity and
general contractible power, ergot in some form or another has
been recommended, but from what I have observed and
learned of its results, it has not generally fulfilled the expectations entertained regarding it. This may arise from the fact
that when the cause of the blood extravasation or effusion is
connected with changes in the minute bloodvessels, it is less
owing to the simple want or loss of functional power in these
vessels than to degenerative or other changes in their textural
structure. From the use of the ordinary astringents, tannic and
gallic acid and acetate of lead, I have frequently seen very good

results   Blood-letting has by some been tried, and, as with
other modes of treatment, differently reported upon , theoreti-
cally this does not seem indicated, the animal having already
been depleted by the local extravasation , in practice, however,
in certain cases where the animals have been young and
strong, not previously weakened by antecedent disease, the
results of blood-letting have been satisfactory   When the
appetite is decidedly defective and exhaustion is imminent,
endeavours must be made to combat the exhaustion, and
render support to the animal by the steady exhibition regularly,
but in moderate amount, of such nutritive materials as good
beef-tea, milk, or raw eggs, which are severally improved by
having added to them a good proportion of such alcoholic
stimulants as port wine, brandy, or ale

When complications occur arising from changes in connection with internal organs, they must be met and combated
in accordance with the symptoms exhibited, never, however,
forgetting the primary disturbed assimilation and hæmal
changes

Respecting the treatment of the local swellings and subcutaneous infiltrations, opinion is somewhat divided as to the
benefits respectively of warm or cold applications   When of
moderate extent, particularly in the region of the head or
limbs, bathing frequently with cold water or some refrigerating
lotion seems to answer well, when these are extensive, involving the greater portion of the limbs or the upper and internal
air-passages, it is probable that warm-water applications are
better   Where the local swellings are of such magnitude that
the extent is seriously embarrassing, it may be needful to make
some effort to lessen these by scarifications, so allowing the
effused fluid to drain off, which may be favoured by fomentation and manipulation , generally, however, free scarification is
not to be recommended, as it is likely to favour the death and
sloughing of the parts cut.

When during the progress of the disease the skin over the
local swellings has become dead, and is removed by sloughing,
leaving unhealthy discharging sores, these are best treated by
attention to cleanliness, and daily washing with some antiseptic and healing wash, as a weak solution of chloride of zinc,
to which has been added a little carbolic glycerine   These

sores, although rather tardy in healing, ordinarily assume a better character as the general health improves; they may, however, from their extent, leave permanent and unsightly blemishes.

CHAPTER XVII.

SCARLATINA—SCARLET-FEVER

Definition.—*A peculiar febrile disease of the horse, usually accompanying or appearing as a sequel to some other general and debilitating disease, and characterized by the occurrence of petechiæ on the mucous membrane of the nose and mouth, and by a mild phlyctænoid or vesicular eruption of the skin in certain situations of the body, and accompanied with sore throat and swollen cervical glands*

Pathology. *a General Characters, Nature, etc*—This febrile disease of the horse, so named from its supposed resemblance to the well-known eruptive fever in man, seems, when we come to examine it more closely, to possess but a faint analogy to that. In man, scarlatina is a specific disease, the result of the reception of a specific virus, which is reproduced during the progress of the affection, which follows a certain determinate course, and as a rule occurs only once in a lifetime

In the horse, it rarely occurs as an independent or idiopathic disease: generally as an accompaniment or sequel of some other and debilitating affection, as influenza, strangles, etc , or when not associated directly with these, it seems to have some ill-defined relation to them   I have observed that when a severe visit of these eruptive fevers, measles and scarlatina, has occurred in a particular locality, that some idiopathic cases of this particular fever of the horse would show themselves, and that more than the average number of horses suffering from catarrhal affections would exhibit distinctive features of scarlatina   It does not in the horse seem to possess the power of propagating itself, only extending by contagion or infection in so far as the primary disease with which it is associated is so propagated ; nor am I aware that it has been produced by inoculation From the fact of its appearance in the great majority of cases in connection with some other disease, its existence is frequently overlooked, or if not passed over, it is regarded as an individual idiosyncrasy in the manifestation of the primary affection, from which, however, there seems sufficient reason that it should be considered separately.

It is not every case of debilitating catarrhal or other disease which develops or is followed by this special and depraved condition, nor can we with certainty predict which shall, save in so far as these are the result of infection or contagion developed from cases which have exhibited similar complications. I have observed that scarlatina has oftener been associated with debilitating diseases occurring during the spring than at other seasons of the year

Although local changes and alterations are largely concerned in the visible and appreciable manifestations of the disease, there is little doubt that the entire system is invaded, and the general functional activity much impaired; that the numerous local phenomena are merely manifestations of a marked constitutional dyscrasia

It may be regarded as a general rule that pyrexial symptoms precede the appearance of the local eruption; also, as we have already stated, that scarlatina in the horse is ordinarily a sequel of some other disease. It will generally be found that the fever of the primary affection has fairly declined ere that of the eruption is developed; this distinct intermittence I have repeatedly noted The eruption or markings occurring in the skin and mucous membranes seem the diagnostic symptoms of the disease; and if there is any specific poison, it is probably here and in this manner that it is expended

From the hairy covering and pigmented condition of the horse's skin, any slight variation in colour is unobservable, while the changes in the character of the eruption are also more difficult to determine. Of this eruption there are several forms In the horse, we have little difficulty in observing that it shows itself in at least two distinctive manners the smooth and the phlyctænoid In the smooth form, the skin, although elevated somewhat above the natural level, exhibits no perceptible change of character, no roughness or moisture; in the

19—2

phlyctænoid or vesicular, we have a number of minute vesicles charged with scrous fluid, which ultimately desiccate and are rubbed or fall of

Whatever is the particular character of the eruption, it is to be remarked that it rarely attacks the whole body, or all those parts of the body where it is ultimately found, at one and the same time The face and head are often first invaded, followed by the limbs, and latterly it may occupy the abdomen and the chest

Although not so distinctly characterized by appearing in successive crops, each separated from the one preceding it by a few days, as is the case in the human subject, this is yet often enough the manner in which the eruption shows itself to attract our attention It is also to be observed that, unlike many other of the eruptive fevers, the elevation of temperature incident to the pyrexial symptoms does not suffer much decline on the appearance of the eruption; while we also find that even after the desquamation of the desiccated exudate, persistent anasarca of the limbs, and more rarely of other parts of the body, remains Although in several of its general features resembling purpura hæmorrhagica, a careful examination of its symptoms, modes of development, and termination would appear to warrant a separation being made between these affections

By writers on human medicine, many varieties of scarlatina have been spoken of; in the horse there seems little difficulty in recognising at least two Essentially similar in their character and nature, these only differ in the manifestation of the severity of their symptoms—*scarlatina simplex* being the mildest manifestation of the fever; *scarlatina anginosa* merely a more severe attack, and where the force of the disease seems expended on the throat and upper air-passages

b. Causation.—Unlike scarlatina of man, we cannot say of this disease in the horse that to its existence in others and to that alone we must look for the source of the disease; for, as already stated, it does not in our patient appear to be produced by contagion in any instance Rather, in searching for the causes of this scarlatina of the horse, must we take fully and carefully into consideration, first, the condition of the patient; and secondly, the nature of the surroundings

The greater number of animal sufferers from this affection are those which, immediately antecedent to their giving evidence of this condition, have passed through some constitutional and debilitating disease.

The entire functional activities of the animal are below par; the system is yet charged with, or at least not entirely rid of, effete and deleterious matters, the result of morbid and excessive tissue-changes produced during previous diseased action If by any means, operating from without, the vital energies be further lowered, or the deleterious materials circulating in the blood be prevented from being eliminated, we can so far comprehend that the extrinsic influences acting in concert with those existing within will most probably culminate in the production of an unhealthy and vitiated state of the blood, and consequently of every other tissue Why this depraved condition of the blood should show itself in this particular and distinctive manner, and not in some others, we may not be able to tell With our present knowledge, we must probably accept this as an ultimate fact until better able to explain many other processes, healthy as well as diseased

In all cases of convalescence from disease, particularly general diseases of a lowering character, it is absolutely necessary, if we would reduce to the minimum the risk of the occurrence of this and other obscure—obscure, I mean, in the sense of their ætiology—blood diseases, that we give particular attention to the enforcement of correct sanitary conditions, and a carefully regulated diet. If the disease is not propagated by contagion we ought to see if its occurrence cannot be limited by correct hygiene From my own experience I do not know, certainly, that there are any indications whereby we may know that any particular animal, recovering from such diseases as strangles, catarrh, or distemper, is likely to develop scarlatina It is seen in cases of recovery from mild as well as from severe attacks, it is encountered in young and in old animals, and in coarse as in well-bred horses.

c. Anatomical Characters. — The structural and tissue changes cognizable to the naked eye, in such cases of scarlatina as terminate fatally, are somewhat similar to those observed in some other blood diseases The blood is darker as a whole than natural, and of greater fluidity, it is also changed in its

chemical propeities, and in the physical characters of its
several constituents, it is less disposed to coagulate   In many
situations of the body the general connective-tissue has a rusty
tinge, while that in intimate association with mucous and serous
membranes is irregularly infiltrated with a jelly-like and more
or less coloured exudate, the membranes themselves being
variously marked with punctated or diffuse patches of a red
colour   The membranes most extensively and clearly marked
with these petechiæ are the mucous membranes of the nose
and mouth, the serous membranes of the heart, and that of the
abdomen.   None of these markings are, however, on examination after death, so bright in colour as during life   The membrane and submucous connective-tissue of the laryngeal and
pharyngeal regions, with the adjacent glands, gives evidence of
at least congestive, probably also inflammatory action, being
largely infiltrated with the products of the diseased process
which has occurred here   With the lymphatic or mucous
follicles scattered over the pharyngeal membrane, and particularly the tonsilar cavities, certain peculiar changes have occurred
chiefly affecting their cell-contents   In some instances these
changes are of a more distinctly destructive character, portions
of the membrane and subjacent tissue exhibiting gangrene and
appearances of removal   In the abdomen the glandular structures, great and small, often show congestion and increased
friability, their textural consistence giving way under very
moderate force

Symptoms *a Of Scarlatina Simplex* —The occurrence of
symptoms indicative of the simple form of scarlatina seldom
occur before the end of the first week of the primary fever
which it may accompany or succeed, and frequently they
are delayed for a longer period   Unaccountable depression,
renewal or increase of febrile symptoms—according as the
previous fever has intermitted or only remitted—not at all
indicated on the previous examination of the animal, with a
slightly swollen condition of the eyelids, are most probably
the features which solicit a more careful examination   The
internal temperature will usually have risen two degrees from
the previous examination ; the pulse, about sixty per minute, is
rather quick and of little volume ; the respirations will not at
this time be much or at all affected   The horse, when caused

to move, will show stiffness from the swelling which exists over
the limb.   On passing the hand over these swellings we may,
in certain situations where the skin is thin and vascular, and
where the swelling is of a patchy character, detect a certain
amount of moisture distributed in a dew-like fashion over the
skin; or if this exuded serosity is becoming dry, the sensation
imparted to the fingers is similar to what is felt on passing
them over a mildly vesicated surface   Very careful examination may detect the vesicles before they rupture and discharge
the serous fluid   More carefully examining the face and head,
to which we are led by the swollen eyelids, there will in all
likelihood be noticed several blotches there and over the region
of the throat, which, although they may not feel dry or rough
to the touch, are yet to the eye rough-looking, from the open
condition of the hair.   In many cases there may be very few
or no elevated patches on either body or limbs, nothing save
some amount of œdema, the only diagnostic symptoms being
those connected with the membrane of the mouth and nose
When the elevated, exuding, or roughened cutaneous patches
are present, the nasal and oral lesions are rarely absent, these
consist of numerous bright red dots or spots scattered over the
membrane both of the nose and mouth   These blood-spots are
most readily observed on the membrane covering the nasal
septum and on the inner surface of the lips, they are variable
in size and form, as also in intensity or depth of colour, not
only in different cases, but in the same case on different days,
or even at different periods of the same day   their size, number, and intensity of colour seem to bear a direct relation to
the severity of the fever, and its advance or defervescence.   At
times there is coalescence of these spots, or a connection of
one with another by rays stretching between them   The
general appearance of the membrane upon which the punctated blood-markings are situated is not in the simple form
much changed in colour   Many of the circumscribed elevations
of the cuticular surface, when of a light colour, and denuded
of hair, show the petechial markings very distinctly, exactly
like those which exist on the nasal and buccal membrane
If the affection to which this scarlatina has succeeded has not
been accompanied with soreness of the throat, such will most
probably now manifest itself, either accompanying the rash or

preceding it   In mild cases, probably a few days—during which
the rash and blood-spotting of the membranes have come and
gone, or the original eruption has disappeared and been replaced
by a fresh crop—are sufficient to establish convalescence, the
cough or soreness of throat is removed, and the animal quickly
regains his former condition

  b Scarlatina Anginosa.—This more severe form of the fever
may start into existence at once, or it may be but the steady
or more rapid passage of the simple form to more numerous,
more complex, and more serious symptoms   In addition to
those already noted as characteristic of the simple form, there
are others more distinctly indicative of involvement of the
organs and structures in the region of the throat   The swellings on the limbs, and the disturbed condition of the cutaneous
surface over the body, are here more extensive and more distinctly marked   The characteristic rash and vesicular eruption of the skin will be found more frequently over the
extremities than the trunk, and, as in the simple form, it is
noticeable as not occurring at once over the entire surface
which it may ultimately cover, but as appearing in successive
crops, or as spreading from separate and distinct centres, until
several patches are united in one   None of these tracts, where
the eruption is shown, are distinctly elevated above the surface
of the surrounding skin, in this differing from the local swellings of purpura   There seems little disturbance amongst the
vessels of the subcutaneous tissue, the serous fluid quietly oozing through the skin, forming minute vesicles, which rapidly
rupture, the contained fluid hardening in very small tear-like
masses   The petechial spots are larger, darker in colour, and
more disposed to coalesce, in many instances by such union,
forming extensive blood-markings or blotches on the nasal
membrane, particularly on that of the septum, while the membrane lying between or amongst these patches will generally
be changed from its normal colour to a dirty yellow.   A similar
disparity as to extent, depth of colour, and tendency to become
confluent, mark the blood-spots on the membrane of the mouth
and tongue, while not unfrequently this latter organ is thickly
furred, and along its inferior surface, particularly at the frænum, there are not merely the blood-markings already noticed,
but extensive effusions of straw-coloured fluid beneath the

membrane and amongst the connective-tissue. Very rarely
have I seen this organ presenting the peculiar strawberry
appearance so characteristic of scarlatina in the human
subject

The chief distinguishing symptoms, however, of scarlatina
anginosa are such as connect it with morbid conditions of the
glands and gland-structures, and other organs and tissues in
the upper part of the air-passages.   There is difficulty in
swallowing, a short painful cough, snuffling or embarrassed
breathing, a generally swollen, infiltrated, and painful condition of the glands and structures in the region of the larynx
and pharynx.

The pulse in these severe cases is characterized by great frequency, is small in volume, and occasionally jarring, while the
respirations are much accelerated.   Both pulsations and respirations vary in accordance with the advance or subsidence of
the general febrile disturbance, which again is in direct relation
to the severity of the anginal symptoms, and to the extent of
the peculiar blood-spots or markings over the membranes, and
the depth of their colouring.

At varying periods during the course of this morbid action
œdematous swellings, not diagnostic, but remarkable for the
suddenness of their appearance, their extent and persistency,
are very apt to occur over the inferior parts of the chest and
abdomen.   In most cases there is a discharge from the
nostrils, usually watery, seldom coloured, and rarely if ever
bloody.   During the continuance of these symptoms the appetite is very capricious, and the condition of the bowels irregular,
rather inclined to be confined.

Course and Termination—In those forms where angina is not
particularly severe, where there are no arthritic complications,
and where the general health has not been hopelessly broken
down by the inroad of the primary affection, of which this is
but the sequel, the distinctive features after repeated subsidence and renewal will have culminated and shown evidence
of decline in six or eight days.   It is seldom that the symptoms
disappear suddenly and at once, or even steadily and gradually;
the usual course they take is that of decline by oscillation—a
considerable improvement to be followed shortly by a renewal
of previous symptoms, these on renewal not being so severe as

previous to their subsidence. The pyrexial symptoms show little defervescence during the continuance of the angina and the appearance of the rash. Following abatement of the fever and decline of the eruption, there is shedding of the hair over the situations where exudation has occurred, and a furfuraceous exfoliation of the scarf-skin; this shedding of the epidermis is not confined to those situations alone, but is to a certain extent distributed over the whole body In severe cases convalescence is often protracted from continued swelling of the glands of the neck, while it not unfrequently happens in such protracted cases that the inflammatory action after apparent subsidence takes a fresh start, and terminates in suppuration in some of these structures, generally those in the submaxillary or brachial region. For some time after all active symptoms have disappeared, general weakness and debility continue marked; there is often much irritability of the heart, and special weakness of the circulatory system, with a tendency to dropsical effusions in the serous cavities of the thorax and pericardium

Diagnosis.—This disease in the horse is apt to be confounded with some other affections which, although resembling it in many features, are yet essentially distinct, the chief of these are eczema, purpura hæmorrhagica, and erysipelas.

From eczema it is distinguished by its general association with some previously existing morbid condition, while whether appearing with such antecedents or not, it is further marked off from the different forms of eczema by the greater systemic disturbance and general pyrexial symptoms developed during its progress, and more particularly by the blood-spots which occur on the nasal and buccal membranes, the accompanying sore throat and swollen glandular and other structures.

It differs from purpura in the general freedom from swelling of the head and the tissues forming the nasal apertures, in the character of the petechiæ, the absence of pure blood-effusion from the nasal membranes, and the character of the cutaneous surface which is the seat of the exudation or eruption In this disease there is no perceptible swelling above the level of the surrounding skin, in purpura, the disturbed cutaneous surface is considerably elevated above the plane upon which it is projected, with a higher-coloured exudate and a tendency to deep and troublesome sloughing

From erysipelas, with which it is most likely to be confounded, it may be distinguished by the absence in that disease of the catarrhal complications, as also of any association with a previously debilitating disease, by the presence of a more sthenic or acute type of fever, by the distinct and uniformly diffused swelling of the erysipelatous limb—the result of inflammatory action in the skin or immediately underlying tissues—this swelling having a distinctly brawny feeling with much heat, and being exquisitely painful. Also in these local exudations in erysipelas there is a tendency to sloughing of the skin, and the formation of troublesome sores, this disposition to form sores is also shown on the membrane of the mouth and nose, where similar blood-markings occur to those of scarlatina

Prognosis.—Although the greater number of cases of scarlatina are of a benign character, it is not safe in the early stages of any to give a decided opinion as to the probable duration or results of the illness. Much will depend upon the previous affection, if such has existed, and upon the condition in which its active symptoms have left the animal

It must not, however, be understood or taken for granted that if this affection should follow a mild attack of some antecedent disease, it will necessarily be mild also, or even the opposite. We can have no assurance of the severity of the symptoms of scarlatina, from knowing what were the nature of the symptoms of a previously occurring disease. Nor are we in a better position to prognosticate the ultimate result, save in so far as an already weakened condition may militate against the animal withstanding any further inroad on its health. Knowing that the course of the illness is likely to be marked by accessions as well as remissions of symptoms, it will be well to watch these for a few days ere any decided opinion is given. If during the first two or three days the swelling and infiltration in the region of the throat do not materially increase, and the animal will take a little food, we may expect a favourable issue. On the contrary, should the angina become more distressing during the earlier days, and the breathing more embarrassed either from the swelling of the upper air-passages or from pneumonic complications, we may apprehend serious results

Of the local symptoms none probably change so much or indicate so truly the exacerbation or decline of the pyrexia, and are thus helpful to us in forming a prognosis, as those connected with the visible mucous membranes, particularly the nasal The spots or petechiæ increase in number, depth of colour, and disposition to coalesce with increase of the fever, on defervescence, they are less bright in colour and fewer in number, seeming to contract rather than extend by diffusion

Treatment —In the treatment of cases exhibiting symptoms indicative of this condition we have termed scarlatina, the marked feature of debility would seem to point to nourishing diet and pure stimulation as most likely to be productive of beneficial results, judged, however, by the results of actual practice, such is rather doubtful. The milder cases as a rule are best treated by what we may term good stable management. The animal should have a comfortable loose box with a fair amount of light, while the food allowed ought to be easy of digestion and of such a nature as will ensure a regular condition of the bowels; water should be allowed in full quantity, in which has been dissolved sulphite or hyposulphite of soda

Where the blood-markings on the membranes are considerable, and the skin-rash and transudation are extensive, together with much pyrexia, but where the difficulty in swallowing is not a marked feature, good will follow the exhibition twice daily of solution of acetate of ammonia with a little sweet spirits of nitre and half a drachm of camphor, given in a pint of linseed-tea or gruel When the throat-symptoms are troublesome and prevent the exhibition of medicines in either solid or liquid form, what we wish to give can only be satisfactorily administered in the form of electuary. The urgent anginal symptoms may further be relieved by employing inhalations of the vapour of hot water, which may with advantage in many instances be medicated by dropping over the material employed in the fumigation such agents as oil of turpentine, tincture of opium, or of iodine, or carbolic acid Externally the throat and swollen glands should be fomented with warm water several times daily, or have heat and moisture applied by means of woollen cloths soaked in warm water and wrapped around the throat, or by the application of poultices, not, it may be, continuously, but for a few hours daily. Where poultices and fomentations have been found inadmissible or difficult of application, I have seen equally good results follow the use of cotton-wool damped with warm oil and retained in its position by means of a cap or hood. When the mouth is disposed to become sour or fœtid, or where there is much submucous effusion with the eruption, it ought to be gargled with a solution of common salt or sulphurous acid, or a mixture of vinegar and cold water, or these may be used alternately.

When the œdematous swellings of the chest and abdomen appear, the exhibition of a moderate dose of laxative medicine, as sulphate of magnesia or soda, which will not unfrequently be taken in sufficient quantities in the drinking-water, or oil, will generally be productive of good; this opening of the bowels not operating, as might be imagined, by hopelessly weakening an already enfeebled system, but seeming rather to confer vigour through its depurative action by the removal from the system of effete and noxious material. It is at this stage, immediately succeeding the action upon the bowels induced by the exhibition of such mild aperients as indicated, or when the anginal and pyrexial symptoms have been much abated and seem not likely to return, that most benefit is derived from tonics, the most valuable of which are dilute sulphuric acid half a drachm, with from twenty to forty grains of sulphate of iron or sulphate of quinine, in twenty fluid ounces of cold water twice daily. Occasionally, when exhaustion is considerable and the food taken is trifling, it may be needful to attempt the exhibition of some general stimulant. When the horse is inclined to take fluids I have found that milk or good ale may be mingled with the water in quantities sufficient to answer the end we have in view. When there is no desire for fluids, and the power of swallowing is not much impaired, this same stimulant may be given as a draught, or alternated with from two to four ounces of whisky or brandy in cold water or linseed-tea, to which may be added raw eggs thoroughly broken down and whipped up, or good beef-tea. Locally the only treatment necessary is at that particular

period when the exudation has become crusted, previous to its
removal in the general furfuraceous desquamation, when a
wash of one part of glycerine to three or four of water or a
mild inunction with vaseline will be found useful, from its
allaying the irritation, favouring the separation of the scales
and crusts, and in preventing the skin from cracking   This
need not be employed oftener than once daily, or in mild cases
less frequently

During the progress of the disease, and particularly towards
recovery, the dieting ought to be carefully attended to   As
the appetite is seldom entirely absent, there will be a disposition on particular days to feed rather freely.   This had better
be guarded against, seeing the digestive organs are not in a
condition favourable to deal with the ordinary supply of food
What food is given ought to be nourishing as well as easy of
digestion, and allowed in small quantities.   Grass or green
food is generally to be recommended ; or where this cannot be
obtained, a few sliced roots will always be grateful ; and oats,
when given, had better be mixed with fresh bran, either in
their natural condition or after being steamed by having
boiling water poured over them ; while linseed-tea may be
substituted for, or added to, the drinking-water.

All cases, even the mildest forms, require considerable time
for the perfect re-establishment of health   Enforced exercise,
with the view of removing the œdema of the limbs, is to be
avoided as likely to induce a return of the febrile symptoms
in an aggravated form.

CHAPTER XVIII

BURSATTEE—BURSATTI—BURSATIE

A DISEASED condition met with and recognised under these
names by veterinarians in India, has, to our knowledge, received attention only in periodical literature   Our journals
have from time to time contained information on the subject,
and we are especially indebted to Messrs. Spooner-Hart,
Western, Phillips, Hodgson, Oliphant, F. Smith, and Burke,
for giving us the results of their experience.   In adding the

present chapter to this work, we cannot lay claim to that practical acquaintance with the disease which is essential to treating of it in such positive terms or with that authority of assertion we could have desired; but the ever-increasing demand for the profession in our Eastern possession is so imminent as to induce us to lay before our readers so much matter relating to the subject as has been afforded us by careful attention to published facts, as well as from information contributed to us personally by observers who have had many opportunities of meeting the affection face to face. This we do in hope that at least we may provide those who intend practising their profession in India with some idea of a condition they may expect to meet with very commonly, and also that united observation may before long solve many of those difficulties which now prevent the explanation of the phenomena on which the production of and alterations in the disease may depend.

The true nature of bursattee cannot yet be said to have been indisputably established, and we shall hail with pleasure every opportunity of increasing our knowledge on the subject; and we feel assured that the scientific energy of many of the members of the Army Veterinary Medical Department, which is frequently coming under the notice of the profession, will embrace every opportunity of elucidating the pathology of the matter under discussion.

The condition may, however, be defined to be a disease yielding to previous experiment no proof of contagiousness or inoculability, characterized by the presence of certain structural changes in connection with external and visible wounds, the subcutaneous tissue, in internal organs, or in each in the same subject. These changes in structure are of slow production. They have a tendency to recurrence at certain seasons, and to the formation of a product called, in its later stages, Kunkur, such sometimes by their extent causing the animal and owner so much inconvenience that slaughter of the sufferer is deemed expedient, otherwise the disease cannot be considered of a fatal nature.

Bursattee derives its name from the fact that those at whose disposal was the nomenclature of Indian diseases had connected its appearance with the season of rains—Bursat, rain.

There seems even now some discrepancy of opinion as to the season of the year at which it is most prevalent We are inclined to think in carefully watched studs it is most frequently noticed to manifest itself from March to May, or that season directly preceding the rainy, though to the casual observer doubtless the condition thus advanced is more conspicuous during the wet season, hence its connection in name with it.

Found throughout the extent of the empire, it is generally allowed that it obtains more largely in northern India It is said to be more common among stabled animals than those at pasture, and among those located on the plains than the inhabitants of more elevated situations Attacking horses in every conceivable condition, opinion appears to favour the idea that the subjects of debilitating influences, such as improper dieting, uncleanliness, etc., are the more frequently affected Thus in well-regulated and carefully supervised establishments it is comparatively infrequently met with, while among the less fortunate portion of the equine community, especially in large towns, it is of common occurrence So that it is probable the civil practitioner will more frequently be brought into contact with the disease than his military confrère.

Native and foreign-bred animals contract the disease equally readily, for imported animals become affected a few months after their arrival in the country

The disease is probably peculiar to the horse Only one case has, to our knowledge, been instanced to the contrary This, that of a donkey, was quoted by Mr Spooner-Hart; but, as hinted by the writer himself, there would appear some reason for suspicion as to the correctness of the diagnosis

In its objects of attack we are not aware of the exhibition of any partiality for particular age or sex, and investigation has not yet given us sufficient information to assert or deny the possession of an hereditary tendency; though by some observers it is believed to be characterized by the power of being transmitted from parent to progeny, and they consequently condemn the breeding from bursattee subjects

To the practitioner the most important features of the disease are the external manifestations occurring in connec-

tion with wounds in which the peculiar product is found It
is not an uncommon occurrence for the material known as
'kunkur' to be met with in internal organs at autopsy of
animals, which, though under trustworthy medical supervision during life, had given no indications of the disease
It is essentially characteristic of bursattee wounds, or, more
properly ulcers, that, after removal by surgical operation,
though cicatrization takes place, there is undoubted disposition to recurrence , but if the excision has been thorough, and
the healing process favourable, a season usually elapses before
we have further evidence *in loco*

The subjects of the disease may be rendered useless in a
variety of ways (see Symptoms) so that the condition must be
regarded as a serious one

Pathology—As we before hinted, some mystery seems still
to shroud the true nature of bursattee, with the natural consequence of much divergence of opinion. To explain the
phenomena involved many theories have been promulgated,
and many views advanced, in several of which, rather than one
alone, there appears to be some progress towards placing
matters in their proper light.

Early in the literature of the subject there is mooted an
idea of its cancerous nature and close resemblance to epithe-
lioma This view has been fostered and enlarged upon by
more recent observers, some of whom assert the growth to be
cancer, and claim for it an intimate relation with epithelial
cancer Reasoning from some anatomical and pathological
characters, and assuming the correctness of the fundamental
premises of the latter, there would seem in many points a
striking analogy

The general clinical features exhibited by cancer (though
what is described as epithelial can scarcely be deemed a
'typical cancer') are in some degree absent in bursattee , for
though 'kunkurs' have been found very rarely in lymph-glands,
I have not met with a satisfactory recorded instance of the
secondary affection of lymphatic structures One of the
earliest observers, who quoted from an extensive experience,
emphatically states we have no true gland-implication While,
referring to epithelial cancer, Sir James Paget says: 'The
lymphatic glands in anatomical relation with epithelial cancer

20

become similarly cancerous in the progress of the disease, and
I think sooner or later in that progress in direct proportion to
its own rapidity, following in the same ratio as other cancers;'
and adds, 'The secondary cancerous elements resemble those
in the primary disease, and the effect may lead to the removal
of the whole of the original tissues.' Further, he speaks most
positively of the involvement of lymphatic glands 'I believe,
rather, no cases reach their natural end without infection of the
glands.' I think, as to these infective properties, the analogy
between cancer and bursattee cannot be said to obtain, as
taking those *internal* lesions which have been found, there is
no proof that they are 'secondary,' and personally we have
been able to meet with no one who has found a bursattee
ulcer (cancerous sore), except in connection with the cutaneous
surface or the mucous membranes lining the natural orifices.
Then, again, we have the formation of the peculiar product
'kunkur,' which identifies, as it were, the disease; certainly
this cannot be considered characteristic of cancer Notwithstanding our willingness to allow that there is a manifest
disposition in the horse to calcareous degeneration of abnormal
tissue-products, we could not even assert that we have found
the majority of tumours to undergo this change, nor can we
recall many instances of ulcers cicatrizing in this manner.

The theory which has received support from others who
have made the disease a special study, ascribes to it a parasitic
nature. This view is upheld by some experienced practitioners, and would seem confirmed by some microscopic investigations recorded in the *Veterinary Journal* for October,
1881 The observer in the last-named found, in connection
with the bursattee tumour, or kunkur, some fungus elements
apparently of a definite character, 'hypal tubes, hymenia
and spores,' the first in organic connection with the brown cells
described by one observer as being special to the growth The
recurrence of the tumours at certain definite periods of the
year is certainly in accordance with the principles of vegetable
life, and seems capable of explanation by the parasitic hypothesis, viewing their return as the 'recrudescence of the kunkur,' when the soil was congenial to the life and development
of the fungus or algæ. Other matters are not so readily reconciled with this view, for instance, those diseases of a cryp-

togamic character of which we know the nature appear to be
highly contagious and communicable, this has not been proved
to obtain in bursattee, though experiments on the point have
not been wanting

We have ourselves seen evidence of the presence of these
low vegetable growths in kunkur but before we can give in
our unqualified adhesion to any theory yet promulgated, many
more of the phenomena concerned in the disease-production
must be made clear

There have been attempts to identify its nature with scrofula
and farcy, but we fail to recognise the special features of
either, so will leave this part of the subject, submitting the
foregoing to the consideration of the reader, in hope that before
long observation will have overcome those difficulties which
are met with in speaking of the condition

The study of the ætiology of the disease is so inseparable
from that of its nature, that to a large extent the same
obscurity enshrouds them both In its propagation, flies have
by several writers been credited with [playing an important
part, but we fail to detect any positive evidence in the deductions presented to us In favour of this view, it has been
argued that the disease appears only in seasons and situations
where flies are most plentiful, also that the application to
wounds of certain materials distasteful to flies is a means of
preventing their assuming a bursattic character As ordinary
irritants affecting certain constitutions, we can understand
flies being exciting objects, and thus providing wounds in
which the peculiar alterations of the disease are manifested,
but this special manifestation, we presume, depends on something more than mere ordinary irritations Should, however,
the cryptogamic nature of the disease be proved, we must admit the importance which the diptera may assume in conveying it from diseased to healthy

It has also been advanced that water is a fruitful dissemi-
nator of the disease, from the fact that certain well-water,
examined microscopically, contained materials of the same
character as that found in bursattee tumours, cells, fungi, etc, as
well as from the increase of the tumours in the rainy season

It appears to us that, at this stage of our knowledge, neither
of these are qualified to maintain the whole responsibility of

propagating the disease. Conditions favourable to the existence of flies may be, and probably are, favourable to the production of those conditions on which the disease depends, irrespective of these creatures. Also, by the irritation they set up, the animal is caused to bite and rub itself so as to produce wounds, in which the special conditions may ensue in those animals so disposed; while materials distasteful to flies may be congenial to the wound in the early stages, by proving antagonistic to the development of the disease. The part claimed for the regular wearing of eye-fringes in obviating the disease, by preventing the attack of flies, may also be due to the exclusion of the element causing ophthalmia, the attendant overflow of tears and consequent abraided surface on which kunkur may develop. And because the water inspected apparently contained cryptogamic debris, cells, etc (a rather ordinary occurrence, we imagine, in water containing comparatively large quantities of organic matter), we cannot assert it as a cause of the disease.

Although bearing no resemblance to those constitutional conditions of an eliminative character, bursattee would appear to us to depend on a state of system not yet defined, which we may call the 'bursattee diathesis,' the method by, or circumstances under, which this is acquired, we still remain ignorant of.

As we have before hinted, its communicability from the diseased to the healthy has not been demonstrated, though experiments have been comparatively numerous and varied; inoculation, introduction of blood, and bursattee matter into the alimentary canal have been attended with negative results. Among animals, the subjects of simple healthy wounds, placed under apparently identical circumstances as regards diet, location (next each other in the stable, etc.), and attendants, it has again and again been noticed that in the one the wounds take on the bursattee character, while in their neighbour, the healing process occurs, naturally leaving nothing on which suspicion of bursattee could rest, and without evidence of having been affected in a previous season.

On what this special condition depends we cannot so far prove, and do not feel in a position to speculate, but its absence in winter when in the tropics all animals are most vigorous, and its apparent preference for those placed under debilitating conditions of sanitation, seem to point to the asthenic rather than the sthenic state as the more susceptible, though we cannot assert that this is apparent in all cases, for, as it has been before stated, animals in every conceivable condition become affected.

The *somewhat* general tendency for abnormal tissue-products in the horse to assume a calcareous character of course is recognised, and the production of hard kunkur is reconciled to it, but this is a very small portion of what has to be accounted for.

The presence of the morbid material (kunkur) in internal organs often found, though by no means invariably, in subjects yielding external manifestations of bursattee, seems, although occasionally involving a considerable portion of the substance of the organ, to be the cause of very little appreciable disturbance. They are never, we believe, met with in an ulcerating condition, but tend to go through the different stages of their development to the calcifying process without ulceration; this disposition seems to be marked in all tumours not in direct contact with the external air. Some observers would suggest that the slight irritation caused by subcutaneous growths induces the animal to so injure itself by biting or rubbing, as to cause abrasion mechanically, and rupture of the outward investing structures, already rendered thin by pressure consequent on increase of tumour.

The manner in which kunkur of the internal organs gains its position is at present only a speculation, and we have no ground whatever in the majority of cases for proving if it be primary, secondary, or indeed independent of other lesions.

Morbid Anatomy.—The post-mortem examination of the subjects of bursattee present to us the peculiar product which characterizes the disease variously distributed, and in various stages of its development in the same subject. The general condition of the body will therefore vary according to the number and extent of the sores, and whether they have been allowed to linger on until they are the pitiable objects which may be imagined from a summary of the symptoms given elsewhere.

The lesions may be found exclusively in connection with

external wounds, in the subcutaneous tissue, or in internal
organs—in two of these situations, or in the whole simultaneously, while kunkurs are frequently met with in internal
organs of animals which have given no indications of their
possession during life. The disease-products are chiefly found
in connection with the fibrous structures. The proportion of
these varies from a millet-seed to that of a filbert or bean.
In the earlier appreciable stage they are recognised as soft
tumours, and if examined histologically are found to be
made up of two kinds of cells—the one apparently having a
tendency to elongate and acquire the characters of stability,
the other exhibits signs of vitality and reproductive power,
having abundant nuclei and nucleoli. In a stage farther advanced palpation detects greater firmness, the section is of a
yellowish-white colour, and the microscope reveals varying
degrees of fibrillation of the stable cells; and between these the
more vital cells are arranged in a variety of forms—according to
some observers in groups, as veritable nidi; according to others,
they are evenly dispersed among the fibres, and are of a brown
colour. This is the condition generally spoken of as 'soft
kunkur'. In the last stage which we shall describe, and it will of
course be understood that no stage is clearly defined, the impression conveyed to the touch is one of extreme hardness. Section
now is not so easily performed; and often we shall find, when
attempting this, that cavities are apparent on its surface—these
are really those parts of the tumour which have not undergone the calcareous metamorphosis, for such is that involved
in production of the true kunkur, if we may depend on some
analyses which have been made, showing them to contain 10
per cent of inorganic matter, principally the phosphates and
carbonate of lime, the cavity being that part of the growth
vacated by the kunkur on the act of section. 'Kunkur' is the
name applied by the natives to a stone used for economic
purposes in India.

In the earlier stages there would seem to be no line of demarcation between the disease-product and the structure on
which it is found; but that in the internal organs acquires, as
it were, a fibrous capsule. Microscopic examination of kunkur
has yielded to different observers widely different results, some
finding everything characteristic of cancer, others of crypto-

gamic growth, others of organic action, as crystals, etc. At one stage of its growth Mr Spooner-Hart has described the tumour as being, to naked-eye appearance, like 'boiled udder'

In internal organs we may find kunkurs embedded in their substance, and when dissected out appearing to have a true fibrous coat. We have records of their having been met with in the lungs, visceral and parietal pleura, bronchial glands, the liver, spleen, mesentery, mesenteric glands, the cæcum, the peritoneum, the prepectoral, parotid, and submaxillary glands, and the submucous tissue of the urethra. These several structures may be variously involved, sometimes to being studded over their surface, and through their substance—or, more rarely, containing a single tumour. On being cut into, sensation will be imparted according to the development of the tumour from, in the early stage, one of undue softness to, in the latter, a feeling of grittiness. In connection with the external and subcutaneous structures the tumours, or sores, will be met with in the situations, and be of the character to be immediately described under symptoms

Symptoms—The more common occurrence of the affection in general practice, where so many matters obstruct observation in the early stages of the disease, and the comparative freedom from it of studs under more perfect hygienic arrangement—including constant medical supervision—may probably, in some measure, account for the scanty information we possess as to the attack of the disease, and the conclusion that premonitory symptoms are wholly wanting. It must, however, be allowed to be insidious and obscure.

The appetite, as a rule, remains in its normal condition, though we have instances of derangement, both anorexia and cynorexia. The temperature from the commencement to termination rarely varies much from that consistent with health. The general constitutional state ranges from vigour to debility, though we believe the latter somewhat predominates ; while in proportion to the involvement of important organs and extent of the sores will be the debility of the later stages

We look for the specialities which characterize the disease to the appearance of the bursattee growths, or kunkurs. These are chiefly noticed in connection with those parts of the body which, from their situation, etc, are most liable to be the seat of wounds from any cause. The subcutaneous tumours are first recognised as soft swellings, apparently underneath and free from the skin, assuming a nodular character, they, however, soon impart the impression of being attached to the skin, and may of course present varieties of consistency—there is little heat or tenderness manifested. In about eight or ten days after the first detectable swelling hardening occurs, the process proceeds until the feeling of firmness of an ordinary fibrous tumour is attained. In a period much depending on the disposition of the animal, or very frequently accelerated by rubbing or biting, apparently induced by the itching, ulceration occurs, and the bursattee sore is manifest. This presents a papillated appearance, and discharges a small quantity of thin puriform material, the edges are slightly raised, and in some cases undermined. On the floor of the ulcer are scattered little hardened eminences—kunkuis—which may usually, by pressure between the finger and thumb, be squeezed out; the sore is of an indolent nature, and manifests little tendency to spread, though this does occur, and we occasionally find the sores becoming confluent. They present an appearance which the term 'vegetative growth' is frequently used to imply, in figure they are frequently circular, but are met with of every variety of shape. The process or product of healing is special. The reparative material invariably assumes in some degree the nature of kunkur; the cicatrix is of a slate-grey colour, and somewhat resembles that of a severe burn. Ulceration and cicatrization may go on simultaneously in different parts of the same sore: the whole scab may be thrown off, and an unhealthy ulcerating surface exposed; or it may become fissured, and through these openings a grumous discharge may issue. They rarely or never heal permanently spontaneously. The edges of the sore are underrun with the bursattee material, and in its extirpation in treatment it is highly essential to recognise this fact.

Though we stated that all parts of the integumentary area were liable to become the seats of the tumours or sores, some, from varying circumstances, appear to be much more frequently affected than others, thus the inner canthus of the eye is often its situation. From here, in aggravated cases, it extends over the face, sometimes involving considerable areas of the locality. As hinted elsewhere, it seems probable that the irritation set up by overflow of tears either provides suitable conditions or exciting cause. The angles of the mouth are also frequently affected, here the bit is credited with a share in its causation. The legs, from the knee downwards, but especially the fetlocks and coronets, are commonly involved, and here some observers have remarked an inclination of the disease-product to assume a character more resembling bone than that found in other positions. The vagina, prepuce, glans penis, and urethra are frequently affected, and the occasional symptom of spasmodic ejection of urine is supposed to depend on the presence of kunkur in the last-named situation; while the growths on the prepuce cause phymosis, and on the glans incapacitate entire horses, and render undesirable property all of its subjects. The site of an old sore always affords soil for the development of the peculiar product of the subject of bursattee, while *fresh* wounds take on this character, which some practitioners assert can be recognised by the red-currant jelly-like material on them, which soon present the small hardened bodies mentioned disseminated on the floor.

When the cicatrized and cicatrizing sores are numerous or extensive they may interfere with function in different ways, as loss of contraction, etc. If the disposition to bursattee is very manifest, it has been argued that it is economical to slaughter at once; our experience has not been sufficient to warrant our endorsing the assertion, and thus incurring for ourselves the responsibility it would involve. Animals, the subjects of bursattee, appear not to be seriously affected by work, and this is taken advantage of. We have been assured that amongst 'cab' horses in the large towns, as Calcutta, there are some loathsome sights of poor horses standing exposed to the attack of flies, dust, heat, etc, but this, we hope, can be but of rare occurrence. At any rate, it will be the duty of the veterinary surgeon to exert himself to prevent such a state of affairs.

Treatment —The uncertainty shrouding the pathology of the condition must also necessarily to some extent involve its remedial treatment; however, experience has put us in possession of facts which render some methods at our disposal rational, and from their adoption we may fairly expect to confer benefit on our client and patient.

Having regard to the condition which is likely to be produced by ulcers of long standing of any character, we must endorse the practice of those who from the first have recourse to general tonic remedies in company with nutritious diet A change of air, also of food, and improved sanitary arrangements, have been found markedly beneficial

However, from what we have stated respecting the comparative insignificance of the constitutional disturbance and symptoms of kunkurs in internal organs, also as in the majority of cases it is impossible until ulceration has commenced to say definitely if this process will assume the character of bursattee—it is not customary to interfere surgically—it is manifest that the ulcer will occupy the bulk of the practitioner's attention.

As simple wounds may become complicated with bursattee, in the management of animals it will behove us to avail ourselves of every means for reducing to the minimum the chances of injuries producing these   Harness should fit comfortably, bits which abrade the angles of the mouth should be avoided, shoes applied so as to prevent striking, etc, etc, while the use of eye-fringes indirectly effect the same purpose

In the early stages of ulceration those who support the theory of its parasitic nature recommend such dressings as contain carbolic and sulphurous acids, and other parasiticides, this course can be open to no objection   While those who credit flies with a large share in its production advise the application to the wounds in the earliest stages of camphor and oil, or other agents distasteful to these insects, and the removal of the patient as much as possible from chance of their attacks.

The ulcer itself should as early as possible be reduced to the condition of an ordinary wound, and then treated as such All vegetating growths and masses of kunkur should be extirpated by means of the knife or the actual cautery, and in carrying this out it is essential that the whole of the 'special' growth be removed, and to this we must bear in mind the tendency of the material to undermine the edges of the ulcer, and to apparently infiltrate a zone outside itself, which should be included in the removal. On pressure this imparts a feeling of extra firmness to the touch. After the operation the sore will frequently assume an indolent character, and will require to be stimulated as its condition may suggest. For this purpose those agents in ordinary use answer very well, such as lunar caustic and sulphate of copper ; while some practitioners advocate the use of alkalies, and others of acids. The whole of these agents in other proportions will of course be equally useful to check luxuriant growths where the wound shows an opposite tendency. A variety of dressings—that is, change from the use of one material to another—appears in certain cases to be followed by some benefit. Cicatrization in most cases is protracted, and of the peculiar character described ; it rarely or never occurs spontaneously, and with the return of the season there is great probability of recurrence in the same as well as other parts of the body.

CHAPTER XIX

DIABETES.

Definition—*A complex morbid condition originating from or closely connected with certain disturbances in the process of assimilation, evidenced by excessive secretion of urine, great and persistent thirst, rapid emaciation and loss of energy ; in one form characterized by the presence of saccharine material in the urine and other animal fluids*

Use of the Term—Unfortunately for the correctness of medical nosology and nomenclature the term *Diabetes* is employed in both human and veterinary medicine to designate two somewhat dissimilar morbid conditions, which although possessing in common certain prominent features, are yet with our present knowledge regarded as in much essentially different

The more malignant and truly systemic of these has, in deference to its most prominent diagnostic symptom, saccharine urine, been termed ' Diabetes Mellitus,' or 'Mellituria,' the other a comparatively less serious malady, generally benign in its results, and in which the urine is marked simply by an increase in its watery elements, being known as ' Diabetes Insipidus,' or ' Polyuria.'

I. DIABETES INSIPIDUS.

Nature of the Affection—This in the horse the more important disorder, because by far the more common, is by many regarded as more truly a functional disorder of the kidneys, and by them placed as a local disease amongst affections of the urinary organs. There are, however, sufficient reasons to warrant its being regarded as something more than this, as intimately related to at least functional disturbance of several of the complex processes in assimilation, and thus correctly viewed as a systemic disorder, and as such we prefer to consider it. There seems strong grounds for believing that both these forms, polyuria and mellituria, are merely symptomatic of several, and it may be differing, functional or structural changes ; and that as our knowledge of the causes and conditions under which these originate becomes more extensive and more exact, so will our estimate of their relations to each other be liable to vary. This disorder is so common amongst horses operated upon and surrounded by certain influences that, although usually a sporadic affection, it occasionally develops truly enzoötic characters.

Although from the mode of its manifestation, and the character of the symptoms developed during its progress, it is perfectly obvious that several steps in the process of food-assimilation are performed in a faulty manner, and that different organs are involved in the general disturbance, we are unable to determine precisely what organ or set of organs are primarily and chiefly affected, nor at what particular stage in the assimilatory process, whether in the alimentary canal, in the gland-structures, or in the blood, the interruption is interposed   In all probability the disturbance exists at more than one point, also that more than one organ is functionally perverted.

Although we may not be able thoroughly to explain its pathology, it is abundantly evident that the disorder consists in more than mere irritation and increased activity of the kidneys; rather that they are acting in response to some influence sent to them, possibly through the blood or some other channel, while by their excessive action they may tend to aggravate the original cause of the disease.

Causation.—A correct and clear statement of the causation of polyuria is somewhat difficult. Probably the direct and immediate cause of the diagnostic symptom, the excessive urination, is to be attributed to dilatation of the renal vessels, the result of paralysis of their coats attendant on disturbed innervation This disturbed innervation may be induced by impairment of the power of vaso-motor nerve-centres, or through irritation of cerebro-spinal nerve-element causing inhibition of vaso-motor power Although, as already said, it cannot be regarded as aught but essentially a sporadic disease, it may yet be observed assuming an enzoötic character In this latter development we are at once brought closely into contact with the inducing factors; in such these must be resident or abiding for the time being in the conditions which operate upon the animals from without, those by which they are surrounded and pressed upon; they must be either those of location or dietary, or both

In other instances, however, and these are the more severe and intractable, the causes seem to proceed from the animal itself, from some constitutional cachexia, which will in this manner develop itself in whatever external conditions it may be placed.

The extrinsic causes are, from what I have observed, specially connected with inferior and damaged provender, oats, or hay. Grain of any kind, when badly harvested, damaged with rain, and allowed to heat or germinate; hay, when similarly damaged by moisture and developing mould, or presenting a favourable nidus for the growth of this and other lowly organized forms, are all fruitful causes of polyuria

It is because of the existence of these agencies on an individual farm, in some particular stable, or over a particular district, that this affection so often attacks several animals at one time. There may be some individual case of improperly secured corn or hay, some unfortunate purchase of damaged fodder, or some extensively operating adverse climatic influence at the particular period of harvesting the crop, which

has operated in the production of a dietary unfit for sustaining healthy activity in connection with the many steps in the
process of assimilation. Certain plants, and forage which
contained these plants, have often been accredited with the
production of this condition This I have not observed, but
rather have I found it to develop in connection with the consumption of various fodders and foods when damaged by bad
harvesting, or where vegetable fungi have largely taken possession of it

During convalescence from many debilitating diseases it is
not unfrequently observed that a very trifling error in dieting,
either as to quantity or quality, will so operate as to develop
the condition of polyuria, the attack generally passing off
when the indigestion which induced it has passed away

Of causes operating from within, and which, when fully developed, are more likely to terminate unfavourably than those
which are brought directly to bear on the animal from without, the chief are excessive tissue-disintegration and imperfect
food-assimilation These conditions may again be regarded
merely as the sequelæ of some antecedent and further removed
operating agency; they may follow the attack or recovery
from some other diseased condition, or they may result from
undue exposure to adverse atmospheric conditions, or from
long-continued and exhausting work.

The products of the excessive tissue-change not only
morbidly influence these excretory organs, the kidneys,
through which they are naturally removed from the system,
but in their entrance into the blood and lymph-channels
induce, through their universal distribution, disturbance and
perversion of power in many, if not in all, the systems of
the body.

Anatomical Features.—In animals which have died directly
from the effects of the disease, as also in others where death
has occurred from other causes while the animals were suffering
from an attack of polyuria, the lesions observed have neither
been numerous nor diagnostic These, when present, are chiefly
in connection with the muscular and glandular systems

In the muscular system we observe want of colour and an
unnatural, soft and flabby condition , in the great glands of
the abdomen there is the same general characters, particularly

that of softness and want of textural cohesion. In the brain and spinal cord we meet with serous effusion in the sub-arachnoid spaces, or else an infiltration of the membranes and connective-tissue belonging to these structures, with a slightly coloured gelatinous material

These effusions and tissue-changes of the great nerve-centres are variable as regards their situation, as also in the matter of their extent and of the amount of the fibrillating matter present, but invariable as to their character that is to say, they are always purely serous or of a gelatinous hyaline material, distributed throughout, or in connection with, the membranes.

Symptoms—The diagnostic symptoms are the excessive urination, immoderate thirst—polydipsia—and impaired or depraved appetite. In addition to these, which sufficiently distinguish the disorder from every other, we have several less important, not so attractive, and probably more variable as to their appearance. The mucous membranes are pallid or dirty coloured, the mouth clammy and sour-smelling, the hair wanting the close, sleek character of full health and vigour, and the skin occasionally scurfy; the pulse, whether frequent or infrequent, is always wanting in volume and tone, while, if put to any exertion, there is evident weakness, and a disposition to perspire. Very often the appearance of the great diagnostic features are not what first draw attention to the horse; he may have simply shown indications of not thriving by want of vigour and sprightliness when at work, by excessive perspiration, or by the existence of a depraved appetite, an inclination to swallow foul material and to refuse his usual food.

Very shortly, however, the immoderate thirst and excessive urination appear, and as these become developed the other symptoms are more confirmed The amount of urine voided is generally increased, and characterized—particularly when the causes seem to be exogenous—by the paleness of its colour and low specific gravity This is accounted for from the excess of water, the absence or relatively small amount of the earthy carbonates, and, it is said, by the presence of free acetic acid Ordinarily, horses' urine has the specific gravity of from 1035; in this condition it is often seen at 1003 However, it has been said—we have not tested the truth of the statement—that the quantity of solid matter voided in a given period of twenty-four hours is not decreased, the quantity of the secretion being sufficient, with even its relatively small amount of solids, to bring the aggregate of these to the normal standard, or even above it.

When this condition exists as the direct result of causes operating from within, as consequent on some antecedent disease, and coincident with excessive tissue-waste, and in some cases with simply imperfect food-assimilation, the character of the urinary secretion is chemically different, it is less watery, and instead of being pale, clear, and of less specific gravity than natural, it is more or less coloured, thick, and of a higher specific gravity. This physical and chemical alternation is probably dependent on the presence in the secretion of a peculiar form of albumen, the product of the rapid and excessive tissue-disintegration going on in the system. In such cases the marasmus and general weakness are also greater, and the chances of a fatal termination much increased.

Course and Termination—In the greater number of cases of polyuria, those which as a rule develop the milder form, and in which the urinary secretion is abundant but of low specific gravity, and where the solid and nitrogenous materials are lessened in amount, the animal may suffer for a very lengthened period before even any apprehensions of serious results become fixed upon the minds of even well-informed attendants or professional men. The conditions of polydipsia and polyuria may continue for some time, and be well known, without exciting much alarm; but at length the muscular system will show undue fatigue on moderate exertion, and cold perspiration will break out over different regions of the body. Languor and want of vivacity are soon followed by impaired activity of the digestive and assimilatory processes, which, if not arrested, speedily undermine the health, and may terminate in structural changes of many organs.

The earliest and most commonly encountered of these are dropsies and effusions in different cavities of the body, and in the meshes of the interconnective-tissue where this is abundant and lax in character.

In that form where the products of excessive tissue-disintegration are being passed off by the kidneys, the progress of the disease is more rapid and somewhat different   Impairment of appetite and rapid tissue-wasting are followed closely by deterioration or poisoning of the blood, from the inability to discharge from the system the superabundant waste, worn out and deleterious materials   The results of this are impairment of the functions of the great nerve-centres from imperfect nutrition   Here we observe no dropsy or effusion, rather paralysis and coma.

Treatment—If saccharine diabetes is invariably, or nearly so, a fatal disease in all animals, this of diabetes insipidus is as truly non-malignant

In every instance, when once the diagnostic symptoms are fairly developed, an endeavour must be made to operate on the animal through the dietary   When, even after a careful examination of the food-supply, nothing can be detected which is likely to induce this disturbance ; when no antecedent weakening disease has existed   when, in fact, no disease-producing factors are capable of detection, it will always be prudent to order for the horse a perfect, or as complete a change as possible of his dietary   At the time this change is being carried through, a little aperient medicine will be useful. Should the desire for foul matter, evidenced by licking the walls or swallowing earth, be marked, it is advisable to place within his reach a lump of chalk, or add bicarbonate of soda to the drinking-water, which ought to be given liberally, if not in unlimited amount, and is improved by mixing it with oatmeal-gruel, linseed-tea, or milk   With a like object in view, viz to correct the unnatural thirst and gastric acidity, some advise the exhibition of clay mixed with the drinking-water , this serves the purpose well, but not so effectually, we believe, as the fluids and salt now mentioned, and is less wholesome.   In the milder cases, this alteration and arrangement of the dietary will often materially mitigate the severity of all the symptoms, if it does not entirely remove them

As a help to our dietetic treatment, recourse is had to such medicinal agents as preparations of iron, arsenic, mineral acids, vegetable tonics, and iodine   Of these medicaments, there is probably none which has yielded such good results as the last.

21

Under its employment, the more urgent symptoms have not only disappeared, but the appetite has improved, and the health has been re-established

When the thirst is great, the animal will take this in the form of the compound solution in the drinking-water, the better form, however, for its exhibition is that of the iodide of potassium, which may be given from two to three drachms twice daily. The beneficial action of the iodine in lessening the thirst and diuresis will usually be exhibited in three or four days, when the amount ought to be decreased, or some of the doses replaced by half-ounce doses of Fowler's solution of arsenic, which is readily enough taken in food or the drinking-water. Some animals are found to receive more benefit from iron than arsenic. This may be given either as the sulphate or the solution of the perchloride in moderate amount, in food or bolus, twice daily.

II DIABETES MELLITUS.

Saccharine Diabetes. Nature and Causation —This, which probably of itself ought to bear the name of diabetes, is truly a systemic disease, appearing to originate in disturbance of function in one or more of the steps in the complex process of food-assimilation. Whether it is entirely during primary, or also partly during secondary, digestion that these changes originate, it is extremely difficult to say. It is certain, however, that although the progress of these changes connected with the derangement of the activities of different organs is no less rapid than their products are dissimilar to those which are met with in health, there is, nevertheless, on examination of these same organs after death, extremely little obvious change

Amongst our patients diabetes mellitus is a rare disease, in the horse, I am only aware of having once encountered conditions in any way analogous to what are accepted as diagnostic of saccharine diabetes.

The agencies and their exact pathological relations which operate in the production of sugar throughout the system, and its excretion with the urine, are as yet more probably matters of hypothesis than capable of satisfactory demonstration. At one time the presence of sugar in the urine was attributed to perverted gastric and intestinal digestion, the blood being, it was thought, directly charged with the material by absorption from the alimentary canal, where its presence was accounted for from imperfect elaboration of starchy and saccharine matters. Further investigation, however, and particularly the elaborate experiments of M C Bernard with regard to the functions of the liver, have caused a partial abandonment, or modification at least, of this theory By these experiments, Bernard sought to prove that one of the functions of the liver was the secretion of a substance which, if not in itself sugar, was at least converted into a saccharine material on meeting some peculiar ferment of the blood in the hepatic veins. Further, that in health, sugar was only found in the blood circulating between the liver and the lungs, that at the latter organs, on meeting with the oxygen of the inspired air, it was chemically changed This chemical change or combustion, it is now thought, is also extensively carried out at the peripheral capillaries in the muscles, largely contributing to force-production

In this way it has been attempted to be proved that the presence of sugar in the general circulation, and its excretion with the urine, must be due either to excessive hepatic or defective pulmonary action

In addition, these experimental inquiries tended to show that this peculiar excretory function of the liver was largely modified by nervous action.

The exciting agent of nervous influence in this hepatic secretion Bernard believed to be the inspired air acting on the pulmonary ramifications of the pneumogastric nerve, by which it was transmitted to the brain, and from this organ by reflex action along the spinal cord and splanchnic divisions of the sympathetic to the liver. With as much if not greater appearance of truth, the nervous influence inducing this hepatic secretion may be looked for as originating in the liver itself, from stimulus supplied to the portal ramifications of the pneumogastric, through medium of blood in the portal veins This seems the more feasible if saccharine diabetes be looked upon as originally only a very peculiar form of dyspepsia, and seeing also that it is most successfully combated on dietetic principles

Feasible, however, as this or any other hypothesis may appear, it must never be forgotten that conclusions arrived at from post-mortem experiments may, when tested by ante-mortem teaching, require much modification In the development of this disease it is highly probable that other and important changes have preceded the appearance of what is generally looked upon as the most characteristic symptom of diabetes—saccharine urine—that this is merely a confirmation of the disease, a passing into the second stage of the morbid process

Symptoms —The increased secretion of urine, with accompanying thirst, are here, as in the already described form, prominent symptoms, they may not, however, if the case has been carefully watched, be the earliest, which in all likelihood are such as indicate simply defective digestion and want of general vigour In all cases of largely augmented urinary secretion, with general disturbance, attention ought at once to be directed to the character of the secretion ; should this be found to be of increased density other tests ought at once to be resorted to, so as to ascertain whether or not sugar is present

In addition to its increased specific gravity, fragrant smell, and sweetish taste, diabetic urine, in certain cases where the quantity of sugar is excessive, will be found, when allowed to remain at rest for some hours in appropriate vessels, to yield a deposit of needle-like, prismatic-shaped crystals of grape-sugar The indications arrived at by attention to any of these conditions being only approximate, definite results are attained chiefly through the employment of two chemical tests, one depending on the reaction of the salts of copper, known as ' Tromer's test,' the other upon the development of the vinous fermentation of the sugar and evolution of carbonic acid, and recognised by the name of the ' fermentation test.'

In employing Tromer's test a small portion of the suspected urine is placed in a test-tube ; to this is added a few drops of sulphate of copper solution, sufficient to give the liquid a slight blue colour Solution of potash is now added, in quantity from one-half to as much as the urine employed ; this will throw down a pale-blue precipitate of the hydrated oxide of copper, which, if there is sugar present, will rapidly redissolve as the caustic is added, leaving the solution of a dark-blue colour. The mixture is now gradually heated to the boiling-point, when, if sugar is present, a yellowish-brown precipitate of the sub-oxide of copper is thrown down; should no sugar be present, a black precipitate of common oxide of copper is deposited.

In the fermentation test a little fresh or dried German yeast is added to a small quantity of the urine; a test-tube, filled with the urine thus treated, is carefully inverted in a saucer containing the remainder, and allowed to remain at rest in this position for some hours, the temperature of the place being maintained about 80° F. If sugar is present the vinous fermentation is speedily developed, during which carbonic acid is evolved, indicated by gentle effervescence, and the presence of the gas at the upper part of the inverted tube; if no sugar is present there will be no effervescence, nor the presence of any gas. One cubic inch of gas so formed will represent one gram of sugar in the urine.

It is upon the existence of sugar or saccharine material in the urine that the diagnosis of mellituria must depend. It is also to be borne in mind that the quantity of sugar present in undoubted cases of diabetes mellitus varies, it being perfectly possible that at some periods of examination none may be found.

Treatment.—In the treatment of diabetes mellitus the ultimate results are as unsatisfactory as the different theories respecting the rationale of the morbid process are conflicting; the most which as yet it has been possible to attain being palliation of the more distressing symptoms. Many methods of treatment have been adopted, and nearly every agent in the Pharmacopœia likely to operate in arresting the great waste of tissue and peculiar sugar-formative process has been experimented with. Some of these have, for a time, given hopes of ultimate success. There has been improvement in the general symptoms, with a diminished quantity of sugar in the urine; ultimately all has become changed, the disease asserting its supremacy with increased vigour, or becoming complicated with other morbid phenomena, most probably with fatal changes of a tubercular character in the lungs.

A carefully selected and strictly enforced dietary, in which

the food given, besides being nutritious, is as devoid as possible
of materials of a purely saccharine or starchy nature, seems to
hold out prospects the most encouraging Of medicinal agents
the most deserving of notice are opium in combination in the
form of Dover's powder; or some of the mineral acids given in
small and repeated doses, either alone or in combination with
some corresponding salt of iron.   Cod-liver oil, both from a
physiological point of view as also from the terms in which its
employment in actual practice has been spoken of, is deserving
of a trial.   It ought, however, to be remembered that there is
a strong probability that every separate case of this disease is
attended with a different series of complications, requiring a
somewhat different management, and calling for a separate
study

The only instance, in a period of over twenty-five years'
practice, which appeared to me truly a case of saccharine diabetes in the horse, was that of a six-year-old agricultural
stallion.   This animal, after having shown for a lengthened
period symptoms of confirmed indigestion and an unthrifty
condition, I was desired to undertake the charge of The
previous history was short and quite reliable he had been
bred upon the farm, was of a rather sluggish or lymphatic
temperament, and had never previously suffered from illness;
he was kept almost entirely for stock purposes, being only
occasionally worked during the winter on the farm.   For some
months previous to being placed under treatment he had
been steadily developing symptoms of ill health, although
his food had been consumed as usual, and his work had been
lightened to favour him, he kept steadily losing flesh, and in
the draught showed want of energy, with a greater disposition
to perspire than was his habit There was also, latterly, an
inclination to swallow clay and foul material, an increased
discharge of urine, and a greater desire for water.   When
examined by me all these symptoms were well marked, and
in addition, it was noted that the skin was particularly unthrifty, harsh, and dry to the touch, with an extra quantity of
bran-like scales being shed from it, and the coat was over the
average length without the usual glossy character of an entire
horse The respirations were slightly abdominal, the pulse
triflingly increased in number, soft and dicrotic.   On being

made to move at a faster pace than natural, there was want of
control over the posterior extremities, he was inclined to keep
his head unnaturally low, was duller than he used formerly to
be, while at times, on carefully watching him, he seemed to
become drowsy, as if coma might be developed, there was
dilatation of the pupils, but perfect sensibility to the action
of light   The urine, to which attention was drawn, was
voided frequently, and in largely increased amount   When
examined in bulk, and as voided, it was muddy, opaque,
and slightly fragrant   when allowed to remain at rest for some
hours, there was a deposit of about 20 per cent of its bulk of
a gelatinous and finely granular-looking material, which, examined more closely, seemed made up chiefly of amorphous
granular matter, some cells, and renal casts   The urine was
examined chemically by Professor Dewar, who stated, that
although unable to obtain sufficient evidence of the existence
of sugar, there was undoubtedly present in the secretion some
peculiar material which acted towards reagents in a manner
precisely similar to sugar   During the time this animal was
under observation—nearly three months—the symptoms varied
somewhat, particularly those connected with the amount and
character of the urine, which, when least opaque and small in
amount, was always accompanied with decrease in the desire
for liquids   The evidence of disturbed nerve-power, and of
true cerebral disease, indicated by want of control over the
movements of the hind-limbs, the partial somnolency, and the
inability to elevate the head without inducing an approach to
syncope, became more manifest for some weeks, after which
they were stationary, or rather suffered some decline   I had
not an opportunity of watching this case to its termination, the
owner parting with the animal, and it being removed from the
district   During the three months this horse was under observation he was at no time perfectly free from symptoms of
ill health, neither was he unfit to perform light work

SECTION IV.

LOCAL DISEASES.

CHAPTER I.

GENERAL NATURE OF DISEASES OF THIS GROUP

THIS group of diseases, as contradistinguished from Group I,
is intended to embrace all which affect the individual structure
of particular parts or organs of the body, and which are
mainly characterized by the prominence of some distinctive
lesion or disturbance in connection with the performance of
certain special functions usually carried on in connection with
a healthy condition of these organs or parts   These diseases
are, in the majority of cases, sporadic, and they may or may
not be associated with such general morbid processes as fever
or inflammation

When diseases of this group are accompanied by constitutional or systemic disturbances, these are usually preceded by
the manifestation of the characteristic local symptoms, and
the general are to be considered as of secondary importance
No doubt local diseases are sometimes met with which owe
their origin to constitutional causes, and where the local disturbance and transformation is so great that the attention is
directed to these, to the neglect of that which has in reality
operated in the production of the more ostensible

The diseases included in this group are sometimes spoken of
as simple or common, in contradistinction to those of the class
in the former group, already examined, termed ' specific '

They have been thus styled because of their having, in common with the specific diseases, certain features or characters
which are taken as the accepted development or recognised
standard of some well-known morbid action , the specific

diseases being specific or peculiar only in so far as they have
this common morbid action, in their case modified in its mode
of development, course, or results, or in their having something added thereto

In this group of diseases we have not to look for any definite or specific morbid condition of the blood; nothing extra
and morbid added to the circulating fluid, and propagating
itself indefinitely in it, or transformed and eliminated in the
diseased local process; nor yet to a peculiar disturbance of the
equilibrium usually subsisting amongst the constituent elements of the blood   The diseased action is simple, uncomplicated, and unattended with the formation or development of
any material capable of continuing in a healthy animal body
a similar disordered process.

CHAPTER II

DISEASES OF THE NERVOUS SYSTEM

GENERAL REMARKS—LOCALIZATION OF NERVOUS DISEASES

ALTHOUGH the functions presided over by the organs or structures entering into the formation of the nervous system are
both numerous and varied, embracing perception, volition,
special sense, motor-power, and common sensation, the list of
diseases taken cognizance of in veterinary pathology as intrinsically or primarily belonging thereto, is less extensive than
that connected with the majority of the other systems or
groups of organs of which the animal machine is made up.
From this alone, however, we are not to imagine that the
diseases of this system are of so much rarer occurrence , the
reason of this paucity in description is rather to be looked for
in the fact that with its physiology or functional activity in
health, the pathology or conditions of action in disease are yet
less fully and accurately known than that of many other
organs and systems   Owing to the absence of psychical influences, the number and variation of diseases originating in
the mass of nervous matter situated within the cranium is
much fewer in our patients than in ourselves

In any consideration of the nature and treatment of diseases of this system, it ought ever to be remembered that the primary or such as seem to have their origin in the nervous centres, and with which we are presently more particularly concerned, are probably less numerous than those which may be regarded as merely secondary or symptomatic, resulting from diseases of other and different organs.

These two varieties of nervous diseases will, as a rule, be found evidencing themselves in a somewhat different manner. In those cases where the nervous structures are primarily affected, the earliest symptoms will be found associated with perverted nerve-force: in the other, or where the interrupted nerve-force is the result of some general or local disturbance, the appearance of the symptoms connected with the nerve-structures will be found to succeed or to appear synchronously with those of the inducing affection

Although our knowledge of the entire nervous system, or of any particular section of it, is even now far from complete, either as to its inherent powers and activities, or its associations, and susceptibilities of acting, or being acted upon by other orders of the animal system, we yet know enough, from the results of direct experiment and careful clinical observation, to enable us to formulate certain elementary propositions, which assist us in making diagnoses of affections of different parts of this important system

Within certain limits, it must be remembered that the ability to localize diseases of the nervous system is absolutely needful for anything like rational or successful treatment We have to recollect that its three great constituent portions, the brain, the spinal cord, and nerves, may be separately or conjointly affected with disease, and that to these associations we must look for an explanation of many of the complex phenomena so often exhibited.

1 The earliest object of our examination in approaching diseases affecting the nervous system is to determine whether the affection is cerebral, spinal, or peripheral, or whether the phenomena exhibited pertain to more than one locality

We presume the **brain-substance** proper to be chiefly involved (a) when perception, volition, and special sensation are affected; (b) when motorial and sensory activity are affected, generally longitudinally and on one side—*hemiplegia;* (c) when muscles belonging to the face and tongue are similarly disturbed; (d) in some rare instances when motorial disturbance occurs in a transverse manner—*paraplegia,* (e) when certain changes discoverable with the ophthalmoscope are observed in the eyes.

The **spinal cord** is regarded as the seat of disease (a) when disturbance of motorial and sensory activities are located in a bilateral or transverse manner—paraplegia—the spasm or paraplegia varying according to the extent of cord cut off from normal connection with the brain, the functions of which are unimpaired, (b) when the functional activity of bladder or rectum is interfered with, indicated by retention of urine and its consequences, or incontinence.

Peripheral nerves are presumed to be diseased when the phenomena of disturbance are confined to a particular muscle or group of muscles, or to a restricted sensory surface. In this way, either motion or sensation, according to the character of the nerve-cord or both, may be impaired Phenomena of this latter character, it may also be recollected, exhibit themselves when disease of nervous centres of a restricted character exist

2. Further than this general association of clinical phenomena with diseased states of the different parts of the entire nervous system, we may in many instances, notwithstanding many difficulties and conflicting opinions, link the symptoms exhibited with particular lesions of distinct areas of the different centres.

a In the **brain**, allowing certain exceptions, we may regard it as tolerably certain (1) that a lesion of one hemisphere is represented by motorial disturbance of the opposite side of the body; (2) that particular injury to the cerebral cortical matter will issue, according as this injury is irritative or destructive, in excitation or paralysis of those movements of a conscious or voluntary character; (3) that disturbance, abnormal activity, or depression of such movements as are automatic or responsive, are indicative of, or will follow, irritative or destructive interference with centres deeper seated than the cortex

Of diseases of the *cerebellum,* we are in greater uncertainty

Although many of the symptoms supposed to be associated with this portion of the cranial nervous matter are probably indirectly induced, it would appear that motor paralysis is not a feature of disease of this part, but rather that it is attended with a peculiar disorder of equilibrium The animal, on making attempts at movement, staggers, with a disposition to fall, and probably also to move in a circle, pressing with its body to any resisting object   Sensation does not seem affected, but there is squinting and spasmodic movements of the eyeball

In lesions of a sudden nature connected with the *pons varolii* and *medulla oblongata*, there is rarely a distinct train of symptoms, a fatal termination being rapid from interference with the functions of respiration and circulation When of a slow or gradually developing character, the indications are often confusing and difficult to decipher, seeing we have here motor and sensory tracts meeting, and the nuclei of origin of several nerves of importance

b Regarding the spinal cord itself, we know if destroyed in its entirety that both motion and sensation are lost posterior to the lesion   Commonly in our patients the disturbance or paralysis includes only the posterior extremities, the lesion being in the lumbar region   When in the cervical region, the anterior extremities are also affected ; while should the injury sustained be situated in the anterior portion, the probabilities are that death will result from interference with respiration and other functions essential to life   Retention of urine or difficulty of micturition may follow a lesion in the anterior portion of the cord, from spasm of the sphincter ; while incontinence will follow injury of the same structure in the loins

In some instances we find that motor-power is interfered with long before sensory, from the fact that the sensory tracts are confined to the superior cornua and the grey matter about the central canal, the outer structure suffering from injury earlier than the deep-seated, which may escape for some time

As regards special tracts of the cord, we find that if one lateral half is completely destroyed, there will be motor paralysis of the same side of the body, posterior to the lesion and sensory of the opposite side; such, however, in a perfect form rarely happens Lesions may be localized in various ways, affecting even very limited areas of motor or sensory tracts of the cord, or they may be confined to particular groups of cells, in which cases motion or sensation, more or less extensive, will be interfered with, or special sets of muscles affected

All these lesions may be irritative or destructive, tending, it is believed, respectively to produce excitation or depression of nervous activity

Another noticeable fact in connection with diseases of this system is, that to a greater extent, probably, than in any other group of organs, we find very serious derangement of function, without being able to associate this with any structural change

CHAPTER III

DISORDERS AFFECTING MOTION AND SENSATION

FROM a consideration of the respective influences which disturbance of these two great functions of the nervous system have upon the value of the animals affected, the comparative rarity of their separate occurrence, with the usual ascendency of the motorial in the compound affection, together with the fact that objective symptoms are those which in all cases most attract our notice, motorial diseases are, to us, always of the greatest importance

I. SPASMS AND CONVULSIONS

Spasms are involuntary muscular contractions, or movements occurring independent of the will In these the nervous force is transmitted in irregular fits of greater or less continuance Attended with painful sensations they are known as *cramp*, when the paroxysms are of short duration, succeeding each other rapidly ; but alternated with periods of repose, they are spoken of as *clonic spasms* When of considerable duration, or terminating in persistent rigidity, they are known as *tonic spasms* These two forms are seen in the horse respectively in common cramp or in string-halt, and in tetanus

Convulsions are muscular spasms of more severity, and affecting a greater extent of structure, but are in their essential nature similar Spasms and convulsions affect all the muscles supplied by the cerebro-spinal axis, and probably also those animated by the sympathetic system.

The term *eclampsia* is applied to a development of muscular spasms or convulsions partaking of the epileptic or epileptiform character, in which the involuntary muscular contractions are accompanied with loss of perception and volition These convulsions are usually tonic at first, afterwards of a clonic character, and are of a more serious nature than ordinary convulsive movements

Causation—All these phenomena of motor disturbance are probably referable to interference with some portion or other of the nervous centres, this interference extending merely to irritation inducing discharges of nerve-force not reaching the extent of destruction of nerve-tissue.

The chief causes in the production of these discharging lesions are—1. *Centric*, as traumatic lesions, or lesions resulting from diseases of the cranial walls, organic diseases of the cranial structures, circulation of impure blood through the nervous centres, or other dynamic changes unconnected with visible alterations, but probably dependent on disturbed nutrition 2. *Eccentric*, or *sympathetic* Here the inducing factor is irritation, propagated from disturbance or disease of a variably situated organ or structure, to a nervous centre It may arise from gastric or intestinal disturbance incident to parasites, to some irregularity of functional performance, or to an injury sustained in a distant part

Treatment—When medical interference is desirable, the indications are—1 To relieve the severity of the existing convulsions, and in all fits of an epileptiform character to prevent the animal doing himself injury 2 To ascertain if there is any condition of an abnormal character of temporary occurrence, as irregularity of dieting, which might operate in a reflex manner in inducing the spasms 3 If any constitutional cachexia or acquired impurity of blood is believed to exist, by good food and tonics to operate against the tendency of the one, and by appropriate medicine to eliminate the contaminating agent of the other.

II. Motor Paralysis—Paresis.

Motor paralysis, palsy, loss of power of motion, although it may occur of itself, is more frequently associated with sensory paralysis, the combined condition being earlier and more distinctly a loss of motion than sensation. It can scarcely of itself be considered as a disease, rather as an indication of such; while in the position of a symptom it occupies an important position in all diseases of the nervous system. In estimating its importance as an indication of tissue-change, regard must be had to various points in its development, such as its mode of attack, whether sudden or gradual, constantly existing or subject to variations, whether affecting a limited number of muscles or very extensively distributed; whether influenced by volition or by causes from without. As our patients affected with serious paralysis are rarely allowed to live long, we seldom have the opportunity of watching changes of trophic and other characters which are observed in man.

According to the situations invaded, and some other considerations, motor paralysis has received certain distinctive names, as—

1. **General paralysis**, in which, although the entire muscles are not invaded, the disturbance is so extensive as to affect both anterior and posterior members, and probably also certain muscles of the trunk. 2. **Unilateral paralysis**, or hemiplegia. 3. **Paralysis of a transverse character, or paraplegia.** 4. **Local paralysis**, when the loss of motor-power is limited to a circumscribed part of the body, a single muscle, or group of muscles

1 **General Paralysis** is only seen in the horse as a temporary condition in certain diseases of the cranial structures, in cerebral congestion, in effusion into the basal ganglia, and in injuries and diseases of the anterior portion of the cord and medulla.

2. **Hemiplegia**, or one-side paralysis, is not often observed in our patients; it is usually the result of some interference with a lateral section of the brain. On the side of the face corresponding to the brain lesion, distinct change in the facial expression often occurs as the result of the loss of muscular power. The angle of the mouth is relaxed, and the lip pendulous,

the tongue may protrude without power of retraction ; there
is difficulty in the prehension of food and drinking of water
Although mastication is impaired, the animal is still able to
swallow. Ability to stand may not be entirely lost, but power
of progression is much affected When motion is forced,
the horse is inclined to hang to the side on which the lesion
exists; and the facial muscles are affected, the limbs of the
opposite side being paralyzed

When of an ephemeral character these conditions may disappear, and the animal regain his power of locomotion in a
few days. Rarely, however, do they recover when ability to
stand is absent from the first

Causation—These are chiefly hæmorrhages from various
causes, and abnormal growths interfering with the nervous
matter of one hemisphere Of the few cases which I have
had an opportunity of watching during life and examining
after death, one appeared to result from hæmorrhage into the
corpus striatum and adjoining nervous structure , the other
was associated with a large cholesteatomatous tumour of the
choroid plexus of one lateral ventricle In such as recover,
the probable cause of the hemiplegia is effusion from congestive action, or some other agency of a transient character

3 **Paraplegia**, loss of motor-power transversely or bilaterally.
This is the form of motor-disturbance which in the horse is
the most common From its almost constant association
with lesions of the cord or disturbance of functions which in
health are intimately related to the cord, it has come to be
spoken of as spinal paralysis

Causation—The agencies which seem to operate in the production of this condition are various, and according to their
supposed situation have been differently grouped They have,
viewed as exhibiting lesions of the central nervous structures,
been spoken of as *centric* or *organic* When appearing apart
from such changes, and in intimate relation with distant disturbance or lesions, or when even these are inappreciable, they
have been regarded as proceeding from peripheral irritation,
and named *reflex* or *functional*

1 As resulting from organic changes, we find in our patients
the chief of these to be—(*a*) Lesions, as fractures or disease of
the bony segments of the vertebral column, involving damage

to the cord , (b) lesions, or disease of the cord itself. 2. Functional paraplegia, or paralysis proceeding from peripheral irritation, is represented probably by (a) loss of motor-power in connection with altered conditions of the blood either directly poisoning it or rendering it of inferior nutritive quality , (b) reflected irritation or propagated neuritis, from intestinal, uterine or other disturbances

Symptoms.—In both forms of paraplegia the loss of control over voluntary movement may as to its development be sudden, gradual, or slow. When of the organic form, its advent will depend upon the rapidity with which the lesions interfere with the integrity of the cord, while, when established, the loss of motion is usually permanent. In functional paralysis the suddenness of its appearance depends much on the virulence of the disturbing agent entering the blood, the contiguity of the seat of peripheral irritation to the spinal centre, and the previous health of the animal , when developed, this form of paraplegia may be subject to conditions of remission.

Treatment.—In any attempts at treating paraplegia it is chiefly the functional, or form connected with peripheral irritation, that is likely to make any improvement , while the indications to be followed are—(a) Removal of all conditions likely to induce local irritation of visceral or other organs, or blood-contamination , (b) the employment of such general remedies as will establish constitutional vigour , (c) local applications of a stimulating nature to nerve-structure or muscles of the limbs

4. Local Paralysis.—This variety is not much encountered in the horse; and although it may, in some instances, owe its origin to disease at the origin or connection of the nerve with the central nervous matter, it is more usually a consequence of direct injury from external violence, or from pressure exerted on the nerve by some abnormal growth or badly fitting harness. The most common manifestation of this form of paralysis which concerns us is, impairment of function of one or more branches, on one or both sides of the face, of the chief motor nerve of the facial muscles, the portio dura

Symptoms.—The indications of the existence of this condition are a lax and pendulous state of the mouth and lips on one or both sides, inability to seize food from want of prehen-

22

sile power in the lips, an awkward manner of drinking, and some irregularity in mastication

Treatment —The objects aimed at in all treatment of local paralysis, whether extensive or limited, are to restore the genetic force of the supply nerve, so that muscular contractility may be resumed, and to obviate any tendency which may exist in the tissues acted upon to destructive changes   The first of these must all be moulded by the causes in operation in the production of the nervous disturbance—which, in the common instance noted, is pressure by head-gear—the latter by appropriate local remedies

III DISORDERS OF SENSATION

In our patients, from the inability we labour under to appreciate subjective phenomena, disturbances or aberrations of sensory power are placed more beyond our recognition than impairment of motor energy.

Hypœsthesia, blunting of common sensation, and *anœsthesia,* complete loss of it, are conditions usually encountered with the accompanying state of motor paralysis, they seem, if less readily developed and less distinctly marked than the co-existing state of impaired motorial activity, to be intimately associated with it in mode of production   In their distribution, when appearing, they present modifications as to localization precisely alike, and may, for the sake of distinction, be similarly named   *Hyperœsthesia,* exalted sensibility, we sometimes observe in certain diseases of the skin of the horse, and probably also in some affections of the nervous system, organic and functional.

CHAPTER IV

DISEASES AFFECTING THE CEREBRAL CIRCULATION.

THE diseases directly connected with the cerebral circulation in the horse, although less numerous than in other of our patients, are yet important enough to call for consideration Under this grouping of disturbance of the cerebral circulation we will consider—1. Cerebral disease attendant upon an over-

supply of blood, or the opposite, in the vessels of the brain—
cerebral congestion and anæmia, 2 Cerebral thrombosis and
embolism, 3 Cerebral hæmorrhage

Without entering into the consideration of conditions, both
admitted and disputed, in connection with the cerebral circulation, it will be well to recollect, as enabling us to understand
many morbid phenomena, that one peculiarity is the absence
in the true cerebral circulation of free anastomosis, save of a
capillary nature In this way we account for, and can better
understand, the largely distributed but limited areas of structural change which occur in the brain substance from plugging of minute vessels, or from escape of their contents

I. Cerebral Congestion—Megrims—Vertigo—Staggers

Pathology *a Nature of the Affection*—These different
terms, and probably some others, have all been applied to that
condition, which is certainly the most frequently occurring, of
the purely cerebral diseases of the horse. It is not, however,
perfectly clear that these different names have always been
employed to indicate precisely the same affection, or that each
of them is looked upon by all as indicating the same morbid
action The terms *vertigo* and *staggers*, particularly the latter,
have probably been more frequently used to indicate the existence of those symptoms merely—without reference to the conditions to which such symptoms point, or from which they arise
—associated with any cerebral disturbance exhibiting obtuse-
ness of perception, and a deficiency of control over the voluntary
movements of the limbs In this way have those truly gastric
disturbances, which by sympathy or reflected action induce disordered cerebral function, come to be grouped and spoken of
along with the more purely cerebral diseases

By the term **megrims, or cerebral congestion,** we would desire
to indicate that particular cerebral disturbance in the horse,
usually sudden in its onset, and of very temporary duration,
but liable to recurrence, marked by much excitement, perversion or impairment, not merely of perception and special
sensation, but also to some extent of common sensation and
voluntary motion, these vertiginous symptoms occurring, in
the greater number of cases, where the animals are actually
engaged in draught, working in the ordinary neck-collar

Another set of cases very apt to be confounded with these, from the similarity of the symptoms exhibited, are those of cerebral disturbance, met with in all classes of horses, irrespective of the nature of their employment, whether in or out of draught, but owing their origin to very different causes, viz organic changes in connection with certain cerebral structures

b Causation —Hyperæmia of the brain-structure may occur from more than one cause It may be associated with general plethora, with increased cardiac power or action, with disturbed vaso-motor activity, or with any interference with the general arterial or capillary circulation, as a result of which more blood is sent to the cranial structures—*active hyperæmia* Or it may follow as the result of interference with the natural escape of blood from the cranial vessels—*mechanical hyperæmia*

There seems little doubt that the latter is the main factor in operation here, that all those cases of megrims or cerebral congestion occurring in harness-horses—excepting, of course, such as may be associated with organic lesions of the brain—are most rationally accounted for by attributing them to obstructed venous circulation, occasioned by the pressure of tight or badly fitting neck-collars No doubt the pushing of an animal beyond his natural pace in going up a hill immediately after a full meal, or exposure to the rays of a mid-day sun, may all have a tendency to hasten the appearance of the symptoms, or aggravate them when occurring; but none of them, individually or taken together, independent of the collar-pressure is sufficient to produce this vertigo This view, however, is not acquiesced in by all, many regarding it as inflammatory in its nature, and the result of the operation of other general or local inflammatory inducing agencies This we cannot understand, seeing that neither in its mode of origin, termination, nor any part of its course, is there resemblance to inflammatory action Again, it has been said, were this collar-pressure the true cause of its origin there would be many more cases in harness-horses than actually do occur This does not appear so clear and incontrovertible as some would have us to believe ; for it ought to be borne in mind that it is, even amongst harness-horses, a small minority which have so peculiarly formed necks, or carry their heads in such a style that, with even an indifferently fitting collar, they run the chance of cerebral congestion from impeded venous circulation , while, as corroborative of the truth of what has been stated respecting the action of the collar, there is the certainty that animals which have been subject to attacks of megrims when working in the ordinary collar, have enjoyed perfect immunity from such seizures when worked with a strap or band across the breast   This is a fact recognised not in this country only, but wherever horses are employed for draught

With respect to those cases where symptoms of cerebral disturbance similar to those attendant on megrims are met with in animals not driven in harness, there need be little hesitation in attributing such to lesions of certain structures of the nervous centre contained within the cranium, which will be noticed immediately.

c. Anatomical Characters.—As cases of cerebral congestion do not often from this obstruction of the circulation terminate fatally, so we seldom have an opportunity of observing the altered state of the cranial contents   When such have been examined, the indications of the hyperæmic state seem generally distributed throughout the entire extent of the cerebral structures   The venous sinuses and vessels of the pia mater are loaded, giving the latter a dark or opaque appearance, while the grey matter of the brain, on being cut with a knife, exhibits over the cut surface a greater number and larger size of blood-spots than usually appear, and is as a whole somewhat redder than natural   When the congested state has been one of repeated occurrence, the vessels are enlarged and tortuous

Symptoms—The symptoms indicative of this congestive action and brain-pressure are invariably sudden in their appearance ; there is no premonitory warning   the animal slackens its pace or suddenly stops , there is a shaking of the head as if some object had dropped into the ear, or the motion is upwards and downwards ; less frequently the head is turned to the side   The vessels of the face and throat are distended, the eyes stare, the nostrils become dilated, the breathing rapid or stertorous, the fore-legs are occasionally placed widely apart as if for support; the cervical and facial muscles exhibit a rapid twitching action, while the skin is damp from perspiration   Occasionally the attack proceeds no further, relief being afforded by the collar being displaced forward, when the excitation steadily subsides and the animal proceeds to his work. When, however, the symptoms increase in severity, the muscular tremors are more extensive, excitement is greater, and the fury becomes uncontrollable; the animal plunging forward or rearing, falls prostrate on the ground. When down, the paroxysm rarely lasts long, the cause being removed during the struggling by the displacement of the collar and the establishment of a free return of blood from the brain

Treatment—In the management of cases of megrims the natural indications are, first, to remove the pressure from the jugulars by pushing the collar forward and thereby permitting a free return of the blood from the cranium, second, to allay the cerebral excitement and restore the natural tone and calibre of the vessels by dashing cold water over the head and face. Those cases which are complicated with gastric and other disturbances must have these functional conditions specially attended to While, should the formation of the neck or manner of working be such as to render recurrence troublesome, the ordinary neck-collar must be dispensed with, and a breast-strap used instead.

II CEREBRAL ANÆMIA

That this and other disorders of the cerebral circulation mentioned occur in the horse there is little doubt; it may be less frequently than in man, but still more so than in other of our patients.

Causation.—Anæmia of the brain-structure may be noticed both as a general diseased condition and as affecting portions or limited areas of the cerebral structure. In the former development it is usually in conjunction with conditions the opposite of those mentioned as connected with hyperæmia. 1. In states of general anæmia, 2 With enfeebled cardiac power and action; 3. With extensive local interference with blood-supply, the result of intercranial hæmal obstruction

Anatomical Characters—There is unnatural pallor, both of membranes and brain-substance. The latter is also often damp and œdematous; and on making a section of it the free surface is marked with fewer and smaller blood-spots than in a natural condition. In many instances, particularly of local anæmia, there may be noticed occlusion of small vessels and alteration of brain-structure

Symptoms.—The indications of general cerebral anæmia which may be observed in the more attractive of the forms are such as are associated with a general weakened condition, in this way forming part of the usual train of symptoms developed in general anæmia. Early exhaustion under any work, general pallor of visible mucous membranes, disposition to syncope, impaired vision with constantly dilated pupils, with, more rarely, want of perfect control over movements—such may be noticed in young horses badly dieted, too early put to work, and where sanitary conditions are adverse. In partial anæmia the symptoms are neither diagnostic nor attractive, they are usually such as appear in association with plugging of vessels, alteration of structure, and morbid growths, and varying according to the locality in which the condition is situated.

Treatment—Only when the diseased condition is general and dependent on general causes may we expect to treat with hope of success. By attention to hygiene, good easily digested food, light work and plenty of fresh air, we may improve the quality and nutritive character of the blood. Of medicinal agents the most approved are tonics, such as preparations of iron combined with vegetable bitters

III. CEREBRAL EMBOLISM AND THROMBOSIS

The plugging of minute cerebral vessels with emboli, or as the result of thrombosis, is probably of greatest interest in a pathological point of view as the direct inducing cause of cerebral softening. Emboli, when occurring in the cerebral vessels, seem to owe their existence mainly to the previous occurrence of morbid depositions in connection with structures acted upon by the blood-stream, as in some aged subjects with warty valvular disease of the heart and some forms of pulmonary thrombosis. Thrombi, again, have probably a more extensive source of origin, chief of which are a diseased state of the inner coat of the vessels, an unhealthy condition of the blood itself, and a disturbance of the relations which in health ought to subsist between the tissues and the circulating blood.

As the result of either embolism or thrombosis there is impaired or destroyed nutrition over a more or less extended area, while the symptoms which might during life lead to the recognition of these states are only such as point to peculiar changes of a chronic nature in connection with brain-substance, chiefly the condition known as softening

IV. CEREBRAL HÆMORRHAGE—APOPLEXY

Nature and Causation.—Intercranial hæmorrhage from rupture of vessels of membranes or of brain-substance, usually spoken of as apoplexy, from its most distinguishing and diagnostic symptoms, sudden loss of consciousness, and disturbance of motion and sensation—disorders which may at the same time arise from other causes than hæmorrhage, as congestion or serous extravasation—is, apart from external violence, rather rare in the horse.

When unassociated with injury, it will be found to be directly dependent on structural changes in the minute vessels of the cerebral structure, or to changes in the brain-substance acting upon the vascular canals, disturbing their usual relation to surrounding textures, and so disposing to extravasation

Anatomical Characters—Neither in amount nor yet as to exact situation is cerebral hæmorrhage characterized by aught like similarity, and upon the variations on these points in chief depends the character of the symptoms   The principal situations in both idiopathic and traumatic hæmorrhage are—
1 Into the substance of the brain; 2 Within the ventricles;
3 In connection with and between the membranes of the brain

The first and the last are in the horse the most frequent of occurrence, the internal hæmorrhages occurring in cases where the causes seem to reside in the brain, the meningeal in such as result from violence.

The appearance of extravasated blood is usually that of a mass or clot, which, if recent, maintains its true blood-characters; but when existing for some time is variously changed both as to colour, consistence, and its relation to surrounding textures.   After some time it separates into fibrinous and serous portions, undergoes gradual change of colour, may have granular pigment or hæmatoidin crystals, and become encysted by a formation of cell-elements tending to form a capsule.   In other instances inflammatory changes may be established, and softening of contiguous structures or an abscess may result

Symptoms.—As we have no power of obtaining information in the case of our patients from a knowledge of subjective phenomena, the first indications are usually sudden and obvious interference with cerebral functions, loss of consciousness, common sensation and control over voluntary movements, the disturbance of motor-power is usually more complete than that of sensation   In the slighter instances of blood-extravasation, the loss of control over voluntary movement may, although general, be incomplete, or it may be limited to certain sets of muscles—a form of hemiplegia. When extensive the motorial power may be completely lost, the animal falling to the ground in a state of profound coma, while when laid there, certain convulsive movements may be executed by particular muscles or sets of muscles   Although these in a general sense may be regarded as representing the indications of cerebral hæmorrhage, apoplexy proper, it must never be forgotten that in moderate cases of blood-extravasation the symptoms vary in accordance with the parts of the brain-substance which are the seat of the effusion   In all, however, their accession is sudden, and in the more extensive fatal in their results, chiefly from the impairment of the vagus power and pneumonic complications   With the less extensive effusions, should the symptoms not show progression or fresh exacerbation after the second or third day, a certain amount of hope may be entertained of recovery, with, it may be, impairment of some local activity

Treatment.—When the truly apoplectic symptoms of coma, with more or less impairment of motion and sensation, occur in connection with appreciable or non-appreciable causes, the ordinary resorted to practice of blood-abstraction ought to be carried out with much caution, and only under particular conditions, otherwise, from our present knowledge of cerebral functions, and the influence of blood or serous extravasation on the normal operation of these, we are disposed to think it is better to trust to less dangerous remedies and the recuperative powers of the animal body   When the sudden disturbance of consciousness is attended with local superficial venous engorgement, stertorous breathing, and a full and rather strong cardiac action in young and previously healthy animals, blood-letting is indicated   When the opposite conditions obtain, the most which we are warranted in doing is to place the animal in as favourable a position as possible, with the head rather elevated ; attend to the general comfort, allow plenty of fresh air, with cold water to the head, friction, and woollen bandages to the extremities.   Where shock has been considerable, and collapse is imminent, stimulation may be usefully employed through means of enemata, attention in all cases being given to relieve the bowels, which are likely to be confined   In all the severer attacks, however, of cerebral hæmorrhage, there is little chance of recovery ; while a rapidly fatal termination is to be preferred to recovery with partial paralysis, and a decided tendency to recurrence

CHAPTER V

ACUTE CEREBRAL INFLAMMATIONS

Synonyms—Encephalitis—Cerebritis, Inflammation of the Substance of the Brain , Meningitis—Inflammation of the Brain-coverings

Causation—Cerebral inflammations of every type chiefly occur in the horse—1 As the result of direct violence sustained from without, as injury to the bones of the cranium , 2 From disease of these bones ; 3 From exhaustion and exposure, particularly to the rays of the sun ; 4 As the result of certain specific fevers ; 5. From the entrance into the system probably of some specific virus, as in cerebro-spinal fever.

Anatomical Characters—The greater number of cases of cerebral inflammation which I have had the opportunity of examining have been those where the diseased process followed as a result of injury or of bone-disease.   In these the appearances were tolerably uniform, in a few less plainly marked than might have been expected considering the severity of the symptoms exhibited during life   The membranes of the brain were opaque and thickened, the vascular much congested, and seemed to contain fluid amongst its meshes; the dura mater in portions adherent, through the medium of fine organized deposit, to the inner surface of the cranial bones; there was also, in some situations, a trifling amount of puriform matter mingled with the connecting structures. The latter condition I attributed to the damage sustained by the walls of the cranium and other structures from injury or bone-disease. The appearance of the brain-substance varied much—in some scarcely at all altered in colour, save where an isolated capillary seemed plugged, presenting a distinct spot amidst the general white cerebral matter; in others the blood-specks and general redness were very distinct, and the consistence, particularly of the grey matter, much impaired. In several the inflammatory appearances were specially located in connection with the seat of bone-disease, and there the membranes were dark-coloured, soft, and thickened, seemingly disposed to remove as sloughs.

Symptoms.—In almost every attempt to detail and describe inflammatory action occurring in connection with those parts of the nervous system contained within the cranial cavity, much time and care have been bestowed in endeavouring to distinguish between the symptoms which indicate disease of the coverings or membranes of the structures, and the substance proper of the organs themselves.

From a scientific or pathological point of view this is both interesting and necessary, and probably in many cases is capable of attainment both in a general sense and also descending so minutely as with tolerable certainty to indicate the particular part of these several structures invaded. Practically, however, such power in diagnosis is of less value than might at first sight appear, seeing there are very few cases of inflammation of the meninges of the brain which do not quickly extend to the brain-substance, and probably also many of an opposite character. The results of the most carefully conducted observations and experiments seem to point to something like the following as the symptoms we may usually expect to meet with when the two different textures, meningeal and cerebral, are severally the seats of inflammation.

When the membranes are primarily affected there is suddenness in development of symptoms, local congestion, excitement with muscular spasms or convulsions, succeeded by subsidence or arrest of normal nervous activity.

Invasion of the true cerebral structure, on the other hand, is less active in development of symptoms, is marked by no frenzy or excitement, but from the first exhibits lowered or depressed functional activity, impairment at the outset of some special nerve function.

The marked excitement and uncontrollable fury so often spoken of as characteristic of cerebral inflammations I have rarely or never encountered, and where exaltation of cerebral function showed itself, it was only for a short time, to be succeeded by an opposite state, a lowering of these below the normal standard

No doubt inflammatory action, when showing itself in connection with the encephalic structures, is much modified by the nature of the tissue in which it originates, as well as by the extent of textures invaded

In the early stages of inflammation of the cerebral structures in all animals during which there is much vascular derangement, and particularly when the meninges seem more largely the seat of this morbid action, there is a great likelihood to be excitement, delirium, or convulsions, the severity of these determined by the extent of tissue invaded. This hyperactivity of cerebral function is not constant or continuous, but paroxysmal in character, liable to be brought on or seriously augmented by any untoward noise or disturbance to which the animal may be subjected. The constitutional fever is well marked, the temperature raised, skin and mouth perceptibly hotter than natural, there seems pain in the head, which the animal cannot bear to have roughly handled; the eyes are staring and bloodshot, with pupils contracted, the pulse frequent and hard or sharp, respirations irregular, and sometimes accompanied with a moan; bowels confined. The animal is restless and uneasy, moving from side to side or around his box, the body sometimes damp from perspiration. Occasionally muscular twitchings and general or local hyperæsthesia are symptoms well marked.

Succeeding this stage of increased nervous irritability and vascular excitement, which is generally short-lived, is that of nervous aberration and depression, indicative of more extensive involvement of the true nerve-structures The fever subsides, the temperature of the body is lower, the pulse diminishes in frequency, is less sharp or hard ; the breathing becomes stertorous, the delirium or excitability gradually declines, and special sensation lessened until consciousness is lost in coma more or less perfect. With the subsidence of the restlessness the horse will, if capable of maintaining the standing posture, do so listlessly in one position, the head lowered, the eyes glassy, with pupils dilated, while control over voluntary movement is much disturbed The disposition to preserve the position of the limbs as they may be placed is not unlike the condition which prevails in catalepsy

From the commencement the appetite is capricious, with discharge from kidneys and bowels less in amount than natural

The partial muscular twitchings or general convulsions are not present in every case, and are usually most attractive as the termination is approached At this period the animal is almost certain, unless carefully watched, to do itself injury by violent and unconscious tossing

Diagnosis—Acute inflammatory diseases of the cerebral structures have to be distinguished from some other disturbances general and local, attended with nervous derangement Many who have given attention to the diseases of animals appear to have confounded these with symptomatic cerebral derangement attendant on indigestion, in which the exaltation of nerve-function is so great as occasionally to result in fits of ungovernable fury True phrenitis is, however, essentially different from any disturbance of cerebral function connected with gastric derangement. No doubt during development symptoms in both classes of affections touch very closely upon each other, or confusion in description would not have so often occurred In the majority of instances the history of the attack will guide us much in determining the character of the disorder In that of sympathetic cerebral disturbance it will point to some dietetic error ; in the other there are no suspicions of such, but rather of some local lesion. The purely cerebral disturbance is comparatively a rare affection ; the other is common under certain conditions.

Fever is a distinct character of the one, unassociated with gastric derangement, in the other it is not. When taken early, the symptomatic form is capable of removal by ordinary treatment the other does not yield readily to medicine

Treatment of Encephalic Inflammations—From the earliest period to the present time, this class of inflammations has been generally treated by a vigorous carrying out of the entire course of the so-called antiphlogistic remedies Now, however, with our altered views of the nature of this process, and the relative importance of the different phenomena of which it is made up, the carrying out of this method in every instance is regarded as rather doubtful, while we know that in actual practice there are encountered many cases in which indiscriminate depletion and a rigorous enforcement of a lowering dietary are productive of results anything but desirable. Generally in those cases resulting from injuries, or where congestion is a marked feature, or excitement and febrile disturbance are high, especially when unconnected with any zymotic or constitutional disease, blood-letting is indicated, will be well borne, and is likely to relieve the urgency of these symptoms When, however, the exalted nervous and muscular activities, indicative of cerebral disturbance, occur during the course of some grave constitutional disease, bleeding is generally unadvisable, badly borne, and attended with disastrous results

During the earliest stages, those of excitement, marked benefit will sometimes result from the employment locally of ice, cloths saturated with cold water, or some evaporating lotion Early attention to the digestive canal is absolutely needful, and promptly unloading it by means of a cathartic is in all cases attended with benefit

Having placed the animal in as quiet a situation as it is possible to obtain, and being satisfied that the bowels have acted, or are likely to respond to the medicine given, the continued febrile symptoms are most successfully combated by the use of salines, as nitrate or chlorate of potash, given separately or combined, or alternated with full doses of acetated liquor ammonia; any of these are taken readily enough in the drinking-water Freedom from disturbance in all these cases is absolutely essential to success in treatment, and this, with correct sanitary conditions, ought to be strictly carried out.

Should the appetite not be entirely gone, any food which is offered ought to be light, unstimulating, and in itself of such a nature as will tend to keep the bowels in a moist condition. Excitement and fever will often subside, and consciousness return, while defective motor-power or impaired special sensation still continues. In these conditions, benefit is likely to result from the application of a smart blister to the pole; while should improvement manifest itself, the blister ought to be repeated, and the bowels kept moist by laxatives or appropriate dieting

In cases which assume a decidedly chronic character, a somewhat different line of treatment seems indicated, which will be referred to when considering these cases specially.

CHAPTER VI.

CHRONIC DISEASES OF THE CEREBRAL STRUCTURES

APART from the disorders of an active character already noticed, we not unfrequently encounter departures from health which are gradual in development, sometimes decidedly chronic. Chief of these are probably—1. *Disease of cerebral membranes and structure, marked by obvious tissue-change; 2. Adventitious growths in connection with cerebral structures; 3. Dropsy of the cerebral organs—hydrocephalus*

I. CHRONIC DISEASE OF CEREBRAL MEMBRANES AND STRUCTURE, MARKED BY OBVIOUS TISSUE-CHANGE.

a Chronic Meningitis.—In some instances of repeated or long-continued cerebral congestion, in certain recoveries from cranial injuries and acute inflammatory action, and in others where no previous disease could be detected, horses have been found, on examination after death, to exhibit evidence of changed meningeal structures, conveying the impression that such changes had existed for some time previous to death, and that they were most probably the result of inflammatory action.

These changes consist in thickening of the membranes

generally, adhesion of the outer to the cranial walls, and of the inner to the brain-substance, together with a variable amount of a variously organized exudate, either partly fibrillated or in some instances undergoing softening This alteration of membranes and existence of inflammatory exudate may be variously distributed , often most conspicuous at the base of the brain, involving the origin of certain of the cranial nerves, occasionally in the sulci, and more rarely in the ventricles.

b **Slow Changes in Brain-Substance—Cerebral Softening,**—The alterations which we encounter in the intimate cerebral structures are chiefly those of change in consistence and colour of circumscribed portions of the mass This alteration in textural integrity varies from an almost imperceptible softening to a condition of marked diffluence, and in colour from pink to a dirty white

The chief causes of this change are probably different grades of inflammatory action, or impairment of nutrition from defective blood-supply, following embolism or thrombosis

Symptoms —The indications of either of these conditions in any of their different forms are not, as a rule, attractive or diagnostic They are rarely connected with excitation or intensification of cerebral function, usually with the opposite ; while depending upon the situation and extent of such changes will be the nature and extent of the interference with special function and activities

II ADVENTITIOUS GROWTHS IN CONNECTION WITH CEREBRAL STRUCTURES

Like every other organ, the brain and structures contained within the cranium are liable to become the seat of certain morbid growths or deposits referable to general or constitutional causes, or certain local changes, and in consequence of which various of the functions exercised by the encephalic structures are more or less impaired

Anatomical Characters—The chief of these adventitious growths or tumours in the horse are *cancer*, *glioma*, *cholesteatoma*, *parasitic and other cysts, and osseous growths* only indirectly connected with the brain

Cancer in the soft form, either diffused or as a separate growth, is in rare instances observed in both the membranes and substance of the brain. When it is met with it is usually as part of a general infective condition rather than as a primary diseased state of these structures. Whether it is rapid or slow of growth depends much upon the form which it takes, and the general condition of which the cerebral change is merely symptomatic

Glioma—This is the term applied to an abnormal growth in association with the connective-tissue of the cerebral matter, the neuroglia. Both in its general appearance and intimate structure, it seems simply hyperplasia of this material; at least, there is in its composition an extra amount of this, having mingled with it certain peculiar cell-elements much resembling those of sarcoma of the smaller-celled variety.

Its existence, of varying extent or bulk, I have encountered on several occasions in connection with the cerebellum. In no case was the tumour well defined, but it shaded off gradually into the healthy surrounding structure; the extent of the growth, and its steady development in several of these instances, inducing recurring disturbance with perceptible thinning of the cranial bones.

Osseous Tumours.—These, when associated and interfering with the cranial structures, are usually as growths springing from, or which have sprung from, the inner table of the cranial bones, chiefly the temporal. In form they are rounded and nodulated, often attached by a well-defined pedicle; their physical appearance when large—and they have become detached, occupying the brain-space, the cerebral matter having been removed through absorption arising from their pressure—has sometimes caused them to be regarded as specimens of ossified brain-substance. In intimate composition they are of the nature of dense, compact bone-structure, ivory-looking, and free from the ordinary bone-cavities or canals, very much resembling the dental-like growths more frequently seen attached to the outer table of the same bone, and, like them, may owe their origin to perverted development of dental pulps.

The most frequently observed adventitious developments in the brain of the horse are probably those known as concentric amylaceous corpuscles, or cholesteatomatous growths, found in connection with the vascular structures or choroid plexuses of the lateral ventricles. The intimate structure of these growths

23

is slightly variable; usually they are composed in greater part of the fatty material cholesterine, arranged in plates closely packed in layers, combined with amyloid or starch-like bodies, a very limited amount of serum and fine connective-tissue; the greater part of this latter being disposed of as an investing capsule

These abnormal growths develop rather slowly, probably appearing first as simple hypertrophy of the villi of the plexuses, and, although they may attain a considerable size, they do not often, under ordinary conditions, cause much inconvenience.

Symptoms—While some of these growths are injurious in virtue of and as part of the operating agency of a general diseased condition, the greater number appear to injure more from the alteration which their presence induces in the surrounding portions of the brain-structure, while it is undoubtedly certain that several, as those of the choroid plexus, may exist for a lengthened period without entailing any obvious disturbance   Violent or great exertion in all animals in which these tumours exist is liable to be attended with cerebral disturbance—uncontrollable excitement, impairment or loss of consciousness, and control over voluntary movement, similar to what occurs during fits of megrims from cerebral congestion

Treatment—The management of these cases with a view to ultimate recovery is of course hopeless, but with careful treatment of animals so affected and the judicious apportioning of their work, making it gradually progressive in severity, very satisfactory results may sometimes be obtained

III HYDROCEPHALUS—DROPSY OF THE BRAIN

Hydrocephalus, or a collection of fluid within the ventricles, in or beneath the arachnoid, or in both situations, although usually appearing as a congenital disease, may be developed at any period of the animal's life. The consideration of this affection is of less importance to the veterinary surgeon than the practitioner of human medicine, as well from the comparative rarity of its occurrence in our patients as from the acknowledged futility of its treatment when present.   Congenital hydrocephalus is to us chiefly interesting from two considerations   first, the apparent connection which seems to subsist between this intra-uterine malformation and some constitutional predisposition or cachexia, most probably the scrofulous, in one or both parents; and second, because of the difficulties such cases offer during the course of parturition. When occurring at a more advanced period of life it is, in all those cases which I have observed, of a subacute rather than decidedly chronic character, and seemed to be intimately associated with a previous attack of inflammatory action.

Anatomical Characters.—The greatest amount of fluid I have invariably found in the lateral ventricles, not in connection with the membranes, which of themselves give very distinct evidence of increased vascular action, the condition of congestion extending to the vessels of the bones. The arachnoid I have observed to be opaque and somewhat thickened, particularly over the inferior surface of the brain, where it will often be found clogged with the results of inflammatory deposition. The quantity of fluid, which is of a pale and watery character and slightly turbid, varies much; I have not, however, met with a greater amount than eight ounces. In such cases, the progress of the disease and accumulation of fluid has operated in destroying the septum naturally existing between the ventricles, raising the corpus callosum, and thus throwing the normally distinct cavities into one large sac, the superior walls of which appear gradually to be undergoing a thinning process.

Symptoms.—The symptoms simulate, or rather are similar to, those of inflammation of the encephalon combined with pressure. In the first stage there is fever and increased irritability, this generally lasts a few days, when it is followed by the second stage, of diminished consciousness and sensibility; which, if not relieved, passes gradually into the final and fatal stage of paralysis with convulsions.

Treatment.—In all these diseases of a chronic nature affecting the contents of the cranium, little can be done in the direction of cure beyond the strict enforcement of correct hygienic conditions, a careful protection of the animal from all disturbing influences, and combating adverse symptoms as they occur. The greater number are benefited by a judicious use of tonic and even stimulant medicines, alternated with certain alteratives and diuretics.

CHAPTER VII.

DISEASES OF THE SPINAL CORD AND ITS MEMBRANES.

General Remarks.—The diseases of this part of the nervous system are as difficult to understand in many of their manifestations, and in their investigation are surrounded with obstacles as great, as those pertaining to the brain proper These difficulties are not of one class or one sided ; they are difficulties as respect time and opportunities for experiments and research, as well as intelligence and fitness for the investigation If many of the doctrines hitherto taught relative to the diseases affecting the cerebral nervous structures are, at the present time, justly regarded as nearly in a transition stage, certainly nothing more definite or flattering can be affirmed concerning those of the spinal cord.

The amount, as well as exactness, of the knowledge possessed respecting the structure and functions of this part of the nervous system has always had a powerful influence in determining the views held, not merely regarding the diseases to which it is liable, but also the value we are to place upon many of the most prominent symptoms, and the inferences which may be deduced from these

Our present knowledge leads us to regard the cord not as a mere aggregation of nerve-trunks, nor yet as a simple extension of the cerebral matter contained within the cranial case, but as an important and independent nervous centre, as well as being intimately connected both in structure and function with the brain proper, and the nerve-cords which issue from or run into itself

From the similarity which exists between the ultimate structure of the cord and cerebral nervous centre, we would naturally anticipate a close resemblance in the character of their diseases, and the alterations which these structures show on after-death examination The healthy functional activities, however, of these centres being different, the disturbed or morbid actions which originate from these, to which we give the name of disease symptoms, are modified accordingly From the extent of discrepance which exists amongst experimenters regarding the functions of the different parts of the cord, it follows as almost a necessary sequence that we shall have considerable variety of opinion in the interpretation of such symptoms as are met with in morbid and disturbed conditions of this particular part   Although quite true that what are more properly regarded as surgical lesions, the results of accidents and injuries, figure more largely than aught else, and are more generally recognised as the immediate causes of spinal affections with our patients, still it seems unwise, because incorrect, to shut our eyes to the fact that other causes are ever in operation to destroy the integrity of function and structure here as in other organs

I CONCUSSION OF THE CORD

Although not aware that any who have given their attention to the diseases of our patients have particularly noticed the occurrence of concussion of the cord, I am yet satisfied that such a condition, if not a common one, does occasionally occur   The few cases which I believe to have come under my notice have all been in hunting-horses, and have resulted from leaping where the drop was considerable, and the animals apparently were not expecting it   The symptoms of injury were manifested at the time by a deficiency of power to move onwards as usual, this being more marked on pulling the horse up and again moving away   In no case did they completely lose the power of their limbs , but the morning following the appearance of these symptoms, on being led from the stable, a marked stiffness of the loins was noticed, and a want of control over the movements of the hind limbs, to such an extent that the points of the ilh—the projections of the haunch—were apt to be brought in contact with the sides of the doorway, and the fetlocks to be knocked against each other   Although, in some cases, the animals might be able to move at a walking-pace in a straight line, the want of control was very obvious when they were pushed into a faster pace, or made to turn or move in a backward direction   In a few, pain was exhibited on manipulation being carried out along the dorsal and lumbar spines , a greater number, however, seemed to suffer from the opposite state—hypæsthesia —and when laid on the ground there was difficulty in rising. That this was not a muscular lesion seemed indicated by the absence of swelling, the trifling amount of pain on handling the parts, by the existence of diminished sensibility in the limbs, by the mode of its production, and the rapidity in many cases of recovery.

The treatment pursued was, rest with perfect quietude, the exhibition of a little laxative medicine, and the application two or three times daily, for an hour at a time, of rugs which had been wrung from hot water. Recovery was in a few cases rapid, in others the animals were not fit for work for several weeks; in none, however, did the symptoms return.

II SPINAL INFLAMMATION—SPINAL MENINGITIS—MYELITIS—INFLAMMATION OF THE CORD AND ITS MEMBRANES

Definition—*Inflammation of the spinal cord and its envelopes.*

Varieties, Nature, and Causation—The structures contained within the spinal canal, the cord, and its coverings are, in common with the analogous contents of the cranial cavity, liable to inflammatory action, which, when occurring, may terminate in resolution, or in alteration of tissue, and the production of heterologous and additional elements. Although, in the great majority of cases of inflammation affecting the cord and its coverings, it is extremely difficult, if not impossible, accurately to distinguish the relative extent to which the morbid process has invaded those different structures, it is, nevertheless, highly probable that the one may be much diseased while the other is comparatively healthy. Sometimes, even with the animals which occupy our attention, it is possible to form in those cases a wonderfully correct idea of the chief seat of the localization of the diseased action.

Spinal inflammation is the term ordinarily employed to indicate inflammation more or less actively distributed in both cord and coverings; *spinal meningitis* being used to indicate a similar process occurring in the meninges or membranes of the cord; and *myelitis* where the inflammation is confined to the substance proper of the cord. For our present purpose it will be sufficient to regard the phenomena of inflammatory action in connection with the structures contained within the spinal canal as associated with, or representing the condition recognised under, the term spinal inflammation; and this condition may be conveniently regarded as exhibiting itself in either an acute or chronic manner

Acute spinal inflammation may result from—1 Violence, and external injury of any kind , 2 Disease of the bony segments of the canal; 3 Exposure to damp, and extremes of temperature, particularly when exhausted by overwork; 4. It may start into existence unconnected with appreciable causes When occurring from injury or violence the connection between cause and effect is not difficult to trace; while, when the injury is severe, the rapidity with which the process of inflammation progresses, and the extent and nature of the structural changes which follow, may be said to preclude all chance of recovery Of course the cases of spinal inflammation included in this category are chiefly such as must be regarded as purely surgical, and the lesions are primarily such as interfere with the integrity of the cord, either by fracture or displacement of the bony segments of the canal, resulting in compression, directly by the displacement of the bones, or indirectly through the presence of the products of the inflammation which has been started in the vascular structures of the cord. When not directly traceable to external violence, the great majority of the cases of spinal inflammation which have come under my notice have apparently had their origin in exposure to wet and cold when suffering from fatigue and exhaustion They have been either harness-horses, which have been driven rapidly rather long journeys, and carelessly allowed to remain for some time exposed to damp and cold, or heavy draught animals treated in a similar manner. I have not observed that any age or breed, provided the exciting causes named were in operation, seemed more particularly predisposed to the affection than another Besides these adverse agencies operating as factors in the production of this disease, there must be taken into consideration such rather inappreciable and ill-understood influences as are spoken of under the terms of heredity and localization of particular or specific poisons.

Anatomical Characters.—Changes occurring in the cord, the result of inflammatory action, are greatly diversified both as to character and extent. In some instances, even after a careful examination, marvellously trifling changes are to be detected, unless we allow our preconceived ideas to overrun our calmer

judgment   Where these alterations are undoubted they vary
from simply increased vascularity and appreciable thickening of the membranes, from adherent gelatiniform amorphous
exudations, or increase of the serous slightly coloured fluid, to
distinct induration of the meninges, and complete destruction of
the integrity of the intimate texture of the cord, which may
be not only pulpy but diffluent, and exhibiting serious alterations in nerve tubes and cells, with the existence of other
elements, corpuscular, etc , the products of the diseased action
These changes, when occurring in the nervous tissue, are
usually most marked in the centre or grey matter of the cord
where the tissue is more vascular   This peculiar softening, or
ramollissement, although by many regarded as a condition
peculiar to nerve-structure, would seem to have nothing
specific connected with it, save so much as attaches to the
tissue which is invaded by ordinary inflammation

Symptoms —Acute inflammation of the structures contained
within the vertebral canal may or may not be anticipated by
premonitory symptoms   As far as experience teaches it would
seem that such are more generally to be observed when the
inflammation is distinctly associated with the membranes of
the cord, and most likely to be absent when this morbid action
is exclusively or more extensively confined to the substance of
the cord itself   Occurring prior to the paralysis, or loss of
control over the voluntary movements of the limbs, the great
diagnostic symptom in all cases, although its appearance may
in some be delayed, is spasmodic or clonic contraction of the
great muscles connected with the trunk and limbs   The animal,
we may be told, has been suddenly seized with cramp of his
hind limbs; but this cramp, we may observe, is not unconnected with constitutional disturbance, as in the condition
ordinarily recognised by that term   The limbs are lifted
rapidly from, and as rapidly placed upon, the ground and
although the movement evidently causes pain, the animal does
not seem able to control or discontinue it   At this early stage
there may be intervals of calm, and freedom from muscular
spasms; only, however, to be succeeded by exacerbation of all
these functional disturbances   Perspiration plentifully bedews
the body, the animal is restless, but the very movements he
executes only intensify the pain and muscular spasm.   This

constitutional disturbance and excitement may continue for some hours, seldom exceeding twelve, when, partly from pain and exhaustion, but more probably because irritation of nervous matter has been succeeded by its destruction, our patient falls to the ground. In the recumbent position there may at first be apparent relief, the muscular spasms, however, often return; and in fatal cases steadily increase in frequency and severity until the power of movement is gone.

During all this time the animal is extremely sensitive to the approach of anyone, seeming to dread being touched; and, although sensation is very much impaired in the limbs, appears, by his expression, to suffer acutely elsewhere.

With the occurrence of these symptoms of disturbed motor and sensory functions, which are, of course, the most characteristic, there are others more or less attractive. In the more severe cases the appetite is much impaired, or wanting altogether, although both gruel and water may continue to be partaken of freely. The pulse is accelerated and hard, the temperature elevated, and the respirations tumultuous. The bowels are irregular, and the urine voided is often altered both physically and chemically.

In other cases we fail to observe any symptoms of illness until our attention is arrested by the sudden and unexpected interference with the powers of locomotion, thus serving to indicate that the diseased condition is fairly established ere we are aware of its existence. In such instances the impairment of motor-power is very rapidly progressive, an hour or two being sufficient to incapacitate the animal from maintaining a standing position, or to return to that if laid on the ground. Although paralysis may have been the first developed and most prominent symptom, the probability is that following this at a very short interval will be muscular spasms, which are, however, neither so severe nor so long continued as in those cases where they are the earliest observed phenomena. In the majority of the cases thus affected, sensation is rarely ever entirely destroyed, pain being felt on pricking the limb or tail, as indicated by the putting forth of a certain amount of effort to remove the part interfered with from the irritation.

Whenever the appetite is destroyed and the pulse much altered, with other symptoms of constitutional disturbance, there is always expression of pain, haggard countenance, and repeated tossings when in the recumbent position

This latter form of spinal inflammation, insidious in its progress, or at least, although sudden enough in its demonstration, not ushered into existence, nor marked during its continuance, by much exhibition of violence, evidence of pain, or muscular contraction, tonic or clonic, is that development which is less likely in its special location to be associated with the meninges proper than with the intimate texture of the cord itself, being more truly *myelitis* than *spinal meningitis*

In addition to these forms of inflammation of the spinal cord and its membranes, appearing suddenly and pursuing their course rapidly until they reach a height previous to decline—or what is more commonly the termination, until death—we are aware that in the horse there are exhibitions of slow or chronic forms of the same diseased action

Chronic inflammation of the meninges and substance of the cord does not commonly terminate in death; more frequently the termination is that of impairment of function to such an extent that it is more profitable as well as humane to destroy the animal than persevere in treatment   One manifestation of chronic spinal inflammation, in which most probably at first the meninges are more largely involved than the intimate cord-structure, has, as its most diagnostic feature, persistent tonic and clonic contractions of certain muscles or groups of muscles; a condition   often regarded as a form of rheumatism or modified tetanic spasm, which, when affecting the muscles of the neck and anterior parts particularly, has been spoken of as 'the cords.' Here the spasms are not rapidly developed, nor are they of great intensity; often insidiously progressive, but rarely for a lengthened period so severe as largely to interfere with the working powers of the animal   Should this state of disturbed muscular contractility not quietly subside, either through judicious treatment or by the natural failure of the morbid process, and through the restoration of the inherent powers of the organism, a change usually creeps over the manifestation of the phenomena

In place of hyperæsthesia and excess of muscular contractility, a certain amount of pain and difficulty in executing particular movements is exhibited, and with the great general rigidity of masses of the muscular system, there is less disposition to lie down, or when down, a greater difficulty to rise these conditions gradually but steadily passing into more or less well-marked deficiency of muscular power and paralysis, earliest and most marked as paraplegia Complete paralysis of the posterior extremities is often well enough observed in its gradual progress and development, from difficulty to turn rapidly or in a limited space, disposition to stagger against doorways in passing through them; inability to move backwards in or out of yoke, trailing of the limbs, and knuckling over on the fetlocks, or bruising of the one from blows with the opposite foot, to complete inability to use the limbs either as organs of support or locomotion.

Chronic inflammatory action of the structures contained in the spinal canal does not, however, in all cases pass through the same phases of disturbed activities, in some seemingly the diseased condition has existed for some time ere symptoms indicative of spinal changes are obvious, or at least obvious enough to direct our attention to the seat of the lesion In- stead of first exhibiting spastic contractions or exaltation of special function, we may at once find decided failure of muscu- lar power Such cases are probably those in which the pure nervous structure of the cord is more largely invaded than the membranes The extent of the paralysis, the first and probably the only attractive feature of this condition, varies with the exact seat of the spinal lesion, while from its appear- ance until completely established, the interval is not usually great, exhibition of impairment of motor-power being rapidly succeeded by complete paraplegia

Diagnosis —There are many cases in the horse in which, as in other animals, the difficulties of distinguishing between diseases of the brain and spinal cord are great, seeing that both conditions may be followed by a somewhat similar train of symptoms In arriving at a correct diagnosis, we are assisted by many considerations, and by a careful observation of collateral phenomena We must give attention to discover if previous indications of pure cerebral disturbance have ever been observed, or if the animal is subject to megrims or epilepsy. An endeavour may be made to determine if alteration in the position of the head as to elevation, or disturbance of it rudely

by force, has any influence in determining the appearance or intensification of the existing symptoms   We must not be misled
by the appearance of the eyes, seeing that similar changes may
follow spinal as pure cerebral disease   Careful manipulation
over the various regions of the spine will sometimes yield a
little information, or the history of the case may afford more

Treatment—When it is evident, or when we are satisfied
that active congestion exists in connection with this portion of
the nervous centres, treatment should at once be directed to
diminish the congestion, and prevent, as far as possible, active
inflammatory action   With this object in view, it is advisable
that particular attention should be directed to the condition of
the bowels.   As they are usually confined, purgatives are
indicated   Should aloes—the best purge, in most cases, for
the horse—have been exhibited, it had better be followed by
the daily administration of salines in the drinking-water.
Bleeding may in some, or in many, instances be indicated, but
must not be carried out where paralysis exists.

Should local pain be an attractive feature, the repeated
application of hot-water cloths or poultices will usually be
productive of relief   These may be medicated with belladonna,
or, following their removal, may be succeeded by a large belladonna plaster   In addition to the purgative and repeated
administration of the salines, there is at this stage, when the
hyperæmia of the cord is more likely to exist, a probability
that benefit will result from the employment of such agents
as experiment proves have a controlling power over the
calibre of the vessels of the cord, chief of these agents are
belladonna and ergot of rye; the former as the extract, the
latter as the æthereal tincture, may be exhibited to the extent
of from one to four drachms daily

The employment of stimulants, ordinary or special, internal
or external, must not be had recourse to during the stage of
active congestion, or at least we may say they appear contra-
indicated, and practically they are worse than useless   When,
however, there is good reason to believe that this condition
has subsided, and indications of defective nervous power still
exist, stimulation both externally and internally is indicated
As an external stimulant, there is nothing equal to the actual
cautery.   This is to be employed fairly over a considerable

length of the spine on both sides, but no cantharides to be used with it. In internal use, following the subsidence of inflammation, strychnine, either as strychnine or in the preparation known as Easton's syrup, given twice daily, combined with some alcoholic preparation, in many instances answers well Along with these medicaments due attention should be given to secure good dieting, correct sanitary conditions, and quietude Occasionally very well-marked cases of spinal disease will, under patient and judicious treatment, exhibit marked improvement, although it must be confessed that they are ever to be regarded as serious affections

III. Sclerosis of the Nervous Centres.

The condition now known by the term sclerosis—hardening —of the nervous centres, to which investigation has of late years been much directed in human pathology, has received less attention from veterinary authorities than it deserves. From what opportunities I have had of attending to diseases affecting these structures, I feel satisfied that both in the cranial and spinal centres this is a condition which in the horse oftener exists than has hitherto been allowed.

Situation, Nature, and Causation —The cases which have come under my observation have been pretty equally distributed between the cerebellal structure and that of the spinal cord ; I have not observed it in connection with the cerebral centres proper. The animals have all of them been adults, none that might be regarded as worn out from age, but such as had during their life been engaged in rather hard work, and in no way deteriorated by other depressing sanitary conditions. In some instances, I am aware that the animals exhibiting the changes indicative of this condition have belonged to families in which there were known to exist several sufferers from ill-defined nervous affections, chiefly associated with the development during life of muscular spasms, usually of a choreic character

Whether or not in its nature inflammatory, the condition as presented for our observation in textural changes is essentially an extra development of the connective-tissue peculiar to masses of nervous matter, the neuroglia This in addition to abnormal conditions previously existing, or which have only lately been called into existence in ultimate nervous elements, tends by pressure on these to interfere with the due performance of nervous function.

Of the agencies which operate in the production of these changes we know little or nothing definitely, they may probably be grouped as—1 Heredity, an ill-defined disposition to develop, under certain external influences, peculiar trophic changes of nervous matter 2 Overwork and exhaustion, particularly when combined with exposure to adverse climatic influences 3 It may follow as a sequel of other diseased states, as certain fevers, or inflammatory action involving the particular localities of the nervous centres, afterwards exhibiting the sclerous changes

Anatomical Characters—The more obvious appearance of disease in nervous sclerosis is the occurrence of greyish patches or circumscribed tracts of varying extent, I have noticed them in greatest amount in connection with the lateral lobes of the cerebellum in the horse—in some they appear as enlargements of the entire tissue affected, in others no alteration in bulk or form is appreciable. They are of varying degrees of toughness, firmness, or hardness, exhibiting, where incised, many of the characters of common fibrous tissue Over the outer surface of these patches the pia mater is often firmly adherent

Examined more minutely, the extra development of the ordinary connecting tissue seems to have separated the nerve-tubes, which in well-marked instances appear pressed upon and shrunk, the true myeline matter being in diminished quantity, while in the grey matter the cell-elements show deviation from the normal character

Symptoms—These in all cases depend upon the locality of the sclerous changes I have observed that they to a greater extent include disturbance of motor than of sensory power although both are ultimately affected Rarely does paralysis in any form suddenly show itself, rather is the aberration a loss or co-ordination of movement of the muscles of the limbs When the sclerosis existed in the cerebellum the animals showed a disposition particularly to gyration in movement, with spasmodic action of the muscles of the eye-ball All these disturbances of nervous function are, in cases of sclerosis of the spinal cord, apt to be complicated, rarely rapidly culminating in serious want of power over the voluntary movements, but steadily marked by the existence of aberration of the controlling function

Treatment — Although it is probable that sclerosis of the cord, or other parts of the nervous centres, is rarely recovered from in the sense of perfect restoration to structural integrity, it is nevertheless true that the condition is more capable of amelioration by judicious management than many other diseased states of the system. I feel tolerably certain, judging from observations made during life and examinations after death, that several instances of this change have, by attention to proper apportioning of work, the occasional use of preparations of bromine, iodine, iron, arsenic, or nux vomica, together with good food, been enabled for considerable periods to be generally useful. Under this management there was an arrest of distressing symptoms which did not again show themselves for more than twelve months.

IV SPINAL HÆMORRHAGE AND MORBID GROWTHS IN CONNECTION WITH THE CORD

The first of these conditions is chiefly a surgical lesion, the result of injury. In rather rare instances, from disease of the vessels, hæmorrhage may take place, either into the substance of the cord itself, between the membranes, or outside the investments. When the intimate cord-structure is the seat of the effusion, or where the blood extravasated is considerable, paraplegia is likely to occur suddenly; when slight, the indications are more likely to be excitation of function first, whether or not this is followed by depression or paralysis.

Of adventitious growths the chief are exostoses or bone tumours, and malignant growths, as melanosis and true cancer. In some cases the existence of these may be determined by manipulatory examination

The symptoms attending their presence vary according as the morbid growth is directly connected with the cord-structure, or only affects this by its contiguity. Besides local pain exhibited on manipulation, there is ordinarily muscular disturbance succeeded by paralysis. The symptoms rarely reach their height suddenly, and even when appearing are subject to

periods of remission and accession. When once the functions
of the cord are in this way interfered with, there is small
prospect of ultimate recovery, or even of restored usefulness

---

CHAPTER VIII.

AZOTURIA—NITROGENOUS URINE.

Definition—*Azoturia is the term applied to a complex morbid
condition or assemblage of symptoms intimately associated
with or dependent on disturbed assimilation, the most characteristic features of which are certain musculo-nervous phenomena, particularly clonic or tonic spasm of the great muscles
of the posterior part of the trunk and limbs, and the discharge
of high-coloured nitrogenous urine*

Pathology   *a Nature and History*—It is no less curious
than interesting to observe how, in the naming of systemic
diseases, we cling tenaciously to those chief and characteristic
local lesions in which the general or constitutional state has
terminated, and upon these bestow consideration and attention,
to the exclusion of the larger subject of the disposition or
condition to which the local changes may be owing   In this way
our ideas, not merely of the nature of these diseases, but also of
the principles which ought to regulate our actions in their prevention and treatment, have been correspondingly dwarfed and
localized   Acting in this manner we examine and hang over
the nodules and caseations met with as concomitants or
sequels of tuberculosis, the effusions and changes of pulmonary
tissue in the specific lung-fevers of both horses and cattle, and
on the urinary secretion or state of the kidneys in both those
conditions recognised by the names of *diabetes* and *azoturia.*
As a natural result of such doings, we often miss teachings
which a more extensive observation of phenomena would
place us in the way of receiving, and by attending to which
our ideas of many diseases would be truer and more comprehensive, because founded upon a more extensive observation of
facts and conditions ; and our grasp of the same would be firmer,
seeing we should have more material and that better impressed
upon our minds

The condition recognised by the term *azoturia*, or nitrogenous urine, although in our day freely spoken of as something new or strange, has apparently been well enough recognised by many who have preceded us. In many of the published records of disease, affections apparently of this character have been confounded and grouped with others, which, although somewhat similar in many of their features of development, are yet in true character and origin essentially different.

As respects the nature of this disturbance, in as far as consequents are related to antecedents, there is probably not much disagreement. All seem pretty well satisfied that it is the result of an over-supply or presence in the system of nitrogenous material, and that to this plethora of these albuminous or azotized ingredients are to be attributed those phenomena so characteristic of the affection. It is when we come to speak of the manner or mode of action by which this superabundant nutritive material operates in the production of the results we call symptoms, that we arrive at divergence of opinion and puzzling explanations.

There seems little doubt that for some time antecedent to the development of the distinguishing features of the disease, the muscular spasms, or paraplegia, and altered urinary secretion, there have been changes and disturbances occurring in the complex process of assimilation in one or more of the steps which exist between the passage of the chyle from the intestine and the period when it is fitted for serving the purposes of healthy pabulum. It is certainly obvious that whatever the pathological changes may be, and however they are carried out in the disease, that the muscular elements of the body are very largely, probably more largely, affected than any other structures. Whether these tissues and elemental structures are primarily affected through the contact of abnormal and unwholesome nutritive material acting upon and destroying their inherent power of contractility, or whether we are to look to the poisoning of the nerve-centres directly, or to the influence of the operation of reflex action, for the occurrence of the clonic or tonic contraction and ultimate paralysis of the muscles affected, seems rather doubtful. We may, however, with safety regard the uræmic condition of the urine—one of the diagnostic symptoms of the disease—as

24

a result of the pathological changes which have taken place
While, from the necroscopic appearances, the hyperæmic, and
altered state of the gland-structures, it seems not at all an improbable theory or mode of accounting for the changes to
regard the excess of albuminoid materials which enter the
system through the exercise of peculiar dietetic conditions as
altered or broken up at the gland-structures, from whence the
extra urea may proceed to join the blood-stream, from which it
is again separated by the kidneys

   To uræmic intoxication or poisoning, the result in all animals
most probably of retained effete materials, which by disturbance of function in some steps of the assimilatory process are
prevented from undergoing the changes requisite for their final
removal, this peculiar condition bears some resemblance. However, although it may resemble uræmia in the character of
certain of the symptoms exhibited, such as the action developed
in connection with the phenomena of disturbance of the great
nerve-centres, it seems somewhat to differ from that in the
causes which produce the uræmic condition of the fluids, and
probably also in the mode of production.   In uræmic poisoning we may have the major part of the symptoms intimately
associated with or dependent on the cranial nerve-centres
being chiefly involved, marked by coma, rapidly developed, and
more or less profound, with stertorous breathing   Of cases
of azoturia simulating this form of uræmia we see fewer than
of the other more resembling epileptic spasms, which are always
developed suddenly but are of varying intensity, in which the
muscular system is largely implicated, either directly through
defective nutrition of muscular tissue, or from disturbance of
nerve function from direct or reflected irritation, or probably
from both   It is of this latter mode of development that the
cases of so called azoturia most frequently present themselves,
sometimes the forms are combined, and we have coma with
muscular spasms and convulsions   •

   It is nowise essential to the development of symptoms of
uræmic poisoning, nor to the appearance of azoturia, that the
urine be suppressed, nor does the mere presence of urea insure
the existence of uræmia.   Rather are we led to infer that the
existence of the nervo-muscular phenomena, so characteristic
of both uræmia and azoturia is dependent on the existence in

the blood of certain noxious materials, which, from some disturbance, have remained unbroken up and unremoved, or which
have resulted from peculiar changes of received or existing
elements In azoturia the cause of the existence of this deleterious agent, whatever it may be, does not in any case appear
to be resident in the kidneys, but is clearly one of assimilation
in some of its complex processes, and is undoubtedly intimately
associated with a form of mal-nutrition, with the entrance
into the system, and into the blood, of material highly charged
with the materials or power of determining or forming azotized
or nitrogen compounds

In considering the rationale of the process of the entrance
and passage through the system of a superabundant supply of
albuminoid materials, their change, degradation, and formation
into other compounds, which from their character are eminently
unfitted for fulfilling the function of healthy nutrition, there
seems to us nothing impossible or improbable in supposing
that the diagnostic feature of musculo-nervous disturbance may
originate in part both from disturbed innervation and from
perverted nutrition

The extreme suddenness of the seizure, the difficulty of
imagining that the great masses of muscle involved could be
affected otherwise than by being acted upon and influenced by
nerve-power, together with the rapid rise of temperature, and
the oftentimes quick subsidence of these muscular phenomena,
are so far presumptive of primary disturbance of nerve-force
being the inducing factor. On the other hand, if we believe that
for some time prior to the violent exhibition of these symptoms
diagnostic of this condition, there has been gradually developing
an altered, perverted, and depraved condition of the nutritive
fluids of the body—fluids which have all the time of this change
or alteration been circulating through blood and lymph channels,
with the purpose of supplying the needful nutriment to the
various tissues, we can hardly suppose that muscular tissue, so
largely irrigated with nutritive fluid, should not, to some extent,
suffer in its nutrition from unhealthy pabulum Still, if this were
the only mode, or even the chief one, through which unwholesome and poisonous tissue-nutriment was operating, it might
be expected that its operation would be gradual rather than
sudden and violent. Besides accounting for musculo-nervous
24—2

phenomena on the ground of hæmal contamination, either from
the presence in the system of effete tissue-elements or their
further change, the chief of which has been supposed to be urea,
and its hurtful influence when resolved into certain ammonia
compounds, we may not unreasonably look for an explanation of
these in the changed character of the blood, owing to peculiarities
in the primary digestion, to its influence on cerebral nutrition,
the induction of brain œdema, followed by brain anæmia, and
consequent disturbance of muscular and nervous function

That this condition is not one which has newly appeared in
our day we should expect to find, seeing that the phenomena
of diseased actions of a similar nature in like circumstances
must ever remain the same, however differently these activities
may be interpreted In Mr. Percival's 'Hippopathology' it
will be found that, under the term 'albuminous urine,' there
is an account of diseased conditions and records of the manifestations of diseased action, which give the impression that these
were cases which we now regard and speak of as azoturia.
From this author's quotation from the *Veterinarian* for 1836,
where one of these cases is reported, it will be observed that the
symptoms there noted are quite characteristic. ' " In October a
bay blood mare, then running in the mail, began to fall off in
condition, in consequence of which she was turned into a loose
box, where she rapidly regained flesh and spirits. A fortnight
afterwards she was taken to exercise previously to being put to
her former work She appeared in perfect health, and very
playful , she had hardly proceeded with her rider about half a
mile when she suddenly stopped, began sweating, without any
apparent cause, and was with difficulty led home."

' Mr. Clayworth—the gentleman who reports the case—was
sent for, found her sweating and trembling, scarcely able to
turn in the stall, the muscles of her back and loins in a state
of spasm, tail quite stiff; kept looking at her flank and appeared
in violent pain,' dropped her hind-legs in going forward, but
her loins did not appear tender when pressed upon About a
pint of fluid was drawn from her bladder with the catheter, of
the colour and consistence of linseed oil ; after that the same
quantity, thicker, and of the colour of porter , and a third
portion of the colour of whey These urines were passed in
succession, the catheter remaining all the while in the bladder.

That the urine resembling oil was albuminous there seems little doubt; that the portion resembling porter was mingled with blood, subsequently and slowly trickling from the kidney, appears probable; but why this should suddenly change and become like whey I must confess I do not pretend to offer an explanation.'

Thus it is perfectly evident that this disturbed state of the process of assimilation, culminating in the conditions of muscular spasm and altered urinary secretion, was well enough known to Mr Percival, whatever interpretation he might give to these phenomena, for no one reading the notice we have transcribed, and at all conversant with the affection, can have any doubt that the case reported is one of what is now designated *azotised urine*. In the record of this reported case, amongst other salient features, it may be observed that particular stress is laid upon the suddenness which marked the change of colour in the urine in a very short period.

At one time, and with some observers, this condition was curiously enough believed to be confined to mares, or at least in them to be much more frequently encountered than in stallions or geldings. This however, is in a great measure disproved, as neither sex, breed, nor age, provided the animals have reached maturity and are stabled, seems to grant immunity from an attack. I have observed that it is more apt to seize upon animals rather handsome, well shaped, and good thrivers, than others differently constituted; that it does not, or very rarely, attack horses roaming at large in the fields, whether young or old; also that in all cases it is more apt to occur under favourable conditions succeeding a period of rather smart or active work followed by enforced idleness.

b. Causation.—There seems sufficient and readily enough obtainable evidence that the true and ultimate causes of this interesting but serious disorder are dietetic; that the symptoms exhibited are the result of the passage into the system of an abnormal amount of albuminous or nitrogenous material; and that to certain changes which these albuminoids undergo when present in excess, and when brought into contact with other materials and under the influence of certain surrounding agencies, must be attributed the whole of the complex phenomena which characterize or are attendant upon the disordered condition. I am well enough aware that this, or any statement, may not explain every symptom, or do away with all that is puzzling in the varied changes which occur in the process of assimilation during the development of the disease

Besides the reception of an extra amount of nutritious material while the body is in a state of quiescence, it seems, if not absolutely needful for the appearance of the symptoms diagnostic of the disease, to be at least highly provocative of it, that this condition of enforced idleness and liberal dietary should be followed by resumption of work moderate or severe, or even exercise, that, in short, a certain amount of movement or activity of function of the different organs of the body be called for

I have observed that the use of certain articles of dietary seems more disposed to be followed by an accession of those symptoms characteristic of the disorder than others; that in particular, feeding in large proportion with vetches, tares, and the leguminous foods generally, are very apt to induce this condition Indeed, upon examination, it would appear that all, or nearly all, cases of azoturia which I have encountered in the Border districts over a number of years, have been directly traceable to full feeding with materials of this class

The largest number of attacks amongst agricultural horses is during the autumn, at the period of harvesting the corn crop. At this time the horses are kept longer in the yoke, and are usually liberally fed with ripe tares. The feeding is not confined to three or four stated diets, but is continuous, so to speak; for in addition to receiving oats or mixed grains at regular intervals, the ripe tares are laid before them the whole time the carts or waggons are being unladen. Should the state of the weather interfere, and the animals be detained in the house, which they usually are, all the time having the same full dietary rich in the leguminous materials, at the end of the week, or even less, when again put to work, the probability is that cases of nitrogenous urine, or uræmic poisoning, will show themselves At one time, judging from what I had observed, I was of the opinion that this operation of working, following the rest and repletion, was necessary to induce the toxic condition Further experience, however, has satisfied me that such is not imperative, that animals may become affected in this manner when remaining in the stable, provided the extra supply of nutriment of this particular kind is kept up. It seems quite sufficient for the development of this disease that the materials supplied be in full quantity, of rich character, particularly of a highly albuminous or nitrogenous nature, and the horses kept from work or exercise

The system seems incapable of utilizing this extra amount of nutrition received, either as a reserve upon which it might at some future time draw, or as pabulum to be consumed in the performance of the different functions of animal life This material enters the system and circulation, and at some step or steps in the complex process of assimilation or manufacture of received material into blood, or pabulum fit for appropriation by the various tissues, it undergoes certain changes, the resulting products, instead of being either healthful or innocuous, prove actually deleterious, poisoning the tissues when it ought otherwise to yield health and power

The great characteristic features of the disease, the uræmic condition of the urine, the exaltation and ultimate loss of function of particular parts of the voluntary muscular system, and the extensive disturbance of the nervous system, are all related more or less directly to the superabundant supply of a particular nutritive material, and to the disturbance or perversion of function, not very well understood, at some points of the assimilatory process The uræmic state of the urine is probably the simple result of the pathological condition of the blood, and accounted for on the recognised physiological or functional power of the kidneys to separate, as urea chiefly, certain chemically formed materials, here probably imperfectly changed albuminoids, and to pass them off in the urine.

The musculo-nervous phenomena may owe their origin either to directly perverted and disturbed nutrition of both muscular and nerve tissue, or to perturbed and diseased nerve-power operating through reflex action.

When developed in lighter animals, and those employed for fast work, the same general causes seem to be in operation which we have already indicated as observed in agricultural horses

It has been noticed by some writers as being more likely to

occur in mares than geldings This statement I am disposed
to corroborate to a large extent , and although I have not in
many of these instances of females been able to affirm that its
appearance was contemporaneous with the period of œstrum,
still there appears nothing incongruous or improbable that it
should be so

Mr Williams, in his work on 'Veterinary Medicine,' accounts
for this, which seems admitted, on two grounds : (1) That mares
are, when in this condition, often detained in the stable for
some days; (2) that at this period they are in a highly excitable
condition, and more apt to suffer from spasmodic diseases
In lighter harness or carriage horses the first explanation is
tenable enough , but in agricultural animals it cannot be said to
obtain, as I am not aware that any attention whatever is paid
to them at the period of œstrum The other is quite satisfactory, and might be enlarged upon by stating that, as a rule, the
female is more susceptible of nervous excitement than the male

c. *Anatomical Appearance and Characters of the Urine* —
The structural changes observable in such cases as terminate
fatally, when viewed apart from the history of the appearance
of the disease and development of the symptoms, may not be
particularly diagnostic ; they are, however, usually extensively
distributed The blood is dark in colour, semi-fluid, partly
coagulated in both sides of the heart , there is general congestion throughout the body, in the glandular system of the
abdomen particularly so, the spleen and liver often simulating
the after-death appearances of anthrax The great muscles of
the loins and haunches are in some instances heightened in
colour, and the interconnective tissue stained with coloured
serum The great nerve-centres may or may not give evidence
of hyperæmia The bladder frequently contains urine of a
dirty, grumous coffee colour, with a similarly stained condition
of the lining-membrane

The very obvious changes which the urinary secretion has
undergone have constituted these a diagnostic feature, so much so
as to have warranted the founding upon this peculiar condition
the name by which this generally disordered state is recognised

In an examination of this secretion it is needful, for the
correct appreciation of its characters, to do so immediately, or
as soon as possible after being voided.' This is the more

needful, as in all cases where urea is present its unstable nature
is, when the examination of the urine is deferred, apt to lead
to incorrect conclusions in the matter of its composition, and
the extent to which this particular compound is present. In
density it is generally high. The colour has often been regarded as due to blood, or the colouring matter of blood. Examination with the microscope, however, fails to detect the
existence of either entire or broken-up blood-globules The
solidification which the urine undergoes on the addition of
nitric acid, which has often been deemed indicative of the
existence of albumen, is, so far, a mistake, being due evidently
to the formation in excess of nitrate of urea, and the absence
of albumen is further confirmed by the non-coagulation of the
liquid on the application of heat. If albumen does exist, it is
certainly not in the form generally met with either in the blood
or urine.

The crystals of the nitrate of urea may be easily produced
and examined by placing a little of the urine on a glass slide
or in a watch-glass, and either adding an equal quantity of
pure nitric acid to this, or first rendering the urine more concentrated by heating previous to the addition of the acid,
when the dark-coloured, rhomboid crystals of the nitrate
will show themselves in a few minutes. It is to the dark-
coloured urea, or rather the salts of urea, that the urine in
bulk chiefly owes its alteration in colour rather than to the
colouring matter of blood, although there are instances where
this has been encountered, as also granular matter and epithelial cells from the urinary tubes. These latter can only be
considered as adventitious, and are certainly not characteristic
of this disease. The dark colour and excessive quantity of
urea present in the urine is, as a rule, most readily detected at
the commencement of the disease. This is, however, not
invariable; for if carefully observed, it may be noticed that in
many cases in the earlier stages of the disease, and while the
constitutional disturbance is most marked, and the animal
exhibiting much pain, the urine is comparatively little altered,
and that not until the pain is alleviated, and the systemic disturbance less evident, does it put on its peculiar and distinctive physical and chemical characters

Without the body, and probably also in its natural conduits,

this urine is given to rapid chemical changes ; the products of
this change may possibly have much to do with the production
of many of the toxic symptoms characteristic of the affection

Symptoms —These are invariably of an extremely sudden
and urgent character, there is no warning or premonitory
indications of either disturbed digestion or innervation, rather
the opposite, the animal immediately preceding the attack
being in the very acme of health and vigour.

Although horses laid aside from work or active exercise and
regularly fed may have an attack while stationary in the
house, the greater number of seizures are in animals where
this rest and steady good feeding has been succeeded by work
or exercise , that is, the period of a probable seizure is on being
taken from the stable for exercise or work following some days
of idleness   On removal from the stable, the animal may proceed a very short distance—I have seen them travel only a
few hundred yards, at other times a few miles—when, seized
with an unaccountable lameness or difficulty in moving the
limb or limbs, generally the hind ones, they are with difficulty got into their own or some convenient stable , or they
may suddenly reel, lose control over their posterior extremities,
and come violently to the ground   Many of these very sudden
attacks, unless we bear in recollection the possible occurrence
of this disease and know the history of the case, are apt to be
at first mistaken for some lesion of the spine or muscles of the
back or loins   Other cases, not so suddenly developing the
musculo-nervous symptoms, may, in the earliest stages of illness, give indications of colic , they are restless, pawing with
the fore-feet, inclined to perspire, and exhibit a disposition to
lie down   It is when attempting to do this that we generally
observe the feebleness and want of motor-power in the hind-
limbs   Very shortly the more specially characteristic symptoms
show themselves,if they have not been observed from the outset
These are tremors and spasmodic twitchings of the great muscles
of the loins and gluteal region, ultimately settling into tonic
contraction or more or less perfect loss of power , together with
discharge of brown or coffee-coloured urine in normal or extra
amount

In the greater number of cases, in the early stages, the pulse
will vary in frequency from sixty to seventy per minute, and

in character from weak and feeble to rather strong, the temperature ranging from 103° F. to 105° F. In the slightly affected cases the appetite will not be impaired, and the bowels may be natural. In the severely seized the animal is prostrate, perfectly unable to rise, will neither eat nor drink, but continues to make ineffectual attempts to rise, and struggles violently with his legs until completely exhausted. In these latter there is occasionally indications of cerebral disturbance, partial coma, with much engorgement of conjunctival membranes

During the time they remain recumbent also in many cases which have been placed in slings, there are periodic fits of straining, ejectment of small quantities of dirty-coloured urine, or constant and involuntary dribbling of it from the passages.

Course and Termination—All cases, even those which at the first seem very much alike, do not comport them or proceed to a termination exactly similar. Some, as already noted, are struck down at once as by apoplexy, they struggle violently for a few hours, become comatose, and die, others, after the abatement of the more severe symptoms, make no further progress, and, although they may be perfectly conscious and have a fair or good appetite, never regain the use of their limbs, and either keep the ground until other complications carry them off, or they are destroyed as unfit for further use. In the majority of cases that do not terminate fatally, and where the urine gradually recovers its natural condition, either with or without the employment of medicinal remedies, the muscular spasms steadily lessen in severity, and the power of movement is restored, the horse in a few days appearing in its usual health without any impaired functional activity. Some, again, there are, where the natural condition of the urine is restored with removal of the unnatural muscular contraction, but where defective action, or perfect want of power in certain muscles, or sets of muscles, continue for some considerable time, these, however, as a rule, under appropriate treatment may be expected to recover

Restoration of healthy character to the urinary secretion is sometimes unattended with perfect or ultimate recovery; this is the more probable where cerebral symptoms continue persistent after this local diagnostic feature has disappeared

I have repeatedly noticed where cerebral complications continue after restoration of healthy character to the urine, that other nervous disturbance, probably related to the functions of the cord, is also persistent—at least there is frequently, accompanying the impaired cerebral functions, persistent and severe muscular spasms or contractions

Diagnosis —The only diseases in the horse with which this affection may be confounded are *anthrax* and *cerebro-spinal* fever. From the former of these it may be differentiated —1. By the constancy of lameness or defect of motor-power in the hind-limbs, which in anthrax is rarely or only occasionally exhibited; 2 The comparative frequency of this affection and its special liability to follow rest and liberal dieting, 3 The presence in anthrax of the specific organisms, the bacillus anthracis, and the power of propagation by inoculation, 4 The rarity of recovery in anthrax as compared with azoturia. From cerebro-spinal fever it is distinguished— 1 By the physical and chemical characters of the urine, 2 By the non-coincidence of the appearance of cerebro-spinal fever with conditions of rest and peculiarities of diet, 3 By the greater constancy in this disease of morbid lesions in connection with the organs of assimilation as contrasted with those observed in the great nerve-centres in the other.

Treatment —In those cases where the loss of muscular power is so great and so suddenly developed that the animal is unable either to move or maintain the standing position, prognosis is unfavourable So long as the animal is able to stand, although unable to execute any movement, there is always some prospect of recovery When neither violence nor excitation are features of the case, but there exists simply muscular spasms and defective motor-power, together with disturbed urinary secretion, it is better to place the patient in a stall than in a box, taking precaution that everything which is done to him be carried out without hurry or excitement. In further assisting the case, the first and probably chief point is that of favouring secretion, with the view of eliminating from the system that which we believe to have produced and to be maintaining the largely-distributed functional disturbance This is most readily done by operating upon the alimentary canal, for, in addition to being easily

accessible to medicinal agents, it is, as regards secretion, the
most potent and far-reaching in its influence of any organ in
the body To ensure an active movement and complete
emptying of the bowels there is nothing so good as a full dose
of aloes. It is better given in bolus than solution, seeing we are
more certain of the quantity given , it annoys the animal less,
and it acts quicker ↗ Should there be much irritation or fever,
good will result from the administration every two or three
hours of a little saline febrifuge, as liquor ammonia acetatis
with chlorate of potash ↗ This will in all likelihood be taken
in the drinking-water, which should not be restricted, and
thus obviate the necessity of drenching, which in such conditions is to be avoided if possible.

Should the muscular spasms be severe they will most likely
induce irritability and restlessness, in which cases I have seen
much benefit from the local use of warmth and moisture,
carried out by means of woollen cloths wrung from warm water
and laid across the loins I am aware this treatment is rather
looked upon unfavourably by some , but, from experience, I am
compelled to view it in a different light It seems to relieve
local irritability, to soothe and calm the system generally, and
in this way favourably influence the course of the disease In
cases where the horse is unable to stand, it will be needful to
ensure his safety, as far as possible, by having him laid in a
comfortable and roomy box or shed, and by taking precautions
that, in throwing himself about, damage is not sustained When
thus prostrate it is always advantageous to remove the urine
at intervals through means of the catheter, by which also the
bladder may be washed out with tepid water It will generally
be needful to assist the animal in attempts to drink, and to obtain a change of position at least once in twelve hours In
cases that do well, following the action of the cathartic and the
discontinuance of the febrifuges, a little diuretic may be given,
alternated with a bolus composed of some vegetable tonics :
as—℞ Pulv Nux Vomic, ʒss to ʒi . Pulv Gentian Rad., Pulv.
Zingiber, aa ʒii ; Terebint Venet, Pulv Lini , aa q s M. fiat
bolus In the course of three or four days, unless the first dose
of opening medicine has acted excessively, it will be advisable
to give a little more aloes Should there be weakness and want
of appetite after the first dose of purging medicine, it is good to

allow a little stimulant, as sweet spirits of nitre, or some of the
common preparations of alcohol; even when prostrate a continuance of this is often productive of good

When incapacity to rise continues after the third day, and
the appetite is not entirely absent, it will be advisable to
attempt to raise the animal, either by placing slings under the
body or other appropriate means   At this stage also the
employment of friction to the muscles of the limbs with soap
liniment, continued at intervals, is deserving of trial

In the greater number of instances which are not of the
worst type, and which do not terminate fatally in a short time,
recovery or distinct symptoms of amendment are likely to
follow the action of the purgative   During convalescence
much care is always needed—first to prevent overloading and
disturbance of the digestive organs, and second, by the
judicious use of medicine to restore tone and healthy action to
the entire system

CHAPTER IX

PARAPLEGIA ENZOOTICA—ENZOOTIC PARAPLEGIA—GRASS STAGGERS

Definition—*A general or systemic disorder appearing as an
enzooty amongst horses fed largely on ray or rye grass at a
particular period of its growth, and characterized by much
disturbance of innervation, particularly by impairment or loss
of motor, and more rarely of sensory, power of the posterior
extremities*

Pathology   *a. General Characters and Relations to some
other Affections*—Many diseased conditions, both in horses and
other animals, have received the name of staggers, probably from
the fact that the most distinguishing feature of these several
affections is disturbed motor-power in certain muscles, or sets
of muscles   This want of ability to regulate movement through
defective muscular action may in a general way be said to
proceed either from direct and primary disease of nerve-centres,
or from disease or disturbance of these centres, originating not

within themselves but from without, and in them appearing as a secondary or propagated affection

Besides this condition now under consideration there are at least four distinct diseases which have been, and are still, recognised by the indefinite term 'staggers' 1. *Mad Staggers*, probably encephalitis , 2 *Epilepsy*, a disease probably of varying cerebral origin , 3 *Megrims* or *Vertigo*, usually arising from an irregularity or disturbance of the cranial circulation, which again may originate from many causes , 4 *Sleepy* or *Stomach Staggers*, otherwise known as gorged stomach The last of these is the one with which the affection now spoken of is most frequently confounded, and like it is a disease of the nervous system, only in a secondary or propagated manner, having its origin in some other organ than the brain or spinal cord, and in connection with other structures than the tissue of nerve-centres.

This stomach or sleepy staggers, otherwise named 'coma,' or 'immobility,' the characteristic symptoms of which are apparently connected with involvement of the cerebral nerve-centres, as distinct from the nerve-centre of the spinal cord, is, I believe, to be regarded as a somewhat different disease from enzootic paraplegia, the one now engaging our attention In taking this view of these conditions I am aware that I am diverging from the opinions entertained by several who may be considered authorities These abnormal states seem to differ from each other in several particulars, such as—1. In their origin ; 2 In their symptoms, development, and termination , 3 In their anatomical appearances ; 4 In the means by which they are successfully combated

In the condition differentiated by the term 'stomach or sleepy staggers,' the character of the food which seems to operate in its production is of less consequence than the amount of it, particularly if it is of a pultaceous and rather indigestible nature Enzootic paraplegia rarely or never occurs on any food save rye-grass, and that only under certain conditions of its growth

In sleepy staggers cerebral symptoms are the diagnostic feature of the disease, coma and loss of consciousness in proportion to the cerebral involvement With enzootic paraplegia spinal, not cerebral, symptoms are the diagnostic feature ; coma does not exist except in a few of the most severe cases, and then only very slightly The symptoms of illness in those cases where the cerebral structures are affected are, as a rule, developed very rapidly, in the condition where want of muscular power of the posterior extremities is the diagnostic symptom, the evidences of disease are gradual in development.

The after-death appearances in the one affection, that where the cerebral symptoms are dominant, are congestion or inflammation of the cerebral membranes, with the attendant results of such morbid activities In the purely paraplegic form the chief or only lesions of the nervous system are associated with the cord, which in many cases is the opposite of hyperæmic Blood-letting, in the form with marked cerebral symptoms, is invariably productive of good , in enzootic paraplegia it is attended with the opposite results

This form of reflex or sympathetic paraplegia, with which we are now dealing, besides arising less, or probably not at all, from the quantity of food taken, being dependent for its origin rather on its character or speciality, is occasionally extensively distributed, but only where horses are depastured on young grasses, or lands where the rye-grass is more abundant than other forage plants, and at a particular stage of the growth of this plant, and is in some years more troublesome than others The subjects of its attacks are not of any particular breed or age ; and we find the disease both in stabled and in pastured horses, provided they are exposed to the one disease-inducing factor, feeding on this particular-conditioned rye-grass. The usual season of its occurrence varies a little with the earliness or lateness of the grass , it is generally encountered from the latter part of June to the end of August, and is probably more frequent in warm and dry seasons than under opposite conditions

Although undoubtedly in one sense a disease of the nervous system, as the disturbance of innervation indicates, it does not seem to originate from the nerve-centre, the cord, but from peripheral irritation or influence consequent on the action of some noxious material present in the alimentary canal While, again, there seems no doubt that the disturbance of the functions of this nerve-centre will react in further disturbing and impairing digestion, seeing that those parts or organs of the animal mechanism concerned with the fulfilment of this function are sufferers equally, or at least proportionately with the extent to which they are dependent for their nerve-supply from the same centre, with other organs, as those of locomotion, which are more visibly disturbed

In examining this matter, it may be noted as a somewhat curious circumstance, if the true cause of this enzootic paraplegia is feeding on specially conditioned rye-grass, that this peculiar disturbance of innervation should only show itself in the horse In the explanation of this immunity many facts and circumstances require to be taken into consideration.

Both cattle and sheep are sufferers from disturbed innervation connected with dietetic causes, and largely from feeding upon grasses in particular conditions of growth and during certain seasons of the year, and although some seem to regard these morbid states in ruminants, marked by characteristic symptoms, as precisely similar to this disease which we are now considering, I am rather doubtful of such similarity. Acute diseases of these animals intimately associated with or resulting from dietetic causes, are all, or nearly all, apparently referable to changes in connection with the cerebral part of the system, and paraplegia alone is not a diagnostic feature of them It must be remembered that cattle as a rule are rarely placed on these particular pastures—the young grasses or seeds, as agriculturists term them—where this disease exhibits itself in horses · they are generally alloted older and rougher grazings, while, when they may be located where rye-grass is abundant, they feed in a very different manner. The horse is disposed to top the grass, to eat the flowering stems almost entirely to the exclusion of the foliage of the plants ; the ox has the opposite taste, and crops both foliage and seed-stem, while if he seems to have a preference it is for the leaves, not the stems of the grasses.

In the case of sheep, again, they rarely crop the flowering or seed-stem, but keep closely to the root foliage. While it ought to be remembered that ruminants of all kinds seem to have a greater power of resisting the poisonous influence of most vegetable substances than solipeds.

b Causation.—The characteristic feature of the disease, the impairment or loss of power of voluntary movement in the organs of locomotion, particularly of the posterior extremities,

25

points to disturbance of function, or inability to exercise it in
connection with certain parts of the nervous system, probably
with the nerve-centre or centres in the cord, or with the nerves
themselves   That this disturbance is owing to a diseased condition primarily existing in the cord or great nerve ganglia
there, does not appear at all probable; the supposition is nega-
tived—1. By the fact that the condition of paraplegia can be
produced at will by the operation of influences acting not
directly but indirectly on such centres   2 By the readiness
with which this disordered functional activity disappears under
appropriate remedial measures; disturbance when dependent
on primary diseased nerve-centres being not thus readily influenced   The most likely mode of accounting for the condition of disturbed innervation is that which regards it as
arising from peripheral irritation or influence, this influence
being conveyed to and acting upon the nerve-centre which in
health ought to originate or determine the controlling force
necessarily connected with the performance of certain activities,
or by impairing the power of those media by which this force is
conveyed

The irritation and toxic influence on the nerve-centre and
nerve-conducting media can here only be produced apparently
in two ways—1. From the excess in the alimentary canal of
ligneous material, which, by its indigestibility and powers of
irritation, so influences both nerve-centres and media of nerve-
power conduction as to impair or destroy the regulating and
conducting influence   2 From the specific toxic influence
exerted by rye-grass when ingested at some particular stage
of its growth, and under certain conditions   This latter seems
the more probable hypothesis

What the particular toxic or paralysis-producing principle
contained in the rye-grass at this time is, or how it is produced, if not actually and of itself contained in the grass,
and at what stage in the digestive process, it is impossible to
say   In some of its features the result bears a certain resemblance to ergotism

Although the evidence, both from clinical and post-mortem
examination, is tolerably conclusive that this special form of
paraplegia does not owe its origin to mere engorgement of
either stomach or intestine with food, it is at the same time

indicative that its true source is to be looked for in causes dietetic, also that, although green food of various kinds may under certain conditions be provocative of various diseases, and amongst these of diseases associated with the nervous system, yet this special nervous disturbance is only induced by feeding upon rye-grass, and that, too, at a particular stage of its growth, and when the plant has either developed within itself, or possesses the power of developing when taken into the animal system, a specific disease-producing agent The idea which attributed this, as well as many other somewhat obscure abnormal conditions, to atmospheric influences is sufficiently answered when it is known that the disease may be eradicated by removal of the particular food-material we consider the true inducing factor, when, to all appearances, atmospheric and other influences remain as before

The particular period when the grass seems likely to induce this disturbed innervation is when, the flower having been developed, the stem becomes somewhat dry and hard-looking, and the seed is being matured. Some have thought that it was through a process of fermentation after the grass had been cut that the poisonous element was developed, this, however, cannot be, seeing it operates in conditions where fermentation could not possibly have existed—it produces effects when the plants are eaten while grown in the fields as well as when cut. Lambs are sometimes sufferers from this condition, rarely or never their dams The probable reason of this seems to yield another item of evidence corroborative of the statement that it is the grass when in the transition stage which is the cause of the disturbance That the ewes and older sheep are not sufferers while grazing on the same pastures where their lambs may be affected, seems capable of explanation by knowing that sheep do not incline to feed on the tall seed-stems, but rather on the more lowly-growing and succulent plant-leaves, lambs, however, not confined to the grass entirely for their food, are disposed, more in play than with the object of obtaining so much food, to nip off the tops of the seed-stems of the rye-grass, this I have repeatedly watched them doing.

c Anatomical Characters —Opportunities to make after-death examination in cases of enzootic paraplegia are not numeious, for although the disease is common enough, in some seasons very common, and although hundreds of cases may pass through the practitioner's hands, and in different ways receive treatment, the mortality is never great ; none, indeed, dying where the animals have been observed early, and have received the benefit of professional advice. All cases that afforded the opportunity of a post-mortem examination had been severely seized from the first, and were unable to stand when advice was obtained, or very shortly afterwards came to the ground   While alive, they all exhibited a certain amount of cerebral disturbance ; in this they were unlike the great majority of the affected, where symptoms of cerebral involvement is not a marked feature.   In no case have I ever observed any great and well-marked organic lesions, in many I have been much disappointed at not seeing, as I imagined, very satisfactory causes for the symptoms shown during life, far less for the fatal termination.   The state of the digestive organs is variable, sometimes the stomach is full, at others both this viscus and the intestinal canal contain little ingesta ; the only approach to disease being trifling congestion at separate and detached portions, but chiefly in or near the stomach.

The lungs are invariably congested, partly from the position in which the animal has been laid both before and after death, and partly from the existing cerebral conditions.   In some instances there may be noticed cerebral congestion, while I have fancied that in the lumbo-sacral region the cord was somewhat softened, the membranes injected with an extra quantity of slightly coloured fluid, at other times no abnormal conditions of the brain or cord revealed themselves, certainly not hyperæmia, rather the opposite.   Other abnormal appearances which I may occasionally have met with in either thorax, abdomen, or pelvis I believe not to have been essentially connected with the disease itself, but rather accidental

Symptoms.—These are gradually developed, not, as in paralysis, from primary cerebral disease or mechanical injury; neither have we the dull, listless condition, gradually passing on to somnolence and coma, characteristic of brain involvement, consequent on gastric engorgement or indigestion.   In this particular form of paraplegia the affected animals are first of all observed as deficient in control over their voluntary movements. In a day or two this muscular weakness increases, they reel or stagger with the hind extremities, and there is danger of their falling, especially if caused to move round in a limited space. They are likewise disinclined to lie down In very severe cases there is an anxious expression of countenance, and partial loss of voluntary power in the fore extremities Although there is from the first, and until convalescence, impairment of the power of voluntary movement, there is perfect consciousness, no somnolence, the animal continuing to stand without exhibiting any excitement or nervous disturbance when handled The appetite is unimpaired; the bowels rather confined; urine normal, both as to amount and composition

Unless the case is advanced, or the seizure a severe one, the respiration is undisturbed, while the pulse, both in volume, character, and frequency, is normal, temperature sometimes a little elevated. When carefully observed in the more severe cases, the animals are very indisposed to come to the ground, to prevent this they generally rest themselves with the side or buttocks against the wall, or some resisting body They do not place their head against the wall, neither do they rear or attempt to get into the feeding-trough with their fore-feet Muscular spasms or twitchings will occasionally develop themselves, and, in rare instances, symptoms of cerebral complications, with these latter the prognosis is unfavourable When the ability to maintain the standing position is lost, and the animals are laid upon the ground, muscular movement is usually excessive, the limbs are moved automatically, consciousness becomes impaired, the breathing stertorous, and death not long delayed Although these symptoms are tolerably constant and uniform, they are yet subject to some variations, chiefly as to their rapidity of development, or their intensity in individual cases

Treatment—In the management of these cases of enzootic paraplegia it is ever well to remember that they are intimately associated with deranged digestion, that they owe their existence to the ingestion of a deleterious article of food, and that, consequently, the earliest treatment which is called for is their removal from those influences which seem to produce the disordered condition I am satisfied that many, even when severely seized, require nothing further to ensure their recovery than a complete change of dietary. Many animals I have seen receive no further treatment than removal from the pasture where they were grazing to another of a different character— a change from rye-grass ripening its seed to old land and natural grasses not seeding—and this change has been suffi- cient to ensure recovery.

In addition to the complete change of dietary, it will in all cases expedite the cure if a smart dose of purgative medicine is given whenever this change is undertaken. When this medicine is administered it will of course be necessary to remove the animal to the stable if in the field; while if green, succulent food, of a character different from what he has been receiving, cannot be obtained, good hay, with a few steamed oats and bran, will do equally well.

When it is determined that the horse shall be returned to the field if removed from there, care must be exercised that he is not again under conditions as to food-supply similar to those from which he has been taken.

In young and vigorous animals some recommend the em- ployment of blood-letting as being likely to relieve the more urgent symptoms.

From what I have observed in cases of cerebral disturbance associated with or resulting from simple indigestion, or im- pacted stomach, where coma, amaurosis, and stertorous breath- ing are present, this may with confidence be carried out. In these it may be observed that the breathing becomes tranquil, and consciousness returns gradually but steadily, and keeping pace with the abstraction of the blood. Here, however, in enzootic paraplegia, where there is rarely unconsciousness, or at least very trifling indication of the cerebral structures being involved, instead of being beneficial, blood-letting is likely to be followed by undesirable results. Should the bowels not in due time respond to the medicine given, unless the symptoms are becoming aggravated, it is better to wait for two or three days before another dose is administered. A free action of the bowels is, however, above all things to be desired, for by this channel we remove materials which, if retained, will certainly further intensify the disturbance. Having secured a moist condition of the canal, it is advisable to keep it in this state for some days by means of the food, while succeeding the exhibition of the cathartic, good will generally result from the administration daily, or twice daily, of a ball containing aloes, assafœtida, gentian, and ginger, or some similar tonic and stomachic agents. In cases where weakness of the posterior extremities continues after the action of the purgative has subsided, and after they have received for a few days the medicines mentioned, it may in some instances be needful to apply a moderate stimulant or blister to the loins or the poll.

A regular daily application of soap liniment may serve for the former situation, but cantharides will be needful for the latter. However, a little patience is often better than injudicious haste in such cases, and a little time and perfect quietness are to be preferred to meddlesome interference. Unless the horse is weak from being previously in low condition, a second dose of laxative medicine, followed by some diuretics, a week or more after the first, had better be given before he is put to work. If, however, the physical strength of the animal does not seem good, it will be better, instead of the second dose of purging medicine, to continue the ball first recommended, or to alternate it with another somewhat similar, composed of aloes, iron, gentian, and ginger, or aloes, nux vomica, and gentian. In some animals of peculiar temperament, and where there seems much danger of their damaging themselves, it may be advisable, either before or after the exhibition of the purging medicine, to place them in slings, by which they are steadied, kept at rest, and prevented from injuring themselves. This, however, is only needful in exceptional cases.

As a rule it will not be found that recoveries from this affection are protracted. Unless complicated with some other disease, or, what is very serious, a previously disordered nervous system, amendment is usually observable in from one to two days after removal from the deleterious grasses, or certainly following the action of the purgative; the steady restoration of function to complete control over the movements of the limbs being usually completed in from seven to ten days.

When restored to health there does not appear to be left any weakness, or disposition to again become affected, unless placed under the influence of similar agencies.

CHAPTER X.

SATURNINE EPILEPSY AND PLUMBISM—LEAD-POISONING.

Definition.—*A peculiar disturbed condition of several animal functions, chiefly those of innervation, digestion, and loco-motion, consequent on the introduction into the system of certain salts of lead, either through the drinking-water, the food, or through the pulmonary mucous membrane of such animals as are exposed to the action of vapours containing lead*

Nature and Modes of Manifestation of the Abnormal Phe-nomena.—In considering the different forms of lead-poisoning, and the modes in which these manifest themselves, it is well to remember that the metal itself has been differently represented as to its action on the living organism and its powers of combination and change. In its pure or simple metallic form it is not generally considered poisonous. The compounds, however, which it forms with certain acids are decidedly noxious, and may prove destructive to life. If, how-ever, lead in the metallic state may with impunity be con-veyed into the stomachs of horses and other animals, we are also aware that in the alimentary canal it is susceptible, by the action of certain acids there present, of forming compounds which, from their solubility and inherent toxic character, speedily find an entrance into the blood and other fluids, and through these channels spread change and death through every organ and tissue.

The assemblage of morbid phenomena induced through the introduction of lead in some form into the body may not inappropriately be regarded as an enzootic disease, seeing that the conditions favourable to inoculation with the metal are largely monopolized by particular districts.

As a sporadic affection it is encountered in various and widely differing situations, wherever animals have access to lead or compounds of lead, as on grazings where bullet-spray from rifle-butts, or the refuse of paint-shops or manufactories of materials containing lead may be found, being conveyed there through mingling with town manure.

The manner or form in which lead or its compounds, when

received into the system, shows itself, is not always the same. This divergence of symptoms and difference in the mode in which the toxic action of the received material is exhibited depends on many and varying conditions, such as the form in which it is absorbed, the quantity taken into the system in a given time, and also, probably, on individual susceptibility.

The forms of lead-poisoning may be variously divided and considered, having relation either to the mode of the entrance of the poison, or to its visible toxic action. For our present purpose it will be sufficient to regard these in accordance with the results exhibited ·

1. As acute lead-poisoning, or saturnine epilepsy, in which the action of the toxic agent is accompanied with coma, delirium, or convulsions. This is the form which in cattle has so often been confounded with reflex paralysis, the result of gastric derangement

2. Chronic lead-poisoning, or plumbism, due probably to smaller doses and a longer continuance of the hurtful element. Here the characteristic symptoms are not so markedly connected with disturbed innervation as with perverted digestion or locomotion.

From observation and registration of facts, it would seem that in direct proportion to the rapidity with which the system is charged with the poison, so is the intensity and marked speciality of disturbed innervation. Also that in every form the hurtful agent is conveyed throughout the entire body. This is proved by chemical examination, which demonstrates the existence of lead not only in the blood, but in varying proportions in nearly every organ of the body. This character of affecting or becoming located in differing degrees in different organs and tissues of the body is distinctive enough both in the acute and chronic form. between these various organs and the empoisoned blood there seems a varying degree of selective affinity, some imbibing and retaining more than others. By these investigations we are also tolerably certain that lead, having entered the body, is detained for an indefinite period in peculiar combination with the different elemental textures of organs ; that it may be detected in the tissues and secretions weeks after the animal has ceased to receive any of the offending material, only leaving the body during the natural changes which regularly occur in every tissue

Causation and Modes of Induction.—The causes of plumbism in any form are of necessity the entrance into the system of lead in its metallic form or in some of its various compounds, either alone or in association with other materials. That metallic lead may be conveyed into the digestive organs without any hurtful results following may be allowed; that it may, and often does, by the combinations and forms which it then assumes, prove the original factor from which serious derangement and textural change may proceed is equally certain Before these undesirable results can follow from the ingestion of the metal, some changes must occur by which the compounds, formed through the action on the metal of the natural and other fluids in the stomach, are rendered capable of transmission into the blood and lymph-stream, and thus carried to the various organs and tissues of the body What the exact compounds of the metal are is somewhat doubtful It is thus far certain, however, that by the action of the different fluids on the innocuous and insoluble metal there is produced a hurtful and necessarily soluble compound of lead, which may only be developed in this form prior to a further and more perfect transformation

Probably the steps in the chemical change are not more uniform than are the ultimate products themselves. The modes by which lead and compounds of lead enter the system vary somewhat With cattle they are often directly conveyed into the stomach in the form of refuse fabrics containing lead compounds, or as the unmixed compounds themselves. With horses this is less likely, as they are decidedly averse to partake of unnatural and extraneous matters, alone, or when mingled with their food

I have, however, met with several serious cases of lead-poisoning in horses, some of which terminated fatally, from the animals, in mischief or in play, picking off and swallowing putty containing a considerable amount of red lead, which had been used in executing certain repairs connected with the water-supply of the yard where they were located. In another instance the offending agent was newly painted wood-work, which, by assiduous licking and gnawing over a period of two days, induced a smart attack of colic and deranged bowels in two colts.

Sometimes the mixing, steeping, or cooking of food in vessels which may previously have been employed to contain preparations of lead, or which are in part covered with the metal, are sources from which spring much derangement of function, or even fatal results   Many years since I encountered a rather curious and, in this direction, an instructive case   A gentleman dealing in horses had for several weeks, and often more than once in each week, to request professional advice and attendance for one or two horses regularly affected with abdominal derangement and pain.

In addition to advice and treatment of the animals as respected the immediate illness, inquiry was made as to dietary, and the probability of any noxious material being mingled with the food, but no positive information could be obtained.

· One article of diet which they, the animals regularly ill, were alone of all the other horses receiving, because of their being somewhat low in flesh, was boiled beans. Although nothing faulty could be discovered with this feed, it was advised to be discontinued, as apparently not suiting these particular animals   On being stopped for a week, the attacks of illness disappeared   The owner, however, thinking he would have another trial, the cooked beans were again resorted to.   On the second day of the resumed feeding, one animal of the two was again taken ill   On this occasion an examination was made of the beans, the vessel in which they were boiled, and the accompaniments, when it was found that the lid of this vessel, a good-sized fixed or standard article, was covered with sheet-lead, and also that the beans, when cooked, were mixed with bran, and allowed to stand in a vessel lined with lead   Further, it appeared that the cooking was always carried out with a supply of common salt, more being added when the mixing with the bran was executed.

Believing that the vapour of the boiling water, the common salt, and other materials in the beans, had so acted upon the leaden cover and vessel in which they were stored, that a soluble and deleterious compound of lead was the result, which, mingling with the food, acted detrimentally on the horses receiving it, the beans were not discontinued, but ordered to be cooked in another vessel without a leaden cover, and when cooked were mixed and kept apart from association with lead. From that time this same food was consumed without any ill effects or indications of acting as an abdominal irritant.

Although it has not yet been established so clearly in the case of horses as of man, that certain waters kept in contact for any length of time with leaden pipes or cisterns may contract plumbeous impregnation, and thereby act injuriously on them, there is no doubt that they are as liable to such influences as human beings, and the water they drink is as likely to be contaminated as that which is used for household purposes. Although it is usually believed that rather hard water is less likely in storing to be impregnated with lead compounds, the absolute truth of this may not be counted upon, seeing there are certain very pure waters which have but a trifling action on lead, and others of a high standard of hardness which possess decidedly solvent powers.

Symptoms   *a. Of Acute Lead-poisoning.*—The indications of poisoning by lead in all forms have, whenever occurring, and in all animals, much in which they resemble each other. In those instances in our patients where the amount introduced into the organism is large, at least as respects the time occupied in its introduction, or where the form, from its ready solubility, is quickly distributed and appropriated by the different organs, the form in which the symptoms of poisoning exhibit themselves is usually that of acute lead-poisoning, the so-named saturnine epilepsy, associated with convulsions, delirium, or coma. The occurrence of the symptoms is quickly following the reception of the poisonous material, there being no premonitory indications of failing health, as in some of the chronic manifestations.

Following impaired appetite and a somewhat haggard expression of countenance, with staring eyes, and injected conjunctival membrane, we observe a rather copious discharge of saliva, with occasional protrusion of the tongue. The position of the animal is often characteristic, the limbs being drawn together under the body, the head depressed, the back arched, and the coat rough and staring. With some the cerebral dis-

turbance is even more marked, and the animal is either comatose or dashes or thrusts his head violently against any obstacle
which may offer itself Examined carefully we will observe
muscular twitching or spasms largely prevailing, both in the
cases which are still able to stand and in such as are paralyzed
The pulse in all is rather variable. sometimes, as in ordinary
cerebral congestion, less frequent and full; at others it is increased in number, of little volume and hard; the breathing is
quickened, and the temperature slightly elevated In all cases
the bowels are inclined to be confined, even while they exhibit
a certain amount of irritability Colic, or symptoms of abdominal pain, do not appear as prominent features. Where
the illness is ushered in by the gradual developing of symptoms,
it is found that, although the indications of cerebral disturbance are not strikingly manifest at first, they shortly follow in
conjunction with epileptic spasms and muscular twitchings

b *Symptoms of Chronic Lead-poisoning* —Between saturnine
epilepsy and true plumbism there are many stages or gradations.
in the one, the symptoms of illness may be developed so rapidly
and steadily that a fatal termination is reached in a few hours ,
in the other, unmistakable indications of the ingestion of lead
may exist for months This latter condition is peculiar to certain
districts, or at least to animals placed under peculiar surroundings, where the metal is furnished to them in small quantities
and over a lengthened period It is observed in the neighbourhood of smelting-works, where minute particles of lead or its
compounds are distributed in an impalpable form over pasture-
lands , and in cases where the same quiet but steady introduction of the metal into the bodies of animals has obtained
through a contaminated water-supply

In this form we find in the aggregate the same symptoms
that are observed in the acute, only somewhat changed as
regards the prominence and distinctiveness with which certain
of these are developed In the acute form the cerebral occupy
the most prominent position, and completely overshadow the
others , in the chronic form, although the nervous are never
removed from our view, those connected with digestion and
locomotion are more particularly brought before us These are
chiefly impaired or capricious appetite, an unhealthy, rough-
looking state of the skin and hair, falling off in condition,

with an irregular and irritable state of the bowels In certain instances there is a peculiar blue line along the alveoli of the incisor-teeth, within a quarter of an inch of their exposed necks; this is generally regarded as diagnostic, although probably not invariably present In a short time the indisposition to move becomes more evident, and if in the field, the animal is usually found standing with the head depressed, and limbs drawn under the body, while the muscles over various regions are irregularly affected with peculiar twitchings

In the horse, roaring is early recognised as a distinctive symptom, probably from paralysis of nerve-tissue inducing imperfect muscular action. In cases where the symptoms have continued for some weeks, confirmed paralysis of the extremities, particularly of the hind ones, is apt to be established, together with chronic swellings of certain of the joints of the limbs, and a peculiar contraction of the flexor muscles of the fore-limbs, or want of power of the extensors, the result being that the animal is disposed to stand on its toes, or in progression to knuckle over on the fetlock In this we see an analogy to the slow poisonous action of lead in man, where the extensor muscles of the upper extremities become paralyzed in a greater or less degree On examination these paralyzed muscles give us the idea of their having undergone certain atrophic and degenerative changes In addition to all these indications of lead-poisoning we must never neglect the chemical examination or search for the metal, the detection of which, either free in certain organs or combined in various tissues, is at once the most convincing proof of the cause of the unhealthy activities

In the *Edinburgh Journal of Medical Science* for 1852, the *Veterinarian* for 1864, and the *Chemist* for 1855, will be found certain very interesting facts and observations in connection with lead-poisoning, both as an acute and chronic affection, which are well worth perusal.

Anatomical Characters —1. In the more active manifestations of saturnine poisoning the muscular system throughout the entire body usually presents a blanched and softened appearance. The blood is fluid, indisposed to coagulate, and given to stain textures wherever brought in contact with them   Previous to making a more minute examination, we observe in many instances, on opening the abdomen, that the bowels generally, and less frequently the walls of the cavity, are extensively marked with ecchymoses and suggilations, also that there exists a varying amount of fluid The glands of the abdomen, the spleen, liver, and kidney, are more or less changed in appearance ; they seem swollen, as if filled with blood, and on being manipulated feel soft In some cases the appearance of the liver particularly has been noted as the opposite of this, being pale in colour, and feeling somewhat hard

The lining membrane of the alimentary canal, from the stomach to the large intestine, exhibits considerable alteration of structure, varying both as to extent and degree. It is either swollen, soft and pulpy over considerable portions from infiltration into the submucous layer, or there are isolated patches of varying size exhibiting blood-extravasations, or more extended tracts, where, from the character of the effused products, inflammatory action seems to have been active. The muscular tissue of the heart is soft and flaccid, and the blood in both ventricles fluid; the endocardium not ecchymosed, but stained, the lungs congested, and blood in pulmonary vessels fluid, with the bronchi full of frothy mucus In all the acute cases which I have examined, the brain and its membranes have been congested, with a variable amount of fluid in the lateral ventricles and subarachnoid space   Not only have the vessels of the pia mater seemed full and distended, but on cutting into the cerebral substance minute vessels were visible, where in health none could be detected

2. In the instances of plumbism, or quiet impregnation of the system with the metallic compounds, the tissue-changes are essentially similar. The only organs which appear to offer any variation are the great nerve-centres. Here neither the brain nor its membranes exhibit a condition of congestion ; in many instances the indications are of an opposite character, the brain-substance being paler than natural, and rather softer, as if containing more fluid, and in a state of defective nutrition The local swellings in connection with the joints are made up of a collection of subcutaneous and super-periosteal effused material, of a hyaline structureless nature, with, in certain

instances, an augmentation of the swelling, from what appears rarefaction of the epiphyses of the bones entering into the formation of the joint. While the blood-markings and suggilations found in the acute form on the mesentery and the outer surface of the intestine may not be present here, the state of the internal mucous membrane of the canal is somewhat similar. The stomach and intestines present detached patches of ecchymosis, or larger tracts of inflammatory action, while the cul de sac of the cæcum and pouches of the colon have occasionally patches of their tissue in a sphacelated condition

The glands of the abdomen are more rarely in an engorged and hyperæmic state than somewhat altered in colour and consistence. I have noticed them to be softer than natural, and of a dirty clay colour; others have spoken of them as of a singularly blue appearance.

Diagnosis—That acute lead-poisoning may be mistaken for some gastric and enteric disorders, accompanied with paralytic symptoms—particularly in cattle—is a fact well known to most practitioners of veterinary medicine. Some confusion, again, may occur as respects the differentiation of the chronic form and severe articular rheumatism. In correctly diagnosing either of the forms of disease resulting from the ingestion of lead, the history of the cases will materially assist us

We are aware that these gastric disturbances simulating the acute form are chiefly, if not entirely, connected with feeding upon grasses or food of a particular character; while in this disease the nature of the food is immaterial, the only essential being the presence of the poison in one form or another

Although the nature of the disturbed innervation in both these morbid states is wonderfully similar, a careful analysis of the symptoms exhibited will give a speciality in each. In lead-poisoning the epileptiform fits and muscular twitchings come more frequent, and are upon the whole better marked, as well as the champing or grinding of the teeth, the discharge of saliva, and the tucked-up condition of the abdomen, than where these phenomena are coincident with primary gastric derangement, however occurring

In the chronic form of lead-poisoning the data for forming a correct diagnosis are more numerous and more reliable.

From chronic articular rheumatism, with which it is most likely to be confounded, it may be distinguished by the presence of the distinct paralytic features, the irregular recurrence of the muscular spasms and twitchings, and the more distinctive indications of disturbed nutrition

In articular rheumatism we have also the character of the local swellings to guide us, their disposition to change situations, and the acute and persistent pain wherever it is located.

The assistance in diagnosis to be obtained by Faradisation —the passage of an electric current through the affected muscles—so helpful in doubtful cases in the human subject, has not, so far as I am aware, been made applicable in our practice; it might, however, be useful

Treatment —In treating the acute form of lead-poisoning it would appear that a larger amount of success generally attends our efforts in the case of the horse than of cattle. This may in some measure be accounted for from the fact that, in the ruminant, the material ingested is usually in a solid form, difficult, if not impossible, to be broken up or passed on, and extremely likely to lodge amongst the ingesta which is always, notwithstanding the action of purgatives, remaining in the pouches of the rumen

The agents inducing the morbid action are, in the horse, less frequently of the solid form, and their nature is usually such that they may with more certainty be chemically acted upon, or got rid of by maintaining a somewhat lax condition of the canal

In all cases where we know, or suspect, that lead-compounds have been ingested, our main object, until satisfied that these have been removed, or their power to injure destroyed, must be directed to the exhibition of agents believed to be capable of preventing the formation of soluble compounds of the metal, or if these are believed already to exist, to neutralize their action, at the same time that the natural evacuant function of the bowels is excited and maintained. Having these ends in view, we generally adopt as a purgative the sulphate of magnesia or soda, to which sulphur and dilute sulphuric acid have been added. These agents are used with the view of converting the lead-compounds existing in the canal, into

26

the comparatively insoluble compounds of the sulphate and sulphide

When abdominal pain is troublesome, relief may be afforded by the addition of tincture of opium or belladonna to the draught, or by occasional doses of morphia administered hypodermically While, should these means fail, I have found good to follow the exhibition, every two hours, of one ounce of sweet spirits of nitre, four ounces acetated liquor ammonia, and one drachm each of camphor and extract of belladonna, given in gruel ; and the application to the abdomen of woollen cloths wrung from hot water

Having given what we consider a fair dose of the saline purge, it is better to wait a reasonable time for a response than to repeat the dose too soon The acid, and probably the sulphur, had better be repeated every three or four hours for one or two days

As soon as the bowels have been placed in a moist condition, they ought to be kept so for some days by the continuance of the saline laxative, which may be taken in sufficient quantity to produce this effect in the drinking-water

Should the symptoms not become aggravated in two or three days, good hopes may be entertained of a favourable issue Following this, supposing the bowels to have acted freely, benefit will accrue from the exhibition twice daily of such tonics as gentian, quinine, or nux vomica

In the chronic forms of lead-poisoning, the results of medical treatment will entirely depend upon the length of time the animal has been under the adverse influences, and the consequent extent to which the different organs and tissues have become impregnated with the poison In the majority of these cases the constitutional strength is so undermined, and special organs have become so much injured, that reasonable hope can scarcely be entertained of restoration to health

When the treatment of these is undertaken, it is based upon a somewhat different principle ; the noxious agent is not now chiefly, or even largely, located in the gastro-intestinal canal, but, having entered the circulation, has become resident in and attached to various organs and tissues, so that any treatment to be adopted must proceed with the view of acting upon it as it is found there, of changing its form, attracting it from its situation and combinations to again enter the circulation, and thereby become subject to elimination through the ordinary channels. For this purpose experimentation goes to show that the properly regulated exhibition of iodide of potassium has a wonderful influence in determining and favouring this result

When this remedy is adopted, it is advisable both to precede its administration by the magnesian sulphate in full doses, as also, at different times during its use, to act upon the bowels by the same medicine, in combination with the acid mixture already recommended

When, however, the animals are so severely affected that the joints are much swollen and the muscles are paralyzed, the results to be obtained by treatment are not worth the expense of carrying it into execution   While, in the management of any case, either of the acute or chronic plumbism, in addition to whatever medical treatment is being carried out, it is necessary that the animal be removed from the originally operating cause, the reception of the lead into the system

---

CHAPTER XI

TETANUS—LOCK-JAW

Definition —*This is the term applied to that disease of the nervous system characterized by involuntary, painful, and continued or tonic spasm of more or less extensive groups of voluntary muscles, and probably also certain of the involuntary, these spasms, during their continuance, being marked by periods of exacerbation and of repose.*

Pathology   *a Nature and Causation* —The exact nature of this diseased condition, of which we are chiefly cognizant by the disturbance of muscular function, and in which, like some others affecting the nervous system, the lesions observable after death are neither very obvious nor uniform, is not yet placed beyond dispute   By many the characteristic phenomena of increased and sustained muscular contraction is explained

26—2

on physiological principles ; in many respects a not unsatisfactory manner of arriving at an understanding of the pathology
of tetanus, although failing to explain every phenomenon
The power of reacting on motor-nerves—? e, of generating an
impulse within itself, on reception of a centripetal impression,
which resides in the spinal dynamic matter, and which Dr
Todd named polarity—is that which in this view is regarded
as the origin or cause of tetanic spasm

This power is subject to very great modifications, both as
respects its susceptibility of being excited by stimulants,
and the extent and force with which it is exerted   In ordinary
circumstances the voluntary muscles are, as a rule, exempt
from its influence, but in certain diseases they are so acted
upon or overpowered that the will has little or no control over
them

Considering these facts, and reasoning on this principle, it is
thought, by those who hold this view, fairly well established
'that the phenomena of the tetanic condition result from an
exalted polarity of the centres supplying the parts affected.

' In cases of traumatic tetanus the exaltation of the polar
state commences in the afferent nerves of the seat of the
wound , if the tetanus arises from cold, the exalted polarity
commences in the nerves of common sensation, distributed to
the exposed part ; from the periphery thus irritated the condition is propagated through the nerves to the centres, and
the effects on the muscular system show to what portions of
the nervous centres the exaltation of the polar force is communicated

' This, however, does not afford an adequate explanation of
the production of tetanus, and it is well known that it is impossible, even by severe mutilation, to produce tetanus in the
lower animals ; whereas a slight accidental injury (as when a
nail penetrates a horse's foot) will often excite the disease in
its worst form   It would seem that some particular state of
the system, probably some peculiar condition of the blood, is a
necessary precursor of this malady   Hence no doubt, its
greater frequency in warm and unhealthy climates, in over-
crowded and badly ventilated hospitals, and among ill-housed
and ill-fed subjects   That tetanus may be produced through
the blood is shown by the results of the administration of

strychnine, which imitates the tetanic symptoms in a very striking manner, so that you may at will develop the phenomena of tetanus in an animal by giving him strychnine, or injecting it into his blood, but you cannot cause it by external injury.'

The fact, so well known to all veterinary surgeons, that numbers of animals may be subjected to treatment in every respect similar, whether this treatment be exposure to vicissitudes of weather, imperfect location and bad sanitary conditions, or a particular method and time of performing an operation ; or that they may be the subjects of accidents in all essential particulars alike, and yet that of these numbers only a small proportion, and possibly the most unlikely subjects according to our powers of judging, become affected with tetanus, seems to point to some peculiar individual susceptibility then existing to this special excitability and disturbance of nervous power in the animals thus acted upon

What this special susceptibility may be, or what conditions are needful to be complied with, even supposing the susceptibility to be present ere the state of so-called exalted polarity, evidencing itself in those fearful muscular spasms characteristic of tetanus, is reached, we do not know.

From the fact that conditions precisely similar to those exhibited in tetanus may be induced by absorption through the blood of certain materials, particularly strychnine, many are inclined to regard this disease as essentially and primarily a blood affection On this hypothesis the true cause of tetanus is regarded as some morbific agent which, being received into the animal system, finds its way through the blood to the spinal centre, for which it has a special affinity, thus disturbing, by malnutrition, its normal dynamic action In corroboration of the correctness of this view we are referred to what is stated as being well known, viz, that the herdsmen of the provinces bordering on the River Plate have been long acquainted with the fact that tetanus is transmissible from animals to men through eating the flesh of the former when these have died from this disease This statement, we suspect, requires confirmation, and, even if confirmed, we have to remember that these individuals are exceptionally situated as regards dietetic conditions, not at one particular period, but generally through their whole life. I have certainly known dogs receiving, as a chief portion of their food for a considerable time, the flesh of horses which have died while suffering from tetanus, and cannot recollect any evil results occurring amongst these, nor yet any cases of tetanus attributable to this circumstance.

Although the condition of the cord, the nerve-centre apparently chiefly or solely involved, is usually regarded as in a condition of undue excitation, some pathologists have considered a condition of depression as that which more truly and satisfactorily explains the phenomena.

All our domestic animals are liable to become subjects of this perverted nervous activity; of these, horses and sheep are the most susceptible.

I am not aware that the statistics of tetanus enable us to speak with any amount of confidence as to the greater or less susceptibility of particular breeds of horses, or the periods of life at which these seem, under favourable inducing influences, most liable to its invasion. Preponderance of evidence seems to favour the opinion that a high temperature of itself, or suddenly alternated with one much lower, is more favourable to its appearance than the opposite, or where the range of the thermometer is less extensive and less liable to sudden changes.

It is spoken of under two forms—*Traumatic*, following the infliction of wounds or injuries, and *Idiopathic*, that which arises from causes internal, or which to our senses are inappreciable. Each of these may be met with in forms acute as well as chronic.

In our patients the appearance of tetanus, apart from appreciable causes, is a much more frequent occurrence than in the human subject. Considering that, as far as we are able to discover both these forms of tetanus, the traumatic and idiopathic are precisely alike in their nature, development, and general and special results, it would probably be more correct not to attempt any such division.

The apparently exciting causes of the so-called traumatic form of the disease are wounds of all kinds, more particularly when inflicted in dense tissues largely supplied with sensibility, and injuries apart from wounds, as fractures or bruises. It also follows such operations as amputation of the tail and castration The period of accession is various, sometimes early, often delayed, seldom occurring later than twenty days after the reception of the injury.

During the course of my experience the apparently most fertile source of traumatic tetanus has been the occurrence, not of extensive wounds, but rather of such as might at first appear comparatively trifling Most of these wounds were of a character to induce pain, being chiefly severe punctures amongst the muscles of the croup, thigh, fore-arm, or feet, situations where the structures are all bound by strong and unyielding tissues , or when merely superficial or little more, as broken knees, and saddle-galls, were, from their situation and liability to abrasion and irritation, acting as a steady source of disturbance

As respects docking—nicking, it is hoped, is now unknown —and castration, which more frequently than any other operations are followed by tetanus, I do not think that we can with certainty indicate the individuals in which the disease is likely to ensue, nor yet say with certainty that any one mode of performing these operations is, of all others, to be chosen as being perfectly free from such disagreeable consequences Still, I am free to confess that the greater number of cases which I have seen following these operations have, in the case of docking, ensued where ligature and severe cauterization were employed to arrest hæmorrhage , and in castration, when the operation was carried out by means of caustic clams

Regarding the appearance of tetanus apart from wounds or injuries, very appreciable causes are exposure to extremes of climatic influence and to fatigue, more particularly if these are associated with insufficient food and improper sanitary conditions Intestinal irritation, either from the presence of foreign and indigestible material, or intestinal parasites, I am satisfied in certain cases is capable of inducing the diseased action , uterine disorders are also similarly blamed—of this, however, I cannot speak corroboratively, but see no good reason to doubt its truth That cold and exposure suddenly encountered have a determining influence in the production of tetanus we occasionally see exhibited on an extensive scale in the case of newly-shorn sheep, where should a lowering of the temperature and boisterously wet weather immediately succeed the shearing operation, it is no uncommon circumstance to find a considerable number of animals, on the subsidence of the storm, suffering from tetanus Horses clipped in cold weather, and incautiously exposed immediately afterwards, are also sometimes similarly affected ; while one of the most commonly observed results of young animals being partly submerged in wet ditches, and remaining struggling in such a situation until completely exhausted, is an attack of tetanus

b . Anatomical Characters —Like many other diseases of the nervous system, the evidences of tissue-change are in tetanus, in the majority of instances, neither characteristic enough nor sufficiently uniform to enable us to speak positively regarding them. The brain proper will generally be found free from structural change

The spinal cord is frequently spoken of as showing evidence, both in its meninges and intimate structure, of congestion, alteration in colour, and other particular changes of the intimate nervous elements , but whether these latter are primary or dependent on nutritive and vascular derangement has not been determined   Much stress has been laid on the appearance and condition often presented by the afferent nerves of the part in which the injury has been sustained in such cases as follow wounds Distinct patches or spots of inflammation, or congestion—neuritis—with, at the same situations, a perceptible increase in volume, and these conditions continued along the course of the nerve to the spinal cord, have occasionally been well made out in many carefully conducted post-mortem examinations of both men and animals Congestion and inflammation of the ganglia of the sympathetic nerve in different parts of its course both in the trunk and neck, mentioned by some as nearly always present, I am disposed, both from the examinations I have attempted myself, and from a perusal of the records of most careful examinations made by others, to regard as extremely doubtful,

Both from the negative and positive information afforded us by such examinations, there seems sufficient evidence to satisfy that the phenomena of the tetanic state do not depend on anything approaching the inflammatory condition of either the cerebro-spinal axis or the nerves. This conclusion is also strengthened when we are aware that the same absence of inflammatory lesions is characteristic of those cases which have succumbed from the action of such poisons as strychnine, where also, during life, identical phenomena were exhibited to those met with in this diseased condition

Throughout the course of the alimentary canal there is sometimes exhibited ecchymoses and inflammatory patches; these are very variable in extent and situation. The lungs and upper portions of the air-tube are also, in many cases, in a similar condition

Symptoms—Although, strictly speaking, the term 'tetanus' indicates involuntary spasm and rigidity of the greater number of the voluntary muscles, it is ordinarily employed to indicate all forms of the disease, irrespective of the extent of the group involved. When the muscles of the face and neck are chiefly affected, resulting in persistent closure of the jaws, from which we have the characteristic name Lock-jaw it is spoken of as *Trismus*. When the muscles of the back and loins are the structures disturbed, producing an elevation of the head and neck, and bending of the loins downwards, the condition is termed *opisthotonos*. *Emprosthotonos* is the state of muscular contraction directly opposed to *opisthotonos*, viz, bending of the body and neck forward, with arching of the spine, while *pleurosthotonos* is the name given to the bending of the body in a lateral direction, in obedience to lateral muscular contraction

Amongst our patients, if we except the condition known as trismus, none of these separate forms of the disease are common. Rarely do we find the muscles of a particular region alone affected, there being most frequently involvement to a greater or less extent of all the voluntary muscles, resulting in the production of the condition ordinarily recognised by the general term *tetanos* or *orthotonos*

From the outset to the termination of the disease the symptoms may be said to be diagnostic. The earliest are generally in connection with the action of the muscles of deglutition and mastication. The animal is observed to grind his teeth in a peculiar manner, with a rather profuse secretion of saliva, which appears about the angles of the mouth. There seems a soreness in the region of the throat, occasioning a difficulty in swallowing, with stiffness of the back part of the neck, and slight protrusion and elevation of the nose

On approaching him for the purpose of examination he is easily excited, and twitching of the facial muscles may be observed ; while, should the hand be brought in contact with the nose or lips, or an attempt be made to open the mouth, the head will be rapidly elevated, and the eyeballs spasmodically withdrawn within the orbit from the action of the muscles of the ball; at the same time the membrana nictitans is rapidly projected over the surface of the eye   The breathing is very early accelerated, but the pulse is not at first materially increased in number, although altered in character, being rather hard and incompressible   The temperature in milder cases is not much elevated, while in the severe, and such as terminate fatally, it may give very high readings   In the earliest stages of the disease, or it may be all through the seizure in less acute cases, the ability to open the mouth is not entirely gone, the movement being only limited, in severe cases this movement becomes rapidly restricted until the jaws are completely locked

This ability to open the mouth all through the disease serves as a very good criterion whereby we may judge of the mitigation or increase of the spasms , although, as a rule, earliest observed in the facial and cervical muscles, and those of deglutition and mastication, this spastic condition rapidly shows itself throughout the entire muscular system   When fully developed the position of individual parts, as the head, tail, and limbs, is regulated by the more powerful muscles which act upon them   The neck and head are much elevated, the nose persistently protruded, with nostrils dilated and immovable, the angles of the mouth somewhat retracted, the eyes watchful and brilliant, with continual retraction of the eyeballs within the orbit, and a rapidly recurring protrusion of the cartilago-nictitans over the globe   The muscles of the back feel, as well as look, rigid , the tail is elevated, and steadily agitated by a tremulous spasmodic movement   The limbs, forcibly extended, are kept wide apart , and any attempts at locomotion are performed with difficulty, and with a peculiar straddling stilty gait and evident pain   The bowels are confined, desire for food and water is never entirely absent, while attempts to eat are often followed with aggravation of symptoms

During the course of the disease, although the muscular spasms are continuous and not intermittent, there will yet be noticed regularly recurring periods of exacerbations, and more rarely of remission These exacerbations are easily induced— the slightest noise, the sudden flashing of light into a previously darkened stable, hurriedly and roughly opening a door, a sudden attempt to take hold of the animal, in short, rough or rapid movement in any way, or even talking loud, are sufficient to develop the most distressing paroxysmal spasms During all these accessions the animals appear to suffer intensely, the breathing becomes laboured, and the body damp from perspiration, while in severe cases they may stagger, lose their equilibrium, and fall to the ground. The pulse, not much affected at first, or rather firm and incompressible, gradually loses this character, becomes rapid, small, and feeble, death appearing to ensue from continued spasm of the muscles of respiration, or general exhaustion consequent on the continued excitation of the nervous system and want of nutrition, or it may be that spasm has seized on the muscular fibres of the heart

Course and Termination—Although of more frequent occurrence in some districts, and during certain seasons, than in other localities and at different times, tetanus may everywhere and on all occasions be regarded as a serious and rather fatal disease Occasionally of a mild character, and occupying in the passage through its various phases a rather lengthened period, it is ordinarily observed of a type which may be regarded as either acute or subacute In the former, cases which are characterized from the accession of the diagnostic symptoms of tonic muscular spasms to their full development, by rapidly recurring exacerbations, febrile disturbance, high temperature, much restlessness and pain, the percentage of recoveries is exceedingly small

When, however, the tetanic spasms do not undergo marked augmentation during the first week, general disturbance not being excessive, nor the temperature above 103° F., restlessness and pain not being attractive features, the prognosis is favourable It is not a common feature of tetanus that, during its continuance, partial recovery should take place, to be succeeded by renewed or intensified motorial function. The usual character of development is that of quiet but steady progress—in

cases which terminate fatally—with symptoms of gradually
increasing severity. In those where a favourable termination
is reached, the muscular spasms may appear for some time
perfectly stationary, and at last slowly decline, perfect functional tone being only reached after a lengthened period

Treatment —Very many of the cases of tetanus which we are
called upon to treat are, from the outset, evidently hopeless ;
these rarely survive long enough to give any therapeutic
agent an opportunity of acting upon the system.

In all cases where remedial measures are intended to be
carried out, the first matter demanding attention is the securing of a box, dry and well ventilated   It does not, in this
disease, require to be well lighted—indeed, it is preferable, if
not absolutely needful, that it should be dark—but above all, it
ought to be removed as much as possible from noise or disturbance of every sort

Having carefully placed the animal in this quiet and rather
dark box, we ought to impress upon the attendant, that all
merely meddlesome visiting or interference with the sick
animal, that all rough handling, noisy demonstrations, or anything which excites or disturbs the patient, tend most effectually to retard its recovery

Unless the bowels are already in a lax condition, it is advisable in every case to exhibit, if possible, a moderate dose of
purging medicine

If the bowels can be once moved, they may generally be kept
in a natural or soluble condition by sloppy mashes, to which
have been added treacle or linseed oil , these the animal will
generally take without any trouble, unless the case is very
acute   While, even when no cathartic medicine could be
administered, I have seen the wished-for results obtained by
this system of dieting

If the case is one of traumatic tetanus, the wound ought to
be carefully examined, and any portions of foreign matter or
animal tissue which, from necrosis, is acting as an irritant removed, and a good poultice, medicated with some such material as opium, belladonna, or cannabis indicus, applied over
the wound or injured part.   In cases of tetanus from docking,
it has been proposed to re-amputate ; practice, however, does
not favour this procedure—rather the reverse.   In addition to

perfect quietude, correct sanitary conditions, and careful nursing, the medicinal agents which I have found productive of any benefit have been belladonna, prussic acid, tincture of aconite and bromide of potassium. Chloroform I have tried largely, but have invariably found that although tranquilizing the animal while under its influence, the spasms and muscular tonicity have appeared with greater severity on returning consciousness

Of the Calabar bean, from which, on its introduction, great results were expected, I can speak with very little more confidence. Lately, chloral hydrate has received much attention, and, from what I have seen of it, believe it is deserving of further trial and close attention, until its use in these particular cases is established.

The employment of external applications, as mustard, sheepskins, ice-bags, etc, to the course of the spine, do not, from their results, warrant us in recommending them with certainty of benefit, but rather in particular cases as matters of experiment, and certainly, the less such applications partake of an irritating character, the more likely are they to be productive of good

The best form in which to administer belladonna is probably that of the extract, while, if it is too firm in consistence, it may be readily made softer and more adherent by grinding it along with a little treacle and acetated liquor ammonia, in this condition it is introduced into the mouth, smeared over the tongue, or placed amongst the molar teeth without causing the animal any annoyance. The quantity given during the day varies from three scruples to three drachms, according to size and age, and is to be administered at intervals of three or four hours, rather than given at once

The hydrocyanic acid and potassium salt are taken without trouble when mixed with the drinking-water or soft mash, the former is better kept constantly before the animal, but never in too large quantities, so that we may regulate the giving of the medicines. From sixty to two hundred and forty minims of the medicinal acid, B.P., may be allowed in the twenty-four hours and from two to eight drachms of the potassium bromide

A very safe and all but needful precaution, when we possess the facilities, is at the very outset of the disease to place the

animal loosely in slings By this means we secure its support
during the severity of the seizure, while at the same time we
do not irritate or annoy it by adjusting these appliances when
the susceptibility to be excited is greatest; we also, by this,
avoid the nearly invariably serious consequences which result
from the patient falling to the ground during a paroxysm of
spasm In a great number of instances the animal is disposed
to partake of food, which may be allowed him in moderate
quantity, and of such a nature as will tend to obviate the tendency to constipation.

—

CHAPTER XII

CHOREA

Definition.—*This term has been applied to an irregular convulsive action of different voluntary muscles of a clonic
character, particularly affecting those of the extremities, and
also in rarer cases of the neck and anterior regions; these
movements are either altogether or to a great extent beyond
the control of the will*

Nature and Causation.—The history of this disease in man is
a curious record of superstition, and of the influence of the
religious or spiritual element when brought to deal with the
wondrous phenomena of bodily disease. In our profession,
from its age and the comparatively recent date at which correct
scientific pathological inquiry has been brought to bear on
animal diseases, we have been spared much of this. Still, we
are probably not more settled in our opinions regarding the
true nature of this and many other diseased conditions of the
same system, than when priestly exorcism, frantic dances, and
authorized processions to some saintly shrine were the orthodox methods of relief prescribed for sufferers from chorea.

Probably, when our instruments and means of investigation
are more refined, we may be better able to deal with such a
subtle and strangely adaptive structure as nerve-tissue At
the present time, even amongst those who are most entitled to
be heard on the subject, there is far from being unanimity of

opinion as to the true nature of chorea, or the agencies which operate in its production. By many it is regarded as simply functional derangement of the great nerve-centres, perverted nerve-force, the result of many and divers influences, or of whatever may produce nervous dynamic disturbances ; others, again, appear rather to view it as the result of a prior deteriorated or poisoned condition of the blood, the exact nature of which is as yet undetermined ; while a third class accept the entire phenomena as merely concurrent or accompanying symptoms of certain peculiar blood crases as the rheumatic, or of such general abnormal conditions as are found in connection with cardiac or renal diseases

In our patients, with the exception of the dog, the horse is probably the greatest sufferer from various forms of nervomuscular phenomena, chiefly attractive through the convulsive action of a clonic character of certain classes of voluntary muscles, which, by almost general consent, we have agreed to designate by the term 'chorea' That this particular form of nervo-muscular disturbance is correctly described as of a choreic character, or as bearing a close resemblance to the abnormal condition known as chorea in man, there is little doubt ; that it is identical with it, I do not believe. Like chorea in man, it is more frequently seen in young than in old animals. Unlike this disturbance in him, however, it does not seem in any instance to exhibit a disposition to disappear spontaneously, or under the influence of medicine

If in some of our patients we may safely regard this disturbance as the sequel of, or in some way closely connected with, certain specific fevers, in the horse any such ordering of its causation is rarely possible. Over a considerable number of years I have only met with one case in which any such connection seemed to exist, and this might safely be regarded as merely a fortuitous coincident. The animal was suffering from a serious attack of influenza, from which it ultimately died, and during the continuance of the fever well-marked symptoms of chorea in both anterior and posterior extremities showed themselves, and continued until death. These choreic spasms had either a concurrent existence with the fever, or they were much aggravated by its occurrence, as they had not been previously noticed. The animal certainly had only been in the possession of its then owner for a few weeks On examination after death, along with other thoracic complications, the pericardium showed much structural alteration, apparently the result of acute inflammatory action The chief factor in the development of this nervo-muscular disturbance in the equine sufferer seems hereditary predisposition If not born with the disease visibly manifest, the ultimate sufferers seem at least to have inherited the tendency to develop it very early in life and under very trivial causes. Apart from this congenital tendency, adverse influences, as overwork, defective sanitation, and improper dietary, exert a very trifling and merely secondary power When established, they undoubtedly tend to its aggravation

Whether in all these forms of nervo-muscular disturbance spoken of as choreic the immediate cause is to be looked for in change in the nerve-centres or nerve-cords, or whether the different manifestations have separate and varying lesions upon which they are dependent, it is, with our present knowledge, impossible definitely to affirm

To me it seems more in accordance with fact and observation to regard the seat of the change or disturbance in those more truly choreic manifestations in the horse spoken of under the term of 'shivering,' and other names taken from the more attractive symptoms, as located in the cerebral ganglia rather than in the cord In these instances the spasms are not continuous, which it is probable they would be if the cord alone, or chiefly, was the seat of textural change Also we find that the muscular aberrations are always disposed to develop themselves whenever will is put forth to execute movement, excitation seeming to spring from the cerebral rather than the cord-centres Other nervo-muscular disturbances confined to individual muscles or groups of muscles, chiefly of the limbs, such as 'string-halt,' which, in default of more perfect knowledge, we are content still to regard as in their nature choreic, may, with less danger of error, be regarded as dependent on particular interference with functional activity either of the peripheral nerves or of the cord-centres

Anatomical Characters—After-death examinations, both of men and animals, although disclosing morbid conditions common to several diseases of the nervous system, do not tell us of any structural alterations which must be regarded as specially characteristic of chorea. In several such examinations I have found that many and different lesions of the textures connected with and entering into the composition of the nerve-centres were easily discoverable. Chief of these may be mentioned as thickening of the serous covering of the brain, effusion in the sub-arachnoid cavity of brain and cord, visible changes of texture, chiefly of a sclerous character, with vascular injection of the cord, and particularly of the central ganglia of the brain, the optic thalami, and corpora striata.

Symptoms—These are chiefly motorial, and, even when most severe, do not seem productive of pain or weariness. The muscular spasms vary much both in frequency and severity. They may only occur at long intervals and on particular occasions, as when the animal is excited, which in all cases seems to produce an aggravation of the contractions; or they may exist, although rarely in the horse, in uninterrupted sequence, scarcely modified when the animal is at rest. They may in their manifestation scarcely attract attention, so little do they disturb the natural movement of the parts acted upon by the affected muscles; or they may be so severe as visibly to impair movement and impart a most singular appearance to the member acted upon.

Amongst horses, as already noted, choreic manifestations almost invariably show themselves as an independent affection not as a sequel of some other diseased condition. The spasms chiefly exhibit themselves in connection with the muscles of the back and posterior parts. Appearing often early in life, this nervo-muscular disturbance does not in the horse, as in many other animals, exhibit with age a tendency to disappear. The muscular spasms, or twitchings, are in him, as a rule, less developed and more liable to be overlooked, than in some other animals, and may only be observed when he is moved in certain directions, so as to call into action a particular set of muscles.

In the most commonly encountered manifestation of this diseased condition, from the peculiar tremulous nature of the muscular contractions, the affected animals are very generally designated 'shiverers.'

In examining horses suspected to be affected with this

27

choreic manifestation, various methods, according to circumstances and opportunities afforded, are employed to elicit the
characteristic muscular contractions   Of these, the most
usually adopted and successful are, in the stable, for the
observer to place himself behind the animal and cause him to
pass from side to side of the stall, when most likely, if subject
to choreic spasms, the affected limb or limbs will be detected
by being lifted from the ground higher and more rapidly than
natural   They are also projected slightly backwards, accompanied with a slight amount of motion in the tail, and a
tremulous movement of the muscles of the haunch, being kept
somewhat longer suspended in a hesitating manner, and rather
rapidly replaced on the ground   If the horse is taken by the
head, either in the stable or out of it, and made to move directly
backwards, the probability is that, if a sufferer from chorea,
the same spasmodic movements will be executed

Seldom is the state of spasm, if slight, observed when the
animal is trotted straight forward ; but it may be detected on
his being turned rather rapidly round   In many instances the
characteristic twitchings of the muscles of the loins, thighs,
and of the erector muscles of the tail, are markedly visible
when the animal is engaged in the act of drinking   Although
the muscles of the hind extremities are in the horse the especial seat of the peculiar clonic contractions characteristic of
choreic disturbance, cases will yet be met with in which these
phenomena are associated with the muscles of the neck and
anterior extremities   When appearing in these, the symptoms
are marked by the same irregularity as respects their severity
and periods of recurrence as when seen in the more ordinary
situations

Treatment.—As the causes which seem to operate in the production of this disturbance of nerve function, of which the
symptoms recognised as choreic are but the natural expression,
are not in every case exactly similar, so it is but natural to
expect that the moderation of the symptoms, or their removal,
may be looked for from the employment of means varied rather
than similar

With horses, although any remedial measures which may be
employed are rarely productive of such beneficial results as
follow their use in other animals, the lines of treatment indi-

cated are much similar, viz, the removal of all causes likely to induce systemic disturbance or irritation ; the controlling and directing of any constitutional cachexy which may seem connected with the animal ; the strict enforcement of correct dietetic and sanitary conditions; a careful apportioning of work, together with the use of some tonic medicinal agent Of the latter there does not seem to be anyone in particular possessed of specific action in every case, which most probably is the reason why a rather considerable number of agents have each individually been so highly recommended by different practitioners and experimenters

CHAPTER XIII

EPILEPSY — FITS

Definition —*A complex diseased condition of the nervous system, evidencing itself in sudden and generally total unconsciousness, accompanied with tonic, and, later, clonic convulsions These fits or paroxysms, besides being sudden in their occurrence, are likewise of variable intensity and uncertain periods of duration and recurrence*

Nature and Causation — This disease, difficult to define, and in its nature as yet imperfectly understood, is encountered in all our patients, less frequently in the horse than some other animals

It is only through a considerable laxity in the use of terms that the complex and convulsive phenomena, which constitute nearly all that we know of this condition, come, in their various forms of manifestation, to be grouped together and regarded as a distinct disease, seeing that these are met with under varying and very different states of organs and tissues Of these the most commonly observed are 1 Organic disease of the cerebral structures, as inflammatory action in cerebral matter and membranes, adventitious growths, various tissue and other changes 2 Lesions of the cranial bones, which tend to produce irritation of the contained structures 3. Changes in the blood itself or the blood-conduits within the cranium, by which the proper nutrition of the cerebral structures is interfered with 4 Reflected or propagated irritation from other

27—2

and, it may be, distant organs in a state of disease and disturbance   5 In cases where no obvious cause can be made
out, as an idiopathic affection so called or functional disturbance, to which only it is probable the term 'epilepsy' ought
to be applied

From the circumstance that the greater number of animals
suffering from epilepsy have, on examination after death,
shown no structural changes considered sufficient to account
for the symptoms exhibited, many have come to regard these
disease manifestations in idiopathic epilepsy as simply and
essentially the result of a certain peculiarity in the putting
forth of the nervous force, and to speak of it as disturbed
functional activity, the localization of which by the demonstration of specific textural changes in intimate nervous elements,
or elsewhere in nervous tissue, has not yet been made out

Although it seems pretty certain that epileptic seizures may
result from various lesions of the nervous system, and highly
probable, also, from influences out of this system, but operating
on it extrinsically, either through nervous connection and association, or by means of the blood, still the main features in connection with these paroxysmal attacks, the loss of consciousness
and disturbed motorial activity, seem to direct our attention to
particular parts of the nervous centres, as the grey matter and
central ganglia of the brain proper, together with the upper or
anterior part of the spinal cord, as the situations most likely
to exhibit textural changes. Many examinations which I have
made of animals dying while suffering from an epileptic seizure,
have satisfied me that in numerous instances extensive and
apparently chronic disease of the membranes of the brain were
prominent features, and doubtless intimately associated with
the various attacks These changes with as much truth may
be regarded as the result of the repetition of these seizures as
the cause of their existence

In every case where local tissue-changes are met with,
whether these changes be congestive or inflammatory, or extend
to increase, loss, or structural change of tissue, always to connect such exclusively with merely intrinsic and local phenomena is unphilosophical and short-sighted They can only
be properly understood either in themselves or their connection with other phenomena, when regarded as parts of a

whole, as results of the general or systemic declaration of some wide-spread morbid condition, and probably this is the light in which not only epilepsy but several other of the diseases affecting the nervous system ought to be regarded.

Experimental researches prove that epileptic or epileptiform seizures are capable of being induced by various and particular interferences with certain portions of the brain-structure, and of the anterior parts of the spinal cord, as also by removal of the kidneys From this we may be guided not to look upon one, and only one, cause as sufficient to induce the peculiar convulsive attacks recognised as epilepsy or epileptic but rather to give each individual case a careful consideration, as well during the intervals between the paroxysmal seizures as while these continue

From all that has been accomplished in this direction we are assured of this, that, as yet, neither the cause nor the exact elemental changes connected with true or idiopathic epilepsy have been satisfactorily demonstrated Although in many instances of epileptiform seizures, obvious textural change may be detected, there are still very numerous cases where these same phenomena are exhibited apart from de- tectable structural or elemental change in nervous matter, and that, should change be discoverable, it has still to be determined whether such is primarily of the true nervous elements or of some others associated with them

Symptoms—The severity of the epileptiform fits being liable to so much variation, the train of symptoms is necessarily in some less distinctly developed than in others The premoni- tory warning or aura, indicative of the approach of a fit, so well recognised in man, we, in our patients, are of course unable to appreciate or turn to advantage, although, from certain ex- periments, there seems sufficient reason for believing in the existence of such in animals other than human In horses under observation, the first indication of the fit is usually in- terference with motorial activity, a staggering gait, an unmean- ing stare, champing of the jaws, followed by rapid loss of consciousness, and falling to the ground in convulsions In slight cases, the convulsive movements after the animals come to the ground are of the most transient nature and feebly expressed, confined, it may be, to one limb, or the muscles of

the facial and cervical region, when, after having been laid on
the ground for only a few seconds, the animal starts to its feet
and moves on as if nothing had happened

More generally, however, the unconsciousness is prolonged,
and the convulsive movements are severe, and, as we are apt to
forget the insensibility to pain, distressing to look upon

The head is moved rapidly backwards and forwards, the
jaws undergoing a lateral movement, so as to produce grinding
of the teeth, or they may, in the act of champing, abrade and
wound the tongue or lips, around which frothy saliva contiues
to collect   The eyelids are either open to their full extent or
partly closed, with the eyeballs distorted and the membrane
injected   The limbs are tossed wildly about, while the muscles
of the trunk, acting in concert with those of the cervical
region, occasionally produce that bending of the body in a backward direction characteristic of opisthotonos   The muscles of
respiration, acted upon in a similar manner, result in inducing
stertorous breathing, or such a fixed condition of the walls of
the chest that respiration seems for a time suspended

The heart's action is tumultuous, with a pulse extremely
variable in character, and at times intermitting, while occasionally both fæces and urine are voided involuntarily.

Having reached a crisis, the muscular rigidity becomes
relaxed, consciousness is in a measure restored, and the animal
regains its feet, exhibiting, however, much depression, or maintaining for some time a stupid semi-comatose appearance,
which, in the more severe cases resulting in a fatal termination,
is but imperfectly recovered from ere the animal is plunged
into another paroxysm.

Treatment.—This resolves itself into the double condition of
(1) immediate, and (2) prospective

1 *The Immediate Treatment* or means to be employed
during the seizures are all such as are calculated to shorten
their continuance or mitigate their severity. Of these the
most important are to give the animal every opportunity to
benefit by a free and uninterrupted circulation of fresh air, by
the removal of all obstructing objects, either upon or immediately surrounding it   Cold water may be freely dashed over
the head, and such precautions as seem needful employed to
prevent the creature doing itself harm.

Bleeding, which may be resorted to in such cases as are evidently associated with plethora, and a congestive state of the vessels of the head, is not to be rashly adopted in every instance.

2 *Prospective Treatment*—In every case where the convulsive fits are separated by a considerable interval of time, attention ought to be directed to the animal's general health, so that the recurrence of these may be less frequent or ultimately disappear. As irritation of the bowels is in some animals intimately associated with the occurrence of these fits, we ought to be certain that the canal is in as healthy a condition as possible; any irritant, whether proceeding from improper food or the presence of parasites, ought to be removed. While, should the use of anthelmintics and purgatives not be absolutely needful for this immediate purpose, their employment will nevertheless be perfectly safe and not at all counter-indicated, seeing that by their derivative action they will tend favourably to lessen cerebral pressure and congestion. Of medicinal agents, those most likely to be beneficial are the bromides of potassium and sodium, the preparations of the Calabar bean, and, in rather chronic cases, the salts of silver, zinc, iron, and arsenic.

In those cases appearing as the sequel of certain febrile and other diseases, and where the nervous system seems below par, a decidedly tonic and invigorating system of treatment is most likely to be attended with favourable results. The food ought to be nutritious, but easy of digestion, and given with regularity, so as to avoid repletion; the animals ought to be well housed, and allowed or compelled to take a reasonable amount of exercise daily in the open air; put cautiously to work, and undue excitement avoided.

CHAPTER XIV

DISEASES OF THE RESPIRATORY ORGANS

PHYSICAL EXAMINATION.

THE diseases of the great organs of respiration and circulation, the lungs, the air-tubes, the heart and great bloodvessels, and of the thorax generally, are recognised by certain symptoms.

local and general, and in addition by certain physical signs indicative of aberration of healthy function and structural change. These physical signs being individually and collectively much relied upon, it will be needful, before proceeding to consider in detail the diseases to which this class of organs is subject, to give them a short review.

Methods and Objects of Physical Examination.

The different physical modes of examination by which an endeavour is made to estimate either the healthy or diseased condition of the thorax and its contained organs are—1 *Inspection of the form of the thorax*, 2 *Mensuration*, 3. *Palpation;* 4 *Percussion*, 5. *Auscultation*, 6 *Succussion*.

These several means of obtaining information relative to the condition of the chest and the organs contained therein, or of confirming opinions formed in the observation of vital symptoms and general states of the constitution, apart from which, even when most carefully noted, they will ever be fruitful sources of error, are not equally applicable to every disease of those organs. Being, however, of such general application in our day, it behoves us to understand how much we may expect to receive from these, and the best means by which these methods may be cultivated.

Of none of these means of strengthening our diagnosis of thoracic disease—particularly the two most frequently employed, *auscultation* and *percussion*—can we obtain a competent knowledge by reading, however carefully, any description of them ; far less can they be mastered so as to give us reasonable grounds for resting on them for support. They must be assiduously and carefully wrought out by ourselves by actual employment on the living animal. The condition of the chest and of the contained organs in healthy animals ought, first of all, to be our study, so as to familiarize our ear and eye with the normal sounds, condition, and appearance; when sufficiently acquainted with these, diseased conditions may be attempted, ever in any doubt having recourse to the examination of the healthy.

With this, as with every separate method of investigation and means of obtaining knowledge of the phenomena of

disease, we must be careful not to allow ourselves to be
guided entirely, to the exclusion of the knowledge and results
which may be offered to us by other means of examining these
cases.

We will first examine the character and general application
of these several physical modes of investigating the condition
of the thoracic organs, and afterwards, shortly, their applications to the different parts of the respiratory organs, with an
estimate of the information which may thereby be obtained in
health and disease.

1 Inspection.—By this mere 'act of looking,' cognizance is
taken of the general form, and also of the movements of the
chest

2 Mensuration, Measurement of the Chest —This is not had
recourse to in the practice of veterinary medicine, not because
we have other and better means of determining the altered
capacity of the thoracic cavity, but more probably because we
have not yet considered it needful to descend to such minute-
ness in diagnosis as has for a lengthened period characterized
the practice of human medicine in respect to diseases of the
thoracic organs

When we desire to apply measurement to the horse's chest,
the double tape is preferable to the single, as it at once gives
the indication if there exists an appreciable difference between
the two sides, as well as any increase in the total capacity at
different measurements

Besides the circular measurement, which ought to be taken
at least at two if not three points, the others which are most
useful are—(a) The distance from the posterior point of the
withers to the commencement of the cartilages of the false
ribs; (b) From the point of the elbow or third rib to the same
point, (c) From the posterior edge of the shoulder to the
margin of the last rib.   These measurements ought to be made
on each side of the chest at the same place, and at the same
stage of the act of respiration

3 Palpation.—This is the term we give to the application
of the hand to any particular part so as to ascertain its
condition of tenderness, heat, power of resistance, and also
impulse imparted by movement of some internal organ.

4 Percussion.—This is understood to consist in striking or

tapping on the surface of the body with a view to determine
the healthy or morbid condition of the parts beneath   The
immediate object determined by percussion is the comparative
density of subjacent parts   This tapping or percussing may
be executed by directly striking the chest with the fingers or
hand, or with an object held in the hand, then termed *immediate;* or indirectly *mediately,* when some object is interposed
between the hand, or object held in the hand, and the wall of
the chest.   In mediate percussion the intervening body is
termed a 'pleximeter.' it is generally a piece of thin ivory,
bone, or vulcanite, or the middle finger of the left hand may
be used for the purpose

In our patients, the most convenient and the simplest mode
of percussion, at least with the larger, is 'immediate,' performed
by striking the surface with the tips of the fingers or the
knuckles of the closed hand.   In carrying out this tapping or
percussing some points require to be attended to.   When the
percussion is immediate, it is desirable to choose for the part
to be struck the surface of a rib where this is possible, and to
strike it perpendicularly, not slantingly; also to deliver the
blow with the same amount of force all over the region percussed, that the sound may be as uniform as possible.   When
an intervening body is employed, whether the finger or a
pleximeter, in 'mediate' percussion, it ought to be applied
closely to the surface and steadily pressed to the parts that
air may be prevented from passing between it and the body-
surface, by which the sound would be modified   In this way
also we compress the subcutaneous fat, rendering it more conducting, and lessen the distance between the surface and the
organ being examined

5 **Auscultation.**—By this we mean to indicate the means
whereby we obtain knowledge of the state of internal organs
by the sound conveyed to the ear; it is listening to the sounds
of the interior by the ear applied to the surface

Like percussion, auscultation may be performed directly and
immediately by placing the ear upon the surface, merely inter-
posing, on the score of cleanliness, a handkerchief or piece of
thin calico; or mediately by the use of an instrument, the
'stethoscope,' which, besides circumscribing the area examined,
assists in conveying the sound from the body to the ear.   Some

experience is needed to use this instrument well, and to obtain from it the maximum of benefit In cases where blistering agents have been employed on the chest, its use is absolutely needful and easily understood.

Each of these methods has advantages peculiar to itself, and either is perfectly efficacious when practised so that the little difficulties and niceties of the art are thoroughly mastered. When immediate auscultation is practised, if a handkerchief is used it ought not to be doubled in case friction between the two surfaces might mislead, and the ear must be placed perfectly flat on the surface to which it is applied In the employment of the stethoscope, the cup-shaped extremity ought to be placed evenly on the skin, and firmly maintained in its position by the ear being closely applied to the larger extremity, it should not be held with the fingers

In all cases we should endeavour to secure for the performance of the operation a place perfectly free from outside noise and the chance of disturbance. To increase the sounds it may in some cases, prior to the examination, be advisable to give the horse a little rapid exercise In the greater number of our cases the direct application of the ear to the chest is better than auscultation by an intervening instrument. In this method the surface covered is greater, the head is steadied by the support of the animal's body, and the ear is brought nearer the objects we wish to examine

So far as examination of the thorax is concerned, the object of auscultation is to examine (a) sounds connected with the lungs and great air-tubes, (b) with the pleura, the so-called friction-sounds, (c) with the heart, and (d) other diseased sounds connected with abnormal conditions of the chest and contained organs

6 Succussion —This is the act of grasping the thoracic cavity between the hands, and by sharply shaking it to cause agitation of its contents and so elicit sound This is only possible in small animals, and in every case has to be carefully performed, not merely from the disturbance it entails upon the animal, but also from the liability there is to confound sounds of the thorax with those of the abdomen produced at the same time

APPLICATION OF THESE PHYSICAL MODES OF EXAMINATION—
SIGNS AFFORDED BY THEM.

It will probably suffice for our purpose of understanding
what these methods of physical examination tell us in investigating the phenomena of disease of the respiratory organs, and
particularly of those contained in the thorax, to regard them
in somewhat of the same order as their description has been
glanced at

I. SIGNS AFFORDED BY INSPECTION AND PALPATION.

These modes of physical examination are chiefly applicable
to the condition of the chest proper; by these we determine
its character as to size, shape, and movements   Any alteration
which may be observable in the simple size or shape of the
chest in the larger animals is so trifling that it may be safely
passed as a source from which information may be obtained as
to the condition of the contained viscera   No doubt there are
some cases in certain of our patients suffering from pneumonic
disease, with effusion of long standing, where an alteration in
form of one side of the chest may sometimes be detected   but
in the horse there is little information of a positive character
to be obtained from change of form in such conditions.

As respects the movements of the thorax, we are able, by
inspection, assisted by palpation, to take into consideration
many of their relations

1. **Alterations in Frequency.**—The respirations may be watched
by the eye, or counted by placing the hand over the false ribs
Their frequency may be (*a*) *increased*, as in certain febrile
affections, when obstruction occurs to the action of the lungs,
or in some diseases of the heart ; (*b*) *diminished*, seen in
certain diseases of the brain, and from the action of narcotics

2. **Disturbance of Relation between the Thoracic and Abdominal
Movements** —(*a*) Thoracic movements in excess from any interference directly with the action of the diaphragm or abdominal
muscles, as in peritonitis, and other structural changes connected with the abdomen ; (*b*) abdominal movements in excess
from causes impeding or rendering painful the action of the
chest-walls, as in pleurisy

3. **Variations of Intensity or Force of the General Movements** —
(*a*) These may be in excess, the animal breathing deeply and
with greater force, more air being changed during each respiration ; (*b*) they may be deficient in force and intensity, less air
being changed during an individual respiration Both these
conditions are observed in diseases of the lungs themselves.

4 **Disturbance in the Rhythm of the Respiratory Act.**—The
chief abnormality here is the prolongation or shortening of
either the inspiratory or expiratory movement. The exercise
of palpation itself is also useful in aiding us, through the
development of local pain on pressure, in diagnosing diseased
conditions of the pleuræ and thoracic walls.

II PHYSICAL SIGNS OBTAINED BY PERCUSSION

A. **Normal Percussion Sounds**—Over the anterior portion of
the air-passages, the sinuses of the head, we find that percussion elicits sounds varying with the age of the horse and
development of these cavities In the young, where the
amount of bone tissue is largely preponderating, and the cavities
comparatively small, the sound is hard and non-resonant ;
as the cavities become enlarged, the walls thinner, with the
quantity of contained air increased, the sound is full, and
resonance augmented.

In health, over the thoracic walls there are encountered
considerable variations in percussive sounds Where the chest
is least clothed with soft tissue, and where the lung-structure
is in immediate contact with the thoracic walls, a moderately
clear sound is elicited ; the sound depending upon the air, or
rather upon the vibration of the air contained in the pulmonary
tissue, and the vibration of the walls of the chest This sound
varies both with the amount of air contained in the pulmonary
tissue, and with the force employed in percussing. When
little force is employed the sound is low, though clear ; when
the force is greater the sound developed is harder, and if the
part struck is over any considerable tract of pulmonary
structure rather resonant. When the animal is in a recumbent
position the sound is distinctly harder and more resonant than
when standing.

In endeavouring to carry out this means of exploring the
chest in our patients it requires us to remember the relative

position, both of the organs contained there, and also of those
in the contiguous cavity, the abdomen, particularly the relation
of these latter to the former   By recollecting these points we
can so far understand the variations of the relative resonancy
observed in the different sides of the cavity, for although the
sounds elicited by percussion of one side may be considered
as tolerably correctly indicating the character of those on the
other, in health this will be found in actual practice not wholly
correct, seeing these are modified by the position of the heart
and of certain of the abdominal viscera   It is also not to be
forgotten that other fortuitous circumstances and conditions
connected with both thorax and abdomen, and organs contained in these cavities, tend to modify sounds elicited by
percussion

As a rule, it may be said that in health the sounds produced
by percussion are most distinct and loudest over those parts
least covered by soft tissues, and where the bronchial sounds
are most distinct   Over the superior portions of both sides in
the horse the sound is clear to the twelfth rib, after this, on the
right side, if the percussion is executed with much force, it
becomes more resonant, of a tympanitic character, as if the
lung, in its intimate structure, contained an extra amount of
air   In all probability this increased resonance proceeds from
the proximity of the arch of the colon

Behind the twelfth rib, on the left side, although by forcible
tapping resonance may be obtained, still it is markedly less
than on the right   so that it is not very far from the truth if
we say that on the right side, in the upper third of the chest,
the sound gradually increases from behind the shoulder to
near the last rib, while on the left side there is a gradual lessening of sound   Over the middle third a good sound is obtainable in both sides very much similar ; the resonance is probably
most marked from the sixth to the twelfth rib, from which it
diminishes to the fifteenth, becoming after this on the left more
resonant, and on the right dull from proximity to the liver.
The lower third gives out a weaker though clear sound on the
right side from the fifth to the eighth rib, when the sound
becomes dull over the region of the liver. On the left, about
the fifth, sixth, and seventh ribs, little sound is heard, from the
space being in great part occupied by the heart, it may, how-

ever, be detected over the eighth, but again declines, and is replaced by dulness over the twelfth or thirteenth rib.

B. **Abnormal Percussion Sounds.**—In abnormal conditions of the thorax and contained organs the resonance, as elicited by percussion, becomes variously modified   It may be (1) *augmented*, (2) *diminished*, (3) *lost*.

1. *Increased* or augmented percussive sound—change in its character—may be general or partial   It is general in cases of extreme pulmonary emphysema, from the amount of air contained in the interlobular structures, and often occurring in quantity in the sub-pleural tissue   Partial increase of sound may follow obstruction, whether from solidification or compression of portions of the lungs, the unaffected being compelled to take in a greater amount of air than natural in discharging extra functional activity, in this way increasing the natural cellular capacity, becoming more dilated, and consequently more resonant on percussion.

2 *Diminished* resonance as a continuous state I have not met with in the horse to any extent, as it is generally so quickly followed by loss of sound. It may, however, occur from any cause which partially obstructs the entrance of the air into the air-sacs, as liquid effusion in the interlobular connective-tissue, or the dissemination through the pulmonary structures of certain diseased products.

3 *Loss* of resonance in the pulmonary tissue is never entire, and its partial or local annihilation may be due to hepatization or to effusion in the pleural sac   When due to the former, the loss of sound will probably have been preceded by the 'crepitation' indicative of inflammatory action   When accompanying the latter, we may have observed symptoms indicative of pleuritis; while in the horse this loss of percussive sound is likely to exist on both sides, beginning at the inferior part of the chest.

III PHYSICAL SIGNS DRAWN FROM AUSCULTATION.

A **Normal Respiratory Sounds**—In health, auscultation over the extended air-passages in the horse discloses at least three typical sounds :

1 *Tracheal, Laryngeal, or Nasal.*—This is the sound common to the large air-cavities of the head, the larynx, and the great

air-tube. By either mediate or immediate auscultation the sound conveyed to the ear over the greater portion of these different sections of the great air-tube during rest is wonderfully alike, consisting of a slight murmur of a soft character, of equal intensity and pitch on both sides of the face, audible during both inspiration and expiration, there being an appreciable interval between these parts of the respiratory act, the latter probably the higher pitched and longer continued. At the inferior portion of the trachea a slight modification of the sound is heard, known as the 'tracheo-bronchial' sound or respiration, caused by the passage of the air to and from the bronchi, it is most distinct during expiration, and augmented by exertion

2. *Bronchial or Tubal.*—This sound is heard in its purity as the tracheo-bronchial respiration referred to as existing at the bifurcation of the trachea at the anterior part of the chest As detected over the superior and middle third of the chest it is less characteristic, and in health is apt to be mixed up with the vesicular sound; in disease there is much less danger of this

In character it is harsher, not so loud, and of shorter duration and intensity than the tracheal, while the interval between the inspiratory and expiratory acts, although still appreciable, is less marked

These tubal sounds are most distinct in the upper third of the chest, least so at the superior part of the lower third where the vesicular sound is loudest. The nearer we get to the root of the lungs, and the divisions of the bronchi, the better is this sound recognised

3. *Pulmonic or Vesicular.*—This sound, otherwise known as the respiratory murmur, is the impression of disturbance conveyed to the ear in the act of auscultation during both inspiration and expiration, between which no interval is appreciable It may be heard when the horse is at rest, particularly if the walls of the chest are not heavily clad with muscular tissue or loaded with fat, and is intensified by exertion or whatever tends to accelerate the respiration It is believed to be the result of the entrance into and exit from the air-sacs of the respired air, together with the dilatation of these, and the peculiarity of their form in relation to the terminal bronchi

There are doubts, however, that this explanation is wholly correct, some considering that, like the tubal, the vesicular sound may originate in the larynx, and as heard over the chest, is the result of conduction and modification

The character of the sound is that of a soft diffuse murmur, and has been compared to the rustling of a gentle breeze amongst green leaves; it is better detected, as well as more prolonged, during inspiration, in expiration it is when heard—which is not always possible—more readily accomplished, and feebler, without the diffuse breezy character   It is heard in its purity at a distance from the greater air-tubes, and where the parenchyma of the lungs is most abundant   The characters of this sound are, in health, subject to variations which require to be noted that they may not be confounded with disease.   It is most distinct in well-bred horses with deep rather than round chests, and where the walls of the cavity are not loaded with soft tissue, also when the animal's stomach and intestines are not distended with food, by which, through pressure on the diaphragm, the thoracic cavity is confined

It is louder or stronger in the young than in aged animals, from the air-cells being more numerous and smaller, and the entire pulmonary tissue being more elastic in nature, this condition of 'juvenile' respiration gradually, with years, gives place probably to a dilatation of air-sacs and weakening of lung-tissue, until the so-called 'senile' respiration is established

In the horse this murmur is distinctly enough heard over the greater portion of the chest—about two thirds—which is exposed for auscultation

Over both sides of the chest it may be detected from behind the scapulæ, or elbows, slightly increasing in force to the tenth or twelfth rib, thence becoming diminished   On the left side in the lower third the pulsations of the heart interfere with its detection

B   Changes in the Health Sounds over the Respiratory Tract due to Disease   1. *Anterior Air Passages.*—In such conditions as engorgement of the pituitary membrane, or where adventitious growths occupy the air-cavities of the head, a more or less blowing or interrupted sound is given out   When the obstruction is very considerable, either from morbid growths or general

28

infiltration of the membranes, these not being much elevated but occupying a considerable space, the sound is of a whistling or sibilant character.

This is apt to be confounded with noise of a similar character originating at some other point of the air-passages, and by propagation, detected at a distance from its place of origin. Generally we may distinguish between these abnormal sounds originating in the upper and lower air-passages by carefully auscultating from the nasal chambers downwards. When originating in the sinuses of the head, they will be found to decrease in pitch as we proceed downwards.

There is a sound often heard in examining horses, of which it behoves us to be cognisant; it is that of a tolerably loud flapping or fluttering noise proceeding from the nasal cavities, emitted when a horse is made to execute rapid movement, sometimes—but we think wrongly—styled 'high-blowing.' This sound, which is heard when trotting or cantering, but disappears, when the horse has settled down to a good and steady gallop, is to be regarded rather as a peculiarity connected with the muscular arrangement of the nostrils, probably the actual noise is the result of flapping or quivering of a voluntary character of the false nostrils. It may be intermittent, but usually disappears when the animal has been galloped for some time It ought not to be regarded as unsoundness

In laryngeal disease, where we have a lessening of the orifice, there is an audible increase in pitch and duration of the sound.

When the mucous membrane is considerably inflamed, with infiltration of the submucous tissue, considerable tumefaction and lessening of the cavity of the larynx, with an extra amount of mucus on the membrane, we have a soft humid sibilant râle or whistle ; this sound, it may be observed, is of an intermittent character, being most distinct when the amount of mucus in the larynx is greatest, and less observed when by coughing the mucus is dislodged.

Another sound of a somewhat similar character, but not moist, a dry sibilant wheezing or whistling sound characterized by its steady persistent nature, is indicative of a narrowing of the aperture of the larynx, it may be from compression, distortion, or approximation of the cartilages or vocal cords, the result of nervous disease

Alterations in the tracheal sounds are chiefly the result of the presence of adventitious materials in the tube. Where liquids and mucus have been poured into the bronchi, the natural sound is modified to a mucus râle, or probably it may be more of a sibilant vibratory character depending on the nature of the contained material. In some cases of asthma a mild wheezing or vibratory noise may be plainly heard along the whole tube.

2. *Lower Air Passages, Thoracic or Chest Sounds*—The abnormal thoracic sounds distinguishable are eithersuch as may be viewed merely as altered normal sounds, or as sounds added to the ordinarily existing ones, and of a different character.

The vesicular or true pulmonic sound is liable to modification—(*a*) *As to its duration or intensity*; (*b*) *As to its extent or area over which it may be heard*; (*c*) *As to its rhythm or regularity*; (*d*) *As to its quality or character*.

a. Changes as to Duration or Intensity (1) *Augmented*—In this there is simply an exaggeration of the natural vesicular sound; it may be extensive or complete when it is spoken of as general, and as partial when the increase is circumscribed; there is no variation in pitch or alteration in character.

A general increase in the respiratory murmur will result from any cause which for a time increases the act of breathing; it is observed in febrile disturbance *per se*, or when occurring as a symptom of other diseased conditions.

The term 'supplementary' respiration has been given to increased vesicular murmur over the whole or part of the lung-surface, consequent on the exclusion of air by the existence of some obstruction from a neighbouring portion of lung-tissue. When heard over portions of the thoracic cavity, where in health it is not usually encountered, it is indicative of the infiltration or solidification of pulmonary tissue, which thus becomes a better conductor of sound.

(2) *Diminution* in the intensity of the respiratory murmur may, like the opposite condition, be general or partial. General diminution depends on many causes, and these are often such as are not directly connected with thoracic changes; very often with diseased conditions of other and distant organs, which, by nervous and other influences, operate indirectly on the activity of the pulmonic function. Of this class are the

28—2

numerous cerebral disturbances, marked by diminished respiratory activity   Also, it may exist in consequence of certain mechanical interferences or obstructions by which the normal expansive capability of the chest is lessened

(3) *Suppression or Absence of the Respiratory Murmur* — This may be permanent or intermittent, and is an accompaniment of conditions similar to what are encountered in diminution of respiration   It is valuable as a sign of pleuritic effusion and lung-consolidation

b· Alterations as to Extent or Area of Lung-structure over which the Respiratory Sound is Heard —These may include an extended or diminished area, according to the expansion of lung-tissue and condition of the thoracic walls

c Modifications as to Regularity or Rhythm.—The disturbances in the regular or rhythmic movement of the respiratory murmur which may be noticed in the horse are ·

(1) The oscillating or jerking, in which the respiratory murmur is interrupted or broken in various ways, seen in certain stages of pleuritis

(2) The unequal, where the one part of the act, that accomplished during expiration, is unequally prolonged, bearing a marked disproportion to the inspiratory action. This is often detected over the middle section of the thorax in emphysema of the lungs

d. Alterations as to Quality or Character—The changes which we group under character of the sound are various; these, besides being altered in sonorousness, pitch, and regularity, have other peculiarities attached to them, all rendering them of importance in directing our diagnosis of disease. In character we may have the respiration—

(1) *Harsh or Rough* —This is simply the respiratory murmur of a higher pitch and of greater intensity, with the soft breezy character replaced in part by a blowing sound   It is more prolonged in expiration than inspiration.

This sound seems to indicate moderate changes of consistence in lung-tissue, as trifling compression in the early part of bronchial and pneumonic inflammations.

This harsh or broncho-vesicular respiration, if not gradually subsiding and replaced by the normal vesicular murmur, steadily becomes fainter, and is replaced by another sound

(2) *Bronchial or Tubular*—This is the sound normally heard in connection with the larger air-tubes, only now unusually marked and hard, where in health it is absent. It is the characteristic sound of absence of vesicular murmur, the result of condensation The existence of this tubal sound in pulmonic tissue, following upon harsh respiration, is indicative of the blocking up of the small bronchi and air-sacs with the products of the morbid action, but it also tells that the air-conduits somewhat larger are still pervious It is also met with apart from condensation of lung-tissue, being sometimes heard as an accompaniment of emphysema.

Other manifestations of this sound, varying according to distribution and other relations, have been spoken of as *blowing*, from the variation detected in their pitch and intensity.

Also, in rare instances, from the connection of the air-tubes with cavities as abscesses or vomicæ, we have particular modulations of sound, varied in accordance with the impression which they convey to the ear, as *cavernous* or *amphoric* These sounds seem to be formed in accordance with the nature, relative size, and position of these cavities, and their tubal communications.

However, from the physical difficulties in connection with minute and discriminate auscultation in the horse, these variations are not so well established, and have received less attention with us than they have with the practitioner of human medicine.

C. **Rhonchi, Râles, or Rattles**—Besides these alterations of the natural respiratory sounds already mentioned, there are occasionally encountered in pulmonary disorders, and having their origin in pulmonary tissue or air-tubes, a class of sounds known by the name of 'Râles,' 'Rattles,' or 'Rhonchi'

Various classifications of these sounds, according to taste and opinion, have been adopted. With too many and minute divisions there is apt to be confusion.

In further regarding these sounds, we purpose speaking of them by the terms of 'Dry Râles' and 'Moist or Humid Râles, in accordance with the impression which is conveyed to the ear of sound travelling along a dry surface or one covered with fluid.

1. *Dry Râles, or Vibratory Râles*—These owe their exist-

ence to the form or character of the tube, the extent to which
its calibre is lessened by infiltration of the submucous structure, or the presence of plastic material on its surface. They
are of necessity of variable intensity or pitch, and are often
spoken of as—

a Large or Sonorous Râle, or Rhonchus.—This is essentially
a sound of the larger bronchi It is of a low bass note, subject to much variation, the greater tones being in the larger
tubes It is generally heard best at the lowest part of the
windpipe, at the anterior portion of the chest, or behind the
shoulder, often of a vibratory character, as if the air were
playing over some dry adherent mucus, and is transient in its
existence, and of variable intensity It is a frequent accompaniment of the early stages of bronchitis, and if there exists
much infiltration of the submucous tissue, will be more likely
to be permanent; it is heard during both expiration and
inspiration Accompanying this sound we often observe the
sibilant or mucous râle in which the smaller tubes are involved

b Smaller Dry Sound, or Sibilant Râle—This is a higher-
pitched whistling or wheezing sound, of varying duration,
heard during expiration and inspiration, but, unlike the larger
sound, better heard during the latter part of the respiratory
act It seems to owe its existence to essentially the same
causes as the sonorous râle. It is characteristic of the earlier
or dry stages of bronchitis, and is best heard over the portions
of the lung-tissue where in health the vesicular sound is
loudest When extensively distributed it constitutes a matter
of more serious import than the larger sound heard in connection with the great tubes.

2 *Moist or Mucous Sounds or Râles*—These are the sounds
which in a general way we find following the dry in cases of
inflammation of the air-tubes The impression conveyed to
the ear by these moist or humid râles is that of bubbles of air
passing through liquids, and in passing bursting The variations in the sound are connected with the character of these
air-bubbles and the fluid with which they mingle.

Of these moist sounds we speak of at least three or four
variations.

a. The Mucous Râle—By this term is ordinarily understood

the sound which on auscultation conveys to the ear the idea of air being drawn through moderately sized bronchi containing liquid, mucus, blood, or pus, and in its passage producing bubbles of a good size The sound co-exists with both expiration and inspiration. It is the sound present in ordinary bronchitis after the dry stage has been passed and secretion fairly established It is modified as to its intensity and continuance by the character of the bubbles formed and the force with which the air is sent through the tube

This sound may be temporary or permanent, and modified at all times by the quantity of fluid present in the tubes

b Submucous or Subcrepitant Râle —This is to be regarded as a modification of the ' mucous râle.' It is the sound comparable to the passage of air through the smaller bronchi containing a viscid liquid When the bubbles produced are of a minute character, it has been likened to the effervescence occurring in liquids containing gas It may be heard during both the respiratory acts, louder, as a rule, during inspiration It is indicative of established inflammation, with secretion in the smaller tubes, and may be regarded as the intermediate sound found occurring between the ' crepitant ' and ' mucous râle '

c Crepitant Râles —Of these, several variations are noticed We, however, only regard—

(1) *The True Crepitant Râle* —To this reference has already been made, and the sound indicated by this term partly described, when speaking of the changed characters of the pulmonic sounds, under that of ' rough respiration '

It consists of a great number of very minute, sharp, crepitant sounds rapidly elicited, and has not inaptly been likened to the sound developed by rubbing a lock of hair between the finger and thumb close to the ear It is believed to owe its existence to the passage of the air through or to and from the minute bronchi and air-sacs, and by the act of the expansion of these latter The certainty of this is not beyond a doubt, many viewing this sound as a ' friction ' sound, and of pleuritic origin It is heard chiefly or only during inspiration. It is the sound which is usually developed in the outset of pneumonia, although often in such cases we find this pure ' crepitant râle ' much modified.

(2) *Modified or Secondary Crepitant Râle.*—This is the name

which we give to the sound occasionally, not always, heard in the horse's lungs in advanced stages of pneumonia when resolution or return to functional activity appears, after absence of sound from inflammatory changes.

It is not unlike the crepitation râle now noticed, only it is audible during expiration as well as inspiration; is of a slower, softer, and irregularly occurring character, not unlike the bubbling of air through mucus or a similar fluid.

d. Cavernous or Hollow Râles—In addition to these sounds now mentioned, which in various modifications are the ordinary rattles or râles detected in pulmonary structures under abnormal conditions, there are, as indicated when speaking of changes in pulmonary sounds, some others which are neither so common nor so easily recognised in our patients as in the human subject. The chief are probably those known as 'cavernous' or 'hollow râles.' These can only be produced when some cavity, as an abscess, exists, having a free communication with a fair-sized bronchus. The sound heard is either of a *gurgling, rattling, hollow,* or *cavernous* character.

In all cases where these modified rattles could be distinguished, I have always found that the expired air was impregnated with a distinct and often disagreeable odour, and that there was expectoration, at least such as exists in the horse. Also that this cavernous rhonchus has often been associated with the existence in the adjoining portion of the lung-tissue of both 'mucous' and 'submucous râles.'

I have not found it, unless following pneumonic disease of some time standing; indeed, it has always been in connection with gangrene and destruction of lung-tissue.

D. Friction Sounds, Pleural Sounds. *Friction, attrition,* or *pleural sounds* are the names given to sounds only detected in disease, and believed to be associated with the cavity of the thorax, independent of the pulmonary organs. Although it is tolerably certain that in disease sound may be emitted or elicited in connection with the pleural membranes, there is much less unanimity of opinion as respects both the existence of these sounds and the manner of their production than with those we have been speaking of as related to the pulmonary structures. It seems highly probable that it is chiefly, if not solely, during the earlier stages of inflammatory action, or at least when in the course of that action certain structural changes have occurred in connection with the pleuræ, and previous to the more advanced condition of liquid effusion into the cavity, that any sound can be satisfactorily distinguished.

In character this friction-sound has been variously described as a mild or smooth rubbing, grating, or crackling noise. It is not uniformly executed, but seems, when heard, as if carried out by short jerks, appreciated during both parts of the respiratory act, more clearly in inspiration, and ordinarily at the inferior part of the thorax. It may be regarded as a dry sound, seeing it is only recognised prior to the condition of effusion, and becomes inaudible with the existence of fluid in the chest, and may again be heard when the fluid is being removed.

In following out the examination of any such sound, when detected, attention ought to be bestowed upon its intensity, its extent or distribution, and upon its relation to inspiration or expiration.

E. **Other Sounds of Varying Character sometimes Heard in connection with Changes in the Thoracic Cavity** —The conditions which seem to favour the production of these unnatural sounds in the chest, and associated with its contained organs, are (*a*) the presence of a moderate amount of fluid in the cavity of the pleural sac; (*b*) the existence of extensive organizations in different parts of the chest; (*c*) a certain quantity of air in contact with the fluid.

Under such conditions we may occasionally detect certain unnatural sounds, chief of which are *metallic tinkling* and *modified gurgling* sounds.

Metallic tinkling, or the sound indicated by this term, may be tolerably well imitated by pressing the palm of the left hand firmly over the ear, and tapping it smartly with the middle or index finger of the right. It is a sound which is neither heard regularly, nor, when detected, is it of uniform character; some of the notes or impulses are pitched in higher tones than others, as well as more prolonged.

It has been regarded as due to the dropping of fluid from the adherent fibrinous exudations into and upon the liquid contained in the cavity.

The gurgling noises, it has been suggested, are due to the disentanglement of air from the effused material in the form of bubbles, or they may be the result of sounds generated elsewhere, and propagated through the partly condensed and partly fluid contents of the sac.

F Cough Resonance —Some further indications of diseased conditions, as revealed by sound, may in certain instances be obtained by causing the animal affected to cough, the sound of which is propagated through the air contained in the minute air-tubes to the surface of the chest

In health, the sound elicited is of a soft, dull, indistinct character   In consolidation of the pulmonary structures, the result either of hepatization or of compression from effusion, the sound, as heard by the application of the ear over the chest, and resulting from enforced coughing, is somewhat louder and harder, and is communicated to a more or less extensive surface according to structural changes.

In cases following the progress of gangrene, or other destructive changes, where previously the 'cavernous rhonchus' formerly spoken of was heard, a considerable modification in sound is obtained   It is generally of greater resonance, varying in accordance with the extent of the cavity in the lung, and with the nature of its communication with the bronchi and its position as related to the surface.

CHAPTER XV

OF CERTAIN SYMPTOMS ASSOCIATED WITH CHANGE AND DISTURBANCE OF THE RESPIRATORY ORGANS

In addition to the physical signs of change and disturbance in the organs of respiration, there are also presented for our consideration some not unimportant symptoms associated with these organs which will be useful to notice, however shortly These are *grunting, coughing, dyspnœa, roaring, whistling.*

Any, or probably all, of these conditions may exist as temporary infirmities, the result of very varying causes, and of a nature not likely to be persistent, but removable by therapeutic

treatment or surgical interference; or they may be of a permanent character, not associated with any active process, not
likely to pass into any developmental change, neither appreciably influenced in a durable manner by therapeutic agents,
nor of a character susceptible of amelioration or cure by surgical interference.

These latter must all be regarded as constituting unsoundness, or as indicative of states or conditions constituting unsoundness; for although they may not at their first appearance,
or even afterwards, impair the usefulness of the horse, they
certainly detract from his commercial value, and in many
instances render him unfit for specific purposes.

1. Grunting.—The emission of this sound by a horse is
often a matter of considerable importance, seeing it is always
brought under our notice in making examinations of animals
relative to their soundness; it is also in some a symptom of
disease.

When a horse is suddenly startled, either by being struck or
by a feint being made to strike him, or by being rapidly moved
into a different position, he may make a rough grunting noise
during expiration; in such a case the animal is said to
'grunt,' or to be a 'grunter.' The emission of this noise may
be associated with or dependent on disease of the larynx, or,
the larynx being healthy, the sound may be indicative of an
abnormal state of the chest.

In dealing with this noise our chief care is to determine—
(a) Whether it is the accompaniment of some acute affection chiefly of the lower air-passages or of the chest-walls;
(b) Whether dependent upon nervous irritability; (c) Whether
we have to regard it as a laryngeal sound unassociated with
inflammatory changes.

As a pure laryngeal sound, unassociated with any affection
of the chest or nervous irritability, it ought always to be
regarded with suspicion, because, if not of itself constituting
unsoundness, it is indicative of a condition the probable result
of which is permanent deficiency in respiration.

2. Coughing.—Cough is the name given to sound mainly produced in the larynx by the forcible expulsion of air from the
great air-tube.

This laryngeal sound is liable to be evoked by direct irritation to the mucous membrane in any part of the air-passages, but chiefly the throat and larynx, by disordered conditions of both intimate and accessory structures of these organs, by reflex or propagated irritation from disorders in other and distant organs, and by direct nervous disturbance.

In studying cough its general character requires to be regarded—(a) In respect of its mode of attack, whether dependent upon some irritation conveyed to the parts, or occurring independent of any appreciable cause; (b) The frequency of its occurrence, and whether of a few isolated acts, or occurring in paroxysms; (c) Its severity and apparent accompanying conditions of pain; (d) Its quality, whether irritating, barking, hoarse, cavernous, dry, or moist

For our guidance, the chief consideration is its special character or quality; and of this, the more important may be grouped as 'dry' or 'moist'

The moist or humid coughs are, as the name indicates, associated with a damp or humid condition of the respiratory mucous membranes.

This kind of cough is usually attendant on the second stage of congestive or inflammatory action in the middle and lower air-passages, sometimes also of the upper. When the disease is chiefly in the upper and middle portion of the air-passages, the cough is full, sonorous, and prolonged.

In some cases of sore throat, and in inflammation of the lower and more minute air-passages, the full and sonorous character is lost, it is weak and feeble.

The dry cough, with characteristic laryngeal sound, is in its various modifications largely indicative of an irritated and rather dry condition of the mucous membrane, and of the earlier stages of inflammatory action. It is also the cough of propagated or reflected irritation

In the earlier stages of active inflammation of the laryngeal and adjacent structures, it is prolonged and sonorous, becoming, as the disease advances, harder from the increased tumefaction, and then moist when secretion is established During the same stage of the process in the lower air-tubes, the cough is hollow or tubal; while, when the pulmonic structure is much invaded, there is a short, scarcely audible, rather dull cough, resonance seeming to be propagated through the solidifying lung-structure   When the lining membrane of the chest is affected we have a dry, short, painful cough

The spasmodic diagnostic cough of broken wind is dry, at first paroxysmal, becoming in advanced cases solitary and feeble. Associated with this cough, because often observed as a distant precursor of it, is what may be termed the ' nervous ' or ' intermittent ' cough   It is dry, hard, irritating, and characterized by its sudden appearance without assignable cause, and as unaccountably disappearing, to return at some rather distant period

3 **Dyspnœa** —Difficulty or oppression in breathing is frequently enough brought under our notice, and although in the horse this is oftener directly associated with changes occurring in the respiratory organs than any other situation, it is nevertheless a complex phenomenon, largely dependent on other causes   As observed by us, it is usually connected with —(a) Obstruction to the entrance of air into the respiratory organs, whether occurring in the upper or lower part of the great air-tube or its minute ramifications   This obstruction may be the result of occlusion, more or less extensive, of any of the air-conduits by a foreign body , it may follow pressure exercised on these by encroaching growths, or it may be dependent on spasmodic closure   (b) It may follow destructive changes of the pulmonic tissue, air-cells or air-tubes, or both, by which the amount of breathing or aerating structure is greatly diminished, as in consolidation, collapse, or compression   (c) Mechanical and other interference with the expansibility of the chest-wall may operate in a similar manner. (d) An improper or imperfect condition of the inspired air   (e) A pulmonic blood-supply, defective or irregular in amount, impure or impoverished in quality

In all cases of oppressed and difficult breathing we have placed before us for determination the causes of the impediment, and the means to be adopted for its removal   To a solution of these we are directed by a careful observation of such phenomena, and their modes of development, as the entrance of air into the lungs, whether carried out freely or with difficulty , the existence or non-existence of noise during the accomplishment of the act, whether the dyspnœa is constant or only paroxysmal , if there are any symptoms of blood-poisoning; and whether or not the supply of respirable air is sufficient for the animal's wants.

Should these efforts at breathing, which ought always to be regarded as a compensatory action, not speedily restore the proper relation which ought to subsist between the amounts of oxygen and carbonic acid in the blood, we know that other symptoms, and a somewhat different condition, is certain to follow. Certain parts of the nervous centres become functionally inert, and a train of symptoms, comprising various nervous phenomena and blood-changes, recognised as *asphyxia*, is apt to destroy life.

4 **Whistling and Roaring.**—These, although probably in the large majority of instances truly laryngeal sounds, and appearing in connection with acute diseases of the air-passages, or indicative of some impediment to the proper performance of the respiratory act, are, from their frequency of occurrence and the importance of their recognition in relation to the question of soundness, deserving of particular attention.

Under the general term of 'roaring,' we are inclined to group all those abnormal sounds emitted by horses under exertion, and known as 'roaring' or 'whistling,' not because we regard them as in every case but modifications as to severity or intensity of one and the same sound, but merely because they are all deviations in the matter of sound from the condition of normal respiration. In investigating this symptom of abnormal sound, amongst several other questions, attention is particularly required to be directed to the following:

A. Whether it has appeared suddenly as the Sequel of some Acute Disease of any part of the Air Passages.—The fact of the development of this abnormal sound occurring suddenly, and succeeding some acute disease connected with the organs of respiration, is favourable, rather than unfavourable. The defect in such cases may arise from the partial organization or non-removal of certain products of the previous inflammatory action. These products may have been effused into the submucous tissue of the laryngeal membranes, thus constricting the opening of the larynx, and altering the pitch and tone of the sounds emitted during respiration. Knowing the probabilities of the occurrence of this, defects in respiration succeeding catarrhal and other analogous affections, the examination of horses at this time ought to be cautiously proceeded with.

B. If it has developed gradually apart from any appreciable Cause.—Ordinarily this is the condition or history which is presented to us of the unnatural sound, whether arising from lesions of the nasal chambers, or in connection with the laryngeal or tracheal portions of the air-tube.

C. Whether it exists at all times when the Animal is placed under similar Conditions, or only occasionally.

D. Its particular Quality and the Conditions under which it is produced, both during Inspiration and Expiration.—This question of character or quality is an important one. There are many who regard all these abnormal sounds heard during exertion as merely indicative of a more or less aggravated condition of the same disease. In this light 'roaring' is looked at merely as an advanced state or more severe form of 'whistling.'

Others, again, regard the character of the sound emitted during exertion as entirely determined by the calibre of the tube through which the air is passed, and consequently view the higher-pitched and shriller note as evidence of a smaller laryngeal opening, and therefore that an animal which whistles is exhibiting a more advanced stage of the condition formerly recognised as roaring.

In actual practice, however, we meet with many instances of horses which are what is universally recognised as 'whistlers' which have not passed through the stage of 'roaring;' and many so-called 'roarers' which have steadily advanced from one degree of roaring to another, without ultimately terminating as whistlers.

Mr Percival, than whom there was no more acute or correct observer, seems to have entertained the latter opinion, viz., that the high-pitched sound was the more advanced state. He says, reasoning from certain experiments which he made by means of a ligature passed around the trachea of a horse: 'That a certain diminution of the calibre of the air-tube produces roaring; that further diminution or contraction of its area causes whistling. A whistler, therefore, I regard as an intense roarer: a wheezer, I should say, is something short of an actual roarer.'

Of the truth of these results, as far as the nature or character of the sounds elicited, and the relation which these will bear to a tube, organic or inorganic, simply narrowed or lessened in calibre, there appears no reasonable doubt. A mistake, however, seems to be made in regarding the abnormal noise as always dependent on the simple relative area or calibre of the tube through which the air is forced, and neglecting to consider whether the form of the tube or adventitious asperities, prominent angles, or other air-impeding entities, may not possess some material influence in developing the pitch or character of the sound

Although it is very difficult, if not impossible, in words adequately and intelligibly to convey to the uninitiated a true idea of the kind and character of these abnormal sounds, they are, when heard for a few times, so impressed on the ear and recollection that we rarely mistake them afterwards   A horse that is very plethoric, and entirely out of work, will, when put to rapid exertion, blow hard, the respiration will be accelerated, and the animal may be distressed , but the increased sound in the respiratory act, by the rush of air along the air-tubes, is in the key of health ; there is a softness and smoothness about it, although rushing furiously along, which in disease we have not · here the pitch is altered , it is harsh, sonorous, wheezing, or whistling

As a general rule, the unnatural sound is only heard during the inspiratory part of the respiratory act; instances no doubt do occur where this is reversed, or in which it is alike audible during both inspiration and expiration   In very few cases will any noise of an abnormal character be heard when the horse is at rest, or moving at a leisurely pace. The greater number of horses of the lighter breeds do not, even when made to exert themselves, emit a sound so distinctly roaring, loud or harsh ; it is oftener of the character spoken of as whistling, a somewhat high-pitched and prolonged noise.   In the heavier breeds the unnatural sound is more sonorous, harsh, and loud, 'roaring' proper ; between these there are variations depending on the seat of the inducing lesion, its character, extent, and period of duration

E   The probable Seat of the Lesions connected with, or acting as Factors in, the Production of the Unnatural Sound —In correctly determining the seat of the lesions which operate in the production of this important symptom connected with the respiratory act, we are materially assisted in forming a true prognosis of the case. These disturbances or changes, upon which the symptoms of roaring are chiefly dependent, may all be grouped as connected with lesions occurring—(1) *In the nasal passages ;* (2) *In the posterior parts of the mouth and pharynx ,* (3) *In the larynx;* (4) *In the trachea*

1. *The Lesions which are chiefly met with in the Nasal Passages,* tending to the production of the unnatural sound 'roaring,' are—(*a*) Alterations of the calibre of these chambers, the result of injuries, by which the bony walls are depressed, or projections of bone-structure are produced interfering with the movements of the air, and altering the character and pitch of the sound resulting from the current (*b*) Alterations in the area of these cavities, the result of abnormal growths, either directly connected with the membrane itself, or proceeding from the bone-structures forming their boundary walls

2. *In the Posterior Parts of the Mouth and Pharynx*—The abnormalities of these parts connected with the production of roaring are—(*a*) Fibrous growths, or mucous polypi of varying characters and situation Their mode of attachment is somewhat peculiar, being usually very movable, either from the elongation of the mucous membrane to which they are attached, or from the possession of a well-developed neck or pedicle From this we account for the dyspnœa and noise attendant on their presence being so excessive at one time and nearly absent at others (*b*) Roaring will also occur from enlarged glands in the pharyngeal region, and from the presence of pus or mucus, either in a liquid state or when inspissated in the guttural pouches

3 *From Lesions occurring in the Larynx*—(*a*) Certain acute diseases of the larynx proper are attended with an unnatural respiratory sound, diagnostic of inflammatory action proceeding in connection with laryngeal structures. This abnormal respiratory sound will, in acute disease of the larynx, be so appreciable that no disturbance of the horse is needed to develop it. (*b*) Following the subsidence of the acute inflammatory attacks, and when it is believed that the animal is perfectly recovered, unmistakable evidence may be afforded of defective respiration whenever the horse is called upon to perform even moderate exertion Many of these cases will

29

ultimately perfectly recover, and seem to depend upon the non-perfecting of the healing or reparative process in tedious recoveries succeeding previous catarrhal affections (c) By far the most common laryngeal lesion, however, which seems to operate in the production of abnormal sounds—of roaring, specially so called—is a peculiar atrophic and degenerative condition of certain muscles of the larynx, notably the muscles which pass between and attach the arytenoid to the cricoid cartilages posteriorly When these are free from disease, and in the exercise of healthy functional activity, the aperture of the larynx is maintained in a uniform and adequate condition, when inactive from any cause, the opposite conditions ensue   there is narrowing and alteration of form, attended with modification of normal sound during the performance of the respiratory act

The morbid condition usually existing in connection with these muscles, in cases of roaring, is that of atrophy and fatty degeneration , by this their power of action or contractility is destroyed, and the more movable parts of the larynx, the arytenoid cartilages, to which they are attached, approach each other, by which the external opening of the larynx is narrowed, and the edges of one or both cartilages brought into the air-current in its passage to and from the trachea

Although it is not uncommon to meet with this degenerative change affecting the greater number of the muscles of one side of the larynx, or even certain of both sides, it is more frequently confined to those of the left side only, or at least in a more marked degree than the other

What may be the primary or direct cause of this disease of nutrition affecting a particular group or groups of muscles, or why those of the left side should be so frequently diseased as compared with the right, are questions of great difficulty, upon which it is easier to speculate than to offer a satisfactory reply. By some this particular lesion, inducing abnormal respiration, has been attributed to manipulatory interference   Endeavouring, by means of reining, to give to the head an unnatural position, by which the larynx, as a whole, is distorted, the muscles thrown out of action, thereby inducing atrophic changes.   That such treatment may in certain instances induce disease in the parts operated upon, resulting in defective respi-

ration, is possible : but that even such destructive treatment
will account in full for the origin of these unnatural sounds we
scarcely believe   Neither is the explanation which is usually
given of the greater liability of the laryngeal muscles of the
left side to become diseased likely to carry with it universal
conviction   This latter fact is attempted to be explained from
the peculiarity of the thoracic origin of the left recurrent nerve,
from which these muscles receive their motor-power

Its origin being more posterior than that of the right, it has
been suggested that in this way it is more readily and more
largely influenced by morbid actions which occur in the cavity
of the thorax   Now, although roaring is often a sequel of
diseases of the respiratory organs, it is certainly more liable to
follow an attack of inflammatory action in the upper than the
lower air-passages, in the larynx than in the lungs   This result
we should not expect to find if it were perfectly true that the
existence of pulmonary inflammation was largely to develop
laryngeal disease through any influence determined to the
recurrent nerve   From its being somewhat more superficially
situated than the right nerve, pressure exercised from without
has also been regarded as actively operating in the induction
of this defective nutrition with its consequent results   If,
however, pressure does operate in the production of this disturbance of nerve force and sequences, it seems more likely
to do so by acting from within, through textural changes, than
by violence from without

In estimating the agencies at work in the production of
this structural change and functional disturbance, there is one
which facts and observation teach us is widely distributed and
constantly prevailing, viz , hereditary predisposition   The fact
that both stallions and mares, themselves roarers, have begotten
and bred animals which ultimately became roarers, is acknowledged by the more intelligent breeders of horses of all classes.
In my own experience I have met with particular sires, roarers,
whose produce from different mares have in large proportion, at
an early period of life, and apart from any apparent cause, as
disease of the respiratory organs, shown unmistakable evidence
of defective respiration, also, I am aware of mares, themselves
roarers, whose produce by different sires, not sufferers from
this disease, were similarly affected to their dams.

4 *Lesions connected with the Trachea.*—The changes which, in the great air-tube, seem to result in the production of this unnatural respiratory sound are—(*a*) Changes of form or calibre, the result of injury, or disease of the naturally resisting walls by which its integrity, as a perfect air-conduit, is interfered with ; (*b*) Textural changes connected with the lining membrane, as morbid growths, or the partial organization of inflammatory products ; (*c*) Distortion and change of form produced by pressure from without, acting much as in the case of mechanical injury, by causing change of area or lumen in the air-tube

Mode of Detecting this Abnormal Condition or Sound.—Proceeding upon the knowledge that the unnatural sound is often elicited without putting the horse to any very severe exertion, that the essential condition connected with its production is to induce a sudden and rapid passage of air along the air-tubes, the method of startling the animal by placing him against a wall, and making a feint to strike him, is adopted, and generally with success in those animals where the lesion upon which the abnormal sound depends, is fully established. Pressure with the fingers over the body of the larynx, inducing coughing, will also assist us in judging of the condition of this part of the air-tube. Should these methods of testing yield affirmative evidence of the abnormal state of the respiration, it may, when very patent, not be needful to proceed further. In the greater number of instances, however, we find it necessary to put the animal to some severe or rapid exertion, by which the respiratory movements will require to be called into vigorous and prolonged action. In draught-horses this is very readily attained by causing them to drag a good load, at a brisk pace, up an incline, which, if they are able to accomplish without emitting an abnormal noise, the respiratory function may be considered as in fairly good condition.

The same end may be attained, though we do not think so rapidly nor so unmistakably, with both draught-horses and the lighter breeds, by simply causing them to move rapidly, usually at the gallop, for a few hundred yards past the examiner ; this is the ordinary method of examining all horses, while, with animals broken for saddle use, it is the only practicable one

In testing a horse's respiration it is always, especially in the lighter breeds, a safe plan to bustle the animal somewhat, keeping him well by the head, while he is occasionally startled by a smart touch of the heels, to turn him rapidly round, and suddenly to pull him up. When pulled up, the examiner ought always to approach near to the horse's nostrils, the more easily to distinguish if any unnatural sound is given forth during either expiration or inspiration; and, if need be, he should be ready to place his ear or stethoscope over first one part of the air-tube, and then another

If we have the power of choice as respects ground over which to gallop a horse with the view of determining the state of his respiration, preference ought to be given to rather soft than hard ground, and to an undulating rather than a perfectly level surface also that he should finish his gallop going up-hill

Horses slight, or even pronounced roarers, may, if the work is not over-fast or too severe, continue for some time serviceable animals. However, as a matter of professional opinion, all grades, degrees, or conditions of this abnormal respiration must be regarded as constituting unsoundness; nor does it appear that we are justified in having any reservation in our opinion, unless it be in those cases where animals are known to have recently been sufferers from some inflammatory condition of the respiratory organs, in which it will be needful that our inspection should be repeated

Treatment of Roaring—When we remember that the condition recognised as roaring is apt to result from lesions so, different as nasal polypi, hypertrophy of turbinated bones, constriction of the laryngeal opening; from infiltration and induration of mucous tissue, or chronic disease of muscles; from injury or disease occurring in connection with the trachea, etc, we can easily understand that the same treatment carried out with the view of cure in one case will not be advantageous in another; and that ere we can reasonably hope to give even an intelligent opinion as to the probabilities of good resulting from the employment of remedial measures, we must be able to determine the seat and nature of the lesion directly operating in the production of the unnatural noise

When the impediment is associated with depression or

change of the bony walls of the nasal chambers, or with abnormal growths, hard or soft in character, situated there, in addition to the dyspnœa exhibited on exertion there is often, even in moderate movement or at rest, a snuffling character in the breathing, with repeated sneezings and a discharge of mucus of a slightly frothy character, occasionally mingled with blood In such cases of abnormal growths in the chambers we are much assisted in their detection by speculum examination and by percussion

When the obstruction is ascertained to be either an osseous tumour springing from the bony walls of the cavity, or a fibrous growth attached to the soft tissues, known as a nasal polypus, we are always justified in attempting the removal of the offending body when this can be accomplished with a reasonable probability of success

When the lesion operating in the production of the characteristic sound appears to be in the pharyngo-laryngeal region, confirmation of the suspicion may be obtained by auscultation, which during excited respiration will give the sound direct, loud, harsh, and near Having satisfied ourselves of the locality of the lesion so far, we may, by examination with the hand, discover whether any adventitious growth or deposit exists likely to cause the embarrassed respiration These, when existing, must be treated according to the recognised rules of surgery.

When following a smart attack of catarrh, strangles, or influenza, the condition of roaring requires more discrimination in dealing with it than at most other times. All these cases are deserving of being for some time carefully observed, and of having the benefit of medical treatment. Although it is not advisable to throw such animals entirely idle, their work ought not to be hard or oppressive, and the diet should be good, but not carried to repletion

The treatment, therapeutically, which I have found productive of most benefit, has been the daily exhibition of potassium, iodide, and arsenic, the former in drachm doses in the morning, the latter three grains combined with three drachms of bicarbonate of potash, or one fluid ounce of Fowler's solution of arsenic in the evening Both these medicines can be given in the food or drinking-water, and ought to be continued for ten or fourteen days, when a rest may be given, to be again continued for a similar period. At the same time, and while receiving these medicines, smart blistering applications ought to be employed around the throat and larynx, being brought well forward between the branches of the lower jaw, and well up to the aural region.

The best blister for this purpose is an ointment composed of equal parts of common cantharides and the bin-iodide of mercury ointments.

Unfortunately the greater number of the cases of roaring or whistling which we encounter in young horses seem to be the result of the laryngeal lesions muscular paralysis and atrophy. They are certainly, also, the most hopeless as respects treatment.

It is probable that such measures as smart blistering, or the application of the actual cautery, may in some instances be productive of good by arresting atrophic changes, and imparting strength to the weakened tissues. It is said by some that when employed early a fair percentage of recoveries may be expected; while from the fact that benefit has resulted in even a moderate number of instances, they are always worth a trial.

It has been proposed, by operative interference, to remove the offending cartilage, which through muscular paralysis has dropped into a false position. The removal of this, it was thought, might give increased calibre to the air-tube, and thus avoid the harsh and unnatural sound. The cases in which this operation have been carried out have not in this country been so successful as to warrant its general recommendation. It is probable that with many, a steady and judicious employment of a galvanic current might be productive of good. From the limited experience which I have had of this and the operative interference, there seems more likelihood of permanent benefit resulting from the former than the latter.

Very confirmed and severe cases are much benefited, and the animal often rendered capable of moderate work, by the use of a compress or pad fitted to the nostrils so as to regulate the amount of air admitted to the larynx, and also by the use of a tube inserted into the upper portion of the trachea through which ordinary respiration may be carried out.

When the disturbing lesion is an abnormal condition of part of the structure of the trachea, as fracture, partial or entire, of certain of the cartilaginous rings, we may occasionally, by judicious operative interference, restore the displaced parts to a position less likely to interfere with the air-current in excited respiration.

CHAPTER XVI

CATARRH—CORYZA—COMMON COLD

I. ACUTE CATARRH.

BEFORE entering upon the detailed consideration of the affections of the respiratory organs, it will be of advantage to examine cursorily the condition so common all over the country, and affecting horses however located and managed, commonly recognised by the term 'catarrh,' or a 'cold'

This might in some respects, considering the very extensive involvement of many organs and functions, be regarded as a general diseased condition   We prefer, however, to look upon it more particularly as associated with those organs where its most characteristic lesions are encountered

Definition.—*The term catarrh, which has been used to identify this most common affection, is ordinarily understood to indicate an inflammatory condition of the lining membrane of the nasal chambers, of the posterior nasal structures and upper portions of the air-tube.   It is attended with a serous and ultimately highly cellular discharge from the nasal chambers, occasionally with cough or sore throat, and with or without fever.*

Causation.—It seems tolerably certain that various conditions are in operation predisposing animals to an attack of cold, such as—(1) Youth, or want of maturity and stability of organization, it being more frequent in horses before than after adult life, (2) A weak and lax condition of animal tissues, either the result of an inherent diathesis, or acquired through inadequate feeding and bad treatment; (3) Previous attacks of the same affection within a limited period

Of the direct inducing factors the more appreciable are— (1) Exposure to cold and moisture, particularly when previously heated; (2) Contact by cohabitation with animals suffering from the same disturbance

1 *Exposure to the Vicissitudes of Weather.*—This, as well as placing animals in damp stables, or any sudden lowering of the surrounding temperature, has ever, with the most of observers, been considered as the most fruitful cause of colds It does not, however, appear that mere cold, or exposure to cold, is so apt to induce this condition as some have imagined. I am well aware of the fact that a fall of temperature extending to 10° or 20° F. will in a wonderfully short period develop a large number of cases of catarrh amongst horses in any city; this, however, of itself will not account for these results. In those cases, animals so circumstanced are, from the unnatural condition of location in overheated, imperfectly ventilated lodgings, so enervated and weakened, that the influence of a lowered temperature suddenly applied acts detrimentally upon them.

Sudden variations of temperature do not, in animals favourably circumstanced, seem very apt to induce disease. Witness the use of the Roman, misnamed the Turkish, bath, where a cold douche is given after leaving the sudatorium. The application of cold seems chiefly to be dangerous when applied to the previously heated body, exhausted by exercise or fatigue, slowly parting with its heat; so that there seems strong reason for believing that the influence of change of temperature and exposure to damp are chiefly to be feared when the animal body is exhausted by fatigue or exposure to debilitating influences

In some old writings on veterinary matters we find catarrh attributed to obstructed perspiration To this some of our modern authors have taken objections. However, cogent reasons may be adduced in support of the supposition that the symptoms exhibited in ordinary catarrh are dependent on the presence in the blood of a specific animal poison, which, either by its direct presence there, or its special irritation of those organs and structures which naturally are its intended emunctories, is

the direct inducing agent. In this way it is argued the arrest
of the secretion of the skin by exposure to cold and damp
throws back into the blood a material which, either of itself
or by virtue of ulterior changes which it undergoes in the
body, acts as a toxic agent. The mucous membrane of the
respiratory tract seems to be the structure delegated to eliminate this noxious material thrown into the system by the suspension of the cutaneous action through the influence of cold.
The symptoms of catarrh are, in this light, regarded as dependent on the vascular disturbance in the mucous membrane
incident to the eliminatory process, and until the poison is
excreted this disturbance will remain, the purification of the
blood being immediately followed by relief from symptoms of
the derangement of the mucous membrane.

2. *Contact with Diseased Animals.*—In many instances this
is abundantly evident.

The placing of healthy horses amongst those which are
suffering from common catarrh has often enough been followed
by the strangers becoming affected. The same can be said of
the converse experiment, that the placing of diseased animals
amongst healthy has often been followed by the appearance of
catarrh amongst the latter.

Symptoms.—Two forms of catarrh have been described, the
simple and the chronic; and although both are undoubtedly
encountered in the horse, the chronic form, sometimes termed
ozæna, is rare as compared with the ordinary or benign.

In common catarrh the symptoms may be regarded as
(1) Local, (2) General. The local usually precede the general
if these latter are developed, which in the mildest forms they
are not.

1. *Local Symptoms.*—The earliest local symptoms are
sneezing, redness and dryness of the nasal membrane, with a
discharge at first of a thin serous, irritating character, succeeded, after some days, by a defluxion of a turbid, yellowish
colour, irregularly discharged.

With these we have also redness of the conjunctival membrane, with a copious discharge of tears, hanging of the head,
with heat over the frontal sinuses, and pain exhibited when
these are percussed.

From the extent of the Schneiderian membrane, and its per-

fect exposure to our observation, coryza is one of the few disorders in which we can watch the different pathological
changes which take place during the development of the
disease. At the outset of the diseased action the membrane
is dry, red, and swollen, the vessels seem turgid, and the perverted function steadily extends to other vascular structures;
the eyelids become congested, the conjunctival membrane red
from the engorged state of the vessels, which in some instances
seem standing out in relief, and more tortuous than in health.
The posterior part of the nasal orifices and fauces are dry,
swollen, and tender.

For some time, it may be only hours, or it may extend to
days, this turgid condition of the bloodvessels, with consequent swollen and dry condition of the membrane, may continue, but at length these over-distended vessels become relieved by the pouring out of a watery fluid from both eyes and
nose.

With the continuance of the inflammatory action the discharge of the acrid fluid continues for a longer or shorter time,
to be ultimately followed by a change both in colour and consistence; it becomes yellow and thicker from the admixture of
mucus and other cell-structures, and with this addition it
becomes less irritating.

2. *General Symptoms.*—In addition to these local indications
of disease, there may in some be others of a systemic or general
character. The animal is dull, hangs his head, yawns, shifts
his position when standing, the coat stares, or there are distinct
rigors or shivering-fits; the surface temperature is alternately
elevated and depressed, and the internal elevated three or four
degrees. The pulse is more frequent, particularly if observed
during a shivering-fit, respiration much accelerated, with
appetite diminished, but desire for water increased.

With the change in the nasal discharge from a watery to a
mucous character, there is subsidence of the general disturbance, the surface-temperature becomes uniform, the breathing
is more tranquil, listlessness has disappeared, and the head is
raised to its natural position; the thirst diminishes, and the
appetite improves.

Course and Termination.—Ordinary simple catarrh, in the
otherwise healthy horse, is probably the most manageable and

least dangerous of any systemic or local affection to which that animal is liable.

It is generally anticipated that ordinary cases will run their course, and that the animal will be restored to his usual health within a fortnight, although it is not uncommon, even in what we would call good recoveries, that a more or less troublesome cough may continue for some time longer

In some cases, where the posterior nasal cavities are largely involved, where the febrile symptoms are well marked, and where the turgescence of the nasal membrane is not re-lieved by a copious secretion and early passing into the muco-purulent stage, we are disposed to fear prolongation into the air-passages in the chest   This is the more to be apprehended when our patient, after an attack of catarrh, either unaccount-ably or as the result of want of sufficient care, suffers from a relapse.

Another class of cases, not, however, a very numerous one when treated properly from the commencement, is that where the characteristic nasal discharge and other accompanying symptoms of inflammatory action have passed off, but the horse is left weak, with much muscular atony, an unhealthy skin and ragged open coat, with a more or less intermittent or remittent discharge from one or both nostrils   This, if owing to simple relaxation and weakening of the nasal membrane, together with general debility, may without interference, or with appropriate medical treatment and good nursing, entirely disappear   When, however, notwithstanding reinstatement in general health and recovery from all inflammatory symptoms, the discharge from the nasal chambers still continues, the case is likely to prove troublesome, and may terminate in chronic disease of the membrane of the nasal chambers or of that lining the sinuses of the face and cranium, or of the bones themselves.

Treatment—With all the milder forms of ordinary catarrh no treatment is needful beyond rest and a little attention to dietary, while, where it can be obtained, it is always advisable to place the horse in a roomy, light, well-ventilated, but not cold, loose box

In all cases where the pyrexia is marked, it will be needful to give such agents as are likely to moderate this condition

and be conducive to carrying the animal safely through the
fever, while seeing that the throat is in all probability sore,
and swallowing difficult, the most convenient form in which
medicines may be given is dissolved in the drinking-water.
For this purpose the ordinary fever-powder, consisting of two
drachms each of chlorate and nitrate of potash given twice
daily, will answer well, or one drachm of the muriate of
ammonia, given in half a pint of water, morning and evening,
has been found useful. If the throat is tender and the cough
troublesome, a little compound camphor and belladonna electuary, given three or four times daily, may be substituted
for the powders, or allowed twice daily in addition to them.

Both while the nasal membrane is dry, and after the mucous
character of the secretion has been established, regular fumigation of the nostrils with vapour, generated by pouring hot
water upon bran or chaff contained in a nosebag, may with
advantage be employed twice daily.

When the throat-symptoms are troublesome, either from the
difficulty of deglutition or the cough, it will be advisable, in
addition to the exhibition of the electuary, to employ externally
either a mustard-poultice or some stimulating liniment, such as
a compound of ammonia, oil of turpentine, or of cantharides.
Mustard is preferred by many owing to the opportunity which
it affords of reapplication by being rubbed off when dry,
cantharides I have always believed to be less painful and more
efficacious. The temperature of the body must be maintained
by appropriate clothing, which ought to be removed daily,
well shaken, and replaced after the body has been quietly
sponged with water, or water with a little vinegar added. The
condition of the bowels may always where the animal is feeding moderately, be maintained in a proper state by means of
the dietary. Scalded oats with bran, to which is added a little
linseed-oil, will serve this purpose well, or, if the season and
place will afford it, green food is probably preferable to aught
else. When the bowels are decidedly confined, and their condition may not be corrected by the food, enemata of tepid
water or oil are to be preferred to the exhibition of any laxative
medicine by the mouth.

II. CHRONIC NASAL CATARRH

Definition—*A continuous, remittent, or intermittent discharge of a varying character from the nasal chambers, usually unassociated with local inflammatory action, cough, or fever.*

Nature and Causation—Considering the very great number of cases of coryza, or simple catarrh, which are regularly encountered, the percentage of bad or indifferent recoveries, or such as terminate in chronic nasal discharge, is exceedingly small. After protracted and severe cases, and where debilitating influences, either extrinsic or intrinsic, have been in operation, it not unfrequently occurs as part of the general atony, that the secreting membrane of the nasal chambers and upper air-passages requires a longer time than usual to regain its normal tonicity and healthy function, during this time exhibiting as the most marked feature of the unhealthy condition a continuous or intermittent nasal discharge.

Clinically, succeeding the subsidence of the active symptoms of ordinary catarrh, it is usual to regard all continuous discharges from the nasal cavities as cases of chronic nasal catarrh or nasal gleet. These discharges are often as dissimilar in character as they are in the source of their origin.

At the present, however, it is the intention only to speak of such as may be traced to a previous attack of common cold, not that this condition of nasal discharge may not originate from other and, to us, inappreciable causes.

By far the greater number of the cases of chronic nasal catarrh which we encounter are associated with or owe their origin—(1) To lesions of the nasal chambers proper; (2) To lesions of the mucous cavities connected with these chambers.

The first of these classes of cases is, as a rule, the less dangerous, and more likely to yield to medical treatment; they may also be only the earliest symptoms of, and may ultimately terminate in, those of the other group. Although to both of these classes of structural lesions there belongs the one common feature of an abnormal nasal discharge, and all cases, to whatever class they may belong, have been indifferently spoken of as cases of chronic nasal catarrh or nasal gleet it is probably

to those of the first class in particular, and somewhat re-
strictively, that these terms have usually been applied, the
others being recognised by having added to them the name of
the locality from which the discharge is supposed to proceed,
thus we speak of discharge from, or collections of matter in,
the frontal sinuses, the turbinated bones, or the eustachian
pouches

Symptoms —When the causes of the discharge seem specially
connected with changes in the great nasal chambers—nasal
gleet properly so called—it is not common that the original
flux connected with the primary and actively diseased mucous
membrane—we speak now of those cases which succeed ordinary catarrh—has disappeared, usually we find that this has
become for a time less in amount and considerably altered in
character; it is less purulent than when the original catarrh
continued When of some time standing it is of a glairy
starchy character, with occasionally flakes of inspissated
mucus or pus mingled with the more liquid portions, and,
although it may be more plentiful some days than others, it
seldom intermits altogether

When connected merely with lesions of the membrane of
the great nasal cavity, it has rarely a fœtid smell Although
the constitutional disturbance may never be so great that the
appetite is impaired, it is seldom that we do not discover some
slight appearance of impairment of the general health There
is often an unthrifty open condition of the coat, with a scurfy,
unhealthy state of the skin; the animal wants bloom and
vivacity, particularly while at work, and is soft and easily
fatigued with even a slight amount of muscular exertion On
a closer examination there may often be detected a condition
of fulness and induration of the submaxillary glands, while
the pituitary membrane, which in health and during the continuance of the active catarrh was bright pink or of a red colour,
is somewhat altered, being less vascular-looking, of a slate or
leaden hue, with, it may be, a rather soft, blanched, and somewhat thickened and infiltrated appearance.

Treatment —In every case of confirmed chronic nasal catarrh,
until we are thoroughly satisfied that the discharge with which
we are dealing is not glanderous, and not likely to propagate
itself, we must be careful to maintain strict isolation of the

diseased, and the reservation for their sole use of particular stable utensils. In the treatment of these nasal discharges little or no good will result unless the means employed are directed with the view of combating both the local and general diseased condition.

The horse ought to be laid aside from work, and placed on good and liberal diet, and under the influence of correct sanitary conditions. Therapeutically, the most successful constitutional treatment I have found to be the exhibition of arsenic or salts of iron, or arsenic and sulphate of iron combined with yellow resin, given alternately. The arsenic can be very readily administered as Fowler's solution, half a fluid ounce morning and evening, in the food or drinking-water, while from half a drachm to one drachm of the powdered sulphate of iron combined with half a drachm of powdered yellow resin can be given daily in the food. Others, I know, recommend as very beneficial small doses of from one to three grains of powdered cantharides combined with copaiba, made into a bolus with linseed-meal, and administered once or twice daily.

As local applications the astringent tonics of the mineral salts, as the sulphate or chloride of zinc or sulphate of copper, varying in strength from five grains of the zinc chloride to forty grains of copper sulphate to the fluid ounce of water, have been followed with probably as much benefit as aught else. There is probably less merit in the choice of the individual material for this purpose than there is in the mode of its application; the difficulty being in every case to have the liquid regularly distributed over the whole surface of the nasal membrane, so that no part shall escape being bathed with the solution.

This difficulty can only be overcome by tact, patience, and perseverance. The two methods usually adopted are that of its distribution by means of an ordinary enema syringe, or through the use of Rey's nasal funnel. Each of these has its special advantages, and, under certain circumstances, either is efficacious. Besides the irrigation of the nasal membrane with such solutions as indicated with the view to restore tone and healthy functional activity, the use of these same or other agents in the form of atomized fluids or solids is always deserving of a trial, and in some instances is superior to the liquid applications. Such agents as iodine and sulphurous acid may be employed in the form of vapour by sprinkling the solution of either over warm, moist hay or bran contained in a nose-bag. They may also be employed in the liquid form through means of the ordinary spray-distributors. In the form of an impalpable powder, iodoform compound, iodine, or carbolic acid, either of the latter being mixed with a fine powder, as ground liquorice-root, may be driven up the nostrils once or twice daily by means of an indiarubber ball attached to a small tube known as an insufflator. This method of local stimulation I have seen attended with much good.

All cases of chronic nasal catarrh which do not improve under a short course of treatment such as we have indicated, are probably dependent for the continuance of the discharge on extension of the lesions to the mucous cavities having connection with the nasal chambers.

Disease of these contiguous cavities, the sinuses of the head and face, with the posterior mucous pouches peculiar to solipeds, although possessing as a prominent symptom a characteristic nasal discharge, belong more properly to the domain of surgery proper.

CHAPTER XVII

DISEASES OF THE LARYNX

I. ACUTE LARYNGITIS—LARYNGO-PHARYNGITIS—SORE THROAT

Definition —*Inflammation of the soft tissues and mucous membrane of the larynx.*

Inflammation of the larynx pure and simple must, we suspect, be of much less frequent occurrence than a combined and more general morbid action involving the contiguous structures which enter into the formation of the cavity common to both food and air tubes, the pharynx.

As affecting the larynx chiefly, or to a greater extent than contiguous parts, we are acquainted in the horse with the appearance of inflammatory action in at least two forms—
1 *Acute Catarrhal Laryngitis,* 2. *Œdematous Laryngitis*

30

1. **Acute Catarrhal Laryngitis** *Nature and Causation*—
This, the simpler form of laryngeal inflammation, is essentially
catarrhal, being connected with the mucous membrane of the
larynx, and occasionally extending to the trachea   The increased vascularity of the parts is shortly succeeded by slightly
increased secretion from the membrane, which appears somewhat thickened, not so much from submucous infiltration,
as from an accumulation of mucus and certain cell-growths
upon its surface.   This unnatural action is rarely observed
as a condition purely local, usually as an early and often
the most prominent symptom of common catarrh.   It is also
encountered as a symptom of some other diseases, particularly
of the great mucous tract of the air-passages, and of different
parts of the respiratory organs

For its origin it seems, like common catarrh, to be dependent on conditions some of which are directly connected with
the animal itself, as a general weak, atonic state of the tissues,
indifferent food, and the fact of having suffered from previous
attacks of a similar character, others are brought to bear
upon it from without, including indifferent location, overwork,
exposure to cold and damp, particularly when exhausted and
perspiring.   In exceptional instances we have it occurring
from extension of inflammatory action from contiguous, chiefly
anterior, structures

Symptoms—The local symptoms are pain, referable to the
region of the throat, particularly shown when food or water is
being swallowed, or when the throat is manipulated externally.
The animal is inclined, both when at rest and when moving,
to keep his nose rather elevated, so as to straighten the angle
naturally existing at the throat and larynx, thereby relieving
the irritable structures from pressure   The mouth contains
an extra quantity of ropy, rather tenacious saliva ; this is in
greatest amount when the pharyngeal structures are much
involved   Cough is easily provoked on attempts to swallow,
and fluids are ejected by the nasal passages.   At the outset of
the affection the cough is hard and rather sonorous, particularly so if of some time standing ; when, however, the morbid
action has advanced, and secretion is considerable, it is less
resonant, rather suppressed, and emitted with evidence of
pain

There is swelling externally, both in the submaxillary space and over the parotideal region. Nasal discharge although occurring when associated with catarrh, is not a characteristic symptom of laryngitis, and, when present, usually appears towards the termination of the affection.

The constitutional disturbance is more marked in the early part of the affection than in simple cold. Fever, more or less severe, characterizes the great majority of cases of uncomplicated laryngeal inflammation. Disinclination to eat, which is often present, I have regarded as owing to the physical difficulty attendant upon swallowing as much as to the existing fever. Any attempts at swallowing food, unless of the softest character are, during the severity of the disease, provocative of violent fits of coughing, during some of which there seems a fear that the animal may be suffocated; he will stamp with his feet, toss his head violently about, and, if secured in the ordinary manner, will pull vigorously backwards.

2. **Œdematous Laryngitis.** *a. Nature and Causation.* —That we are warranted in regarding this as a distinct and separate form of inflammatory action seems reasonable, whether we regard the usual suddenness of its attack, the speciality of its symptoms, or its often fatal termination. It cannot, in the horse, as a rule, be said to follow a previously diseased condition of the larynx; it may rapidly succeed to what at first seems an ordinary attack of sore throat; it may start into existence suddenly, asserting its specific symptoms and running its course with great rapidity, or it may be met with as the result of the inhalation of hot air or acrid vapours.

b. Anatomical Characters. —In all fatal cases of œdematous laryngitis the structural changes observed are wonderfully uniform well marked, and specially distinctive. The infiltration of the submucous tissue, both of the general pharyngeal cavity and specially of the different parts of the larynx where connective-tissue abounds, is excessive, so much so that occlusion of the opening of the glottis may have suddenly and unexpectedly carried off the animal through suffocation. Both over the pharyngeal and laryngeal mucous membrane we encounter amidst the general hyperaemic condition patches or spots, of greater or less extent, of specially ecchymosed or even gangrenous and sphacelated tissue. The latter condition is

30—2

certainly not so often encountered as that where a considerable extent of tissue is changed to a metallic hue, much swollen and pulpy from submucous infiltration. While occasionally over both the surface of the pharyngeal and laryngeal membrane there may be partially adherent flakes or shreds of lymph, the exact spots where these adventitious products are adhering we find are generally superficial erosions or ulcers

This state of submucous infiltration with serous fluid and varied cell-growths is not, when occurring, confined strictly to the pharynx or larynx, but is found extending forward to the base or root of the tongue, while the entire glandular structures in the vicinity of the throat and of the anterior cervical region are affected in a similar manner

Symptoms—The rapidity with which the general swelling of the structures of the throat, and the special infiltration of the true laryngeal structures, and of the textures in the immediate vicinity, take place, together with the general distress and severity of the fever, are the distinguishing symptoms of this form of laryngitis Sometimes in a few hours, not only is the external swelling considerable, but, from the amount of the laryngeal infiltration, breathing becomes distressed. The heart's action and pulsations are much increased, and the temperature is elevated, while, from the embarrassment of the respiration and the imperfect manner in which the blood is aerated, the membrane of the nasal cavities acquires a purple hue In many there is a certain amount of stupor, or an unnaturally anxious expression of face with occasionally great restlessness, the animal wandering around the box, if such liberty is allowed, with no desire for food, but with an evident desire to be relieved from pain, or from the oppressive dyspnoea.

Should life be prolonged for a few days—for in many instances this form of inflammatory action proves fatal in forty-eight hours—there is generally marked fœtor of the breath, or of any discharge which may flow from the nose, while the diseased action may have extended along the course of the great air-passages to the organs contained in the chest

Course and Termination—In the greater number of cases of inflamed pharyngo-laryngeal structures of the catarrhal type, after a few days of considerable annoyance chiefly from difficulty in deglutition, with laryngeal irritation and cough, the horse will gradually regain his former condition. In a few others there is an evident tendency in the inflammatory action to move downwards, and beginning with what is ordinarily spoken of as a sore throat, may ultimately terminate in disease of the minute air-tubes or of the pulmonary tissue. Occasionally we find this pharyngo-laryngeal inflammation seems to give way to, or is propagated into, that of particular inflammation of the glands and gland-structures in the region of the throat. These cases may terminate in apparently well-developed instances of strangles, and the throat-symptoms may subside as soon as those of the glands are developed, or they may continue while these exist, and only defervesce with the maturation of the glandular inflammation in a well-developed abscess.

In the form of œdematous laryngitis—œdema glottidis—the severer cases give no time for much or extensive textural alteration. For when the laryngeal symptoms are not speedily ameliorated, the probabilities of a rapidly fatal termination from interference with the function of respiration are very great.

In other manifestations, especially such as accompany certain specific fevers, or appear as sequels of these, this œdematous laryngitis assumes a subacute or chronic form, and as such may remain for a rather lengthened period, only troublesome or even attractive when the horse is moved rapidly, or when engaged in feeding.

Treatment — Besides strict attention to location, *i e,* the placing of the suffering so that the influence of cold air or draughts may be avoided as much as possible, with an equable rather warm and moist atmosphere, the only general treatment which we have observed to be productive of much or any benefit is that by which excessive febrile action is mitigated, and the animal steadily supported and guided until the fever has run its natural course. From the irritable condition of the throat and contiguous parts, it is nearly impossible to administer medicine either in the solid or liquid form. If the ability to swallow is not entirely gone, the ordinary febrifuge powders of chlorate and nitrate of potash may be given twice daily in the drinking-water, or probably the form of electuary may be em-

ployed as the medium through which the medicine is conveyed
into the system   Such a mixture as the compound belladonna
and camphor electuary we have already advised for similar
conditions is very good , it may be administered in moderate
quantities two or three times daily, along with the febrifuge
powders

Of local applications, which are always productive of good,
the chief is the assiduous use of the inhalation of hot-water
vapour , this may be simple, and generated by pouring hot
water over chopped hay or bran contained in a nose-bag ; or
it may be medicated by pouring a little of such agents as
chloroform or sulphurous acid, or some liquid preparation of
iodine, conium, or opium, over the material contained in the
bag In the employment of fumigation in cases of laryngitis,
great care is needful in carrying out the details, seeing that
with the extremely irritable condition of the parts there is
great liability to injure the horse, and particularly to induce
needless coughing or suffocation.

Externally, over the region of the larynx, when pain or
swelling is considerable, it is desirable to have recourse to
warm-water applications , these are carried out either by
means of poultices, or, what is easier, by cloths saturated
with hot water and wrapped around the throat, or, as being
capable of retaining for a longer period both heat and
moisture, tow or cotton-wool soaked in hot oil, and retained
by means of a hood or appropriate bandaging   When not
sufficient in a day or two to alleviate the urgency of symptoms,
these local appliances may be removed, and the parts receive a
moderate vesication with a liniment of cantharides ; this, however, I have not found to be so safe or beneficial a practice as
the assiduous employment of heat and moisture   When the
presence of saliva in the mouth is troublesome, either because
of its quantity or quality, the employment of a gargle, as a
solution of alum or sulphurous acid, nitrate of potash, common
salt, or tannic acid, will always be advantageous and grateful
to the patient

Whenever the dyspnœa is considerable, we must not forget
the possibility of suffocation , the animal ought to be watched,
and should the respiration become so impeded that restlessness
and anxiety of the animal are attractive, we ought not to risk

the chance of this, but have recourse at once to tracheotomy.
When this has been accomplished we ought to allow the tube
to remain in the trachea until the laryngeal complications
have perfectly subsided

II CHRONIC DISEASES OF THE LARYNX

The chief chronic diseases of the larynx which attract attention in the horse, viz muscular atrophy and degeneration,
with the existence of adventitious growths and changes of inherent tissue, have already been noticed when speaking of
abnormal laryngeal sounds classed as 'roaring.'

CHAPTER XVIII

DISEASES OF THE LUNGS—PNEUMONICI

General Observations—In observing disease of the pulmonary
structures as presented to our consideration in the living
animal, we find that active inflammatory action is to some
extent mapped out and distinguished by the character of the
tissues invaded, as well as the symptoms attending it. The
structures mainly concerned in the making up of the lung-
substance, the great respiratory bellows, are (1) The great
air-tubes or conduits, *bronchial tubes* which pass on and are
distributed to all parts of the lung-substance, terminating
in (2) The air-cells or sacs, *pulmonary air-cells* or *parenchyma of the lungs*, and (3) The expanded sheet-like membrane covering this structure proper, the *pulmonary pleura*—
this pulmonary pleura, or visceral pleura, forming part of that
serous sac interposed between the lungs and the thoracic walls,
the portion intimately associated with the latter being known
as the *costal pleura*

In the actual occurrence of inflammatory action and its
results, one or more of these separate structures may be involved and exhibit symptoms diagnostic of its more severe or
more extensive involvement than the others. When the air-
tubes, great or small, are the special seat of inflammatory

action, we speak of the process as *Bronchitis*, when the parenchyma, or true vesicular substance of the lungs, is the seat of the disturbance, the disease is called *Pneumonia;* while when the action is chiefly located in the serous membrane covering the lungs, or the thoracic walls, the condition is known as *Pleuritis.*

Very rarely, however, in practice do we find that these several diseased conditions are distinctly and sharply marked out from each other; it is more frequently, if not invariably, the case that they are variously combined and shaded into each other, the morbid condition of one particular structure most probably holding a sufficient prominence and distinctiveness to give to the entire state its leading and characteristic features

It is seldom that in veterinary practice we encounter in any of our patients inflammation of the lung-tissue proper—pneumonia—without at the same time finding the air-tube, large or small, more or less implicated—bronchitis—constituting the condition we recognise by the term pneumonia-bronchitis, or broncho-pneumonia; or when the air-tubes have in a great measure escaped the inflammatory action we find, along with the pneumonia, an inflamed condition of the investing membrane, the pleura, the condition known as **pleuro-pneumonia.**

It is not, therefore, to be expected in the study of pneumonic diseases, as they are presented to us in the living animal, that we will usually observe any one of these separate and distinct structures alone and of itself invaded by the diseased action, we may, however, by attention to the symptoms and phenomena specially distinctive of diseased action in these individually, become the better able to determine how far each is involved in any morbid condition in which they severally participate.

CHAPTER XIX.

DISEASES OF THE BRONCHI

I. ACUTE CATARRHAL BRONCHITIS

Definition.—*Inflammation of the air-tubes, large or small, leading to the pulmonary air-sacs, characterized by a short, troublesome, rather harsh cough, a soft, frequent pulse, and accelerated breathing. Febrile symptoms often, but not invariably, precede and accompany the earlier stages.*

Pathology.   *a. Nature and Causation.*—At one time, in veterinary medicine in particular, bronchial inflammation was, as a rule, mixed up and confounded with the same action occurring in the pulmonary tissue; now we are inclined to pass to the other extreme, of endeavouring to draw a sharp line between this and the other closely related morbid actions taking place in pulmonary structure.   In this we are as likely to fall into error as in the former case.

No doubt there must always exist between inflammation as appearing in the pleural sac, and the same action occurring in the bronchial tubes and vesicular structure of the lungs, the difference in the course and results of this process as exhibited in a serous and in a mucous membrane.

The disease, while consisting essentially in congestion and inflammation of the bronchial tissues, with an exudation over the bronchial mucous membrane into the tubes, in all cases so far of a similar nature, is yet in many instances modified by the conditions as to general health of the animal attacked, the causes which determine the attack, and the extent of the structures involved.

Of the causes which tend to the production of acute bronchitis we may be able to recognise two varieties—(*a*) Those which are of a predisposing character, as constitutional or acquired weakness, previous attacks of bronchial inflammation, cardiac diseases of some time standing, location in certain situations where special atmospheric changes are liable to occur, as prevailing cold winds at particular seasons combined with moisture.   (*b*) Such as are directly exciting, comprising all those connected with exhaustion and sudden exposure to

vicissitudes of atmospheric conditions mentioned as productive
of common catarrh, direct irritation of the bronchial mucous
membrane by various noxious materials, general blood-contamination, as met with in certain specific diseases and unhealthy
states of the system also we may, in special cases, regard
bronchitis as acknowledging an epizootic influence, as seen in
some manifestations of influenza

Modified by causation, locality, and extent, we observe that
acute bronchitis presents some special clinical features which,
in the horse, may be grouped or comprised under such varieties
as—1 *Primary or idiopathic bronchitis,* (*a*) involving the
larger air-tubes, (*b*) capillary bronchitis, bronchitis extending
into the minute tubes 2 *Secondary bronchitis, bronchitis
connected with certain specific and general diseases and other
unhealthy states of the body* 3 Mechanical bronchitis.

b Anatomical Characters.—The obvious after-death appearances in the pulmonary structures of horses which die while
suffering from bronchitis are variable, although probably less
so than the symptoms which they exhibit while alive.   In
animals of full age, but in the enjoyment of previously vigorous
health, which have succumbed to an acute attack of bronchitis,
we find the lining membrane of the bronchial tubes, of all sizes,
of a rather dark venous colour, this colouration may be very
generally diffused, or it may be distributed in streaks or
patches, with rays proceeding from one spot or patch to
another   Occasionally the membrane itself, and in its entirety,
is turgid and swollen, soft and pulpy, with more or less of
differently coloured tenacious mucus adhering to it, particularly in the larger bronchi   The material contained in the
tubes in the earlier stages, succeeding the first condition of
arrested secretion, is chiefly of a serous character, the detached
and partly developed epithelial cells are loaded with elements
simply of a watery character, it is generally slightly frothy,
and in the pharynx and nasal chambers may be coloured from
the colouring matter of what food is being taken   When the
disease is somewhat more advanced the character of the exudation becomes altered, a certain amount of fibrinous material
is mingled with the more watery constituents, and fresh cell-
elements abound, giving it a tenacious pus-like character
When not examined immediately after death, the lining mem-

brane of the larger tube, as also the trachea and larynx, may show patches of a dark greenish metallic hue, a character which, somewhat modified, we almost invariably meet with in those animals which have either, when affected with the disease, been of a special cachectic condition, or, if in vigorous health, have had operating on them serious depressing influences

In almost every instance where the amount of bronchial secretion is great and particularly viscid, we will observe more or less consolidation of lung-tissue; this is generally of a diffuse character, although we occasionally see it also limited to small and circumscribed patches. When occurring extensively this condition is usually associated with acute and rapidly fatal cases. When glanced at hastily, this state of collapse or condensation of lung-tissue, which arises from plugging more or less perfectly of a bronchus or bronchi leading to the parts, may be passed over or mistaken for consolidation, the result of ordinary pneumonia. It is, however, different from that condition both in its general appearance and the manner in which it comports itself when incised or minutely examined. This collapsed lung-tissue is of a dark or dirty violet colour externally; it feels less crepitant than healthy lung-tissue, but more so than the same when suffering from hepatization.

When cut into, it is of a mahogany-brown colour, the extent of this depending upon the amount of blood it contains; the exuded material is a slightly opaque bloody serosity, and may be mingled with pus from the inflamed bronchi. In true pulmonic consolidation the result of inflammation of the parenchyma of the lungs, where the air-vesicles are obliterated through exudation into their interior, we have on incision, or may obtain by scraping, a thick pasty material, chiefly made up of granular elements and various cell-growths generally found in inflammation of parenchymatous organs. If of any time duration, this collapsed and condensed lung-tissue becomes atrophied, the special pulmonary structure seems to be replaced by fibrous material, the whole condensed portion occupying less space than in health. As an invariable accompaniment of the atrophied condition of the collapsed and condensed lung we find vesicular emphysema, this emphysema seeming to compensate for the diminution in bulk sustained by the altered lung-tissue. This emphysematous condition occurs at those parts of the lung-substance away from and not acted upon by the bronchial inflammation

This state of pulmonary collapse, I have observed, is more frequent in cases of secondary bronchitis, such as are associated with certain specific and general diseases, also where the vital powers of the animal seem invalidated by previous disease, or by presently operating vitiating influences; in such the collapse may be extensive, although the obstruction appears small.

General Symptoms *a Acute Bronchitis of the Large and Small Tubes* —In the greater number of its forms of manifestation bronchitis is preceded by febrile symptoms, although in many these may be trivial, and are more commonly such as are spoken of as indicative of a 'common cold;' or the inflamed condition of the bronchial membrane may be ushered into existence without previous indications of illness; in such the pyrexial symptoms will to a great extent be regulated by the extent of the structures invaded

When fully developed we have, in addition to the symptoms of ordinary catarrh, should it follow that condition, a frequent, short, rather hard cough, not markedly painful, with much acceleration of breathing; the horse is dull and listless, not much inclined to move, appetite impaired, and thirst increased. As the disease becomes more confirmed, the cough is more troublesome, occasionally paroxysmal, loud and sonorous, particularly when the larger tubes are the seat of the inflammation; the pulse is increased in frequency and rather soft, the respirations relatively more accelerated than the pulse.

On auscultating the chest the healthy respiratory sounds are found to have undergone considerable modification. When the larger bronchi are specially the seat of the disease, we will, on placing the ear over the anterior part of the chest, at the termination of the trachea, and less so at the upper and middle third behind the scapulæ, hear a tolerably loud, sonorous noise—'rhonchus,' if the inflammatory action is largely distributed through the smaller ramifications, the sound will, where the unhealthy condition exists, be of a higher, shriller pitch—'sibilus' Between these two extreme points there are heard various modifications, according as the large or small tubes are chiefly involved. This earlier condition of the membrane, resulting in arrest of natural secretion and consequent dryness and rigidity of the tubes, is very shortly replaced by an increased secretion and consequent moistness and relaxation. With the presence of liquid in the tubes, and its varying conditions of quantity and viscidity, the sounds become interrupted and modified by the passing of the air through bubbles of mucus, and as these bubbles vary in size and tenacity, so the sounds vary also. In the larger bronchi, where the sonorous rhonchus was heard in the earlier stages, when effusion exists the hard sound is modified to that of a mucous bubbling or larger crepitation, so called; in the smaller we have the moist sibilant râle, or lesser crepitation.

Occasionally the mucus may become so much inspissated that, adhering at some particular point, the hardened material seems to play to and fro by the action of the air passing along the tube, somewhat in the manner of a valve, thus yielding a sharp clicking noise. It is to the relative amount and distribution of these sounds, and to the amount of fluid in the tubes, that we have to attend in arriving at an opinion as to the severity of the attack and the dangers to be apprehended. When the deeper and more sonorous sounds, dry or moist, are in excess of the higher-pitched sibilant râles, there is less danger to be feared than in opposite conditions. In such the disease is chiefly confined to the larger bronchi, while the more extensively distributed and finer tubes are comparatively free. When the smaller bronchi are specially the seat of inflammation, the relative disproportion between the inspirations and expirations becomes more marked; the latter being much prolonged, and the danger in all commensurately increased.

Percussion, when exercised over the region affected, yields no positive evidence of disease, unless over such portions of the lung-structure as from auscultation we find, from the absence of the healthy murmur, to be wanting in functional activity. These portions, from the still existing resonance, we find to contain a certain quantity of air; this condition we judge to owe its existence to the obliteration of one or more bronchi of which we have already spoken, and tending to collapse of lung-tissue consolidation, atrophy, and pulmonary emphysema.

The usually accompanying cough, dry and sonorous at first,

becomes, as the exudation into the bronchi increases, less hard, and with it there is sometimes a discharge into the mouth or through the nasal openings of a ropy, tenacious mucus, tending to give the mouth a moist and gluey feeling   All these symptoms, which are the true pathognomonic indications of the disease, are apt to vary according as the morbid action varies from a very moderate congestion or inflammation of the large bronchi, to severe involvement of the minute and ultimate ramifications, or to collapse of pulmonary tissue and obliteration of air-tubes

  b *Secondary Bronchitis, Bronchitis accompanying certain general Diseases and Conditions of Blood Contamination* — This form of bronchial inflammation is sometimes met with in the horse in rheumatism and glanders-farcy, while in young animals suffering from specific arthritis it is a common complication, and is here found in conjunction with pulmonary embolism. When found in these relationships its symptoms vary little save as respects severity from bronchial inflammation occurring independently and apart from other diseased conditions In such cases the bronchial symptoms do not precede the manifestation of the general or specific disease, but are usually developed during its progress, and seem to depend for their existence on the morbid state with which they are associated.

  c *Mechanical Bronchitis* —This form of acute bronchitis in the horse is not, as in other of our patients, of a parasitic origin, but is generally the result of the contact of some irritant with the membrane of the air-tubes   It occurs by the accidental passage into the trachea of medicinal agents given in the form of draughts, also from the entrance into the tubes of heated smoke, air, or other volatile agents, in the case of exposure to these, as in buildings which have been destroyed by fire   The symptoms exhibited in this form are eminently characteristic of acute bronchial inflammation   They may be of all degrees of severity, from the most moderate irritation, causing merely cough, with the ejectment of a little frothy mucus, and continuing only for a few days, to the destruction of the lining membrane of the tubes as a whole, inducing much distress, with excessive expectoration and discharge from the nostrils of frothy, blood-stained mucus, terminating in asphyxia and death   The symptoms of distress and irritation follow imme-

diately on the action or entrance of the irritant, and are, when
the agent is at all active or the amount and exposure considerable, urgent and rapid in development. The accelerated
breathing is at once established, with the characteristic rhonchus and sibilant sounds. It is deserving of notice that this
mechanical irritation is occasionally followed by a condition
which otherwise must be considered rare in the history of
bronchitis in the horse, viz., that known as *plastic bronchitis*,
in which, as the result of the diseased action, well-formed casts
of the tubes may continue to block these, and induce further
pulmonary disease for a lengthened time

Treatment—It is seldom that we are called upon to advise
regarding the management and medical treatment of our
patients during the incubative or very early stage of disease,
from which we lose the opportunity which human physicians
so often have of making an endeavour by free use of anodynes
and stimulants to cut short an attack of bronchitis. Generally, when seen by the practitioner the horse has the bronchitic
attack fully established. Here the only correct line of treatment is that which is directed to safely guiding the animal
through the fever, to watch complications as they occur, and
to moderate excessive irritation

When laryngeal inflammation is an accompaniment the
administration of medicines is always attended with difficulty,
and must be conducted with care. The compound camphor
and belladonna mixture already recommended in somewhat
similar affections will be found both grateful to the irritable
pharyngeal membrane, and capable of being compounded so as
to moderate febrile action. In addition to the moderate use of
this two or three times daily, from four to six drachms of
chlorate of potash may be allowed daily in the drinking-water
When the condition of the throat and upper air-passages does
not interfere with the exhibition of medicine, a draught composed of four fluid ounces solution of acetate of ammonia,
one fluid ounce sweet spirits of nitre, or the same quantity of
aromatic spirits of ammonia with forty grains of camphor and
one drachm of extract of belladonna, or half an ounce of
syrup or tincture of squills in ten fluid ounces of water, will
be found advantageous exhibited twice daily, while, if desired,
a little of the electuary may be used between these draughts

To favour the exudation from the bronchial mucous membrane in the dry stage, and to assist its discharge when secreted, it is always desirable to have recourse to the inhalation of the vapour of hot water, which in cases of much irritability is improved by being medicated as previously directed

In the greater number of cases this inhalation, executed once or twice daily, with the administration of the medicines mentioned, together with good and careful nursing and giving attention to maintaining for a few days at first the temperature of the box nearer 60° F than 50° F —never, however, neglecting to see that a sufficiency of fresh air is permitted to enter— will suffice to place the animal on the way to recovery

Where the inflammation is rather extensively distributed through the smaller air-tubes, and where the bronchial exudation is excessive, stimulation or moderate blistering of the chest is likely to be productive of good results   In many instances an application of equal parts of soap liniment and tincture of opium employed with smart friction twice daily will produce wonderful results ; it seems to relieve bronchial irritation, soothes when very restless, and confers greater freedom in the respiratory act   When thought desirable to apply some more severe measures, mustard cataplasms, or a cantharides liniment, are the best

The condition of the bowels, although in many cases of bronchitis rather confined, I feel satisfied, if we will only have a little patience, rarely call for the administration of any purgative or laxative medicine more powerful than the daily use in a mash of a few ounces of olive or linseed oil Enemata of tepid water, employed twice or thrice daily, will not harm

When the more acute symptoms have subsided and convalescence seems fairly entered upon, but a troublesome cough still remains, benefit will often be obtained from increasing the amount of camphor and squills in the electuary, and by the application of a little cantharides liniment to the throat

Should weakness or want of appetite be marked features during recovery, a daily administration of some tonic medicine may be needful ; for this purpose there is nothing better than iron in some of its compounds a half drachm of the powdered sulphate, or double this quantity of the carbonate, made into a powder, one or two of which are given daily in the food, is a convenient form. Or a very excellent ball may be compounded of half a drachm of powdered sulphate of iron, the same quantity of nux vomica, and one drachm of powdered gentian, with linseed-meal and treacle sufficient to give bulk and consistence. This may be given daily, or morning and evening, or it may be alternated with another composed of a drachm each of powdered camphor, gentian, myrrh, and ginger.

In the management of cases of mechanical bronchitis, much discrimination is needed. It is futile attempting by heroic measures to cut short the diseased action; we must endeavour to moderate its intensity. The employment of simple salines in the drinking-water, or the exhibition, where this is attainable, of the febrifuge draught recommended for ordinary bronchitis, with an extra quantity of the solution of the acetate of ammonia, are more likely to be attended with benefit. If we can only enable the animal to pass over the earlier stages, and maintain strength enough to enter upon those attended with mucous râle and soft, frequent cough, there will be reasonable hope of an ultimate recovery.

With complementary bronchitis treatment must not be attempted apart from that of the constitutional disorder with which it is associated, and which in all these cases must be regarded as the inducing factor of this bronchial disturbance. While attending to the primary and general disease, urgent bronchial symptoms must not be neglected, but receive such attention as is calculated to relieve these special developments.

Complementary bronchitis, as associated with specific arthritis in foals, I have found a very serious and intractable extra development of symptoms. In these young animals, in addition to the general or constitutional treatment adopted for the systemic disease upon which this secondary bronchitis depends, relief is always afforded by the local application of hot, damp rugs or woollen cloths, followed by gentle friction with compound soap and opium liniment, while the exhibition frequently of moderate doses of stimulants, combined with salines, seems adapted to both this extra development of symptoms and the original constitutional disease.

31

II. Chronic Bronchitis

Nature and Causation.—This condition of chronic bronchial catarrh we meet with in the horse less frequently than in some other of our patients   In him it appears occasionally both as a sequel of acute bronchitis and as an independent affection. It differs from any of the manifestations of the acute by the absence of fever, and the persistence of a hard, sonorous, troublesome cough ; while the discharged or expectorated material is rarely of the viscid, tenacious, cellular nature of acute bronchial inflammation.

When the result of acute bronchitis, the chronic form is more usually attended with defective respiration when the animal is put to rapid movement, than when developing as an independent diseased condition

From the manner in which the symptoms seem to be susceptible of aggravation, the cough and dyspnœa would appear to be largely dependent on constriction of the smaller bronchi, either from partial occlusion, the result of thickening of the lining membrane, or from irregular spasm of the encircling fibres   In isolated instances chronic bronchitis may continue for some time, and at last, on the occurrence of a very trivial cause, terminate in a rather smart attack of the acute form, from which, when the animal recovers, the original chronic bronchial irritation and paroxysmal cough remain Many cases in horses spoken of as chronic cough, if examined carefully, will be found associated with some little difficulty in breathing and impediment in the process of respiration, and are apparently true instances of mild chronic bronchitis. Although fever may not be present in chronic bronchial inflammations, and, with the exception of the local symptoms of cough and impeded respiration, the horse may show no indications of ill-health, we yet find, in numerous instances where this condition is of any time standing, that a steady loss of flesh is not uncommon even when the appetite continues good

Symptoms—On making examination of the respiratory organs of such animals as are sufferers from chronic bronchitis, auscultation may satisfy us that, although somewhat similar to acute bronchitis, the lesions are not of precisely the same nature. There is rarely much, if any, of the dry or moist 'rhonchus,'—the hard and sonorous, or the moist and larger bubbling sound; nor is the pure 'sibilus' or sibilant râle—the whistling and softer smaller crepitation, heard, as in the acute bronchial inflammation. The sound is a modification or mingling of the dry and moist higher-pitched noises, and is rarely heard in the same animal of the same character or quality at different examinations.

When occurring independently of any previous inflammatory condition, this state is usually very gradual in development, and, when established, very persistent in character. Animals suffering from it are exceedingly liable to unaccountable exacerbations of the attendant cough, with wheezing and difficulty of respiration ; they seem also susceptible of being acted upon adversely by atmospheric changes. Although cough is a tolerably constant symptom, it is rarely, and then only as an adventitious circumstance, of a laryngeal character, or connected with laryngeal irritation.

In almost every instance of chronic bronchitis the respiration is so far affected, particularly when put to rapid or rather severe work, that the impediment is usually recognised—from the nature of the abnormal sound—under the term of 'thick wind,' this, as already noted, has the peculiarity attending it that the readiness with which it may be detected, even in the same animal, varies with conditions of time and surroundings. This defect is exceedingly persistent, and liable, from the operation of various influences to intensification of symptoms apart from appreciable causes.

Treatment—Although less influenced by treatment than acute bronchitis, it is nevertheless often much benefited by the administration of such agents as we have recommended for that form. I have found good results to follow from the employment of from one scruple to half a drachm each of powdered camphor, myrrh, squills, digitalis, and extract of belladonna, made into a ball and given morning and evening for a week, and less frequently for a similar period. With this medicine the horse does not require to be laid aside from work; nor need any change in the dietary be adopted, with the exception of the administration daily, with the oats, of one or two fluid ounces of good linseed-oil. In some, much relief is obtained

31—2

from repeated applications to the chest of the compound soap and tincture of opium liniment, or even simple cantharides liniment; this latter to be applied only once, and not repeated until the scurf raised by the vesication is removed   When weakness or want of tone with loss of flesh occurs, the work of the animal ought to be lightened, and such tonics as iron with nux vomica and gentian, or some preparation of arsenic, administered.

CHAPTER XX.

PULMONARY CONGESTION—CONGESTION OF THE LUNGS

Definition.—*A hyperæmic condition of the pulmonary capillary vessels, sometimes attended with extravasation from these into air-sacs, and interconnective-tissue.*

Nature and Causation—Congestion of the lungs, or engorgement of the vessels of the pulmonary tissue by unnatural collection or detention of blood there, may occur in the horse and all animals as a precursor and accompaniment of inflammation in pulmonary structures; also in other local and general diseased conditions, as in some cardiac affections, enteric diseases, arthritic inflammations, and in some special epizootics.

In addition, however, congestion, or collection to repletion of blood in the pulmonary vessels, occurs as an independent and distinct condition, which is that to which we now chiefly refer, and which we mean to indicate when not qualified by any accompanying term explanatory of its origin or association.

When of an acute character, and accompanied with capillary hæmorrhage, it is sometimes spoken of as pulmonary apoplexy.

This state of hyperæmia, or hæmal engorgement, is recognised as *acute*, and *passive*, or *mechanical*   The former is the manifestation which we most frequently encounter and most readily recognise in our patient. Active congestion in the horse is most frequently the result of—1. Increased cardiac action, without or apart from relative resisting power in pulmonary vessels; 2. All agencies which at other times or with other subjects develop bronchial or common catarrh   Passive congestion is encountered under conditions associated with retarded venous circulation or depressed heart-action, as in mitral and some other cardiac disturbances, and in general exhaustion attendant on some fevers and debilitating diseases

Active congestion, the most frequently occurring form in the horse, may be observed to a certain extent, but not to that of disease, accompanying all active exertion   In well-developed pulmonary hyperæmia we have functional activity in excess until this induces impairment, or, it may be, arrest of functional power   When the rate of speed or power with which the blood is driven to and through the lungs is excessive, there must speedily be a certain amount of relief, either by diminished rapidity of circulation, increased cardiac or pulmonary power, or the result is a fatal accumulation of blood in the pulmonary capillaries, terminating in pulmonary inaction.   Rupture, in these cases, is rarely sufficiently extensive to produce even temporary relief   Of this irregularity and stagnation in the flow of blood through the pulmonary vessels we observe many grades or variations as to extent, from the simple turgescence of active exertion, and the somewhat distressed pulmonary condition connected with defective cardiac action, to the perfect engorgement and rupture of capillary structure incident to an excited and continued circulation overpowering both heart and lungs.

Of increased cardiac action operating in the production of pulmonary congestion we have the most striking examples in those instances which follow attempts to hunt raw or unprepared horses.   These examples and warnings, we fear, nearly invariably follow from overlooking the fact that horses are living machines, and that for the comfortable performance of even moderate work they must have their living organism kept in regular action, while for the execution of extra work that organism requires to be in a high state of preparedness   For this latter the animal's powers must be gradually developed and maintained in a high state of efficiency ; he must, as horsemen say, be in fairly good ' condition '   This state of ' condition ' does not consist in the possession of a full amount of flesh, nor yet in a glossy coat, nor even in high spirits , a horse may possess all these, and yet be in an unfit state to undergo severe and prolonged exertion   The muscular system must by steady and at first slow work be gradually accommodated to exertion, while in the developing of the muscular power, properly so called, both the respiratory and circulatory systems become strengthened and rendered capable of performing their work under the exacting conditions of rapidity and continued duration   Unless these points are attended to, no horse, however good in health, and in however high spirits, can be expected to perform an ordinary day's work at an average horse's pace, far less such severe and sustained exertion as we require in the hunting-field, without the risk of pulmonary congestion.

In horses of any class this may occur when put to severe exertion or prolonged work, for which they are unprepared by a certain amount of previous work and by proper feeding   It is common in horses brought from dealers' stables, when sufficient care is not exercised in putting them to the work for which they may be intended.

In the same way, animals suffering from catarrh, or only recently recovered from some respiratory disturbance, are more susceptible of an attack of pulmonary hyperæmia than others

Instances, also, may be encountered in cases of collapse of lung-structure from pressure by fluid contained in the pleural sac, on the sudden removal of this fluid by operative interference.

Further, pulmonary congestion may occur without direct over-exertion in cases where horses are confined to defectively ventilated stables after having undergone active exertion in the open air, this is apparently from a deficiency of respirable air and consequent non-oxygenation of the blood.

Whenever the amount of oxygen or carbonic acid in the blood, or the relationships which ought to subsist between these, are permanently disturbed, the consequences are either asphyxia or apnœa   asphyxia, when the want of oxygen is very marked, and the irritability of the nerve-centres, which require for their functional activity so much oxygen, cease ; apnœa, when the blood is too rich in oxygen and poor in carbonic acid, respiration becoming arrested because of the want of the normal excitant of the respiratory centre

Anatomical Characters—The after-death appearances appreciable by the naked eye in the lung-tissue of horses which have fallen victims to a serious invasion of pulmonary congestion are perfectly characteristic.

There is distension and general engorgement of the pulmonary vascular system with dark-coloured fluid blood, with occasionally irregularly distributed circumscribed hæmorrhagic effusions from rupture of minute and capillary vessels. The lungs are swollen—pulmonary œdema—of a dark colour, firmer than natural; the crepitant character which so distinguishes healthy lung-tissue is not gone, but diminished—it feels to contain more liquid than air. Although heavier than natural, its normal elasticity and spongy texture are not so much destroyed that it will not float in water, in this respect differing from the consolidation of pneumonia, the condition of red hepatization to which in many respects it bears a resemblance. This state of splenization of lung-structure, as the result of pulmonary engorgement has been called from its resemblance in physical character to the spleen, has, when incised, a dark red colour, with occasional spots of a deeper hue marking the points of blood-effusion, and from the cut surface there is an oozing of bloody serous liquid mingled with mucus, and rendered frothy from the entanglement of air. The entire structure is from the engorgement and distension rendered more friable than natural, probably less so, however, than in the more advanced stage of hepatization.

The lining membrane throughout the entire tract of the air-tubes, particularly the bronchi, is heightened in colour, and covered with frothy mucus.

In no parts do we find effusion, save of serous material, the characteristic plastic exudation of inflammatory action being as yet undeveloped.

In the examination after death of animals which have died from pulmonary congestion, a mistake very commonly made by non-professional observers is to regard the dark-coloured, friable condition of acute engorgement, with its softened, damp appearance tending to putrescence, as indicative of a diseased condition of some time standing; whereas we know that the opposite is the direct conclusion to be drawn from these conditions. Darkness of colour, with softness and liquidity of

texture, without the presence of organized or plastic and
organizable exudate, may be accepted as the condition of pulmonary congestion, a state which may develop itself in any
animal previously healthy in less than an hour   Both sides of
the heart, but particularly the right with the large vessels proceeding to and from it, are more or less full of dark-coloured,
rather viscid, but not coagulated blood

The cases of congestion which have terminated fatally connected with other diseased conditions—passive congestion
chiefly—rarely present so characteristic lesions of the hyperæmic state as those which are the result of over-exertion
in perfectly healthy animals   The lung-tissue is in these not
so dark in colour, more crepitant, with a greater quantity of
frothy mucus in the air-tubes, while from the state of the
minute bronchi in particular, we are disposed to believe that a
certain amount of capillary bronchitis is very often associated
with these attacks

Symptoms—In the worst cases of pulmonary congestion,
such as we have referred to as common in horses put to severe
and prolonged exertion in a comparatively unprepared condition, the symptoms are, as a rule, extremely distressing   The
animal is in a state of great disturbance ; he stands with limbs
outstretched, neck extended, head depressed, flapping nostrils,
heaving flanks, trembling more or less over the whole body,
with partial perspiration rolling from him in great drops

These great and distressing efforts, however, are not sufficient to stir the current of blood which moves sluggishly in
the heart, lungs, and great bloodvessels, the imperfect oxidation of which induces stupor and somnolency, with livid nasal
membranes, cold ears and extremities   The continued pressure
may cause rupture of some capillaries in connection with the
air-passages, and we then have a discharge of frothy, blood-
stained mucus from the nostrils   The pulse is small and indistinct ; although the artery feels under the finger tolerably full,
it may be soft and the contents compressible, while we with
difficulty make out the number of its feeble beats, which may
be as many as one hundred per minute.   The superficial veins
are turgid, and stand out in well-defined form all over the head,
and wherever the skin is thin, the heart's action is rapid, jerking, disturbed, and tumultuous, but void of power   In auscul-

tating the chest the healthy respiratory murmur is modified to that of minute crepitation, a sharp or fine crackling sound peculiar to the very earliest stages of inflammatory action, or to that of returning health in resolution.

This sound may be very generally diffused; or we may find cases where it is difficult of detection except over limited portions of lung-structure, the rest giving no sound whatever. In some, a grunt accompanies the expiratory part of the respiratory act

Cases of pulmonary congestion occurring in connection with other diseases, although the symptoms exhibited are seemingly less severe, are more generally fatal than when appearing as the result of over-exertion.

Course and Terminations.—In severe and acute cases of pulmonary congestion, unless the primary determining and sustaining element of the abnormal state, the increased blood-flow and pressure, is withdrawn or arrested, and time and power obtained for the natural resumption of the circulation, the condition of imperfect oxygenation of the blood and the physical obstruction offered to the circulation in the pulmonary vessels rapidly terminate in death from asphyxia and coma. When, under judicious management, the vascular engorgement is arrested, and the power of heart and lungs restored in the function of corrected circulation, the turgid vessels and blood-channels gradually resume their former condition, and with the free course of the circulating fluid, and its regular contact with pure air, the horse may shortly regain his normal state.

Still, it is always deserving of recollection that even this temporary disturbance of function seems not to be possible without leaving a certain amount of weakness and susceptibility to disease. In many instances following recovery from congestion of the lungs we meet with a great susceptibility, under very slight or no appreciable cause, to a recurrence of the same condition, or one equally dangerous, inflammation of lung-structures.

Treatment.—In many cases of pulmonary congestion, even when the seizure is severe, if these be attended to when observed, great relief is obtained by the employment of the simplest means, such as clothing the body and allowing the

animal plenty of pure air   When occurring in the hunting-field,
where of all out-of-door conditions and situations this disturbance is most likely to demand our attention, the rider ought
to dismount, loosen his saddle-girths, and turn the horse's head
to the wind, while he proceeds to smartly rub the surface of the
body.   This, when carried out before the animal has actually
come to a stand, will most probably restore the circulation
through the lungs and unload the engorged vessels   However much blood-letting may be condemned, and however certain it is that in the majority of cases it may be dispensed
with, there are yet situations and conditions where to neglect
its employment were to throw away the chances of a good and
rapid recovery   The situations referred to are where we may
be placed with no possibility of obtaining help from the use of
any medicinal agent ; the conditions, where the animal is not
perfectly pulseless, or where the pulsations are not of a
peculiarly feeble, flickering, nearly imperceptible character.
By blood-letting when the blood-current is still moving on,
we may be able to relieve for a time the over-charged
heart

No doubt those cases which are most benefited by blood-
letting are such as might without any interference recover, and
the more seriously affected are those where its employment is
likely to prove destructive , still, in moderately severe cases,
where we are by situation or other conditions precluded from
employing any remedies likely to be useful, the abstraction of
blood is not to be neglected

In cases both stabled and occurring in the open air, whether
blood-letting is resorted to or not, every attempt must be made
to secure a sufficiency of fresh air and a restoration of the disturbed equilibrium of the circulation by smart friction to the
surface of the body and the extremities, together with the
repeated exhibition of moderate doses of some diffusible stimulant, of which the alcoholic appear to answer best   The attempt
to promote circulation in the extremities may, in addition to
simple friction with the hand or a hay-wisp, be carried out by
the application of a stimulating liniment applied previous to
the limbs being swathed in woollen bandages

I have always found the internal administration of stimulants, whatever these may be, most successful when given in

moderate doses and repeated probably every hour, or every second hour, and when they have been given in combination with such salines as solution of acetate of ammonia

In treating all cases of pulmonary congestion, we must ever bear in mind what has already been stated when speaking of the course of the disease, that for some time after apparent recovery there is a great aptitude to recurrence of the same state, or even the more dangerous one of pneumonia. With the view of guarding against such recurrence, care requires to be exercised alike in the maintenance of an equable temperature in the stable, a due supply of pure air, and of a natural state of the skin, bowels, and kidneys, together with gradual accommodation of the horse to the work to which he may be put when believed to be fit for it.

CHAPTER XXI.

PNEUMONIA—INFLAMMATION OF THE LUNGS.

Definition. — *Inflammation of the true lung-substance, the vesicular elements, and most probably the connective-tissue forming the parenchyma of the lung, and which in its uncomplicated and acute or pure form of development is attended with well-marked pyrexia, which, after a variable period of existence, suffers distinct defervescence even while the structural changes in the lung are decided and unremoved.*

Pathology. *a. Varieties.*— Inflammation in lung-tissue is spoken of under different names, some of which are merely synonymous or convertible terms, others are employed to indicate supposed differences either in the morbid action itself or of its exact distribution as respects the particular lung-tissues involved, or the nature of the resultant products. Thus we speak of—1 *Croupous, exudative, lobar, or diffuse pneumonia,* because of the character of the exudate, which contains a large amount of fibrinous material, and because of its generally extensive distribution through or amongst the pulmonary tissue. 2. *Catarrhal, lobular, patchy, or broncho-pneumonia,* from the non-existence, comparatively speaking, of organizable exudate, and the extent of alveolar and endothelial proliferation so characteristic of catarrhal inflammation of mucous membranes, and because of its limited diffusion as compared with the lobar, being confined to lobules or collections of lobules

3 *Interstitial pneumonia*, when the action is believed to be confined to the interlobular connective-tissue of the alveoli of the lungs, and to result in thickening of the walls of the alveoli and of the interconnective-tissue.

It is also spoken of as *primary pneumonia* when the diseased process appears to originate in or from the lung-tissue, independently of association directly as an inducing cause with any other diseased condition ; as *secondary pneumonia* when the inflammatory state of the pulmonary structures succeeds to, or is believed to proceed from, some antecedent unhealthy condition. It is also styled *specific pneumonia* when accompanying such specific diseases as glanders-farcy.

Of these different forms of inflammation of lung-tissue, it is of the commonly occurring, independent inflammation invading the entire pneumonic structures, ordinary exudative or lobar pneumonia, that we would chiefly now speak ; of that which is *par excellence* pneumonia

It is, however, deserving of notice that the form and character of the diseased action is much modified in those creatures which severally come under our notice, by the variations which we observe in the anatomical structure of the lungs of these individually. In the horse, where the interlobular tissue is comparatively small in amount, the inflammatory action is more truly catarrhal than croupous ; in the greater number of instances the inflammatory products accumulate largely in the interior of the air-vesicles. In the ox the conditions are reversed, the exudative character of the action being a prominent feature.

b. Nature and Causation.—Ordinarily, and by the majority of observers, pneumonia has been regarded as merely a local diseased condition—inflammatory action—with which the more or less highly developed pyrexial state was to be regarded simply in the relation of effect to cause, as truly an expected symptom of the local tissue-change. There are, however, others who regard the entire morbid conditions and changes in a very different, or rather we should say opposite light. With these, the various phenomena observed in the course of any true or sthenic pneumonia are regarded as in reality manifestations of a morbid state of the nutrient material, the blood, the pulmonary tissue-changes being simply the mode through which the vitiated fluid purifies or rectifies itself. This latter explanation of the phenomena has many facts to support it.

In the one view, the pyrexia and other phenomenal occurrences are to be regarded as resulting from the inflammatory-product changes occurring in the pulmonic structures, which must ever be looked upon as the essence of the disease; in the other, all these general and local disturbances and changes, not even excepting the inflammatory-product alterations in the lung-structures, are viewed as the result of the primary vitiation of the blood. In this latter view the pulmonic structures are looked upon as possessing a selective power for the specific abnormal material existing in the blood, and which, by its elimination at the lungs in the form of so-called inflammatory product, relieves the hæmal vitiation, and restores the disturbed equilibrium. In this manner it is proposed to account for the defervescence of the pyrexia, and amelioration of many of the constitutional symptoms and features of the disease. In regarding it as essentially a local diseased action, the causes of which are often occult, or in their mode of action difficult of explanation, the inflammatory product, instead of being regarded as a local abstraction from the hæmal circulation, of a specific contaminating agent, is to be viewed in its development in the same light as swelling and effusion in common inflammatory action of such open structures as ordinary areolar tissue, and to be capable of explanation, as regards its occurrence, on physical or mechanical principles, rather than by reference to what are chemico-vital.

Whichever idea may be embraced, or in future may prove more worthy of support, there are certain facts connected with the development of pneumonia of which we are tolerably satisfied, and in respect of which we have sufficient evidence. We know (1) that there is a period of well-marked pyrexia, which in acute uncomplicated cases runs a determinate course, terminating in or succeeded by (2) a period of less-marked fever, during which lung-consolidation is begun, or at least perfected, to be succeeded, during the same period of moderate fever, by liquefaction of the inflammatory-action products and their removal, chiefly by absorption, and maybe by expectoration

Of the influences which appear to be in operation for the production of pneumonia, some may be regarded as predisposing and others as immediate or exciting. Of the former the most obvious are—1 *Season and locality* It is more prevalent during spring and autumn, when temperature is liable to sudden variations, particularly with moisture ; also in districts where north and north-easterly winds prevail at the periods when horses are changing their coats 2 *Previous attacks of inflammatory and other weakening affections* of the pulmonary structures 3 *Particular states of the general health,* it being more liable to attack animals weakened by some previous general disease, and where the vital powers are somewhat depressed

Of the latter the chief are—1 *All agencies which we observe operating in the production of the allied affections laryngitis, bronchitis, and common catarrh* (a) Exposing animals in a state of inaction to cold and damp after having undergone severe exertion or fatigue (b) Confinement in close, badly-ventilated stables, with foul emanations operating in addition to deficiency of respirable air.

2 *As the result of pulmonary engorgement* This, we are satisfied, is more apt to be the case than is generally supposed, nor do the chances of such an untoward result seem to be confined to a few hours immediately succeeding the congestive attack ; they are in operation for some days In such cases very trivial disturbances, either from irregularities of diet or changes in location, are exceedingly apt to be followed by inflammation in the lung-substance

3 *Direct irritation* is not an unfrequent cause of pneumonia, and may occur (a) through medicinal agents in the liquid form—when attempted to be administered to animals of violent temper, or where, from physical impediments, deglutition is difficult—finding their way into the trachea and minute ramifications of the air-passages (b) From wounds or portions of fractured ribs penetrating the thoracic walls and injuring the contained structures.

4. *The existence of other diseased conditions.* (*a*) Probably the most fertile source of pneumonia in the horse is that of neglected or badly treated ordinary catarrh Here the inflamed condition of the mucous membrane is very apt to extend downwards, implicating the smaller air-tubes; while succeeding bronchitis we most commonly, in such cases, have pneumonia also. This disposition of catarrhal inflammation to extend from the upper to the lower air-passages is often seen when the animals are comfortably housed and well taken care of, but is nearly sure to follow when in ordinary catarrh the animal is in any manner abused or otherwise circumstanced so as to favour the development of pneumonia. (*b*) Following some specific and general diseases, also certain states of blood-contamination In this form of secondary or complementary pneumonia there are many instances where accompanying, or probably immediately inducing, the inflammatory condition is pulmonary thrombosis , this is well exemplified in the pyæmic state accompanying specific arthritis and other septic and infective conditions

5 *Epizootic agencies* Pneumonia may of itself, or as part of the symptoms or development of such epizooties as influenza, call for special attention, where by whatever channel the inducing factor—the so-called epizootic influence or agent—may enter the system, it is so far occult or inappreciable that it is only known by its action and the results which it may induce.

Anatomical Characters.—The general pathological condition of pneumonia may be stated as hyperæmia and œdema of lung-tissue, with a variably constituted fibrinous exudation, chiefly in the air-cells and minute bronchi These conditions of vascular turgescence and exudation are, in the examination of animals which have succumbed while thus affected, presented for observation under somewhat variable characters.

Although it is probable that the very earliest condition of lung-structure when about to become inflamed is that of irritation or arterial injection, indicated by crepitation and harsh respiration, and exhibiting a state of unnatural dryness and a bright red colour, the usually observed appearance and condition at the commencement of pneumonia is rather that known as *The stage of simple engorgement*

This is generally very observable at an early stage in all
diffuse inflammations of the true pulmonary structures, in it
the lung-tissue becomes exceedingly vascular, of a darker
colour than natural, not uniform but mottled; it is increased
in both absolute weight and specific gravity. Its tenacity is
lessened, the texture being more easily broken down by pressure than in health; it is less crepitant or resilient, but is not
altogether void of air, as may be discovered from the feeling
imparted on manipulation, and from the fact that it will still
float in water, and that when incised the fluid material contained in the intimate tissue is of a frothy character. That it
contains as yet none of the true exudate of confirmed inflammation is demonstrated by washing, which to a great extent
removes the exalted colouration. A section of pulmonary
tissue in this condition exhibits enlarged and engorged
capillary bloodvessels, dilated air-cells with varying conditions
of cell contents. This stage of engorgement may, in the living
animal, quietly subside, and the parts gradually resume their
normal condition, or it may develop into the more serious
lesion recognised as *The stage of exudation, red hepatization,
or red softening.* It must be recollected, however, that none
of the variations into which the morbid process of pulmonary
inflammation have been arbitrarily divided are sharply defined
or marked off, but that they imperceptibly shade into each
other. In this exudation stage we have, along with the
serum, an outpouring of the fibrinogenous materials of the
blood, the liquor sanguinis, and a migration of leucocytes and
some red globules into both the air-vesicles and interconnective lobular tissue; the exuded fluid materials coagulate, and,
in so doing, enclose the various corpuscular elements.

The physical appearances and characters of the lung-tissue in
this condition are somewhat different from the previous state of
engorgement. It is rarely so livid in colour, being reddish-brown
or dull red both on the outer surface and when cut into; its
specific gravity and absolute weight are increased; there is little
or no air contained in the vesicles, it does not crepitate on
manipulation; it is extremely friable, the structure being easily
broken down by the finger; it does not collapse when the chest
is laid open, cannot be injected or inflated, and is disposed to
sink in water.

When torn or cut the exposed surface has a soft granular aspect, from the existence of plugs of the solidified material entangling corpuscular blood-elements impacted in the air-vesicles This condition of solidification and friability is marked by many variations in character, not merely from the variations in the anatomical structure of the lung-tissue of the different animals with which we are connected, but also in animals of the same species, from influences some of which are easy enough of appreciation, as period of duration or intensity of the action, and others less obvious and less easily under-stood

If, in the living animal, auscultation be employed over any portion of lung-structure undergoing this condition of red solidification or softening, we will not, as in the stage of en-gorgement or arterial injection, detect any crepitant sound if we are able to detect sound at all, it will be of the character known as bronchial ; the vesicular structure and interconnec-tive-tissue being solidified, while the air-tubes remain perme-able.

This state of coloured solidification, should the animal continue to live, is not the final one ; we have, as a rule, suc-ceeding this, or under certain conditions and influences appearing without its intervention, the state of suppurative or purulent infiltration, recognised as the third or fourth, and final stage of pneumonia, and spoken of as *grey hepatization or softening*. Occasionally a division has been attempted in this condition of advanced inflammatory action by speaking of sup-puration of lung-tissue of the diffuse character, as distinct from the recognised grey softening or hepatization , this is scarcely applicable, for although the variations in this stage are great—in some the cut surface being comparatively firm if pale-coloured, in others the puriform material is so abundant as to ooze freely from the recently cut surface—they are yet both marked distinctly enough from the other stages by the obvious existence of puriform matter appreciable to the naked eye

Although probably in essential structural changes both con-ditions of grey and red hepatization may be regarded as similar, there are yet several particulars in which they are distinctive The most obvious and prominent individual feature of the

32

stage of grey hepatization is the difference in colour, which
varies from a reddish-brown to a grey or yellowish-white, and
appears to be owing chiefly to two conditions, that of pressure
exercised upon the minute bloodvessels by the adventitious
products of the inflammatory action, and the degenerative
fatty changes which have occurred, and are occurring, in the
cell-elements of the product

Besides this alteration of colour from brown to grey, we have
also the continued existence of the impervious character, im
possibility of inflation, and increased density and friability o
the previous stage of red hepatization it wants resilience, and
sinks in water   On incising a portion of lung-tissue in this
condition we find appearances and characters varying from
each other in different individuals, as they vary in all from the
former stage of red consolidation   The granular character
either in a torn or cut surface, is less distinguishable in the
grey than in the red hepatization.   In the horse, in some cases
the previous well-distinguished granular condition of the red
hepatization may still be perfectly distinguished , in other
cases matters are very much similar to what we encounter in
the lung-tissue of bovines undergoing this modification o
pneumonic inflammation, where the grey material is firmer and
of the planiform character, which it maintains throughout the
course of the disease

Although these several conditions of *engorgement, red*, and
grey hepatization, are tolerably uniform and regular, in perfected cases of pneumonia, in the sequence with which they
succeed each other, we have ever to remember that even
this may be interrupted , that cases, for example, may show
themselves where diffuse suppuration is established without
the intervention of red hepatization, and that each is in very
many instances shaded off and imperceptibly passes into the
other, while it may be that some two of these otherwise
distinct states may coexist in the same lung-structure   Also
that there are many cases, chiefly those of secondary pneumonia, occurring in connection with, or as a sequel of, some
other diseased action where these states of consolidation are
much less perfectly carried out, and where the various steps
and changes of the process undergo much modification

Besides these common and usually encountered pathological

changes, there are some others which, in exceptional cases, attract attention, namely: 1. The formation of one or more abscesses. This is probably a rather rare condition, unless we regard the extensive purulent infiltration in the light of a large collection of very small abscesses. When an abscess does exist, it may, by opening into some of the air-tubes, become discharged, or from being perfectly encapsuled, may undergo calcareous or cheesy degeneration. 2. Gangrene, this is certainly not more common than the preceding. By some this condition is considered more likely to follow excess of inflammatory action, but from what I have observed of the condition in the horse, I am disposed to credit peculiarities in the type of the inflammatory action, and depressing or pestilential influences operating upon the animals affected, with the onus of the production of this peculiar change. When occurring, I have not observed that it affects the whole lung-structure which is invaded by the pneumonia; the extent of its inroad is circumscribed, sometimes rather extensive, at others limited. The appearance is that of the so-called humid gangrene, the tissue being of a greenish-brown or metallic hue. It is often marked off from the healthier lung-structure by a distinct line of demarcation, and feels soft and doughy. Accompanying this state I have observed, particularly in foals suffering from specific arthritis, where the pneumonia is a secondary affection, that thrombosis of pulmonary vessels is a rather frequently associated feature. 3. Chronic pulmonary inflammation tending to the development of a form of fibroid or cicatricial tissue, apparently closely connected with the walls of the alveolar cavities and the connective-tissue intervening. The growth of this fibro-nucleated structure may be of such a character and extent as largely to impair the capacity of the air-vesicles, and by its firmness and tenacity give to the lung-tissue the character of cirrhosis or induration. When once established, this is likely to go on increasing, while the structure so affected seems rather decreased in bulk because less dilatable and expansive, the air-vesicles gradually becoming smaller from the steady thickening of the alveolar walls and increase of the fibroid material in the interconnective-tissue. 4. This last condition may further develop into more extensive circumscribed or nodulated portions of indura-

32—2

tion, which, as a rule, have no tendency to undergo ulterior change.

When making examination of lung-structure in animals which have been sufferers from pneumonia, it is not common that the diseased action is found attacking both lungs with the same severity. Bilateral or double pneumonia is rare in all animals; still there is little doubt that in its common form of broncho-pneumonia in the horse it is met with in both lungs, the right being oftener and more extensively invaded than the left.

Symptoms. 1. *General.*—As it rarely happens that in the horse pneumonia is encountered as a pure and uncomplicated disease, we may only speak of those cases where the indications lead us to believe that the true lung-tissue is more largely affected than the bronchial membrane or the pleural covering Seeing that the more numerous attacks of pneumonia are accompanied, or rather preceded, by catarrh, we can readily understand that a very early, if not the earliest, symptom may be cough, which most likely occurs, or has continued for some days, without attracting much notice, until certain well-marked febrile symptoms exhibit themselves There may be occasional rigors, with an open and staring coat; there is disturbance of animal heat, with coldness of skin and extremities, all connected with perturbed nutrition Accompanying these there is languor, capricious appetite, injected, or dull, or rusty-coloured visible mucous membranes, the pulse is increased in frequency, vessels feeling tolerably full, but the pulsations obscure, sometimes small, the temperature elevated from three to four degrees, and respirations slightly accelerated

Although febrile symptoms such as these are generally observed in the earlier stages of pneumonia, it not unfrequently happens that considerable progress has been made in the process, and distinct consolidation of lung-tissue exists ere the symptoms of illness are sufficient to direct our attention to the chest As in many other chest affections, the horse is not disposed to lie, occasionally moving listlessly around the box if at liberty, and inclined to stand where fresh air is finding the readiest entrance

It is deserving of notice that when the febrile symptoms are fully developed, and the pneumonic changes established, these febrile symptoms seem to maintain a distinct corelation to each other, this corelation being a disturbance of that which naturally subsists between the temperature, the frequency of the pulse, and the respirations   When cough exists, which is not always the case, it is at first dry, after some time becoming less so from the exudation which is taking place in connection with the bronchial and pulmonic structures We do not, as in man, find much expectorated material to assist us in forming an opinion as to the condition of the lung-tissue and air-conduits

When gangrene and disintegration of tissue occur we have full indications of such, chiefly from the fœtor of the breath, and it may be also from the debris of the structures undergoing removal being mingled with the matter expectorated

During the continuance of fever in a high degree the urinary secretion is greatly lessened in amount, and altered in composition.   There is excess of urea, probably the direct result of active tissue-change, also a diminution of the salines, markedly of the chloride of sodium , this is a feature particularly noticed by observers of pneumonic inflammation in man, and I have observed it in the horse, although I cannot affirm that in his case it is in direct relation to the state of resolution, or regard its reappearance in the urine as a certain symptom of returning health, or restoration of lung-function   The bowels are rather torpid as a rule, but of such a character as to be very susceptible of being acted upon by purgative agents

2 *Local*—In addition to these general symptoms, those which are regarded as the truly physical signs are in every instance deserving of careful observation and study, seeing that, apart from the assistance which they render us, the differing changes of structure might pass unappreciated   The sounds detected by auscultation, and elicitated by percussion, are both of them in inflammation of the lung-substance much modified

During the earlier stages, those of arterial irritation and that of turgescence, auscultation reveals to us a condition at first of rather increased and harsh respiratory murmur, to be succeeded by weakening of the normal sound , while as effusion takes place, the respiratory murmur, however altered, is replaced by minute crepitation, the true 'crepitant râle.'

This sound much resembles what we have already remarked as occurring in cases of capillary bronchitis, but does not, as there, continue or become modified according to the amount and nature of the mucus secreted and found in the tubes. After a little, as the air-cells and surrounding connective-tissue become infiltrated, the crepitation ceases not again to be heard until a return to health has been established. As the engorgement or effusion into, and consolidation of, lung-structure progresses, and the natural respiratory murmur ceases, the characteristic bronchial respiration appears, and this tubular or bronchial sound is the more distinct, the more complete consolidation of the pulmonic tissue becomes.

Seeing that in pneumonic inflammation we rarely, by percussion over the seat of the disease, are able to obtain aught more definite than a slight amount of dulness, or want of resonance, even when, from other symptoms, we may be tolerably certain that the pulmonary tissue is much diseased, we can only look upon this as valuable in corroborating what we learn by auscultation.

However, when forming our opinion with respect to the existence of pneumonia, it is well, if we would endeavour to avoid mistakes, not to lean too implicitly on any one symptom or class of symptoms, but to observe that each one corroborates the others, to note whether the general symptoms, which usually first attract attention, are confirmed by what may be learned from a physical examination of the chest.

Course and Termination.—Ordinary cases of pneumonia, even those which are complicated with a considerable amount of bronchitis, usually reach the height of the pyrexia in a week, or little more, taking a somewhat longer period ere resolution is well established.

Although we have noted the different pathological changes which lung-tissue usually undergoes, it ought also to be remembered that all these various changes of structure are not necessarily accomplished or gone through in every case ere restoration to health is established. Very many, probably the greater number of those which recover, have proceeded no further than the entrance of the territory of true inflammatory action, the beginning of the stage of red hepatization; others, no doubt, have not only proceeded to consolidation of lung-tissue, but this has been succeeded by softening and purulent infiltration ere resolution has been established.

For the first few days of the earlier stages of the disease, during the continuance of the conditions of arterial irritation and vascular engorgement, the symptoms of febrile disturbance are great and sometimes alarming ; immediately succeeding the defervescence of the pyrexia, which may be within the first week, the respirations become more embarrassed or quicker, although both temperature and pulse may have fallen. Should return to health not show itself by the gradual development of functional activity in the pulmonary vesicular structure, followed by the resumption of the respiratory murmur, the condition of lung-consolidation may continue to advance, and death result from deficiency of aerating pulmonary surface. Or even when partial resolution is established we may have, by the softening and rapid disintegration of tissue and its absorption, a condition of blood-contamination, and a renewal of fever and inflammatory action. In primary pneumonia of a severe type, particularly when associated with bronchitis, there is occasionally exhibited a tendency to the occurrence of metastatic action, in the horse this is apt to assume the character of inflammation of the vascular structures of the feet.

When occurring as a secondary affection, or in conjunction with other diseased conditions, particularly where epizootic influences and surroundings of an evil and debilitating character are in operation, pneumonia is more apt to assume a less certain and determinate course, and is more likely to terminate in destructive changes than in resolution. The inflammatory action is here probably more truly of the patchy or catarrhal type ; there is little or no fibrinous exudation as compared with the pure croupous variety, the chief changes being a filling of the alveoli with cell proliferations, which, in the milder cases, undergo liquefaction and removal, and in those which do not thus terminate forming collections of indurated cheesy material, which may take on further changes of a more stable or fugitive character. These local patches of inflamed and altered lobules may be distributed throughout a considerable extent of lung-tissue, which otherwise gives evidence of previous bronchial inflammation. Often they seem to the eye, and feel when touched, rather firm, although on section they evidently want cohesion, breaking down easily under pressure, and are in their early stages surrounded with a more or less marked area of congestion

In influenza, where pneumonic complications occur, we almost invariably find that if these do not terminate in gangrene we have purulent infiltration of an extensive character, accompanied with much tissue-disintegration; the same results often accompany pneumonia associated with or following common catarrh, when the animals are acted upon by certain septic or depressing influences.

Interstitial Pneumonia.—There is a condition sometimes encountered in the pulmonary structure, recognised as fibroid induration, which in all animals occasionally follows as the result of ordinary pneumonia. The horse is certainly as little liable to this as any animal, but even with him it may occur

In this condition of interstitial or interlobular fibroid induration there is a thickening of the walls of the pulmonary alveoli and intervening connective-tissue, with structures resembling that developed in ordinary connective-tissue which has been the seat of inflammatory action, the so-called cicatricial tissue. By the development of this fibro-nucleated growth, and its deposition in the walls of the pulmonary alveoli and in the interlobular structure, together with the products of endothelial cell proliferation which have accumulated in the air-sacs, the vesicular structures become gradually obliterated, the entire lung-structure affected becomes less in volume, while the feeling imparted on manipulation is one of hardness and density. This progressive consolidation of pulmonary tissue, the result of inflammatory action of a rather slow or chronic character, with a development of fibroid and fibro-nucleated elements in the walls of the pulmonary spaces, and amongst the interlobular connective-tissue, is probably more frequently observed in the ox than the horse; and is in that animal more prone to take on a form of caseation, and other retrogressive changes frequently comprehended under and associated with the condition spoken of as pulmonary phthisis

In the pneumonia of glanders in the horse we may often observe these changes, particularly in slowly progressive cases; in these we will find the alveolar walls thickened, and the

interlobular tissue augmented from the infiltration of a growth
of varying cellular and fibroid characters, the ultimate tendency
of which is to limit and circumscribe the pulmonary alveolar
structure, and thus to interfere with the function of respiration
tion

Diagnosis — When the morbid action is chiefly developed in
the substance of the lungs we have less pain and distress exhibited by the horse than in either bronchitis or pleurisy ; so
much is this the character of the disease that it is no uncommon circumstance to have considerable structural change in
the pulmonary tissue ere we are aware of its existence. From
inflammation of the bronchial mucous membrane pneumonia
is also distinguished by the more regular occurrence of troublesome catarrhal symptoms in the former than the latter. In
bronchitis the cough is generally a prominent symptom, and is
always irritating and attended with pain.

In pneumonia the respirations, somewhat or considerably
accelerated, are never of the distressing or marked abdominal
character they are met with in bronchitis and pleurisy ; and
while in pneumonia they bear no relation in distubance to the
rise of temperature and quickening of the pulse, they do in
pleurisy, and frequently also in bronchitis, bear this relation ,
i e , the respirations increase in frequency in these in direct
relation to rise of temperature and frequency of pulsations.

In pneumonia in the early stages we have crepitation
gradually displacing the natural respiratory murmur, and terminating in loss of sound from consolidation ; in bronchitis we
have the early existence of the dry and sonorous rale, succeeded by the soft or mucous sounds , in pleurisy the absence
of these, or, it may be, the addition to them of a distinct
rubbing sound, together with evidence of pain when the
animal is compelled to move, or smart percussion is employed
over the chest

In pneumonia the pulse is more variable than in either
bronchitis or pleuritis , it is also of less resistance In every
case, however, when forming an opinion as to the existence
and extent of pulmonary inflammation we must be guided not
by one class of symptoms, but all must be carefully observed
and collated with each other, the general with the physical,
and the physical and local with the general

Treatment—As an inflammatory action, developed in connection with organs large in superficial extent and essential to life, pneumonia, like some other morbid conditions, has in its treatment given room for the greatest divergence of opinion and is still likely to do so.

As there are many roads to Rome, so both in medicine and surgery are there many, and, it may be, apparently different modes of treatment, which nevertheless all tend to the same end, the restoration of normal structure and functional activity. In no cases more distinctly, probably, than in pneumonia will it be found that he is the best practitioner who can most readily and fully grasp the differences so regularly met with in the constitutional disposition of the different animals we meet with—the characters and types which diseased action is liable to assume, as well as the effect of surrounding influences upon both animals and disease. There is little doubt that to be treated successfully, pneumonia must be treated individually, and not generically, we must consider the case of each animal separately—(*a*) as to its individual constitution, (*b*) the influences to which it is subjected; (*c*) the form of development or type of the diseased action by which it is assailed. It will not serve our purpose in the adoption of remedial measures to forget the individual patient in a recollection of any particular group or collection of so-called typical cases; such is very useful in enabling us to form opinions from which we may draw certain conclusions, but each case of disease must form for itself matter for our consideration, and must be managed in accordance with its own individual peculiarities, both intrinsic and extrinsic.

In this way, and following such considerations, we find that bleeding—under certain conditions—so much decried in our day, will be productive of good, while in animals specially constituted and circumstanced it will be productive of only serious results; that some are most benefited by salines with mild diuretics; while a third class seem to benefit by moderate stimulation, and a final group accord best with being left entirely to the recuperative powers of the system.

At one time not so long antecedent to our own, the remedy universally adopted in the treatment of pneumonia in all animals was blood-letting. Our most prominent teachers and reliable practitioners not only advised its employment, but its employment under all circumstances and in every condition, giving it as their opinion that anyone called to attend an animal suffering from pneumonia and neglecting to abstract blood was acting in a blameworthy manner. That any remedy, carried out thus unreflectingly, without regard to the many modifying influences which are ever in operation, should, in a not very lengthened period, come to be regarded with distrust, and ultimately with disgust, is not to be wondered at.

Now, although it does not appear that indiscriminate blood-letting, the constant exhibition of tartar emetic, aconite, or calomel and opium, the so-called antiphlogistic system of treatment, is all-potent to cut short an attack of pneumonia, or to promote its rapid resolution, we cannot doubt that cases do occur where the abstraction of blood is not only admissible but attended with much benefit

Whatever may have been the reason for the extensive employment of depletive measures in former days, whether it may be accounted for on the supposition that these morbid actions in which it appears to have played such a prominent part as a remedial measure were of a different type from the same processes now encountered, or whether animal constitutions and activities were so different from those of our day, it is probably not easy to tell

This, however, is certain, that a much less heroic and destructive system of treatment is now found to be productive of more beneficial results

In recommending for adoption what may be considered a rather simple line of treatment, I only state what, from experience, I feel satisfied is a preferable method, both on account of its efficacy in averting fatal results, and shortening the period of the disease

The lines upon which I have found it most advantageous to carry out the constitutional treatment of ordinary cases of pneumonia are

1. Locating the horse in a roomy box, where an endeavour is made to maintain an equable temperature

2 The body-temperature to be regulated by means of friction and clothing. The rugs and bandages ought to be

removed occasionally, and the surface-warmth promoted by
gentle friction with a soft hay-wisp or stable-towel

3. The febrile excitement and the processes of natural
elimination seem most successfully managed by the frequent
administration of moderate doses of saline diuretics and anodynes. I have found much benefit from the administration
three or four times daily of a draught composed of from four
to six fluid ounces of the solution of acetate of ammonia, two
drachms of chlorate or nitrate of potash, one or two fluid
ounces of spirits of nitric ether, with a scruple each of camphor
and belladonna extract in twelve ounces of water. Should
the irritability of the throat or the natural excitability of the
animal prevent the comfortable exhibition of the draught, the
preferable plan is to give the medicine in the form of an
electuary

4 Water, or weak and cold linseed-tea, to be allowed *ad
libitum,* in this may sometimes be given such medicines as
the simple salines recommended for the fever draught

5. The bowels to be kept moist by giving linseed-oil in the
food, or by the use of tepid-water enemata. Sulphate of magnesia in the drinking-water is, in some instances, deserving of
employment for this object.

6 When prostration is considerable towards the latter stages
of the disease, and when by extreme fœtor of the breath we judge
that gangrene and breaking-up of lung-tissue exists, moderate
stimulation is to be steadily carried out The stimulants,
whether alcoholic or ammoniacal, may be given alone with
water, gruel, or beef-tea, or added to the draught already
mentioned, if still receiving this

7 The food given during the course of the disease, and until
convalescence is established, to be light and easy of digestion;
green food, if obtainable, is to be preferred, or, when not procurable, a few sliced roots will do well, with bran and oats well
steamed with hot water, and sweet hay.

The employment of the febrifuge draught and salines ought
to be continued, regulated, of course, by individual symptoms
for some days, or until the pyrexia subsides or the crisis is
reached, which will probably be indicated by a softer and
somewhat moist condition of the skin, a lax state of the bowels,

or a marked increase in the secretion of urine, when they may be administered less frequently

When convalescence has been established, but considerable systemic weakness and inappetence remain, benefit will often be obtained from the administration twice daily of a ball composed of thirty grains of sulphate of quinine, and from one to two drachms each of powdered gentian and ginger

Local Applications—In the local treatment of pneumonia much benefit may be obtained by the employment of heat and moisture through means of woollen cloths wrung from warm water and retained around the chest for some hours daily When removed the parts ought to be well dried, and to avoid the evil results of cooling had better be smartly rubbed with soap liniment, or a compound of soap liniment and laudanum More active applications, as turpentine stupes, sinapisms, or cantharides preparations, have by many been unhesitatingly condemned as not merely worthless, but as likely to be productive of evil results at any stage of the disease

Now, without entering into the vexed question of the mode of operation of vesicants in such internal inflammations, I am forced to acknowledge, as the result of considerable experience, that I have encountered many cases of these morbid actions in the lungs and thoracic structures which have been much benefited by vesication The favourable action of these I have in many instances observed in from twelve to twenty-four hours, the number of the pulsations being lessened by one-third, and the temperature lowered two and even three degrees

It is worthy of notice, that those cases of pneumonia which are of the secondary character, or owe their existence to epizootic causes, are exceedingly obnoxious to blood-letting or other depletive measures , and that there is nothing so sure as that if we bleed and give purgatives, so will we greatly increase the fatality from the disease, while those which may survive are almost certain to make an indifferent recovery.

CHAPTER XXII.

ASTHMA.

Definition —*A peculiar diseased condition, marked by paroxysmal attacks of difficulty in breathing, often with much
distress, and a wheezing noise in the respiration; these
symptoms appearing to depend upon spasm of the encircling
bronchial muscles. The attacks are of uncertain occurrence
and duration; they may pass completely off, or they may be
prolonged into the aggregation of symptoms spoken of as
broken-wind.*

Nature and Causation —That a condition apparently dependent for its production on the existence of tonic or clonic
spasm of the bronchial muscular tissue may be encountered as
a distinct and separate affection in the horse I feel satisfied
That it has not oftener been specially alluded to I believe may
be accounted for from the facts—first, that it bears a close
resemblance in many of its features to what we speak of as
' broken-wind ,' second, because it not unfrequently appears as
a precursor of this latter condition. From these associations
it seems to me that it has usually been mixed up and confounded with that and the terms regarded as synonymous. In
making this separation I believe we are warranted both by the
symptoms and history of many cases, and by the manner in
which they severally respond to or are acted upon by therapeutic agents. That these conditions are dependent on different
or rather dissimilar, pathological states may not be so easy of
demonstration anatomically; still the differences in their
symptoms and development, together with the variations in
action upon them of similar therapeutic agents, seem to indicate
a non-similarity of textural lesions

In pure asthma the attacks are uncertain as to occurrence
and periods of duration, and they are in the same animal
usually separated from each other by considerable, often by
long intervals of time; they are truly intermittent. The same
cannot be said of ' broken-wind,' which, when once established
although marked by remission and accession of symptoms, is
never intermittent

The mingling in description and classification of these two

very different states, through the apparent similarity of their general symptoms, has been rendered easier by the circumstance that the spasmodic affection, 'asthma,' is not unfrequently prolonged into, or terminates in, that of the paralytic condition of the air-tubes and associated lung-structure which we call 'broken-wind;' also that this latter and persistent state may at any time be aggravated by an onset of a further attack of the spasmodic affection, extending to other and additional bronchial muscular structures.

The agents or influences which seem to operate in the production of asthma are very similar to those which are credited with the induction of the disturbance recognised as broken-wind; the chief of these are heredity, direct, and reflected nerve irritation. In many instances these operating agencies seem more occult in the spasmodic affection, and, when existing, less under the influence of treatment. In many I have believed them to be intimately dependent on fatigue and overwork, when in an unfit condition from debility or previously existing disturbance.

Symptoms—These are sudden in their development, distressing while they last, and uncertain in their duration. The dyspnœa, which is of a spasmodic character, so far resembles that of broken-wind that the inspiration is accomplished with greater freedom than the expiration, which is usually carried through in a jerking manner, with a less marked double action than in the latter affection. There is also here a more distinctly wheezing noise during the performance of the respiratory act, greater anxiety of expression, and exhaustion, with less cough, which, when emitted, is not so soft or hollow, but rather short, quick, and suppressed. The peculiar wheezing is very distinctly detected in auscultating both the anterior and lateral parts of the chest; and if emphysema is present, percussion may give an increased resonance. The more distinct or individual features are the suddenness of the appearance of the symptoms, their true spasmodic character, their marked accessions or decline in the same animal over a very short period of time, their severity, and their equally unaccountable disappearance.

When fully developed the constitutional disturbance is considerable, and the existence of fever, as indicated by the

thermometer, is well marked. When cough is at all troublesome, small patches or pellets of rather thick mucus are discharged from the nose, or found clinging to the nasal membrane. The chest, viewed as a whole, shows fixidity of position,
with increased movement of the abdominal muscles. In its
course this spasmodic condition is rather erratic—it may
continue for a few days or extend to weeks; and although it
may disappear, not to return for a considerable time, there are
often seen cases where it slides imperceptibly into that persistent state of peculiar disturbance of respiration known as
'broken-wind,' which, being now continuous, may yet be encroached upon at any period by a recurrence of the previous
acute dyspnœa, to again subside into the persistent state of
steady impairment of pulmonary nerve-power.

Treatment.—In this particular it is found that the condition
which we have regarded as asthma is more unlike that with
which we believe it has often been mixed up, viz, 'broken-
wind,' than in many other points. The former, characterized by
paroxysmal dyspnœa, and, as we believe, spasmodic contraction
of the minute air-tubes, when receiving benefit from medicinal
agents, which is not often, seems more directly under the
influence of agents which are of questionable value in the other.
The chief of these are stimulant anti-spasmodics, sedatives, and
depresso-motor agents, as mixtures and compounds of valerian,
æthers, bromides, chloroform, amyl, belladonna, etc. In the use of
these agents it is often found that what has been productive of
good in one animal will not be equally beneficial in another
apparently similarly affected; and that ere any good results
from treatment are obtained several remedies may have to be
tested. With many, when much distressed from the dyspnœa,
I have found as much good from a mild laxative, in conjunction with a smart vesicant to the sides, as from aught else.

CHAPTER XXIII

BROKEN WIND

WHEN viewing this diseased condition somewhat carefully there is a certain amount of difficulty experienced in giving it a place in any attempted methodical arrangement of diseases

In its most characteristic symptoms it is apparently so intimately associated with disturbed respiration, if not invariably with tissue-changes in the organs chiefly concerned in the performance of this function, that its place seems naturally amongst the diseases of these organs, where we now place it. Viewed again from another standpoint, and with the light furnished us by a study of the causes which seem to produce it, we might, with little violence to the subject, regard it as a disturbance of digestion or of innervation.

Definition —*A considerably disturbed condition of respiration, usually gradual in its development and non-inflammatory in its character, distinguished by distressed and spasmodic breathing, inspiration being executed easily and steadily, expiration protracted, and accomplished by a double effort. The dyspnœa is continued, but marked by remissions and accessions, not, however, intermittent, as in asthma, and is accompanied with a peculiar short, nervous, pathognomonic cough. These features are generally aggravated by association with gastric and occasionally with cardiac complications*

Pathology *a. Nature* —This is one of those diseases of the horse which has given rise to greater divergence of opinion as respects its nature than most others, and it seems very early in the history of the profession to have engaged the attention of those who made these diseases their study. Blaine, writing of it, says: 'It has been attributed to external and internal causes, to a defect and to a superabundance of vital energy; to altered structure of the heart, of the lungs, of the diaphragm, the stomach, the liver, etc It is a lesion with some, nervous with others, and simple distension with a third'

One reason why the opinions entertained as to the nature of the disease have been so different, is the fact that the examinations which have been made of the organs of animals notorious

33

as sufferers during life have yielded no uniform results. Changes of pulmonic structure, the result of inflammatory action, chronic or acute—because these have occasionally been encountered in certain cases of broken-wind—have been laid hold of and regarded as a fruitful source of the disease, as represented, it is believed, by the peculiar dyspnœa. Others, again, have attempted to explain both the disturbed functional activity represented by the spasmodic expiration and the most frequently occurring pulmonic lesion, emphysema, by reference to simple mechanical obstruction to the movements of the abdominal muscles, associated with defective muscular power.

Probably the theories of the pathology of this disease, or, if we choose to call them, the explanations of the mode in which the various morbid phenomena—the exhibition of which constitutes, to the majority, all that is known of the condition—are produced which have attracted and still retain the larger amount of support, may be briefly stated as—(1) That which ascribes all the morbid phenomena directly to structural pulmonic change, chiefly emphysema ; (2) That which attributes these to perverted innervation

1 The minute tissue-changes of the pulmonic structures, the existence of which have been taken as explanatory of the diagnostic features of broken-wind, are emphysema of the lung-tissue, interlobular or vesicular, or both The former of these conditions consists in the presence of air in the meshes of the delicate connective-tissue existing between the pulmonary lobules and the minute air-cells the latter is believed to consist in the dilatation of the ultimate air-cells with air, or the distension of contiguous air-cells with rupture of their intervening septa, and consequent union of two or more in a common cavity

In considering the bearing which these alterations of intimate lung-tissue have in explaining the nature of this disease, there are certain questions which demand from us a consideration and an answer It is needful that we determine whether these emphysematous conditions are invariably present in the lungs of all animals affected with broken-wind; and if so, whether this textural change in its extent bears a direct relation to the severity of the symptoms exhibited during life;

also whether every case of emphysema has been coincident with the phenomena usually understood to constitute broken-wind.

From personal examination and observation, as well as from what I have been able to glean from the experience of others, there seems little doubt that emphysema, particularly the vesicular form, does exist in many horses which have not at any period exhibited symptoms indicative of the condition known as broken-wind, also that a very large number of notoriously broken-winded animals have, on post-mortem examination, shown, in an unmistakable manner, pulmonary emphysema. Another, not such a numerous class, which during life were undoubtedly sufferers from this affection, did not, on after-death examination, give evidence of either emphysema or other structural pulmonic changes Further than this, with respect to the connection and relation subsisting between broken-wind and emphysema of lung-tissue, post-mortem examinations will not permit us to go

This hypothesis was first enunciated in the end of the last century, and was spoken of by the late Bracy Clark as having originated in connection with the post-mortem examination of an animal which had been sent to the London Veterinary College to be destroyed on account of this disease Although when carefully handled it may afford a somewhat plausible rendering of the mode of operation by which these pulmonary lesions may be regarded as inducing factors in the defective respiration, it is not altogether free from objection, while the various phenomena connected with the performance of the morbid respiratory act are, we believe, capable of a somewhat different interpretation

Although we may not refuse to regard the emphysematous condition of the lung-tissue in any other light than as an impediment to the due performance of the respiratory act, as also that probably the extent of respiratory derangement bears a very close relation to the extent of this abnormal condition, there is yet this to be remembered, that if the condition of emphysema with alteration of air-cell tissue and thickened mucous membrane, with an extra amount of secretion in the minute tubes, were the invariable accompaniment of the diseased condition known as broken-wind, then would the relation of these lesions to the pathognomonic dyspnœa and to the peculiar manner in which the act of respiration is executed be more easily understood

However, as it is tolerably certain that many cases during life exhibit all the characteristic symptoms of broken-wind, which on examination after death give no evidence of any of these structural changes, we are compelled to believe that the truly essential factor in the production of the distinctive dyspnœa and diagnostic expiration is not accounted for in these explanations offered of the various phenomena connected with this pulmonic tissue-change

2 Thus, although allowing that these textural changes of the pulmonary tissue may in many instances be accepted as sufficiently explanatory of the various morbid phenomena cognizable to our senses and by our means of observation, it seems that the acceptance of that other idea which regards this condition as essentially a disturbance or perversion of innervation consequent on certain dietetic conditions is more capable of accounting for the many changes both of function and structure, is less liable to objection, and as capable of including and explaining in a great measure these tissue-changes themselves This view of regarding broken-wind— often named asthma of the horse—as a disturbed condition of innervation directly traceable to gastric and intestinal derangement, although not new, has during the present generation been more strongly insisted upon by various teachers and writers on veterinary medicine, and although not universally received by those who have made the subject their study, is that explanation of the causation of the disease which seems most in accordance with observation and experiment Considered as paralysis of lung-tissue of the reflex character, we must look for the origin of the nervous disturbance in the gastro-intestinal tract, where from irritation and the impress of certain influences, partly mechanical, partly chemical, conveyed to the sensory nerves, and through them propagated to the centres of innervation in the medulla and brain, the influence so operating that the impulse or force conveyed through the efferent branches of the same nerve, the pneumo-gastric, becomes disturbed, perverted, or arrested in those structures to which these branches proceed

The contractile tissue of the lung, represented by the encircling involuntary muscles of the minute air-tubes, and which functionally are subservient to the expulsion of the air from the lungs, are dependent for their motor energy on the integrity of the nerve-centres and on the correctness of impressions conveyed to or from these centres The difference in the character and extent of impediment in the execution of expiration met with in different stages of the disease may be accounted for by supposing that at first these muscular structures of the minute bronchi are merely spasmodically contracted , that at a more advanced stage of the disease they become structurally altered, apparently atrophied, with certain changes of a degenerative character

This paralysis of the muscular tissue of the air-tubes, or the arrest of their contractile action induced by gastric irritation, will, in process of time, from the continued action of accessory agencies, as the compression carried out by the abdominal muscles operating on the air retained in the pulmonary alveoli, and aided by certain ulterior textural changes, tend to produce dilatation or rupture of the fine interconnective tissue of the air-lobules, thus permitting the passage of air into the partially destroyed structure.

The ulterior changes to which we refer are those of impaired nutrition of the pulmonary tissue consequent on arrested circulation in the interlobular pulmonary plexuses from distension of the lobes or cells , this disturbance of nutrition in the intimate texture of the lungs, tending to degenerative changes, will render the tissue more liable to be acted upon injuriously by retained and imperfectly expired air subject to repeated compression

It is from regarding the phenomena of broken-wind, or at least the peculiar dyspnœa characteristic of it, as the immediate result of extensive contraction of the smaller bronchi due to tonic spasm of their circular fibres, that the disease has come to be regarded as analogous to asthma in the human subject, to which it certainly bears a close resemblance in many of its features However, if we regard the term asthma as meaning a condition or assemblage of phenomena dependent on spasmodic contraction of the bronchial muscular tissue, we cannot accept this as the true pathology of the condition we call ' broken-wind ' It may, and, as stated previously, often does, seem to usher this state into existence; but once established, the condition of the minute air-tubes would appear to be the directly opposite of a state of spastic contraction. They are paralytically fixed, existing simply as inert conduits which are not capable of acting expulsively on their contents themselves, and only discharge this part of their function in as far as they are acted upon by other contractile agents

The phenomenon of the arrest of the expiratory act, and the second prolonged contraction of the abdominal muscles, one of the diagnostic symptoms of this disease in the horse, is probably better accounted for by regarding it as an extra expulsive effort employed to empty the paralytically fixed bronchi, than as the regularly recurring effort of the animal machine to rid itself of air extravasated or contained in interconnective cellular tissue or dilated air-cells

It is clearly an effort to overcome the existing dyspnœa, and obtain space for fresh atmospheric air ; so that the point to be determined really is, What is the cause of the dyspnœa ? is it difficulty of expiration from emphysema and distended air-vessels, or from some impairment of the normal contractile power of the pulmonary tissue ? I believe it follows more largely and more regularly from the latter cause The cough usually present in all cases of the disease is accounted for much in the same way as we explain the spasm of the bronchial muscular tissue, viz, as resulting from reflected nerve-action, the irritation seemingly proceeding in a great measure from the extra amount of the secretion in the air-passages, and the difficulty to get rid of this

In considering the varied phenomena of this disease, and the relations which they bear severally to each other, as well as that which any one bears to the whole, there ought not to be omitted from our reckoning the changes which so often occur in connection with other organs of the thorax, the heart in particular

These two views of the nature of broken-wind which we have now stated, although probably both true, and the latter more inclusive than the former, I am yet far from regarding as the whole or full statement of the truth. It would appear, viewing this diseased condition in its assemblage of phe-

nomena, that these ought not to be regarded as the expression
of any one constantly existing structural change ; rather that
they are to be accepted, these phenomena, this so-called
asthma or broken-wind, as merely the ordinary expression of
conditions of a rather variable nature It would appear to
be nearer the truth to view it merely as a symptom of several
diseased conditions, in all of which deficiency of contractile
power of the minute air-tubes and of the resilience of the
pulmonic structures is the one abiding condition Simple
emphysema of lung-tissue may induce such a state , disturbed innervation, the result of gastric disturbance and
disease, may prove even a more fruitful source, and be capable
of explaining more Still, I feel satisfied that the entire
assemblage of those symptoms we term broken-wind may
be met with, if not consequent on, certainly concomitant
with, various changes and alterations in pulmonic and bronchial tissue I have encountered such in cases of chronic
bronchitis, with thickening of the lining membrane, and other
textural alterations of the bronchial tubes, this bronchitis
resulting from a previous attack of acute bronchial inflammation Also where these changes were not consequent on antecedent inflammatory action, but developed gradually and
of themselves, or were the sequel of a steadily continued
mechanical irritation

The same may be said of true pulmonary disease, of cardiac
changes, or of centric nervous disturbance

b. Causation—While there appears little conformity even
amongst professional men as to the proximate cause of broken-
wind, there is, curiously enough, a wonderful concurrence of
opinion as to those conditions which, taken separately or together, seem to operate as more remote factors in the production of those recognised phenomena characteristic of, or which
together constitute, the diseased condition

Of these may be noticed—

1. *Heredity*—It is generally admitted to be true that to this
abnormal condition is attached a certain amount of disposition
or capability of propagation from parent to progeny Not that
those who support this idea suppose that the exact paralysis
of lung-tissue is received as an inheritance from parents, but
rather that, born with a certain bodily conformation or tem-

perament, the animals are, under the same conditions and surroundings, more liable to become sufferers from this particular disordered condition than others not possessed of the same congenital constitution.

2 *Breed* —It is rarely denied that broken-wind is peculiarly a disease of our coarser-bred horses, not, probably, because of their breed simply, but rather because of their subjection to influences which may more truly be ranked under the next group of causes

3. *Dietetic* —The most frequent sufferers from broken-wind are our agricultural horses, and others used for purposes of slow draught With these the food is often of a bulky, dusty, or innutritious nature, and where the animals are compelled to undergo exertion immediately succeeding a bulky meal and a full allowance of water

That defective dietetic conditions are largely operative in the production of disease in all animals we can easily enough understand, but that errors either as to quantity or quality should be specially operative in the production of this special disturbance, chiefly characterized by impeded respiratory function and not generally affecting the system, seems not so obvious It is to the special or particular effects of certain foods on particular organs, not to the general results of these foods, that we must turn for the true cause of this abnormal condition

By those who regard the emphysema and other textual changes of lung-structure as the direct and immediate cause of those symptoms which together are taken to represent this condition known as broken-wind, the distended and overloaded stomach is, by its mechanical bulk and pressure on the actively engaged lungs, believed to operate in the production of the pulmonary lesions.

By others the series of morbid phenomena which constitute the disease, although recognised as proceeding from the admitted gastric engorgement, are believed to have been reached in a somewhat different manner, not by physical embarrassment of pulmonary tissue and its subsequent disorganization, but by paralysis of lung-tissue the effect of reflected nerve-action resulting from peripheral irritation.

For many years during the earlier part of my professional

life in the Border counties, the agricultural horses were fed on oats, with hay or oat-straw, the fodder being given *ad libitum* in racks While this, a rather expensive system, was continued, broken-wind was a disease unknown

Some years since the chopping of both hay and oat straw for fodder began to be carried out, and with the extensive use of this, broken-wind became a comparatively common disease

So long as the horses are fed on part oat-straw and part hay, both cut rather long, matters are not so bad ; but when hay alone is used, and cut very short, the effect on horses is most destructive. There can be no doubt that even of the best quality, too much chopped hay is apt to induce broken-wind ; but the most serious results are encountered when the hay cut and given is bad in quality, too much heated, or even too old Here I believe much damage is done by the quantity of dust, which is not only swallowed with the hay, and operates injuriously through the stomach, but also by that which finds its way into the air-passages, and by direct irritation of the parts, further aggravates the disturbance That our lighter breeds of horses are not greater sufferers from broken-wind is entirely owing to the fewer opportunities they have of receiving damage from improper dietary I have seen well-bred animals, when fed on inferior, damaged, and dusty hay, and no means taken either to restrict the allowance or remove the dust and damaged parts, become in a short time distressingly affected with this disorder

4 *Structural Changes, the Result of a previously diseased Condition.*—Organic disease, the result of inflammatory action extending over a greater or more restricted portion of lung-tissue, may give origin to symptoms very much resembling, if not identical with, those of broken-wind. Whatever may arrest the contractile power and action of the pulmonary tissue chiefly resident in the smaller air-tubes, will simulate or induce this disease

Other structural alterations connected with the lungs or heart, tumours, etc, with other obscure diseases of nerve-structure, may of themselves, and directly in certain instances, induce a train of symptoms which may resemble the association of phenomena grouped under the name 'broken-wind'

That it does follow sudden and severe exertion in conditions
of the animal system where the lung-structure is unprepared
for such may be possible, but it is certainly not a common
mode of its production

c. *Anatomical Characters* — The anatomical characters
which are observable on examining animals which have died
while suffering from this disease are rather variable in character, but tolerably constant as to the organs where lesions
are usually met with

The extent of these changes does not seem to have a direct
relation to the severity of symptoms exhibited during life, or
the period over which these have been distributed   The
organs in connection with which we may expect to find alterations of structure are in the thorax—the lungs and heart; in the
abdomen—the gastro-intestinal canal, particularly the stomach

In many instances the examination of the lungs of horses
which have died during the earlier stages of broken-wind has
resulted in the discovery of nothing abnormal; others show
merely a deficiency of resilience, a slight want of colour, and
greater buoyancy when floated in water than normal pulmonary tissue

When the disease has existed for some time, the usual
appearances are pallor, retention to a great extent of bulk, and
indisposition to collapse, with emphysema, vesicular and interlobular   The former of these structural changes shows itself
as small bags or vesicles containing air beneath the enveloping
serous covering of the organs; these are irregularly distributed,
or they may be grouped together at particular situations;
the latter appears as an infiltration and distension with air of
the fine connective-tissue subsisting between the air-vesicles
and minute air-tubes; this air, by pressure, may be passed along
from one part of the connective-tissue to another   The minute
bronchi seem thickened, their walls in some appearing to have
undergone degenerative changes, while the larger air-tubes are
lessened in character from hypertrophy of the lining membrane   The pallor of the pulmonary tissue as a whole is
probably owing to the lessening of the blood-supply as well as
to intimate tissue-change, the interlobular emphysema, by
pressure on the capillary plexuses, having these effects   The
emphysematous condition of the lung-tissue is, as a rule,

more extensive than it appears; its amount is only discoverable by examining the tissue by means of sections made at different situations with a low magnifying power, embracing a rather extensive field, when the vesicles will be observed distended, as also the interconnective-tissue, and by their form pressing upon and altering the shape of those adjoining.

In the greater number of cases the heart is increased both in bulk and weight, the former being more marked than the latter, from the distension of the right side in particular

The stomach in chronic cases is greatly dilated, and the walls attenuated, with less secretion than natural, and having various particles of rather dry food adhering to the membrane Occasionally the intestines seem to partake, although in a less degree, of the same enlarged and dilated character as the stomach, seeming flabby and weak, as if wanting tone, while the contained material appears not to be undergoing a healthy transference into material fitted for assimilation, it is broken down and softened, but is either retained too short a time in the bowel, or the chemical changes are not of the normal character connected with healthy digestion

Symptoms —When fully developed, the symptoms by which this diseased condition is recognised are so well marked and so characteristic that they are rarely mistaken for those of any other disorder, save that which we have designated asthma, and which many regard as the same affection   In many cases, however, where the disease is not thoroughly pronounced, and where we may not be expecting to meet with it, even professional men may overlook symptoms which, when more carefully regarded, are sufficiently indicative of the disease   Those which may safely be regarded as diagnostic are—(1) *The character of the respiration* , (2) *The cough*

1 The most marked and characteristic symptom of brokenwind is the deficiency of expiratory power, shown by the laboured and difficult manner in which the air is expelled from the lungs succeeding inspiration   This difficulty is most observable when the animal is at rest, undisturbed and unexcited   Inspiration is performed easily and rather quickly   In animals slightly affected this rapidity may not be noticed unless contrasted with the succeeding part of the act of respiration ; in advanced cases the rapidity of the inspiratory move-

ment is very obvious, the posterior ribs and abdominal walls
receding from their upward and forward movement by a
simple fall   Expiration is prolonged and difficult , it commences by a sharp contraction and upward movement of the
posterior walls of the abdomen, which is suddenly arrested
when the act is half accomplished, and is immediately afterwards finished by a slow but continuous motion upwards and
forwards of the abdominal muscles, as if attempting to steadily
squeeze the contents of the chest. The expiration is thus a
double movement, not, however, invariably well marked

2. The cough of broken-wind is very peculiar, rather difficult to describe to those who have never heard it, but so
striking that when once recognised it is rarely mistaken.   It
has been described as a sort of grunt, an ejaculation through
the upper part of the trachea; it is short and suppressed, as if
arrested in the performance , of little volume or force, apparently from want of expulsive power, and is often accompanied
with forcible expulsion of gas from the anus   This cough at
the commencement and throughout the continuance of the
affection, is apt to be paroxysmal, and to follow slight exercise,
the act of drinking, or any trifling disturbance   When otherwise in good condition, and under no excitement, coughing
rarely occurs in fits, but is only heard at long intervals and in
solitary barks, arising from no appreciable cause.

Both the condition of impaired respiration and continuous
cough are liable to variation   They are more troublesome
after full feeding and a liberal supply of water   They are
subject to exacerbation with variations of atmospheric conditions and temperature , both extremes of heat and cold,
particularly when the latter is accompanied with wind, are
liable to induce aggravation of the symptoms

Auscultation over the thorax and region of the trachea gives
varying indications of altered conditions   In well-marked
cases, a loud sibilant tracheal noise may be distinctly heard,
standing by the side of the animal, without placing the ear
over the tube   The sounds discoverable by a careful auscultation of the chest vary much in different animals, and sometimes in the same animal on different examinations   In
nearly all cases we will find—(1) A distinct variation in sounds
accompanying inspiration and expiration, the former a cooing

or friction sound, the latter a very indistinct and weak murmur or crepitis; (2) Irregularly distributed sibilant or sonorous râles. Percussion shows increased resonance, not over all, but merely portions of the chest.

Indigestion and a distinctly unhealthy appearance of the whole animal are also indicative of the confirmed cases of broken-wind. The appetite may not be diminished, but the process of assimilation is disturbed, and the food which is eaten seems to be productive of no permanent benefit The bowels are tympanitic, and there is constant borborygmus ; the skin is scurfy and dry, with coat long, rough, and open. On being put to any exertion the animal shows weakness, perspires easily, bowels generally lax, with the discharge of much flatus.

In cases where cardiac complications are considerable, additional symptoms associated with such lesions are more or less attractive.

In a very great number of horses which ultimately become confirmedly broken-winded, the first indications are not those of impaired respiration, but of cough This cough may not at its first appearance be of the true diagnostic character, but is continuous and persistent, at last acquiring the true pathognomonic character and accompaniments.

Diagnosis—In confirmed forms of broken-wind there seems little chance of its being mistaken for any other disease The cough, together with the respiration, are so truly pathognomonic that, having once recognised them, they are not likely to be confounded with the cough or respiration of any other diseased condition

Asthma, as an affection distinct and independent, has been spoken of and described as a condition of perverted function, exceedingly like but not identical with this abnormal condition , it is the one with which it is more likely to be confounded than any other, both from the similarity of the general symptoms and the disposition which the one exhibits to pass into or terminate in the other The condition of lung-tissue as we regard it in these affections, when well marked and fully established, is probably diametrically opposite. In asthma there is contraction of minute air-tubes; in broken-wind there is paralytic and permanent dilatation.

In the former state functional power is often regained, in the latter rarely

Other features of difference have been noted when speaking of asthma

In the very early stages, when the cough alone exists to excite apprehension, I have certainly seen this symptom over-looked, or not understood as a sure prognostication of the results which were to follow, frequently being accepted as merely indicative of some trifling catarrhal condition, or of irritation of the fauces This may be avoided if attention is given to the act, and observation is made of its peculiar sup-pressed character, and its want of energy, with the presence of a sibilant râle, which can often be detected following the cough by placing the ear over the trachea.

Treatment.—Cases of broken-wind are often those in regard to which the advice of the professional man is sought, and although we may not be able to cure—*i.e*, to place the animal in the same position as to his powers of work-doing which he occupied previous to the invasion of the disease—we are yet satisfied that much may be accomplished to relieve the symp-toms which are distressing, and to 'fit the horse for being useful. To accomplish these ends our course must be directed and carried out by means which may be grouped as—
(1) *Dietetic* ; (2) *Therapeutic*

1 *Strict Attention to Dietary* —There is in the horse no condition of an abnormal character which is more subject to the influence of dietary than broken-wind ; and this influence is perfectly appreciable, not merely so long as the affection is confined to what we are in the habit of describing as functional disturbance, but also when it is certainly associated, if not de-pendent upon, structural change in various organs   This influence is not a matter of supposition, it is capable of demon-stration, the symptoms of disturbance being subject to abate-ment or aggravation in strict conformity with the nature of the food and state of the stomach and intestinal canal

The feeding of animals suffering from this disease, to be successful, must be conducted with the object of not overloading the stomach and bowel, keeping these in healthy functional activity with food of an appropriate character and fairly nutri-tious, together with the giving of this food, and also the water which is drunk, at periods which, as related to the work of the animal, will obviate physical discomfort, and not disturb functional action

2 *Therapeutic Treatment* —The amelioration of the symptoms of the disease is secured medicinally by the judicious administration of the greater number of those agents which improve the general health, and which confer tone on the digestive system in particular In this way it is probable that the majority of agents of the vegetable or mineral tonic classes are found beneficial , still there are certain agents which alone, or in combination, have a special mitigating effect on the distressing symptoms With some practitioners nux vomica, in moderate doses and continued for a week or ten days, is said to produce good results

For rapidity of action, ease of administration, and certainty of effect, I have found none superior to arsenic, given in gr i ss to gr ii , combined with bicarbonate of potash twice daily , or a better form is probably that of Fowler's solution, which can be given amongst the food or drinking-water This medicine has a wonderful effect in mitigating the dyspnœa, and in many cases restoring for a time the respiration to a healthy and natural condition Under its administration the cough will disappear, and the horse, enjoying vigorous health, will be able to perform his usual work with freedom and satisfaction All this improvement, however, is not permanent, and will, on the withdrawal of the arsenic, return as before.

The best method of employing this agent, I have found, is that of continuing its exhibition daily in the quantities mentioned for two weeks ; after this period, giving it only on alternate days, or even bi-weekly This moderate administration must be continued until the symptoms of disturbed breathing again appear, when we fall back upon the daily exhibition until these are ameliorated, when the quantity is again diminished by the less frequent doses, or by its withdrawal altogether, the medicine to be again employed when the symptoms are distressing. In this way I have given a horse arsenic continuously for eighteen months, with no apparent results save those of greatly mitigating the urgent dyspnœa attendant on a severe form of broken-wind, and thereby enabling him to work with comfort to himself and pleasure to his owner.

In addition to this or other treatment by specific or ordinary medicinal agents, the exhibition daily, in the food, of small doses of linseed-oil is always deserving of a trial.

In cases where a sudden accession of symptoms occurs from no appreciable cause, or as a sequel of a slight catarrhal attack good in all cases seems to follow the application to the sides of the chest of a smart cantharides liniment, and the exhibition of the usual febrifuge mixture of æther, acetate of ammonia camphor, and belladonna

When the urgent symptoms are relieved, the continuance for some time of such tonics as arsenic and nux vomica are indicated

---

CHAPTER XXIV.

PLEURISY—INFLAMMATION OF THE PLEURA.

Definition —*Inflammation, partial or general, of the serou membrane lining the thoracic cavity, and covering the viscera contained there It is characterized by the early appearance of febrile symptoms and local pain, shown when the horse i moved, or the chest percussed The morbid action is attended with effusion into the cavity of the pleural sac of serous fluid plastic material, or purulent liquid*

Pathology *a Causation* —The appearance of a pleuriti attack may, in numerous instances, be attributable to th operation of influences very similar to those which have bee indicated as connected with the development of pneumonia the greater number of which may be grouped under—
(1) Extension of an inflammatory action from parts connecte with or contiguous to the pleura ; (2) Direct irritation, result ing from injuries, or the existence of certain adventitiou growths in immediate connection with the membrane ; (3) Th action of a rapidly lowered temperature, and other meteoro logical disturbances ; (4) Blood-contaminations, as appear in in certain specific and constitutional diseases.

Like pneumonia, having regard to the mode of its origin, w

are disposed to speak of it as primary, or idiopathic, when arising suddenly, by an apparently direct attack upon the pleura, when the animal has previously been in good health , as secondary, or propagated, when immediately connected with some previously existing general or local disease

1 *Extension of Inflammatory Action from Parts connected with or contiguous to the Pleura* —This we observe to operate in many of those instances of complicated diseases of the viscera of the chest , for, as already observed, inflammation of the several structures entering into the composition of the lungs rarely occurs of a pure and simple character, but is ordinarily more fully developed in some one in particular, with a less distinctive character in those contiguous. In this manner we encounter pleurisy as associated with pneumonia and bronchitis, also with cardiac and pericardiac disease   This disposition to extend in virtue of contiguity of structure is more liable to show itself when the operating agency is of an epizootic character, or connected with previous disease of other viscera and distant structures

2 *Direct Irritation from Injuries and Morbid Growths* — Irritation sufficient to produce pleurisy may follow—(*a*) Wounds penetrating the walls of the thoracic cavity, or the laceration and constant friction occurring to the pleural membrane from fractured ribs , (*b*) Disturbance arising from the presence in the pleural sac of abnormal fluid, or the development in contact with the membrane of cancerous and other growths

3 *The Action of Cold and other adverse Meteorological Influences* —At one time, we may safely say, it was universally believed that the chief, if not the only, inducing factor in the production of pleurisy was exposure to cold, particularly when the animal body had been recently heated by exertion, and when the cold was accompanied with moisture. Now, however, there is a very general belief expressed, by pathologists of human medicine at least, that this idea ought to be largely modified, and that pleurisy, like many other inflammations of serous membranes, is probably more frequently the result of an essentially morbific state of the blood, and that cold and moisture play only a secondary part in its production   This idea has much to recommend it to the consideration of the comparative and to the purely veterinary pathologist , for we are

34

well aware that morbific influences, whether operating intrinsically or extrinsically on animals, are frequently accompanied
with specific inflammations of serous membranes generally
Still we cannot ignore the fact, that in many instances pleurisy,
in the animals which more properly come under our consideration, shows itself in situations and under conditions where its
existence is most satisfactorily explained by referring it to the
direct and immediate action of cold and exposure

It is a tolerably safe assertion to make, that pleurisy is chiefly
owing to the presence in the animal system of some specific
morbific agent, seeing such is often difficult to disprove. At the
same time we are well aware that it not unfrequently appears
as an accompaniment of such constitutional disturbances and
states of ill-health as pyæmia, suppurative arthritis, or suppurative phlebitis; that it is well known under certain not
understood and ill-defined conditions of both enzootic and
epizootic influences

Still, notwithstanding the evidences and the probabilities,
which together are strong, that in many cases of pleurisy succeeding exposure to cold, there exists in the animal affected
some specific diseased condition tending to particular localization of diseased action in special serous structures, it is difficult
to persuade those who have often witnessed its succession in
the horse to severe exertion, attended with subsequent exposure, that this same latter influence was not the chief and
direct agent in the production of this inflammatory state, apart
altogether from indwelling morbid conditions

4. *Blood-contaminations as appearing in certain Specific
and Constitutional Diseases* —The influences and agencies
represented by this last group of causes are, without doubt,
extensive and ever existing, although often inappreciable save
by their results   They include all which are spoken of as
diathetic, dietetic, infective, enzootic, and epizootic, and have
their representative results in association with such diseases as
rheumatism, pyæmia, and some specific fevers.

b Anatomical Characters.—Ordinarily, and in health, the
pleura is an all·but colourless membrane in itself, the colour
which we may imagine it to possess when viewing it *in situ*
being conferred upon it from subjacent textures and vessels.
When involved in inflammation the pleural vessels show them-

selves in a punctiform or radiated manner over patches of the membrane, the endothelium of which is still intact. Very often these newly appearing bloodvessels occur as a number of spots or streaks slightly elevated, and, steadily extending, at length by coalescence give to the membrane the appearance of a uniform redness more or less extensive

In all, save the mildest forms of pleuritic inflammation, the first effect upon the membrane, in addition to turgescence, is probably a state of dryness Very shortly this suspension of secretion is succeeded by an increased exudation of serous fluid, containing more or less plastic and organizable material, the true product of inflammatory action, with the effusion of this liquor sanguinis we have also an emigration or passage from the inflamed vessels of the corpuscular elements of the blood With this activity and change in the vascular structures we have certain alterations occurring in the membrane itself, the endothelial cells enlarge, multiply, rupture, and are shed, and these, mingling with older cell-elements, become mixed with the exuded fluid in the pleural sac The effect of these activities and changes is to give to the pleural membrane a roughened vascular appearance, very unlike its natural smooth and glistening character. This surface rapidly becomes coated with a layer of fibrinous material of a soft, velvety, or reticulated character, from which fluid continues to exude This condition, when occurring over the opposing surfaces of the sac, may, if liquid does not intervene, produce adhesion of the formerly separated membranes, or even when the fluid is not in great quantity, give rise to feeble attachments In some instances there may be little exuded fibrinous material present, but union may occur from the interconnection of the raised and papillated growths of the sub-endothelial tissue.

The effused material contained in the pleural sac is of variable amount, and at first is always turbid, from the quantity of emigrant leucocytes and endothelial cell-elements which probably proliferate in the effused material. When the inflammatory action is both severe and extensive, or when the amount of fluid in the cavity is great, so keeping separate the membrane covering the walls of the chest and the surface of the viscera, union will not ensue until the action somewhat

34—2

abates, and a partial removal of fluid takes place. In many instances, with the continuance of the morbid process in intensity, or even from a comparatively early stage, the same result, the prevention of adhesive action, occurs by the formation and presence of pus, the condition known as empyæma.

The period which may be expected to intervene between the first step of the morbid action and the appearance of the diseased products, effused fluid and the formation of false membranes, it is important to know has to some extent been determined by actual experiment. However, it is always good to remember that a certain amount of variation may exist as respects the course and completion of morbid processes induced experimentally, and such as may be developed without direct or mechanical interference.

From what is learned from symptoms exhibited during life, and comparing these with appearances observed after death, it would seem tolerably certain that vascular engorgement, with effusion of serous fluid, may be expected within a few hours after the onset of the pleuritis. While there is a certainty, from experiments which have been performed by inducing artificial inflammation of the pleura, that exudation of fibrinous material—false membranes—are developed in a certain form in twenty-four hours.

At first soft, granular, amorphous, and very friable, these pleuritic exudations or membranes steadily undergo change, until at the end of the first week they may show vascularity, and a steady and gradual solidification or toughening of their texture, and greater closeness of their attachment to the investing serous membrane. While, as they become supplied with bloodvessels—whatever way these are produced—we have from these a further and fresh exudation of fibrinous material, giving to the entire exudate a stratified character and appearance.

The liquid material found in the pleural sac, as the result of the inflammatory action, is as invariably a sequence of the diseased process as the existence of the solid exudate, the false membrane.

Chemically, it may be said to consist of the same materials as blood, although the relative proportion of these seems to vary according to the age or stage of the process at which it may be effused. In the earlier stages there would appear to exist in the pleuritic effusion a greater proportion of plastic and coagulable fibrinogenous material than at other periods, whilst it is at this time, also that we observe the colour of the liquid is darkest, being mingled with blood or blood-colouring from capillary hæmorrhage

Although there may be a gradual tendency with age for the fluid to become clearer, partly by the subsidence of the heavier particles and absorption of others, while the latter exudate is more purely serous, I am inclined to attribute this difference in character and colour in no small degree to original difference in the effusion itself, which again is closely related to the type of the diseased action

In all cases of pleurisy where the effusion into the pleural sac is considerable, we find that the pulmonary tissue has undergone considerable change. It is of less bulk, not so clear in colour, collapsed, and on manipulation has lost, to a greater or less extent, its resilience ; still it is not like the solidification of pneumonia, it may, as a rule, be inflated, the pulmonary vesicles not being destroyed When incised it is dry and light-coloured, and feels tough, both air-cells and intercellular tissue being free from infiltration or deposit This condition of collapse is chiefly the result of pressure of the pleuritic fluid, probably also influenced by the inflammatory action propagated to the integral pulmonic textures

Pleurisy may attack the membrane lining both cavities of the chest, or it may be confined to one, oftener the right When there is much serous fluid exuded into the pleural sac of one side, we may from the normal perforated condition of the pleural septum, the mediastinum, expect to find it at the same time occupying the other also. This is, however, not invariable, seeing that from the results of inflammatory action, this condition of perforation may be obliterated, and the fluid confined to the side where exuded ; or, in some instances, the liquid product may be enclosed in loculi or spaces formed by the more consistent exudate

Symptoms —In the horse, pleurisy in its acute form is readily known and well marked by several leading features Generally ushered in by some slight chilliness or more perfectly marked rigor, followed by fever, succeeded by quick and careful breathing. Accompanying these symptoms, or following close upon their appearance, may be restlessness and exhibition of pain; this pain seems aggravated by breathing, the inspiratory part of the act being cut short by coughing. A like exhibition of distress is induced by causing the animal to move round, and particularly so when the chest is manipulated or percussed

From the peculiarity in carrying out the inspiratory act by the fixing of the ribs and special action of the abdominal muscles, there is exhibited very early one of the most characteristic symptoms of the disease, a depression or line of demarcation running from the floor of the thorax at the posterior part of the sternum, in an oblique and upward direction, backward to the anterior iliac spine, known as the pleuritic or abdominal ridge

In the earlier stages the pulse, increased in frequency, is concentrated in its impulse, hard and vibratory. The mucous membranes are not altered much in colour, the mouth dry, internal temperature elevated three or four degrees, while the countenance is anxious-looking, expressive of pain, and the expired air is less hot than in pneumonia.

If at this time we apply the ear to the chest we may be able to hear the unnaturally dry membranes, the costal and pulmonary pleura rubbing against each other, and may even, in many instances, by placing the hand over the chest, feel the same movement—the 'friction sensation.' At the same time it will be found that the vesicular murmur is weak, from the imperfect manner in which it is performed. Percussion, when such can be carried out, which is not often, will give no appreciable difference of resonance

Very shortly the sounds heard by auscultation cease, either from return to health, the occurrence of adhesion between the membranes, or the presence of fluid in the cavity

With the occurrence of effusion the more active symptoms of pyrexia and pain subside The temperature may fall a little, the pulse will be less jarring and the appearance of the pleuritic ridge less distinct.

When the effusion is considerable, and the amount is little influenced by the natural absorptive powers of the system, or where the morbid activities still continue, the symptoms, although altered, are more serious

The pulse becomes increased in frequency and of smaller volume, probably eighty to ninety per minute, or irregular, the respirations are laboured, or dyspnœa may be distressing, the flanks heave excessively, and there is a peculiar lifting of the loins. The animal generally stands with his head protruded, the nostrils flapping synchronously with the heaving flanks, while dropsical swellings, appearing first at the inferior part of the chest, extend along the floor of the abdomen, and may ultimately invade the limbs, which usually remain of deathly coldness. That the dyspnœa and imperfectly performed respiratory function are owing to compression of lung-structure from the presence in the pleural sac of adventitious fluid, we are satisfied by auscultation and percussion.

Although the symptoms of acute pleurisy are tolerably attractive and diagnostic, there is no doubt that a latent morbid state of the pleural membrane not unfrequently exists, and proceeds to fatal results without giving much or any indication of structural alterations during life.

The knowledge of these facts ought to warn us that in all cases where indisposition proceeds from rather inappreciable causes, but where, from certain associations, suspicion may be directed to the chest, that the conditions of this cavity are not to be fully comprehended by the observation of rational symptoms alone, that nothing but a careful physical examination can satisfy us of the existence of very important structural changes occurring there.

Course and Terminations.—The period over which an attack of pleurisy may extend and yet terminate in recovery is very varied. The milder cases, where the inflammatory action is not severe, the surrounding influences favourable, and the animal's previous health good, may give evidence of recovery in a few days. The small amount of effusion has, on the suspension of the inflammation, been rapidly removed, and convalescence established within a week from the occurrence of the attack.

In others, again, the action may have been of a more violent character, the animal may have been possessed of less constitutional vigour, or the surroundings may have been decidedly depressing. In such the exudation is more likely to be copious, whether of the form of plastic organizable material or simply serous fluid   Here, after a longer period of convalescence, we may calculate upon a removal of a certain amount of the fluid exudate, we cannot, however, with anything like the same confidence, calculate upon the removal of the organizations, the false membranes and adhesions. These may, and often do, continue for life, and may prove obnoxious in future attacks of inflammatory action

When this almost invariable condition or sequel of inflammation of the pleura is of such an extent as seriously to interfere with the pulmonic function, and when unrelieved by absorption, we speak of the condition as dropsy of the chest, or *Hydrothorax*. When the morbid pleuritic action is from the first very intense, or from some peculiar specificity in connection with the action itself, or the influences brought to bear upon the animal, we have in association with the effused liquid a quantity of pus sufficient to give it a true purulent appearance, the condition is termed *Empyæma*

Diagnosis of Pleurisy.—Pleurisy may be distinguished from pneumonia and bronchitis by the evidence during the earlier stages of its invasion of a greater amount of pain and fever, by the harder and more incompressible nature of the pulse, the shorter and more painful cough   The respirations, which are simply accelerated in pneumonia, are never, unless complicated with the membranous inflammation, of the purely abdominal character we observe in pleurisy   In pleurisy we want the crepitant râle found existing in pneumonia, while when absence of sound is indicated by auscultation, we find that in the pleuritic affection it is the result of the presence of fluid in the pleural cavity, while in the pulmonic it usually arises from consolidation of lung-tissue

When occurring from solidification of lung-tissue, the absence of sound is not equally distributed, the respiratory noise being most marked farthest from the solidified portions, gradually becoming less distinct as the more perfectly obliterated air-cells are reached   When the deficiency or modification of sound is due to the presence of fluid in the chest, the absence or modification takes place, abruptly or at once, at a certain height from the floor of the thorax, indicative of the height to which the fluid has extended

In cases of extensive inflammation of the pleural membrane

we often have paroxysms of pain simulating abdominal disturbance; in pneumonia and inflammation of the mucous membrane of the respiratory organs this is not at all common

Treatment.—In the management of pleurisy, both hygienically and therapeutically, very much the same indications are to be observed as in those cases where we believe the substance proper of the lungs is specially the seat of the inflammation When we have regard to the character of the pulse, its greater resistance and more incompressible nature, together with the presence of acute pain, it is not difficult to understand why blood-letting as a proper and commendable measure in the active hyperæmic stage of pleurisy has more steadily held its position, and been more extensively employed by even careful practitioners, than in the condition of pneumonia

Although it would appear that the employment of venesection in no stage of either pleurisy or pneumonia is capable of arresting the disease, there is at least this to be said for it, viz., that when employed in the very early stages of pleurisy, while the pulse is yet firm and exudation hardly commenced, it has the effect, when carried to the extent of six or eight quarts, of conferring marked and immediate relief

It must be remembered, however, that its employment, even to a moderate extent and in the very early stages, is only admissible when the affection is of a sthenic type, and appearing in an animal in a vigorous habit of body, apparently originating idiopathically, and not associated with any constitutional disease, and where no adverse and depressing influences are in operation With these limitations, experience seems to warrant its employment, and to hold out reasonable expectation of favourable results

In all cases of pleurisy, of whatever character, it is well to give early attention to the locating of the animal A good comfortable box is to be preferred to confinement in a stall, while a sufficiency of body-clothing is conducive to the equalization of temperature and the normal action of the skin The moderation of the excessive arterial action, and lowering of the temperature, seem most readily and advantageously accomplished by the regular and repeated administration of such saline febrifuges as have already been recom-

mended in pneumonia   When this draught is given only
twice daily, one or two powders, containing two drachms each
of nitrate and chlorate of potash, may be administered between
the draughts; these are readily taken in the drinking-
water   When pain is a marked feature in the attack, a moderate amount of some soluble preparation of opium may be
given with benefit, or instead of the opium mixture, Fleming's
tincture of aconite may be administered every three hours
until relief is obtained, or at least until three doses have been
given if no relief has been obtained before   When fugitive
abdominal pain is troublesome, relief is afforded by employing
opium subcutaneously   To effect this purpose, forty minims
of the solutio morphiæ hypodermica B P , containing three
and a third grains of the morphia salt, are to be injected
into the subcutaneous tissue at the point of the sternum
This will usually afford immediate relief, and if not, may be
repeated in an hour   With the same end in view, to relieve
pain, it is desirable, at this stage of the disease, to assiduously
employ heat and moisture by means of woollen cloths wrung
from hot water and wrapped around the chest   In some instances the water thus employed may be medicated with tincture of opium.

In whatever way this is carried out, whether by poultices or
cloths wrung from hot water, the applications ought to be
made at least twice daily, two or three hours continuously;
and on their removal the sides ought to be dried and the
animal clothed, or have some compound soap liniment rubbed
smartly over the parts.

By many the treatment of pleurisy during the first week by
the administration twice daily of half a drachm of opium and
a scruple of calomel, is spoken highly of, but from my experience I cannot recommend this as superior, or even equal to
that already indicated, by saline febrifuges.

Following the defervescence of the premonitory fever, we
not unfrequently meet with cases where the conditions seem
stationary, the temperature, having fallen somewhat, still
remains high; inappetency continues, the secretion from the
kidneys is restricted, the respirations are embarrassed, and the
horse is languid and listless   In such I have invariably found
good to result from a moderate stimulation or vesication of the

chest by the application of a cataplasm of mustard-meal or the use of mild cantharides liniment, of which one application is all that is needful. By this treatment it is a common result to find pulse, respirations and temperature decidedly improved in twelve hours. Strong cantharides ointments, repeated applications of cantharides liniment, or even poultices of mustard, have always appeared to me to be productive of more harm than good at any stage of inflammation of thoracic organs. While, after employing both methods, I feel certain that all the benefits said to be derived from severe and repeated blistering can more surely be obtained by much simpler and less hurtful means.

At this particular stage, the subsidence of febrile action with lowered vital activity, and the presence most probably of effusion in the pleural sac, in conjunction with the stimulation of the chest a certain amount of stimulation internally may with safety be carried out, and for this purpose I have found nothing superior to some preparation of alcohol. From two to four fluid ounces of whisky or brandy added to the draught already recommended to be exhibited twice daily in water is a form convenient for administration. Or in place of one of those bi-daily draughts, one fluid ounce of the tincture or solution of the perchloride of iron in half a pint of cold water may be substituted, and the powders of nitrate and chlorate of potash may also at this time be replaced by drachm doses of iodide of potassium, which may be employed once or twice daily in the drinking-water.

During the earlier stages of the disease the horse may have whatever kind of food he seems most inclined to partake of, the only reservation being that it be easy of digestion and such as will keep the bowels in a natural or rather moist condition. When the febrile symptoms are abated, and exhaustion seems imminent, the quality of the food may partake of a more nutritive character.

By a carefully regulated regimen, and the exhibition of such medicines as we have indicated, it is wonderful what an amount of fluid may be absorbed from the pleural sac. During the employment of these it is often an advantage to give the patient a change ; thus, as an alternate medicine with the iron salt already recommended, sulphate of quinine and nitric acid will be found of benefit in all those cases wheie debility follows the subsidence of more acute symptoms.

In those cases of subacute pleuiisy, or, indeed, in any foim where the liquid effused into the pleural sac or sacs—*hydro-thorax*—does not become lessened or removed by absorption after a reasonable length of time has been allowed to transpire for the restorative powers of the system to come into opera-tion, assisted by the aids which we may have supplied, and when the amount of the effused material is such as to interfeie with the respiratory function, the question of instrumental interference for its removal comes into operation

Although it can hardly be considered a prudent practice, whenever we may be satisfied of the presence of liquid in the chest as the iesult of disease, to have iecourse at once to punc-turing the cavity with a view to its removal, there is also the opposite extreme into which we may fall, that of delaying the performance of the operation until the strength of the animal is so much reduced that collapse is almost certain to follow. The operation itself is a simple one, but is not invariably successful, rather the opposite, it may be that it is often too long delayed, or that, the cause upon which the exudation was dependent still existing, the removal of the adventitious material is followed by the outpouiing of moie   From what I have obseived of this condition in the horse, I feel disposed to think that we are oftener too hasty than remiss, and that in all cases a fair trial for three or four weeks ought to be given to well-considered remedies ere the operation is performed.   By some who have employed them, powdered cantharides from four to ten grains, with digitalis twenty to thirty grains, and nitrate of potash two diachms, made into ball, and given twice daily for a week, or alternated with a ferruginous tonic, have been highly spoken of.

The conditions, general and local, to which we ought to have regard in directing us whether or not we ought to resoit to this operation—paracentesis thoracis—and the stage of the ill-ness when it should be carried out, aie—(1) That the dyspnœa which exists depends upon the piesence of fluid in the pleural sac, that it is dangeious in its extent, and that it is disposed to increase, (2) That all oidinary means, dietetic and therapeutic, have failed to ielieve the distressing symptoms; (3) That the stamina and external surroundings of the patients are such as hold out fair prospects of success.

Having determined upon the removal of the fluid by tapping, the exact spot chosen to puncture is usually the eighth or ninth intercostal space, and midway between the bottom of the cavity and what is believed to be the superior limit of the fluid, this latter being detected by auscultation and percussion The instruments employed are either the ordinary trocar and canula, or the pneumatic aspirator. It is not needful to remove all the fluid in order to ensure permanent benefit, the abstraction of a moderate amount may in some instances give an impetus to the energies and hasten the removal of the remainder When considered needful the operation may be repeated in two or three days.

In all cases where this operation has been performed we will require for some time to be careful regarding the horse's dietary, it ought to be good, easy of assimilation, and such as is not likely to confine the bowels, while moderate but regular doses of some tonic medicine, with an occasional diuretic, are likely to be beneficial, and when the strength has sufficiently recovered, a mild dose of laxative medicine

This is one of those operations which, in the practice of both human and veterinary medicine, has been viewed and spoken of very differently By some it has been regarded as a trifling matter, and as usually attended with a large amount of good, by others it has been unsparingly condemned as one of the most misleading operations which can be performed upon any animal Very much, we suspect, depends on the cases upon which it is performed, their chances of recovery being largely influenced by the character of the disease upon which the effusion depends, as also upon the constitutional vigour of the animals affected, and various other obvious and inappreciable influences In cases such as we have already marked out, we cannot see there is much or any valid objection to be urged against its adoption, while the certainty that apart from some such treatment the majority of these would die, and the probability that from the operation a proportion might be enabled to outlive the morbid conditions, will ever warrant its adoption in all animals.

CHAPTER XXV

PHYSICAL EXAMINATION OF THE CIRCULATORY ORGANS, THE HEART CHIEFLY

In endeavouring, by observation and study of the condition and action of the heart, to obtain some knowledge indicative of general or special diseased states, we may, in addition to the assistance derived from observation of the sounds properly so-called both in health and disease, be further helped if we give attention to the information afforded by simple 'inspection' and 'palpation' By these we may judge of the position of the heart, the force or impulse of the pulsations, the changes of these in the great vessels of the neck, the frequency of the heart's action, and the regularity or constancy of its movements

To succeed to any extent, and to be even moderately accurate in our observations of cardiac action and sounds in the horse, great care is needful to ensure that the animal to be examined is not or has not lately been excited or disturbed, either by exercise or in any way to cause excitement or increase of cardiac function

I. CARDIAC IMPULSE

To determine the impulse of the heart, the hand, or stethoscope or ear, must be placed directly over the cardiac space of the thorax on the left side, and by either or both of these modes the position, the force or impulse, character and rhythm of the heart's action appreciated Allowance must be made for form of chest, extent to which the walls are clothed with soft tissue, and also for the breed of the animal

In considering the cardiac impulse the chief points for examination are—(1) *The position and area of occupation;* (2) *Force and character,* (3) *Rhythm.*

1 *Position and Definition* —The impulse may suffer alteration in position from causes directly connected with the heart-structures, or from changes acting from without the proper cardiac area The chief of these are—(*a*) Displacement of the organ forwards and upwards, from abdominal distension operating through pressure upon the diaphragm, (*b*) Displace-

ment in an upward and lateral direction , this may occur from collections of fluid in pericardium or chest, or from changes connected with the great vessels at the root of the lungs

The space over which the impulse is defined may be enlarged or diminished   It is increased in all cases of cardiac hypertrophy, and those of structural change of the pericardium with adhesions to the costal walls ; also, although of a feeble and muffled character, where pericardial effusion exists

2 *Force and Character* —(*a*) Increased impulse, impulse more forcible and sometimes over a greater space than in health, is detectable in many cases of structural change of the heart itself. It is well marked in most instances of hypertrophy with dilatation and valvular insufficiency, probably the most common form of cardiac disease in the horse In this condition the character of the impulse is peculiar and rather diagnostic ; it is not accomplished by a jerk, but is rather slow and steady, occasionally giving the impression of being double from its being prolonged through both systole and diastole of the ventricle, between which there is a short but perceptible pause   (*b*) Diminished impulse, appreciated by hand or eye, and usually circumscribed as to extent of area of distribution, is due to feebleness of the heart's action, and indicates disease of the muscular structure , in the horse this is usually softening from degenerative changes, or the diminution in force may arise from debility, systemic or cardiac, and where there is thinning of the walls of the heart's cavities , also from the presence of fluid in the pericardial sac   Further, it has been found much diminished where the pericardium had contracted adhesions to the lung-structures or the pleura of the right side

3 *Rhythm* —This may suffer disturbance in several ways. (*a*) There may be irregularity as to character, force, or time , (*b*) The irregularity may have respect to the relation which the impulse ought to bear to the ventricular systole

II AUSCULTATION OF THE HEART

A **Sounds of the Heart** —The sounds proper connected with the heart are understood and, with some differences of opinion I am aware, are accepted as the result of certain movements of the heart or particular parts of its structure in connection with the blood contained in the cavities, and the action of the muscular structure on this The phenomena connected with the action of the heart are in the majority of instances quite distinctive and capable of appreciation, while, for the intelligent comprehension of the changes connected with that action in disease, the more salient points connected with it ought to be borne in mind

The contraction of the auricles is simultaneous ; the contraction of the right and left ventricle succeeds that of the auricles, and is synchronous

The muscular fibres of each part relax immediately following their contraction, and a distinct period of repose intervenes between the contraction of the ventricles and secondary contraction of the auricles Thus, if we start with this interval of repose, the general cardiac diastole, we find that the two pouches are being filled with blood from the great venous trunks When sufficiently full, the auricles contract and send a portion of the blood they contain into the ventricles, and these, immediately contracting, send the blood into the arterial tubes This passage of blood into arteries is a necessary consequence of the contraction of the ventricles, for with their contraction is the raising of the auriculo-ventricular valves which prevent the return of the blood into the auricles ; the blood is thus forced into the arterial openings, the valves of which are opened by the impulse of the liquid When the heart returns to a state of repose the blood is prevented from returning to the ventricular cavities by the dropping of the uplifted valves

By the term *systole* is meant the contraction of the walls of the heart's cavities ; by *diastole*, the respose or relaxation of the same

It is thus that each complete revolution of the heart, or entire performance of its circle of function or action, is indicated by two successive sounds, between which are two intervals of repose The sounds are unlike, and the intervals of silence vary in duration

The first or systolic sound is prolonged as compared with the second, and of a dull character, and is immediately succeeded by a very short interval of silence, followed by the diastole or second sound, short and sharp, followed by a more appreciable period of rest, to which succeeds the systolic sound again

The first sound, whatever caused by, is coincident with the contraction of the ventricles and the impulse of the heart against the walls of the thorax The second sound corresponds with diastole of the ventricles and the recedence of the heart from the side

The natural sounds may in disease be variously modified (*a*) They may be altered in intensity and power, being either increased and prolonged, as in hypertrophy, excitation of the heart's action, and in some blood-changes , or they may be diminished and lessened, as in weakness, atrophy, and degenerative changes of the muscular structure of the heart (*b*) They may be modified in character or quality ; the tones may be high-pitched and clear, or muffled and indistinct (*c*) Their rhythm or regularity may be destroyed, as in diseases of the valves and orifices

B **Cardiac Murmurs**—More strikingly abnormal, however, than the alteration of the natural sounds are those which in disease we find so often added to them, the so-called *cardiac murmurs* These may occur in conjunction with one or other of the natural sounds, or they may altogether usurp their place

From their supposed origin, or the mode in which these sounds or murmurs are produced, they are spoken of as— (1) *Valvular* or *endocardial* , (2) *Pericardial* or *exocardial*

1 *Endocardial or Valvular Sounds.*—These sounds as a class give out a uniform *blowing, rasping*, or *bellows* character, from which impression they have come to be spoken of as bellows-murmurs They are called valvular sounds because of their nearly uniform origin from valvular defect or disease

The chief structural changes from which these bellows-murmurs are supposed to proceed are—(*a*) Simple dilatation of natural orifices , (*b*) Simple contraction of natural orifices , (*c*) Simple roughness of valvular or endocardial surfaces , (*d*) The association of either of the former conditions with the latter

Valvular murmurs, when believed to be associated with any of these conditions, are spoken of as *structural* or *organic murmurs*, to distinguish them from abnormal murmurs not

35

traceable to structural changes, and believed to be intimately connected with constitutional causes, with peculiar states of the blood, or with functional impairment of the heart itself, and named *inorganic* or *functional murmurs*

These murmurs or bellows-sounds being essentially connected with the great valvular orifices of the heart, we can easily understand how each orifice may be the seat of two distinct murmurs—(1) *Constrictive*, (2) *Regurgitative* One with the current, one against it, the blood in the one instance not being allowed a free passage, in the other not being effectually prevented from returning In this way eight murmurs only are possible As I do not, however, believe that with the horse it is possible to separate and differentiate these eight distinct possible morbid sounds, it is scarcely worth wasting time in going through them in detail, but I will merely mention shortly those we most commonly encounter, and of the existence of which I believe it is in many cases possible to satisfy ourselves.

a. Probably the most frequently encountered and most pronounced of these bellows-murmurs is that which may be heard accompanying, or immediately following, or sliding away from the first sound—the ventricle systole, and hence called '*a ventricular systolic murmur*'

This, as will be understood, may have its origin either in the auriculo-ventricular or in the arterial orifices If in the auriculo-ventricular, it is a murmur of regurgitation, if in the arterial opening, it is a murmur of obstruction This sound may thus be indicative of insufficiency, or disease of the mitral valve, disease of the aortic valvular opening, either constrictive or the result of endocardial roughness, also from collections of fibrinous coagula amongst the chordæ tendineæ.

This is ordinarily a murmur of considerable intensity, it is high-pitched and prolonged, particularly so when associated, as it sometimes is, with hypertrophy of the ventricle Its existence has been most frequently noticed by me in cases of insufficiency of the mitral valve consequent upon hypertrophy with dilatation It will also be heard in those instances where, although insufficiency does not exist, there is yet disease of the ventricular surface of the valve, generally in the form of puckering and thickening of the endocardial membrane of the

valve, or that of warty vegetations or excrescences In cases
where considerable collections of fibrinous coagula have been
found in the ventricles, and largely entangled amongst the
chordæ tendineæ, and which from their character appear not
to be post-mortem conditions, this systolic ventricular murmur
has been heard

I have heard it in a horse affected with disease of the
tricuspid auriculo-ventricular valve, there being also less extensive disease of the left side

b When the murmur coincides with or runs off from the
second sound, known as the '*ventricular diastolic*,' it may be
produced in either the auriculo-ventricular or arterial openings It coincides with the dilatation or filling of the ventricles if auriculo-ventricular, it is a murmur of obstruction,
if in the arterial openings, a murmur of regurgitation.

This bellows-sound accompanying the second sound of the
heart seems chiefly indicative of aortic insufficiency from
warty growths situated on the edge of the festoons, and from
a similar condition or a merely roughened auricular surface of
the mitral, or, more rarely, the tricuspid valve

c. When the murmur is continuous during both sounds, or
properly speaking double, it is spoken of as '*a ventricular
systolic and diastolic murmur*,' a condition not of uncommon
occurrence in the horse With the existence of this sound, we
may suspect aortic insufficiency and mitral obstruction

2 *Exocardial or Pericardial Murmurs, or Friction-sounds*
—These are not unlike the analogous abnormal pleural sounds,
and when heard give the impression, varying in character,
tone, and pitch, of friction or rubbing They are synchronous
with the heart's action, and may be systolic or diastolic, or
both, in this way seeming double from the short pause which
occurs between the acts

They are considered indicative of pericardial inflammation
in its earlier stages, or at least without much effusion or
adhesion

They are not invariably continuous, but may disappear after
existing for a few days, probably owing to the occurrence of
effusion, while, when existing, they rarely overpower or mask
the true cardiac sounds

We have to remember always that in disease of other

35—2

organs of the thorax all cardiac sounds become modified or altered

In consolidation of pulmonary tissue, and in case of effusion into the pleural sac, these sounds are, as a rule, intensified; they are somewhat diminished in severe cases of pulmonary emphysema.

CHAPTER XXVI

GENERAL SYMPTOMS AND FORMS OF CARDIAC DISEASE

IN a few forms of heart disease, chiefly such as result from traumatic lesions, fatal results may be reached apart from the development of any very obvious general disturbance. When symptoms pointing to any serious lesion show themselves, they are generally of short duration.

Ordinarily, however, the common acute affections, those largely partaking of inflammatory action, and in which the membranous structures of the organ are chiefly involved, are accompanied with well-marked fever of a varying character. By far the greater number of cardiac diseases marked by more or less extensive structural changes, and which may be said to compose the greater number of the affections, are of a chronic character, and have invariably, in a more or less perfectly developed form, certain general symptoms connected with them.

Languor, lassitude, and impeded respiration, approaching to or actually culminating in dyspnœa when made to undergo any severe exertion, are very general features of such cases. The horse, although perfectly susceptible of being excited, is rather disposed to remain undisturbed; and when engaged in active work, and following its completion, shows muscular weakness, or, it may be, decided muscular exhaustion. The impeded respiration occurring during active exertion or severe work may be, and often is, taken for a defective condition of the respiratory functions, and not attributed to the true cause, impaired cardiac power. It may, however, be differentiated from the same disturbance arising from disease of the respiratory organs by the absence of fever and cough, and from the presence of an unequal, irregular, or intermittent pulse and cardiac action

Many of these cases, while at rest in the stable, give little indication of the extent of the cardiac mischief which exists; but when put to work or rapid movement on unequal or heavy ground, the dyspnœa may be so great as completely to incapacitate for further progression until the cardiac oppression is somewhat removed

Such animals are generally sufferers from valvular insufficiency of the right auriculo-ventricular opening, with dilatation of the same side Others, again, are disposed to exhibit symptoms of what are usually known as fainting-fits, syncope, or vertiginous seizures

These attacks may be developed equally when the horse is at rest and in the stable, as when at work—most probably of more frequent occurrence in the latter condition. Even then they may be distinguished from the ordinary attacks of vertigo connected with cerebral disturbance Their occurrence is generally the occasion of directing attention to the examination of the pulse and heart's action, hitherto unattended to, when most probably both will be found abnormal, exhibiting varying characters of inequality and irregularity of sequence

In cardiac diseases generally we have often indications of the irregularity and insufficiency of the circulatory functions by the persistent coldness of the extremities, and the appearance of œdema, first of the limbs, and at length of the inferior thoracic and abdominal regions, which, although continuous and persistent from the time of its appearance, is often of varying extent and severity

These general symptoms of heart disease, either of its membranes or more intimate structures, occur with different degrees of frequency and severity, according to the characters of the affections and the structures more immediately attacked.

Cardiac diseases in the aggregate are usually regarded as involving either the heart proper, or as confined to the true cardiac membranes and their appendages The diseases of the heart itself may be—(a) Of the nature of functional disturbance; or (b) The result of structural alteration. And both disease of heart and membranes may be acute or chronic.

CHAPTER XXVII

FUNCTIONAL DISORDERS OF THE HEART

I PALPITATION

UNDER this group is intended to be placed such disturbances of the normal activities of the heart as are believed to be unconnected with alterations of structure The consideration of these is chiefly important from the resemblance which disturbance of this character bears to structural change, and from the difficulty which so often exists in distinguishing between these very different conditions

The usual form in which functional disturbance of the heart presents itself to our notice is that of palpitation—tumultuous and irregular cardiac action, sometimes associated with peculiar cardiac sounds, and irregular character of the heart's action and of the arterial pulsations These symptoms, from the frequency of their occurrence and their connection with organic disease of the heart, derive an importance which they would not otherwise command, seeing that of themselves, and apart from this association, they are, as a rule, not of serious moment

Causation—This disturbance of the rhythmic action of the heart and of its functional activity is the result of various causes acting upon the system generally or upon the heart individually (a) It may occur in connection with disease, acute or chronic, of the heart or its covering, inducing defective power, or from obstruction at some of the orifices, which its muscular exertion cannot overcome (b) It is occasionally associated with disease of the lungs, in which the power of the organ is overcome by pulmonary obstruction (c) Changes in the quantity or quality of the blood, as anæmia, plethora, or special contaminations, may induce this disturbance. This latter effect is observed in certain specific, constitutional, and epizootic diseases (d) Influences operating through the nervous system have the power to produce similar results   These may be intrinsic, centric, or reflex   These latter are observed in intestinal disturbances, acute or chronic, with the existence of which they are closely bound up, usually disappearing when they are removed.

The former, besides being in many instances rather occult

and somewhat varying as to their modes of operation, are in the horse of more frequent occurrence than has hitherto been recognised They are in him intimately connected with hard work, particularly work of a fast and exciting character, the excitation and suddenness which attends its execution seeming to have a direct influence upon all animals, although more distinct and appreciable with some than others

In many of its forms nervous irritability or palpitation, although very troublesome and somewhat inexplicable, often seemingly connected with disturbance of the normal relations which ought to subsist between the vagus nerve and the cardiac ganglia, is yet more susceptible of management and successful treatment than the cases dependent upon structural disease of the heart or pericardium, where the opposition offered to the flow of the blood is greater than the power at command to drive it.

Symptoms—Palpitation is ordinarily accompanied with increased frequency and apparent force of the heart's action The action may be regular, or the irregularity may partake of alteration either in force, quickness, or frequency, often passing into the more advanced condition of cardiac failure, intermittency. The irregularity and intermittency may regularly pass through a certain cycle in a given time, or the cardiac action may seem completely confused The palpitation may be continuous, or occurring only at intervals, or in paroxysms, depending upon the causes of its development, or upon some very obvious immediately exciting influences Although actual pain is rarely a marked feature, there are usually observed such general symptoms as anxiety, restlessness, and hurried breathing, while in paroxysmal seizures, dependent on nervous irritability and disturbance, I have observed faintness and actual syncope

In some the arterial pulse will indicate, by responsive throbs, the heart's action; in others the pulsatory wave is weak or feeble, while the cardiac action is tumultuous, or regurgitative action in the large veins of the neck may be the most distinctive feature; this latter feature is particularly the case when the condition has been of some time standing, and the right heart is structurally impaired

Treatment—This disturbance of function and perversion of

cardiac rhythm will of course, when unconnected with alteration of structure, disappear when the causes of its production
are removed   When of a permanent character, and accompanied with other symptoms, as sudden seizures of exhaustion,
syncope, or dyspnœa, then its merely functional character may
well be doubted   In such cases the probabilities are that the
disturbance is the result of organic changes.

In palpitation and disturbance of cardiac rhythm, the result
of anæmia and debility, where the whole volume of the circulating blood may be diminished, or what is more generally the
case, where the formed materials of it are lessened in amount
and the blood is poor and thin, a condition found associated
with serious and wasting diseases, and where peculiar blood
sounds—anæmic murmurs—exist, treatment is usually advisable   In this state, unaccompanied with organic change,
we may speak with tolerable certainty, and give fair hope of
ultimate recovery through the use of good, easily digested
food, together with rest, and the exhibition of tonics, of which
the chief are the preparations of iron   Although this condition often presents itself as a sequel of influenza, we must not
forget the great liability there is in this fever to alteration of
the true cardiac structures.

The same general principles, by whatever means we may
propose to carry into action the details, must regulate our
management of those cases where the disturbance of cardiac
action is the result of perverted or vitiated blood   An endeavour
must be made to discharge the vitiating agent, while the
production and elaboration of healthy blood must be fostered,
so that a normal and pure stimulus may be furnished to the
great central circulatory organ, as well as sound food supplied
to the whole body   For the attainment of this end the same
means as already indicated are to be employed—good food,
correct sanitary conditions, mild stimulants, together with
regular doses of some salt of iron, which may, with advantage,
be alternated with arsenic   The forms of palpitation associated
with dyspepsia and acute indigestion will disappear when the
disturbed assimilation which operates in its production has
disappeared

In the management and medical treatment of those cases of
functional disturbance of the heart believed to be the result of

excited or perverted nerve-power, probably more discrimination is needful than in some of the others They generally
appear suddenly as a rather serious matter, and are often taken
for functional disturbance of an entirely different character.
They are most successfully combated by rest with perfect
quietude, and a moderate amount of opening medicine, followed
by the exhibition twice daily of a ball containing twenty grains
each of powdered digitalis, extract of belladonna and opium.
Where the palpitation is excessive, dilute prussic acid half a
drachm, or Fleming's tincture of aconite five or ten minims,
the former given in cold water, and the latter in bolus, every
two hours until the excessive cardiac action and excitement
has been subdued, will probably be more effectual The rest
and quietude ought to be continued not merely while the
disease or disturbance is under treatment, but for some time
afterwards, so as to avoid a recurrence of the seizures which
we have seen occur when put to work too hastily Palpitation arising from change of pulmonary or cardiac structures
must not be treated apart from a consideration of the lesions
upon which it is believed to depend

II SYNCOPE—FAINTING

This condition, which is essentially and primarily dependent
on failure of the heart's action, followed by the effects of a
defective supply of blood to the nervous centres and arrested
pulmonary action, is rarely encountered in the horse I have
only seen it in a few instances—(a) As the result of uterine
hæmorrhage , (b) Accompanying rapid abstraction of blood in
certain cases from the jugular vein, (c) Upon the entrance of
air into the circulation in blood-letting.
    The treatment consists in the employment of diffusible
stimulants, dashing cold water over the head, application of
ammonia to the nostrils, friction to the surface of the body, and
in some cases an attempt, as in man, might be made, by
pressure upon the large vessels of the neck, to confine the blood
to the central parts

CHAPTER XXVIII.

DISEASES OF THE PERICARDIUM

I. ACUTE PERICARDITIS

Definition—*An active inflammatory condition affecting the fibro-serous investing membrane of the heart.*

Pathology. *a. Causation*—Inflammation of the investing and containing membrane of the heart, although it may appear as a primary or idiopathic disease, depending for its production, in acute forms, upon cold, exposure, and fatigue, is more frequently observed as a secondary or symptomatic affection developed as the result of, or in intimate association with, such conditions as—(1) Certain general diseases and blood-contaminations, particularly rheumatic fever, strangles, influenza, purpura, and many pyæmic and septic conditions; (2) From extension of inflammation from contiguous structures, as the lungs and pleura; (3) From the irritation incident to the development of new formations, as cancer, or the appearance of parasitic growths; (4) Penetrating wounds inflicted by bodies from without, or by fractured ribs.

Of all these causes or influences, probably the most potent as affecting the horse are the rheumatic; while, wherever these are in operation, either in the form of acute rheumatism, or of epizootic catarrhal fever with a rheumatoid tendency, the induced diseased action is very often complicated and accompanied with the involvement of other fibro-serous structures.

b. Anatomical Characters—Not only is the nature of the inflammatory action which seizes on this fibro-serous structure of the heart very various in the intensity of its action and the symptoms which it may exhibit during its development, but the structural changes which accompany, or are the result of it, vary in a similar manner. Although inflammatory action here may, in a general sense, be said to run a similar course to that which is observed in serous membranes generally, it is yet to be observed that its products and textural changes are modified by the constant movement which exists between the heart and its enclosing capsule. In studying these results we ought not merely to confine our attention to the membrane, or the fluid, or other products found in the cavity, but we ought to take into consideration the state of the tissues in contiguity with these The diseased action once started may, in a comparatively short period, subside, and the textures return to their normal condition Usually, however, following the hyperæmic state, a considerable quantity of both serous fluid and lymph are poured out, and are found in varying proportions in connection with the membrane and the sac which it goes to form The quantity may be trifling in amount, and may be readily absorbed; it may be considerable, and by its mechanical presence act adversely on the functional power of the heart, and may even tend to impair the integrity of its muscular fibres. Very often accompanying this fluid there is a greater or less amount of lymph of varying character and consistence, which may sometimes exist in greater amount than the more watery elements of the exudation At other times the power and capacity for organization of this plastic material is greater, or the amount of fluid being less, the surfaces, visceral and parietal, become coated with an adhesive material, by which they become glued together, and these adhesions of a more or less perfect character are extensively distributed over the membrane intermingling with the contained fluid The tendency to exudation of a plastic but only moderately-well fibrillated material is very great in pericarditis so much so, that in all animals a very frequent form which this assumes is that of being completely spread over the heart's surface, but only forming a very loose attachment to the pericardial sac When distributed in this manner it invariably assumes a reticulated or honeycomb appearance, extremely characteristic, and of considerable thickness, though, as already stated, of not much tenacity, and easily detached from the pericardium

Occasionally pus is mingled with the inflammatory products, or they are stained with blood, evidently from the newly-formed vessels in the friable exudate, which have given way, or from the congested and inflamed capillaries of the primarily involved serous membrane

In the acute rheumatic and epizootic cases of pericarditis the muscular tissue of the heart, together with the endo-cardial membrane and valves, are involved to a greater or less extent The muscular tissue seems to undergo a change both in appearance and consistence, it is of a dark or dirty brown colour, and when cut into is easily lacerated, seeming to want cohesion, and having always, from the want of muscular power and tenacity, a tendency to favour dilatation of the cardiac cavities The white spots or patches known as 'milk-spots,' so often seen on the surface of the heart, are usually ascribed to diffuse and patchy pericarditis Their intimate character is not always similar, while their presence is so often observed in hearts where the probabilities of the existence of a previous inflammatory action are very remote, that I am disposed to regard them, if not always, at least in certain instances, as owing their existence to rather different conditions

Symptoms—The indications afforded us, either through the occurrence of constitutional disturbance or peculiar local or physical signs, of the existence of this diseased state of the pericardium are exceedingly variable in their expression, while it is doubtful if there are any of these which in the horse may be entitled to be regarded as diagnostic In certain instances, when unassociated with general or constitutional disease, the symptoms may be decidedly obscure, not at all indicative of the involvement in disease of structures so essential to life as the heart and its covering When occurring associated with such general diseases as rheumatism, influenza, and extensive renal disturbance, the existence of inflammation of the pericardium is sometimes indicated by symptoms not easily mistaken It is seldom, however, if we had merely to depend upon either physical, local, or functional disturbance, that we would be warranted in giving anything like a decided opinion

The much depended upon to-and-fro friction-sound, and the increased systolic bellows-murmur existing in the human subject when suffering from pericarditis, are in the horse rarely heard of such well-defined characters as to entitle us to speak with confidence, and when detected, it is probably owing to the fact that other concomitant circumstances have led us to expect them, rather than from the nature of the sounds themselves

When connected with the sthenic fever of simple rheumatism, or, indeed, when occurring at any time apart from the adverse and preceding influence of some constitutional cachexia, pericarditis is ushered in with considerable febrile symptoms, and a rather hard or harsh pulse, somewhat increased in frequency; there is also pain, particularly when made to change position, the respiration is disturbed, or there may be distressing dyspnœa

When the inflammatory action is moderate in character, when the fibrinous exudate has not been excessive, and the amount of serous fluid secreted is trifling, we may have only moderate constitutional disturbance and inappreciable local signs of disease Of this we are satisfied by after-death examinations.

When, however, the effusion has been considerable, pressing upon and impeding the functional activity of the heart, while the muscular tissue has undergone change with adhesions and organizations of exudate distributed over a large space, we may have a different train of symptoms Fever is still marked, but the pulse is altered, having lost its hard or harsh character, becoming feeble, fluttering, unequal and irregular; we may have both carotid pulsation and jugular regurgitation, with distressing dyspnœa, all indicative of obstruction in the thoracic circulation.

There is also often cough, much debility, coldness of the limbs, with œdema both of these and of the trunk It is always necessary to bear in mind that we must not be governed by a consideration of any one separate symptom, seeing that many of these, both general and local are found accompanying diseased conditions of other organs of the thoracic cavity

In that particular form of influenza-fever or distemper in which the serous and fibro-serous structures of the body are largely involved, and which in particular seasons and certain districts appears as an epizooty, a very prominent and serious complication or symptom is pericarditis Here the symptoms may not at once attract attention to this particular structure as being largely involved, and they are often much mingled with those indicative of the involvement of other structures and organs, both of the thorax and elsewhere

In these cases the physical or local signs of this condition are sometimes very well marked, at others very much disguised They are well marked when there is little involvement of the lungs and pleura, and they are much obscured when these structures are extensively diseased. In all, the general disturbance is sufficient to direct our attention to the state of the heart. There is feebleness and deficiency of tone and force both in the heart's action and in the pulsations; this change of character in the circulatory forces is of gradual but steady development, until the inequality and irregularity terminate in feebleness and intermittency.

The cases of pericarditis which appear to be of a primary or idiopathic character, owing their existence to cold, exposure, and bad treatment, I have observed have all occurred in young horses, animals under two years of age, and which had been much exposed, being unprovided with sufficient shelter during the late autumn or early spring, and inadequately supplied with food. Several of these had shown no symptoms, general or special, of ill-health, and others only a trifling amount of inappetency or a somewhat unthrifty condition of the coat and skin. The lesions observable were the existence of fluid and fibrinous exudate in the pericardial sac, with or without adhesions between the visceral and outer layers of the membrane, and sometimes with much thickening of the entire membrane itself, all which changes indicated considerable inflammatory action, which, as stated, had never been significant or pronounced enough to attract attention.

On all these occasions, upon making careful and minute inquiries, I have found that now when the matter of previous illness has been placed before the attendants, it is recollected that the animal was somewhat indisposed, or at least that some symptoms were shown which, with the death, have received their correct interpretation. Usually these symptoms have been described as lassitude; an open condition of the coat, it may be rigors, inclination to be alone, and when made to move seeming stiff or lame, the exertion causing the animal to breathe rapidly and probably to cough.

Treatment.—In the management of cases of pericarditis it is important to have as clear an understanding as possible of the causes which seem to operate in its production, and of the collateral associations as respects morbid action in the animal in which it occurs.

Pericarditis as a primary and idiopathic affection is rather a different matter from the same condition as a symptom or accompaniment of any constitutional or general diseased condition, and necessarily demands a somewhat different treatment. Also it must not be forgotten that the treatment of the disease ought largely to depend upon the stage of the morbid process and the existing results which have followed that process at the period of our treatment.

If in our diagnosis we feel satisfied that the earlier stages of acute pericarditis—indicated by a tolerably full and hard pulse, much cardiac force and irritability, unaccompanied with constitutional debility or the action of epizootic influences—are being passed through, a fair amount of blood-letting will tend to do good by lessening the congestion of the heart and tending to allay its irritability.

This may even be repeated if the circulatory force, as indicated by the action of the heart and the character of the pulsations, seem to warrant it; but more frequently, even in these rarely met with instances of acute sthenic inflammations of the pericardium, will the results we desire to obtain—viz., to lessen the excitation and irritability of the heart—be achieved by following the first blood-letting with small and repeated doses of tincture of aconite. Where pain is a prominent feature the aconite, if not seeming to afford relief during the first six or twelve hours, may be superseded by tincture of opium given in gruel, along with linseed-oil; while heat and moisture are applied by means of woollen cloths wrung from hot water, and wrapped around the chest for two hours consecutively. When these have been removed, a compound soap liniment containing tincture of opium ought to be smartly rubbed over the sides of the chest. This latter application to be carried out between each fomentation.

When the earlier stages of the diseased process have passed, and liquid is effused in the pericardial sac, a somewhat different treatment is called for. Bleeding is here inadmissible; our endeavours must be directed to give the system such assistance as may enable it to overcome the depression consequent on the effusion, and lead to the removal of the liquid through absorption. Here the application of a smart cantharides liniment to the chest may be expected to operate beneficially, while, instead of aconite, it is highly probable that stimulants with diuretics are called for; these may with advantage be alternated with the exhibition of certain salts of iron, or with iodide of potassium

In some instances in uncomplicated pericarditis, where I have felt satisfied that effusion existed, the system of supporting the animal with a nutritious dietary and the exhibition of mild stimulants and tonics, combined with diuretics, has seemed to be productive of much good, the intermittency and irregularity of the pulse and cardiac action steadily subsiding as the powers of the system were more firmly established

When pericarditis appears to be ushered into existence in connection with or as a symptom of rheumatoid inflammation, or the epizootic fever of influenza, it is always a wiser procedure to direct attention more to the general or constitutional disease upon which the pericardial lesions seem to depend than to the pericarditis itself

Appearing as an accompaniment of acute rheumatism, or where I have observed it in the same relation to meningeal and certain nervous diseases, the means which have proved most conducive to favourable results have been the early and continued exhibition of full doses of bicarbonate of potash, with, where the pain and cardiac irritability were considerable, the addition of full doses of tincture of opium or aconite, together with the local application of heat and moisture through the medium of heavy woollen cloths. In all these cases it is generally advisable, in addition to the use of bicarbonate of potash, to allow full quantities of either sulphate of soda or magnesia, the tendency of these, after a few days' employment in the drinking-water, being to maintain the bowels in a soluble condition

The appearance of pericarditis during the development of influenza will rarely call for a great alteration in our treatment of that disease. The probabilities are that the animal will require a more steadily continued stimulant course of treatment than would otherwise be needful; while, if the chest has not already been moderately blistered, benefit will result from the use of a good mustard-meal poultice or a moderately active cantharides liniment. Where the condition of hydro-pericardium remains persistent, not seeming disposed to yield to such remedies as we have adopted, there is no reason why an attempt ought not to be made to remove the fluid by puncturing the pericardial sac.

II HYDRO-PERICARDIUM—DROPSY OF THE PERICARDIUM

The state of pericardial dropsy, although it may follow as a result of a mild pericarditis, is usually dependent on other causes for its existence, being in most instances a distinct part of general dropsy

Its anatomical characters are somewhat different from those of inflammatory action The fluid contained in the sac is purely serous, there being no fibrinous organizations or adhesions.

Rarely during life are there any symptoms indicative of the state, excepting those connected with the general disease to which it owes its origin

As the condition during life is merely one of supposition, and only determined by an after-death examination, treatment of it can only be entertained as part of that which is applicable to the general disturbance of which it forms part, or on which it is dependent for its existence.

CHAPTER XXIX.

ACUTE CARDIAC INFLAMMATIONS.

I. ACUTE ENDOCARDITIS WITH VALVULITIS.

Definition.—*Inflammation of the serous membrane, the endocardium, lining the cavities and covering the valves of the heart.*

Pathology. *a Nature and Causation*—Inflammation of this internal serous lining of the heart, although we may conceive of its existence as an independent and primary condition, is yet rarely presented to us in the horse, or probably any animal, apart from an appearance in some contiguous or analogous structure, or association with some general or constitutional disease, or some septic state of the blood.

It has by many been stated to be a condition more fre-

36

quently encountered than any other cardiac lesion, and to
exceed in frequency the same morbid alteration in the investing membrane and sac of the heart. If by this it is meant to
be stated that endocarditis of itself, and apart from other
diseased conditions, is of more frequent occurrence than associated with a similarly diseased state of other cardiac structures, I can hardly agree to it. If, however, its occurrence
with pericarditis be considered, and the combination of the
double inflammatory action be regarded as one, I am quite
prepared to endorse the finding that endo-pericarditis is the
most frequently observed of cardiac lesions When occurring,
as it usually does, associated with the same morbid state of the
other serous structures of the heart, it may be safely regarded
as a more serious condition than pericarditis, not so much from
the immediate results of the diseased action as from the
ulterior consequences of the structural changes incident to
endocardial inflammation.

Moderate pericarditis may subside, and no permanent
textural changes of a serious nature follow Moderate endocarditis probably rarely disappears without leaving changes in
connection with those fibro-serous structures the valves, which
are liable to steadily increase, and finally seriously impair the
functional activity of the heart

Appearing as a symptomatic condition, the primary states
with which it is connected may all be conveniently grouped as
those in which the blood is charged with some unhealthy or
poisonous material It is particularly observed in rheumatism,
several specific fevers of an enzootic or epizootic type, in
pyæmia and many forms of septic infection

The idea that the irritation inducing it is directly conveyed
to the membrane by the contaminated and heated blood is
neither chimerical nor without facts to support it

b. *Anatomical Characters*—Rarely are we fortunate enough
to see the endocardial membrane in its first stage of hyperæmia
and heightened colour Usually it has passed this, presenting
an opaque, cloudy, and swollen appearance

Where heightening of the colour is observed, we must not
forget that such may be the result of simple imbibition of the
blood-colouring matter, as well as the natural sequence of
inflammation. The results of this disturbed activity are, in

the majority of cases, most distinctly visible near the orifices of the heart, and in connection with the valvular structures which guard these.

This preference in endocarditis for seizing on the valves and their appendages, the chordæ tendineæ, is characteristic of all forms of the diseased action, but chiefly of that where it is developed in association with rheumatism and rheumatoid inflammations This may be so far accounted for when we consider that the cardiac valves are in part made up of white fibrous tissue, which seems peculiarly the seat of the specific inflammatory action

The form in which these results develop themselves is to some extent determined by the anatomical formation of the valves, they being constructed in part of fibrous tissue peculiarly disposed between duplicatures of the membrane. When inflamed they become thickened in two ways, first from augmentation in bulk of their intimate structure, and second from aggregations of a warty character, by proliferating cell-elements on their outer surface and free margin, these latter being steadily added to by the deposition of fibrinogenous material from the blood with which they are bathed.

These excrescences are of variable size and form, generally numerous, situated, as we have said, both upon the surface of the valve, its free margin, and its intimate texture In some cases they partake of a cartilaginous or calcareous character, these materials being deposited sometimes in layers, at others in points or masses

The continued existence or repetition of the inflammation, and the increase of these warty growths, tend to restrict the cardiac orifices and interfere with the action of the valves They may undergo certain changes, as softening and disintegration, or they may be removed in whole or in part The portions thus set loose may mingle with the general current of the circulation, and in this way may be carried to distant parts of the body and find a lodgment in tissues and organs, obstructing the blood-supply in these, and inducing paralysis or minute and destructive changes, terminating in general disturbance and death

Symptoms —The symptoms by which endocarditis may be detected, or by which it may be differentiated from pericarditis, are in our patients, particularly the horse, chiefly general, or symptoms of functional disturbance   There is fever, and, when existing in association with rheumatoid inflammation, exacerbation of existing pyrexia with obvious cardiac disturbance. Although tumultuous and rather energetic action of the heart, and feeble irresponsive pulsation in the arterial wave, noted by some as diagnostic of endocarditis, may not be so regarded in every instance, it is yet a very common, indeed too common, symptom to be ignored.   There is in the early stages of endocarditis less probability, in auscultating the chest, to hear the attrition or friction sound, spoken of as sometimes possible to be heard in pericarditis, and a greater probability in the purer forms of the disease of detecting murmurs of a soft or cooing character.   As the morbid condition becomes established there seems a marked tendency, greater than in pericarditis, to venous regurgitation and dyspnœa, particularly when disturbed even to a trifling extent   Although in some animals considerable information may be obtained in respect of the condition of the endocardial membranes from the character of the various true cardiac murmurs, we are less assisted by these, in the study of this affection in the horse, than in any other.   Here these endocardial sounds are often so disguised by their combination with other varieties of abnormal sounds, developed consecutively with exorcardial disease, a not unfrequent accompaniment of the other condition, that little reliance can be placed upon auscultation in forming our diagnosis.

By some it is said that the existence of clonic spasms of the superficial muscles in the anterior part of the body, associated with dyspnœa, is more generally indicative of endocardial inflammation than any other symptom.   That these spasms are frequently present during the course of the disease I believe is quite true; that they may be regarded as diagnostic is doubtful; while the disturbing action is only in the undisturbed animal a marked feature when valvular structures are seriously involved

In studying the symptoms indicative of disease of the endocardium we ought never to forget to note particularly the systemic or general conditions with which any established cardiac disturbance is associated   In all cases where rheu-

matoid inflammations exist, or where certain septic states of the
blood are present, and where undoubted cardiac disturbance
shows itself, either by peculiar and tumultuous action of the
heart and blood-flow in the vessels, or where abnormal sounds
may be detected in connection with the functional play of the
organ, we may be pretty certain that a diseased condition of
its fibrous and fibro-serous structures is going on; the difficulty
may be to determine whether the exocardial or endocardial
disease is in ascendency.

Inflammation of the endocardium, as it largely affects the
valves of the heart, is usually followed by structural changes
connected with these, also as a sequel of this valvular change,
with dilatation and alteration in the capacity of the cavities of
the heart, and with the consequent attendant symptoms of
certain of these changes, weakened cardiac action and dropsical
effusions in different parts of the body

Treatment —The most important features of endocarditis,
both as respects frequency of occurrence and severity of
attack, are, as already noticed, associated with its connection
with rheumatism, rheumatoid inflammations, and some other
states of blood-contamination In the treatment of this inflammation in such conditions it will be better to concentrate
our attention on the constitutional or general disturbance than
on this cardiac lesion, which is better regarded as a sequel or
symptom of the primary and more extensive, while it will
be found that in direct proportion as the general diseased
condition shows itself amenable to treatment, so will the
local and secondary morbid action in cardiac structures be-
have itself

In a general way it may be said that treatment of a nature
much similar to what has been recommended for pericarditis
is to be carried out here, probably, in endocarditis, the good
results of blood-letting, even in the earlier stages, are less likely
to be unmixed with evil than in inflammation involving the
other great fibro-serous membrane of the heart Bleeding may
give temporary relief, but is apt, by lowering the tone of the
heart's action, to favour the production of fibrinous excrescences on the valvular and tendinous structures of the cardiac
cavities   For the same reason the employment of direct
cardiac sedatives, although indicated where the irritability and

pain is great, is to be carried out with watchfulness and care. Following the employment of a moderate blood-letting where blood is abstracted, and also where blood-letting is not carried out, full and repeated doses of salines, as the bicarbonate of potash, alternated after some days with iodide of potassium, will be found most useful.

Should debility or exhaustion set in, stimulants must not be withheld, but are best administered in small or moderate doses, and often, and where little food is taken, are judiciously combined with good gruel or beef-tea. The acute and highly developed symptoms attendant on endocarditis are, however, less to be feared than the concurrent or consequent valvular lesions, with the usual attendant change of cardiac structure and restriction of cardiac orifices. When resulting from pyæmia and other blood-contaminations the same general principles must guide our treatment. The cardiac lesions must be made subordinate to the primary and inducing

II. ACUTE MYOCARDITIS—CARDITIS.

Inflammation of the true muscular structure of the heart, there is little doubt, does occur, if not throughout the entire organ, at least in a circumscribed and superficial manner, in certain cases of peri- and endo-carditis, where, from contiguity, the muscular fibres participate in the morbid action progressing in the investing membrane. Like the inflammations occurring in these membranes it seems also to owe its existence to pyæmic and septicæmic conditions, in which states the deeper-seated textures are more likely to be involved, and the termination to be the formation of abscesses and fatal destruction of tissue.

The anatomical characters in the few cases which I have seen were darkening and softening of the cardiac structure, the intimate elements of which were moistened with slightly bloody serous fluid and pus.

The symptoms of this condition, which are not diagnostic, are chiefly weakened and irregular cardiac action.

One of the few cases of secondary carditis which have come under my observation is interesting, as showing the extent to which serious changes may occur in connection with the muscular structure of the heart without specially attractive symptoms

The animal was a three-parts bred two-months old foal, it had been attacked with strangles; the abscess had matured and suppurated in the submaxillary space But shortly after this it became the subject of pyogenic fever, disseminated abscesses occurred at various parts chiefly in the course of the vessels of the pectoral limbs, which, after some little time, healed, and the patient appeared to be doing well

On the occasion of one of my visits, while standing looking carefully at the foal, which was with the dam in a large loose box, it seemed to me to be lame of both fore-limbs, on being made to move across the box it suddenly commenced to breathe rapidly, dyspnœa in a short time being very marked, and before I left the place the animal died

On making an examination of the carcase, several small localized collections of pus were found in different situations in the course of the lymphatic vessels of the anterior limb of one side The viscera of the great serous cavities appeared healthy, except the heart and investing membrane, the pericardial sac contained a little bloody serous fluid, and was slightly ecchymosed on both visceral and parietal layers of the membrane, the muscular structure being of a darker colour and softer than natural On incising the wall of the left ventricle there was laid open a considerable abscess, which contained laudable creamy pus, around the abscess the muscular fibres were darker, softer, and more friable than natural

No other collections of pus were found in the chest. In addition to this condition of the muscular structure of the heart there was also rupture of one of the fleshy pillars of the ventricle, and of the tendinous cords attached to it; these appeared to have been of recent occurrence, and probably accounted for the death

CHAPTER XXX

CHRONIC DISEASES OF THE HEART

I. ENLARGEMENT OF THE HEART—HYPERTROPHY AND DILATATION.

Definition.—An unnatural development of the muscular walls of the heart, augmenting its bulk by increase of the muscular structure, and generally accompanied with increase of the cavitary capacity

Meaning of Terms.—Enlargement of the heart, increase of its bulk from increase of the muscular structure, and dilatation of one or more of its cavities, has in the horse attracted the attention of the majority of observers for a lengthened period; but attempts to connect these changes with particular symptoms exhibited during life have, from anatomical and other difficulties, been sparingly attempted, and not always successfully

The auricles or ventricles may severally be the seat of this extra growth, or the venous or arterial heart may each in different cases be more particularly involved. The superior cavities or auricles are much less frequently the seat of this enlargement or increase of their walls, and probably the left ventricle is more liable to the change than the right.

When affecting the heart sectionally or in parts, we speak of it as partial hypertrophy; when the entire organ is involved, as general hypertrophy. Cardiac enlargement may be regarded as resulting from two general conditions 1 Increase in bulk of the muscular walls; 2 Increase of cavitary capacity—dilatation.

As these conditions rarely exist uncomplicated, but are variously related to each other as to extent, the state of enlargement has been named in accordance with these relationships 1. *Simple hypertrophy*, when the increase in bulk is unassociated with alteration of cavities 2 *Simple dilatation*, when there is increase of cavitary capacity without increase of bulk of muscular tissue in walls, or with thinning of these. 3 *Hypertrophy with dilatation—eccentric hypertrophy*—when there is increase of muscular structure with increase of capacity of cavities; sometimes the hypertrophy is in excess of the dilatation, at others the dilatation is greater than the hypertrophy. 4 Another form is mentioned by some, but its existence is doubtful, apart from congenital malformation; *i e*, *hypertrophy* with diminished cardiac capacity—*concentric hypertrophy*

Causation —Hypertrophy, with or without dilatation, may in a large view of the causation be regarded as a compensatory condition, and as the effort of the main organ of the circulation to overcome some existing obstacle.

1. It may appear in what may be regarded as an idiopathic form in animals which have for a lengthened period been subject to continuous and severe exertion In horses which have been hunted for some years simple hypertrophy, or hypertrophy with dilatation, is of frequent occurrence, not appearing suddenly, but gradual in development

2 It is attendant on direct obstruction to blood-flow (*a*) occurring at the cardiac orifices and large vessels, chiefly at the mitral and aortic openings, (*b*) in the pulmonary circulation from structural changes in lung-tissue, as in bronchitis and emphysema, (*c*) occasionally in the systemic circulation, from impediment in different organs, particularly when suffering from fibrosis and other changes in peripheral vessels.

3 Dilatation with hypertrophy is very liable to occur from internal pressure during systolic relaxation, when, from aortic or mitral insufficiency, regurgitation takes place

4 Enlargement of the same character may arise from weakening of the muscular structure following inflammatory action

Anatomical Characters—Of these, the chief are increase in weight and increase in bulk, the relative extent of these being in proportion to the ascendency of hypertrophy or of dilatation

With many, change of form or shape of the organ is a conspicuous feature, the character and extent depending upon the parts actually affected, ordinarily it is more globose than natural In the intimate structure, unless degenerative changes have occurred, the appearance of the muscular substance is a darkening or heightening in colour, and either an increased development of the minute fibres, or the production of new ones

Symptoms —In many cases of simple hypertrophy, and where it has been gradualy developed and purely compensatory, no indications, general or local, may exist to point to these structural changes   When the hypertrophy is considerable and in excess of the dilatation, the general symptoms usually observed are at first a full, rather hard, strong pulse, which after some time, as dilatation increases, becomes altered to one much smaller and feebler, even while the cardiac action is bounding. The impulse of the heart is increased, it is sometimes slow and prolonged, the sound may be more intense, but less distinct and sharp; it seems to hang in delivering the impulse and in the production of the sound, which is distributed over a great extent laterally.

The impulse of the heart in cases of considerable hypertrophy is often so great that it may be observed at a little distance from the animal, and is distinctly felt when the hand is placed over the cardiac region

Percussion, although in some instances indicating the greater space occupied by the hypertrophied and dilated organ, is not to be depended on as affording much information.

As dilatation increases and is in ascendency to hypertrophy, the impulse of the heart becomes feebler, although neither the sound given out nor that which is elicited by percussion may be less clear   The pulsations are lessened in frequency, smaller, more feeble, unequal, irregular, or intermittent, with occasional dyspnœa, particularly when excited.   In advanced cases there is coldness of the extremities and a tendency to œdema or general dropsy.   With other observers I have noted when the right side in particular has been the seat of dilatation, that the peculiar movement in the jugular vein, known as the jugular venous pulse, is most frequently noticed.

There is always less danger and fewer distressing symptoms attendant upon dilatation of the heart, accompanied with hypertrophy, than when the opposite condition exists.

So long, therefore, as hypertrophy keeps pace with the increasing capacity of the cardiac cavities, organic change of the organ may not be suspected; when the dilatation becomes in excess of the increase in substance the impairment of function rapidly becomes obvious, the performance of even moderate exertion being attended with difficulty

From the records of veterinary medicine, both in this country and abroad, many wonderful instances of dilatation of the heart may be gathered Both Mr Percival in his ' Hippopathology,' and Mr. Gamgee in his ' Domestic Animals in Health and Disease,' drawing from these records, relate some very significant and well-marked cases Some of the cases mentioned by the latter I had the opportunity of examining, and can vouch for the reality and accuracy of what is there stated

II ATROPHY OF THE HEART.

Unnatural lessening or loss of the substance of the heart, as well as increase and augmentation, is observed in the horse and other of our patients   This abnormal decrease may, as with the hypertrophic state, be particular or general ; it may involve only portions, or affect the whole. It may occur without alteration of the cavity or cavities ; or it may, as with the opposite state, be attended with thinning of the walls and dilatation of the cavity—the former known as simple, the latter as eccentric atrophy The frequency with which the several cavities of the heart are usually affected with atrophy has by some observers been stated to be the opposite of that which holds good in the condition of hypertrophy, the auricle being more liable to atrophy, the ventricles to hypertrophy.

The anatomical characters are lessening of bulk and absolute weight, with often undue pallor of the muscular tissue, which is occasionally suffering from degenerative changes.

The symptoms, general or local, are not diagnostic. There is much weakness, with feeble cardiac impulse distributed over a restricted area.

III FATTY CHANGES IN THE HEART.

Of the diseased conditions affecting the intimate structure of the heart dependent on fatty changes, we have in the horse, as other animals, two forms—(a) *Fatty infiltration*, or deposition upon and amongst the muscular fibres of oil or fat in the form of ordinary fat-cells or adipose tissue ; (b) *Fatty degeneration, or metamorphosis*, in which fat or oil particles take the place of the true muscular elements in the minute tubular elements of the tissue. Although not recognised as of so much importance because occurring less often in our patients than in the human subject, these conditions are still, with many animals which come under our notice, a very serious matter, and of more frequency than is believed. When occurring, they are often associated with other unnatural states, specially with dilatation, partial or general, of the cardiac cavities, and with this operate prejudicially by largely impairing function, and offering facilities for other lesions which may prove rapidly fatal

a Fatty Infiltration—In many of our patients, where their treatment has for some time been highly artificial, where, in particular, from a want of exercise sufficient to maintain the system in a healthy and vigorous state, there is a disposition for the excess of nutriment to be stored throughout the different structures of the body in the form of fat, we find that the heart, in connection with many other organs, participates in this accumulation of adipose structure. In these cases, in addition to the ordinary situation of fatty tissue around its base and at the origin of the great vessels, it is found that this tissue insinuates itself amongst and between the muscular fasciculi and ultimate fibres Although this condition is not what is meant when we speak of fatty degeneration proper, it is yet highly probable that by this intermingling of fat with the muscular fibres these may be impoverished, injured, or paralyzed, or it may even be the active means in the production of that more serious state—

b Fatty Metamorphosis, or Degeneration—Here, in addition to simple atrophy of the fibres and loss of their functional power in consequence of the atrophy, we have a removal of the sarcous elements, and their replacement with fat granules or globules and other amorphous material, the result of the disintegration of the intimate muscular elements

By this degenerative change the integrity and action of these are ultimately destroyed, nor can they be again restored

The great majority of cases where this true fatty degenerative change—not the mere infiltration of the substance of the organ with fat—occurs, are those also where thinning of the walls with enlargement of the cavities exists, resulting in the condition of a truly weak heart, very unfit even to carry on

ordinary circulation, and totally so to act with safety in cases
of severe exertion

When examining a heart thus affected, we may observe,
both on the surface beneath the lining and covering membrane, and throughout the interior of the substance of the
walls, variously distributed pale or buff-coloured spots, also
that the entire substance feels softer than natural

Examined more minutely, we find that these paler patches
are the changed muscular fibres, in which the healthy transverse markings and nuclei are absent, and that their place is
occupied by fat or oil globules, with some other amorphous
material.   The muscular structure is found in a great measure
to have lost its tenacity, it is more brittle, and seemingly less
capable of resisting any strain which may be put upon it.

Any clinical phenomena which may attend either of these
conditions cannot be said to be diagnostic, they may indicate
disturbance or textural alteration of the heart, but not such as
will lead us, apart from other information, to hazard with any
degree of safety an opinion as to the existence of such changes
Both conditions, of fatty metamorphosis and fatty infiltration
of the heart's structure, may occur in the heart individually
and separately, or they may be associated with similar changes
and deposits in other organs and structures of the body

IV RUPTURE OF THE HEART

This lesion, although not what may be properly termed
chronic, seeing it is always of sudden development, is in many
instances but the natural result of some antecedent diseased
condition In any instance, either apart from minute structural change, or as the result of certain degenerative processes,
it is a rare lesion

The immediate causes of cardiac rupture, from the records
of such cases as have been reported, and from my own experience, I am disposed to regard as over-exertion, and concussion or shock, these latter usually the result of a fall or of
violence applied directly to the chest-walls

Mr. Percival, in his 'Hippopathology,' gives one instance of
rupture of the right auricle in a horse immediately succeeding
a hard-contested race   From my own experience I must corroborate what Mr Gamgee, in 'Domestic Animals in Health

and Disease,' states with regard to these lesions, that their usual situation in the horse is at the conus arteriosus of the left ventricle, where the tendinous ring uniting the great aorta with the ventricle is the structure which is found to have ruptured. The only cases of this lesion which I have encountered were in this particular situation; both were aged animals, previously in the full enjoyment of health and apparent vigour, nor after death could I on examination detect any structural changes at the seat of rupture, which we might have anticipated would have led to this

In both animals death occurred immediately after a short but sharp drive, they were placed in the stable apparently well, and shortly afterwards were found dead.

As illustrative of the fact that violence applied to the chest-wall may cause rupture of the heart, there is quoted by Mr Gamgee a case reported in the *Veterinarian* by Mr Parker of Birmingham, where a pony, in running away with a gig down a hill, came violently in contact with the wheel of a cart, striking it with his right shoulder. The animal came to the ground, from which he was never able to rise, and was shortly afterwards destroyed. On being examined after death the pericardium was found ruptured on the right side, and contained a quantity of coagulated blood; there was also a blood-clot attached to the base of the right auricle, which was here separated from the ventricle. The ribs and investing muscles were uninjured.

I have also, on one occasion observed rupture of another portion of the heart-structure, which is probably not at all common, and which, in the instance referred to, was associated with suppurative disease of the true muscular structure. The rupture was that of one of the fleshy pillars of the ventricle and of some of the tendinous cords attached to it. This was in the case of the foal already mentioned as affected with myocarditis associated with pyæmia. The integrity of the fleshy pillar seemed impaired by the progress of the contiguous inflammatory action.

In anatomical characters there may be some differences both of situation and form of rupture, which will have an important bearing upon the suddenness with which a fatal termination is reached.

V ADVENTITIOUS GROWTHS OR NEW FORMATIONS IN CONNECTION WITH THE HEART

In addition to the structural changes, either of extra development of muscular tissue or minute elemental changes, we find that the heart is liable to become the seat of various morbid growths or new formations, which may directly or indirectly terminate fatally

The most commonly occurring may be classed as—(1) *Growths of parasite origin,* situated internally or externally (2) *Cancerous* or malignant growths (3) *Fibroid tumours*, or cardiac polypi , (4) *Vascular tumours*

Adventitious growths or new formations of any of these several varieties, in the influence which they exercise upon the animal health and in their tendency to produce fatal results, as well as the urgency of the symptoms which accompany their existence during life, depend probably more upon their situation in the cardiac structures than upon their extent or even their intrinsic character

Thus it is easy to understand that a comparatively small tumour, or amount of adventitious deposition, situated in either of the cavities of the heart is more likely to be productive of serious or fatal consequences than a more extensive or more malignant growth in connection with the external and free surface of the organ   Even the exact situation of these growths, when occurring either within the cardiac cavities or on the outer surface of the heart, has an important influence in determining symptoms of illness, as also the ultimate results A very small tumour, if interfering with the valvular sufficiency of any of the cavities, is a more serious matter than a more extensive growth situated apart from these structures , in like manner, interference with the great vessels at the base of the heart by the presence of fibroid or other tumours is more likely, by interfering with the free course of the blood to and from the heart, to be productive of functional disturbance and other changes, than would be the case if the same growth existed at the apex

The chief parasitic growths found connected with the heart are hydatids, or echinococcus cysts, which, although I have encountered them in cattle and sheep, have not come under my observation in the horse Single parasites, wandering individuals of the *Strongylus armatus*, I have found in the pericardial sac of young horses, their presence having evidently been the immediately inducing cause of pericardial inflammation and some other structural changes

Occasionally, in decidedly cachectic subjects, the heart may become the seat of malignant or cancerous growths, the appearance of which may usually be regarded as the sequel to a general invasion of the system by cancer, although it is perfectly possible that these malignant growths may appear primarily in the cardiac structures previous to or apart from their existence elsewhere

In some instances dilatation of the cardiac veins beneath the endocardial membrane may become so extensive and assume such a form as to be viewed as vascular cardiac tumours The most frequently encountered cardiac growths are probably the fibrinous, often situated in the interior of the cavities of the heart. In speaking of these fibrinous growths, or cardiac polypi, we must not forget that there is a danger of confounding these with the existence of fibrinous coagula, or thrombi, often found in the cardiac cavities, and which, although they may be of ante-mortem formation, are yet distinct from the true polypi which have obtained a true and intimate connection with the muscular walls When present, the fibrinous growths seem to arise from the muscular tissue beneath the endocardial membrane They may reach a considerable size without their existence being suspected during life, and seem, from their anatomical structure, to steadily increase in growth through attraction and incorporation of fibrinogenous and lymphoid materials When examined carefully, the interior and portions closely connected with the peduncle are evidently more perfectly organized and fibrillated than the outer and more superficial parts These growths, although found in the hearts of horses, seem, from the recorded cases, to be more common in cattle, I have met with them in both animals, and their existence has struck me as most likely to have arisen in consequence of limited endocarditis, and that they steadily increase in bulk from the deposition over the original seat of some inflammatory exudate of fibrinogenous or plastic and lymphoid materials, which in certain states of the blood are specially abundant.

As a general rule none of these different varieties of abnormal growths may, with any degree of certainty be diagnosed during life; many animals may be sufferers from such and give no indications of illness, while, where symptoms of cardiac disturbance have been observed, these have as often been referred to other and very different states. Their existence has only been discovered after death, which, in all probability being sudden, called for an examination. As we are unable to diagnose the existence of these abnormalities, and as they so often, even when existing seem to cause no inconvenience, it were needless to speculate as to treatment

VI. AFFECTIONS OF THE VALVES AND ORIFICES OF THE HEART.

The natural as well as unnatural cardiac sounds have already been alluded to, and to a certain extent described (Chap XXV.) What are now to be taken up very shortly are certain definite organic lesions productive of the 'murmurs' or abnormal sounds associated with obstruction or regurgitation of the blood in its passage through the orifices of the heart.

Causes and Results of Valvular Disease.—The greater number of the diseased conditions which are observed as connected with the lining membrane of the heart and of the valves are probably the direct result of inflammatory action, common or specific. These are usually augmentation in bulk of the minute textural elements entering into the composition of the valves, or depositions on the surface of the membrane, in this way causing thickening and puckering of these structures, while the depositions, once established, possess a disposition rather to increase than diminish. Or the valve-structures may become the seat of warty excrescences of an atheromatous or calcareous character

The common results of any or all of these changes upon the valves are—1. To thicken corrugate, and render more bulky the otherwise fine web-like structure, and thus obstruct the flow of blood—*valvular obstruction*; 2 By the thickening and puckering to contract the valve upon its base, and leave the orifice insufficiently guarded — *valvular insufficiency*

37

These conditions may exist separately, or they may be combined

Situations and Symptoms of Valvular Disease—In the diagnosis of disease affecting the valves of the heart, attention must be directed—1 To the physical or local signs of disturbance; 2 To the physiological or functional indications.

In our patients, particularly the horse, the power accurately to discriminate the different physical signs, which are those of abnormal sounds and murmurs, is in a great measure taken from us by the formation of the chest and pectoral region The close approximation to the chest of the pectoral limbs, and their peculiar formation, so cover and shield the heart, that anything like nice or correct auscultation is impossible

The abnormal sounds or murmurs which may be heard in many forms of valvular disease, or of abnormal states of the blood, vary much; sometimes soft and cooing, at others harsh and rasping; sometimes accompanying or following the natural sounds, sometimes so developed as to obscure them or take their place It is further worth remembering that disease of the endocardial membrane, the valves and the orifices of the left side of the heart, are of more common occurrence than those of the right Also that disease of these structures of the left side chiefly affect the arterial pulse, rendering it unequal as to character or rhythm; while those of the right side give more distinct indications in the venous circulation, being often attended with the jugular irregularity known as the jugular pulse; while effusion into the natural cavities and the general connective-tissue, the attendant dropsies and anasarcous swellings of cardiac disorders, are more common in disease of the structures of the right than of the left side.

Probably the most common seats of disease of the valves and the orifices of the heart in the horse are in connection with the mitral or aortic valvular apparatus Disease of these structures in both situations may in character be either insufficient or obstructive, commonly it possesses the double feature. When the defect in the aortic valves is of the distinctly obstructive character, preventing the free passage of the blood into the great arterial conduit from the ventricle, the murmur, or abnormal bellows-sound, if heard at all, will be during the systole or contraction of the ventricle; when both obstructive and insufficient, preventing the flow of the blood from the cavity and permitting also its regurgitation, the murmurs will be both systolic and diastolic.

The pulse in the first of these conditions—of simple aortic obstruction—is not materially altered, although the heart's action may be forcible. In the other—where valvular insufficiency exists in addition to obstruction—it is jerking, wanting in the regular swell or sustained wave of either health or hypertrophy, the blood feels shot past the finger in separate masses

When the valvular structure between the ventricle and auricle of the left side is diseased, either impeding the passage of the blood into the ventricle, or permitting of regurgitation into the auricle, there is usually a tendency to pulmonary complications, with cough, dyspnœa, and general distress, particularly on excitement or severe exercise, while the pulse is markedly irregular and unequal both in force and volume. Murmurs of both systolic and diastolic character may be heard, but not generally, and in none are they to be depended on

To determine the systolic or diastolic character of a murmur, the pulse, during auscultation, ought to be noted either at the jaw or the fore-arm. If the sound is systolic, it will of course be heard synchronously, or nearly so, with the pulse; if diastolic, it will not be synchronous.

The general or functional symptoms of this form of cardiac disease may be regarded as mainly owing directly to disturbance or obstruction in the pulmonary capillary system, or in that of the systemic circulation With disease of the valves of the right side, the auriculo-ventricular, is usually associated dilatation of the right cavities, often of itself the only abnormal condition, and the direct result of pulmonary obstruction, or both may be encountered following mitral disease

Here, although we may not by physical signs or sounds be able to satisfy ourselves of the altered condition, the effects produced on the circulatory system, particularly the venous, are quickly and often distinctly marked As the direct result of venous turgescence, or internal pressure, we have a tendency to general dropsy, shown by accumulations of fluid in the serous cavities and spaces of the connective-tissue throughout

37—2

the body, while the immediate effect on the venous system is exhibited in the regularly occurring venous pulsation in the jugulars.

In estimating the general or systemic symptoms accompanying different forms of chronic valvular disease, it is well to recollect that after some time all of these are prone to produce or to be attended with capillary disturbance, and thus largely to simulate each other.

This peculiar hæmal obstruction is chiefly indicated by such general symptoms as—1 Distressed breathing, passing on to confirmed and serious dyspnœa when the horse is much excited, made to move rapidly, or undergo severe exertion. 2. Palpitation and irregular action of the heart, discoverable by auscultation 3. Irregular, unequal, or intermittent action of the circulation, both arterial and venous 4 Anasarcous swellings, usually appearing first in the extremities, and ulti mately extending to the inferior portions of the chest and abdomen This is associated with accumulations of fluid in the great serous cavities, particularly of the pleural and peri cardiac sacs 5. Pulmonary complications, as congestion bronchitis, or hæmorrhage. 6 A peculiar anxious and dis tressed expression of the animal's countenance, with occa sionally symptoms of coma or vertigo, indicative of cerebral disturbance. Of these it is probable that the most diagnostic in the earlier stages are the peculiar and urgent dyspnœa, un associated with primary pulmonic disease The palpitation and irregular condition of the circulation are followed later by the appearance of dropsical effusions The occurrence of these in combination, or of any one in particular, ought at once to call for a careful examination of the state of the heart

Treatment—In the management of all these cases of struc tural disease of the heart it is obvious that the most which can be done is merely palliative, our efforts being directed to the moderating of the abnormal cardiac action, and to th combating of untoward symptoms as they arise.

With us it is not often, as with the practitioner of huma medicine, an object to prolong life when our patients are man festly unfit to serve the purpose for which they are adapte and maintained.

In the great majority of cases attention to dietary an

general tonic treatment, with, in cases of special cardiac irritability, the use of such agents as seem to possess a special
power of influencing the heart's action, are the indications we
require to follow, and from which the greatest benefit may be
expected The different preparations of iron, combined with
the common vegetable tonics and diuretics, or with such agents
as nux vomica or digitalis, are those chiefly employed

The prognosis in all these cases is certain as to the ultimate
results, but may not be determined as to time ; the animal
may continue to work for a longer or shorter period, but, as
the disease progresses, usually succumbs suddenly, and oftener
from the rapid progress of some of the secondary affections
than from the original disease

VII CALCIFICATION OF THE HEART.

Of this peculiar and rare condition of the muscular substance of the heart we know little ; cases, however, are recorded
of its existence One is mentioned by Mr Percivall as having
been met with in the practice of the late Mr Henderson,
London The only history attached to this is that the animal,
in an emaciated condition, dropped dead while at work in a
dust-cart Of another mentioned in the *Receuil de Médecine
Vétérinaire* for 1840, it is recorded that, although a young
animal, he was unable to work from recurring and persisting
attacks of exhaustion and dyspnœa, and that death appeared
at last to result from an attack of pneumonia In both these
instances it was the right auricle which had undergone the
calcifying change

CHAPTER XXXI

DISEASES OF THE PERITONEUM

I PERITONITIS.

Definition —*Inflammation of the serous membrane lining the
cavity and covering the viscera contained in the abdomen.*

Pathology.—Although of all our patients it is probable that
the horse can tolerate least of all interference in any way with

the serous membrane of the abdomen, even in him pure and simple inflammatory disturbance, apart from disease of other organs contained there, and external violence or traumatic lesion, together with certain general diseased conditions, is rather a rare occurrence   While, both from the similarity of the symptoms attendant upon this condition when it does take place, and those of a like diseased action in the bowels in particular, as well as the frequent amalgamation of these, there is little doubt that the two conditions have often been confounded

a Causation —1 *In an idiopathic* form, as the result of cold and exposure, an active, subacute, or chronic attack of inflammation of the peritoneum may assert itself, not, however, save in the last form, so frequently as is generally imagined.   As subacute or chronic peritonitis, it is rather frequently met with in young horses which have been badly treated as respects location and dietary, these cases it will generally be found have been exposed during inclement weather, and upon a food-supply inadequate in every respect to serve the requirements of the system.

2 *From Contiguous Irritation* —In this form the inflammatory action is either circumscribed or diffused, confined to a small area in immediate connection with the originating disease, or distributed throughout the peritoneal sac.   The cases which originate in this manner are propagations of the same action from disease of organs in or connected with the abdomen, as irritation or inflammation of the bowels, liver mammary glands, or even propagated from the structures o the chest.

3 *From Blood-contamination* —This secondary or symp tomatic peritonitis we encounter in some general diseased con ditions, in certain specific fevers and other constitutiona disturbances   In some of our patients, more particularly than in the horse, a peculiarly troublesome development of peri tonitis is found associated with the puerperal state, which probably, in addition to its merely irritative character, is pos sessed of specific properties, and capable of propagation

4 *From Causes Traumatic* —The production of peritonea inflammation from injury to tissue, the result of mechanica violence or operative interference, is probably of more fre

quent occurrence than in association with the general and often inappreciable agencies previously noticed. It may follow the infliction of wounds penetrating, or non-penetrating, of the abdomen, the performance of castration, the surgical treatment of hernia and some other diseased conditions.

5 Besides agencies strictly traumatic and operating from without, peritonitis of a dangerous and most frequently fatal character *follows abdominal ruptures and perforations* The chief of these in the horse are rupture of the gastric or intestinal walls, rupture of the liver and spleen, either of their intimate structure or of an abscess or hydatid cyst which they may contain, bursting of similar accumulations in the pelvis or gland-structure of the kidneys, of the bladder from over-distension, or of collections of matter in natural situations or in adventitious products

b Anatomical Characters—With the full development of the disease there is heightening of colour of the peritoneal membrane, with perceptible increase in its thickness from effusion amongst and gemination of its ultimate elements, together with extension of the same activities to the free surface of the membrane

Rarely do we find this redness and hyperæmic condition of the membrane of a uniform character, certain portions of it having definite relations to particular organs being more disposed to the unnatural action than others. Its usual appearance is that of spots or streaks of greater or less extent scattered over a variable surface, having a disposition to increase by coalescence

In some instances where the activity of the process has somewhat subsided, or where it never has been so active, there may not be much redness, thickening being the only or the most distinctive feature

With the early alteration of the free surface of the membrane effusion of serum is a usual concomitant · this effusion may be small in amount, or of such a quantity as to constitute abdominal dropsy. The condition of considerable effusion with much thickening of membrane without heightening of colour is commonly observed in those cases in young horses, the result of exposure and insufficient dietary. In the more active forms we find that the effused material is not entirely of a watery character, but that more or less of a varying-conditioned fibrinous material is associated with it.

The variations in the general character and plasticity of this fibrinous exudate are distinctly seen in the different ways in which it comports itself at one time it will be found forming a loose coating over the parts diseased, or causing adhesions between the coils of the intestines, or between these and different parts of the abdominal walls, at others, particularly when fluid is in great amount, instead of adhering to the walls of the cavity, it is found in loose portions floating in the fluid, with which are mingled varied forms of cell-growth, epithelial and pustular, as also colouring matter of the blood. These latter adventitious materials are rarely absent in the effusion we encounter in the peritonitis of the puerperal state.

The condition of thickening and increase in bulk which the effusion and cell-proliferation give to the membrane, parietal and visceral, tend much to alter its physical character of cohesion, it being more easily lacerated of itself as well as more readily torn from the structures which it covers.

Symptoms—These vary much, both as to their character and severity, nor may we with certainty, from suspecting the cause of the disease—*i.e.*, whether traumatic or proceeding from agencies more hidden—predict the course or the character which they will develop. When occurring as an independent affection it more frequently assumes the subacute or chronic form, with a rather slow and insidious development of symptoms. The patient is restless, lying down, resting uneasily, repeatedly turning his nose to his flank, and although not showing so much pain by violence of movement as in many less serious bowel disturbances, has yet an anxious and wearied expression of face.

When following injuries and wounds inflicted in surgical operations, or in cases following abdominal perforation and rupture, there is usually more demonstration of internal pain, pawing with the fore-feet and restless moving of the hind ones, even when there is no lying down and rolling, which latter symptom occurs less frequently than with severe and serious bowel affections.

The appetite is much disturbed, the respirations quick and catching, with a frequent, small, and rather hard pulse, and elevation of internal temperature. Manipulation of the abdomen, or friction, usually well borne in simple colic, is both in inflammation of the bowels, and in peritonitis, provocative of more distinct manifestations of pain.

Course and Termination—Unless the extent of the membrane involved is small, and the diffusion of the morbid action is early arrested, the course, although not so rapid as enteric inflammation so-called, is generally steady, and ultimately fatal.

Instances of patchy and circumscribed peritonitis do frequently, judging from *post-mortem* evidence, terminate, after moderate change of textural integrity, in a return to normal functional activity. The amount of fluid effused, being small, is removed without having given evidence of its existence, and before producing further serious complications.

Treatment.—In the majority of cases, and in every stage, peritonitis is rationally treated upon the same lines which are applicable to inflammatory action affecting the bowels. In particular instances of strong, previously healthy animals unaffected by depressing influences in the early stages of the disease, and where the cardiac action and character of the pulse is favourable, blood may be abstracted with benefit. The active and dominant symptom of pain must in all instances attract the greatest share of attention, and is most surely mitigated by the administration of opium, or opium combined with aconite. One or both may be exhibited in gruel, with salines, as the solution of acetate of ammonia, or more certainly, in the case of the opium, by the subcutaneous injection of a morphia solution.

Even when the bowels are confined there is no necessity of making attempts at once to incite their movement, but the reverse. As thirst is often considerable, water or gruel may be freely allowed containing salines in solution.

With the employment of blood-letting and the exhibition of opium internally, the early and steady application to the abdomen of heat and moisture is to be recommended, while, when these applications are withdrawn, the use of soap liniment combined with tincture of opium, or of turpentine stupes, is deserving of a trial.

In the second stage of the disease, whether the pain has been removed or not, I have often believed that benefit has

resulted from the administration every three or four hours of
half-drachm doses of powdered digitalis and camphor in a
little spirits of nitric æther and solution of acetate of ammonia,
with milk or gruel as a vehicle; while linseed-tea, or water
with salines dissolved in it, is freely allowed as drink

In the cases of chronic peritonitis, when satisfied that such
exists, their treatment is somewhat different   Essentially less
active, the morbid process is most successfully combated, both
as to progress and results, by treatment which is largely tonic,
by wholesome dietary, and correct sanitary conditions   Seldom
if ever, in the instance of young horses sufferers from this
form, will depletion need to be resorted to, while any restlessness and fugitive abdominal pain which may be shown are
best treated by such medicines as have been recommended for
the second stage of the acute form—viz, spirits of nitric æther,
with digitalis and camphor   These, it is probable, will require
to be continued for some time longer than in the acute manifestation, and are usually advantageously followed by good and
nutritious food, mild tonics and diuretics, careful location, and
freedom from exposure until fully reinstated in health   In
many instances, along with the use internally of the medicines
mentioned, I have seen much good follow the application to
the abdomen of a smart cantharides liniment

II MORBID GROWTHS IN CONNECTION WITH THE PERITONEUM

In the horse, both hydatid cysts and malignant new formations, the latter of more frequency than the former, are encountered connected with the peritoneum   When appearing,
cancerous growths are chiefly, as secondary developments, associated through contiguity with some organ where the diseased
condition has appeared as a primary, or at least as an earlier
development   Of more frequent occurrence, however, than
these are growths of an innocent nature   They are chiefly
fatty, and show themselves in connection with the folds of the
membrane, the omentum, and the mesentery   Fibrous tumours
also have their situation in the same position, and occasionally
a compound growth of gland-structure with adipose and fibrous
tissue   These may prove troublesome or dangerous by their
mere bulk, interfering with functional activity of particular
organs   The smaller, which are also frequently pedunculated,

are probably more dangerous, from their liability through their free necks to become entangled around and cause strangulation of the intestine.

These unnatural growths, even when troublesome, may only be guessed at , they cannot be diagnosed. The symptoms to which they give rise are only indicative of some interference with or change of a particular organ or structure, not of the character of the interfering agent.

Any treatment having reference to the existence of these can only resolve itself into that of dealing with the symptoms which they through their character, position, and relation to particular functions and organs may develop

III. Ascites—Dropsy of the Peritoneum.

Definition.—*A collection of serous fluid, usually of gradual accumulation, in the cavity of the peritoneum.*

Pathology.—The presence of fluid to an abnormal extent in the abdominal cavity has, ever since animals were examined after death with a view to the obtaining of information regarding conditions of disease evidenced during life, been a recognised fact long prior to any attempts to formulate its symptomatology.

a. *Causation*.—That this localized dropsy may occur as an active abnormal condition, independent of structural changes save such as are connected with the peritoneal membrane, is abundantly evident   In these it may be regarded as a sequel of chronic peritonitis, probably resulting, as has already been said, from cold, exposure, insufficient food and shelter, operating upon the young rather than the adult, they being the animals more particularly exposed to these influences

More frequently, however, ascites may be regarded as a passive condition, and developed in connection with disease of other organs, chief of which are—(1) Disease affecting the walls or valvular structures of the heart, tending to venous obstruction, and often accompanied with œdema of the limbs or general anasarca ; (2) Functional disturbance, or textural alterations of the liver, by which the free passage of blood in the portal vein is obstructed ; (3) Renal diseases, which are often complicated with cardiac disorders , (4) Enlargement and other structural changes of the spleen ; (5) Adventitious deposits and morbid new formations on the omentum and

some other situations, these acting often mechanically by
pressure upon large or small venous trunks. I have also
observed that aged mares which have had several foals are
rather liable to suffer from ascites, probably from repeated
pressure of the gravid uterus upon the great abdominal veins.

  b. *Anatomical Characters.*—In a few cases where the presence of the fluid seems unconnected with any actively existing
disease, there may, apart from the dropsy, be nothing abnormal.
A greater number will show, as the sole lesion in any way
associated with the ascites, a thickening, more or less extensive,
of the peritoneal membrane. This latter state is usually quite
distinctive in those cases of subacute peritonitis which have
been mentioned as happening in young animals which have
been exposed and otherwise indifferently treated. Most frequently, however, several organs give unmistakable evidence
of disease and varying structural change.

  The peritoneum may exhibit traces of active and recent inflammatory action, the liver or spleen may be enlarged,
atrophied, or otherwise texturally changed; morbid growths
may be connected with these organs or scattered over the
membrane, free or attached, or the heart may exhibit hypertrophy with dilatation of its cavities and weakening of its
walls, or other changes in some way obstructing the general
circulation.

  The quantity of fluid in the cavity is occasionally very large,
amounting to many gallons; it is usually entirely serous, of a
straw or greenish colour, in some particular instances it will
contain shreds of lymph.

  Symptoms—When unassociated with some diseased condition more pronounced in character, the indications of ascites
are usually occult, insidious in development, and sometimes
spread over a considerable period of time. At first there may
be little attractive and certainly nothing diagnostic. The
animal is dull and spiritless, and if in the field there is a desire
to be alone, appetite impaired, general aspect unthrifty, with
indications of a badly nourished body. Watched more carefully, or examined more minutely, we may notice that it is disposed to rest much, not, however, with comfort; the hair is
overgrown, and the abdomen becomes gradually pendulous.
The pulse is weak and rather frequent, with, in some cases, a

blanched appearance of the visible membranes   As the disease
becomes confirmed the symptoms first observed may become
more pronounced, or others may be added to them. In
numerous instances, as the dropsy advances, œdema of the
limbs and lower parts of the body become troublesome   We
must never forget, however, that the character and relation
of the development of the symptoms to each other are largely
modified by the inducing factor of the dropsical condition,
the urine, which is always scanty and usually loaded, being
charged with biliary matter when the liver is much diseased,
and with albumen when the changes are chiefly situated in
the kidney   A certain amount of confirmatory evidence may
also be afforded us by palpation and percussion, while the concurrent symptoms of disease of other and important structures
or organs, which we know are largely concerned in its production, must not be overlooked.

Treatment.—In the successful management of ascites very
much depends upon our correct appreciation of the causes
which are operating in its production   In the great majority
of the cases appearing in young horses not stabled, and which
have been recklessly exposed and otherwise badly treated,
nothing is likely to be productive of good without first removing them from the operation of such untoward influences;
following the providing of sufficient shelter and good food,
much benefit will always result from efforts to improve the
general tone of all the tissues and promote absorption of
the fluid by the cautious exhibition of preparations of iron,
with occasional diuretics.   Where the bowels are confined,
moderate doses of aloes may be administered at long intervals,
or sulphate of soda may be steadily given until its laxative
effects are developed   At the same time the animals must
not be continuously confined, but exercise ought to be taken
as they are able to bear it

Where cardiac disease is known or suspected to exist in
connection with the ascites, a system of treatment essentially
tonic and occasionally eliminative by acting on the bowels, is,
what seems indicated.   When albumen exists in the urine,
and renal disease is suspected, diuretic medicine ought to be
withheld, or sparingly employed; here iron, in the form of the
solution or tincture of the perchloride, or the sulphate com-

bined with dilute sulphuric acid, and alternated with solution of iodine or iodide of potassium—the one in the morning, the other at night—are likely to serve our purpose better The removal of the local œdema may be facilitated by fomentation, smart friction with simple oil, and moderate exercise.

In cases where the amount of fluid is great, and producing much inconvenience, or where its amount is not perceptibly lessened by the use of medicine, and particularly when associated with cirrhosis and other structural diseases of the liver, paracentesis or tapping the abdomen and withdrawing the fluid by means of the trocar or aspirator may be adopted, and even repeated at regular intervals Rarely, however does this afford permanent relief, the immediate inducing cause being constantly in operation

<hr />

CHAPTER XXXII

DISEASES OF THE ALIMENTARY TRACT, STOMACH, AND INTESTINES

GENERAL REMARKS AS TO THEIR IMPORTANCE AMD CLINICAL CHARACTERS

WITH certain breeds of horses, and in particular districts of the country, there is probably no class of organs the diseases of which are of more importance to the veterinary surgeon than those affecting the alimentary canal Their importance arises from the frequency of their occurrence, and the fatality of their results In many agricultural districts they are not only the diseases which most engage his attention, they are those also in which his largest death-rate is found In addition, they are particularly deserving of the attention of the professional man, seeing they are those diseases over which he is able to exercise the greatest and most certain preventive influence, chiefly through the carrying out of a properly regulated dietary

Diseases of the digestive organs are largely modified and influenced in much relating to their appearance and development by many causes and conditions Although there is little doubt that particular breeds and special constitutional peculiarities of horses to a certain extent determine the frequency or otherwise of diseases of this class of organs, still I am rather inclined to place the chief cause of the production of these to the credit of agencies operating from without, to causes dietetic. It is certainly true that agricultural horses, and those of the heavier and coarser breeds, are greater sufferers than others, this, however, is probably not because they are constitutionally more disposed to suffer from these disorders, but rather that they are differently operated upon by causes from without, that they generally receive in the matter of their food-supply less attention than their more fortunate fellows

The relation of work to the occurrence of these diseases is also deserving of notice as having a marked influence in their production

We find that exhausting labour followed by full feeding is exceedingly apt to be succeeded by disorders of the digestive apparatus. The lowering of the vital powers consequent on fatigue is in all cases adverse to the healthful performance of digestion Where the work of horses is irregularly distributed, there must of necessity be an irregular distribution of alimentation, while, as the consequence of the enforced fasts and continued work, the food is frequently given at the particular time when of all others it ought to be withheld

Irregularity of work associated with irregularity in the feeding of horses is everywhere a fruitful source of diseases of the organs specially concerned with digestion

In our different patients there are, it is to be noted, varying degrees of susceptibility to contract disease exhibited by different portions of the digestive apparatus; this varying susceptibility may in some instances be feasibly accounted for, in others there seems some difficulty

Of our two chief patients, the horse and ox, the former is more subject to disturbance of the intestinal, and the latter to disorders of the gastric portions of the canal This speciality for locality of derangement may in great measure be accounted for on anatomical grounds.

In the horse there seems little doubt that the number and character of the entire class of the diseases of the alimentary canal are largely influenced by causes under our control;

that where a correct dietary, with work duly apportioned to age, capabilities, and other conditions, is carefully carried out, comparatively few diseases of these organs occur; and that where the dietetic conditions and arrangements respecting work are bad, they are most prevalent and most likely to terminate fatally.

Clinical Characters—In nearly all disorders of the digestive organs general symptoms, when such are present, are less attractive and less diagnostic than the local and objective ⁃ In one group of disturbances of these organs, both symptoms and lesions, if connected with what are more properly the digestive organs, are also largely and often more distinctively attached to other, to distant and to different organs; that although truly, as respects their origin, dietetic affections, they may with equal correctness, having respect to their symptomatology, be spoken of as diseases of other systems, depending upon the prominence of particular phenomena appearing during their course and development

Very commonly it is found in acute disturbances of the digestive organs, and where both symptoms and lesions are chiefly confined to these, that resulting from the sudden interruption of the digestive process, with the bulky character of the contained food prone to rapid chemical changes, very serious inconvenience is experienced, and shown by unmistakable symptoms from flatulent distension of different portions of the canal

In all, the inclination for food and water is more or less altered; while, when the disturbance is chiefly gastric, eructation and regurgitation, with, more rarely, expulsive efforts at discharge of ingesta, attract attention

The disturbance in the true intestinal portion is ordinarily more marked with restlessness and pain, while irregularity of action, exhibiting itself in the direction of constipation or diarrhœa, is frequently a prominent symptom. As enabling us to arrive at a satisfactory diagnosis, an inquiry into these conditions, with an examination of the discharges, and manipulation carried out externally and internally, are absolutely needful

CHAPTER XXXIII

DISEASES OF THE MOUTH, TONGUE, AND ASSOCIATED GLAND-STRUCTURES.

ALTHOUGH it is probably chiefly under the province of surgery that the greater number of the affections of the mouth and contiguous structures in the horse ought to be grouped, seeing they are mainly the result of injury inflicted wittingly, or through maladjustment of bits, etc, there are yet several disordered conditions which, as they may appear unconnected with violence sustained from without, or in the ordinary process of mastication, more properly demand some notice at our hand.

I. CONGESTION OF THE BUCCAL MEMBRANE.

A turgid and somewhat hyperæmic state of the buccal membrane, to an extent which seems to interfere with the process of mastication, and even to induce a slight amount of fever and general indisposition, is a matter of common observation   As the condition known to our fathers under the term ' *Lampas*,' it occupies a rather prominent place in all their descriptions of equine ailments   Its frequency of appearance in nearly all classes of horses, particularly the young, may be accounted for when we have regard to its symptomatic character, and the very numerous conditions with which it appears associated as an accompaniment or symptom

Causation—It chiefly results from—(1) Direct irritation of the buccal membrane and contiguous structures   (*a*) From the contact with bits and other means of restraint ; (*b*) From the action of certain substances and food materials ; (*c*) From dental changes, natural or abnormal.   (2) From disturbance of the alimentary tract, gastric or intestinal

Symptoms—The principal symptoms indicative of this state are local ; the general are rather exceptional   That which is likely to attract attention more readily than aught else in the earlier stages is a disposition to slaver more than usual, both when at work and in the stable, particularly when feeding. When an examination is attempted there is shown disinclination to have the mouth touched ; and however quietly the

38

fingers are passed between the lips there is tenderness, particularly when the bars and interdental spaces are pressed upon. When the mouth is opened the membrane may seem somewhat heightened in colour, but more certainly it gives the impression of a puffy or swollen character, markedly so along the palatine surface, while behind the incisor teeth the membrane is so much tumefied as to be on a level with the cutting surface of the teeth. When the cause is gastric or intestinal derangement, and severe or of long continuance, the probability is that the appetite will be impaired, with general languor, a slight amount of fever, and some other special indications of general or gastric disturbance

In aged animals, when associated with unnatural dental activities, we find added to the common symptoms of local congestion those of disturbed mastication, specially indicative of disease of the teeth

Treatment —This ought in great measure to be regulated by a consideration of the causes which operate in the production of the congestion   The heroic local treatment formerly carried out through removal by the actual cautery of the buccal membrane and tissues, bounded by the second or third ridge or bar of the palate, is, we trust, now a method of the past. In a few instances the utmost extent of local manipulation warranted is that which is represented by free scarification of the tumid membrane.   Where local irritation is directly operative through improperly applied bits or mouth-gear, these must for a time be removed, and greater care exercised in their replacement ; should normal dental changes seem to be mainly concerned in its production, these must be watched, and any untoward results obviated by local or general soothing measures. Where abnormal dental conditions are in existence judicious surgical interference must be brought to bear, in order that such may be rectified.   The greater number of dyspeptic cases which are attended with buccal congestion require most probably constitutional treatment ; in these a moderate dose of laxative medicine, with afterwards some cooling salines, will suffice, along with attention to a properly regulated regimen, to place the animal, both as to its digestive organs and the membrane of the mouth, in accord with the outward conditions of its life.

II Stomatitis—Inflammation of the Mouth

Definition.—*Inflammation of the mouth, of varying forms and degrees of violence.*

Under the generic term *stomatitis* have been gathered several, and somewhat differing, forms of inflammatory action invading the mouth. According as the lesions attending this morbid action have been viewed, so have separate designations been given to the processes. In the horse, the chief, if not the whole, of the different manifestations of the inflammatory process may conveniently be viewed as—(1) *Simple or catarrhal;* (2) *Vesicular,* (3) *Pustular.*

Ætiology—The causes which operate in the induction of the several forms of stomatitis are in part predisposing, as—(a) Age, being more frequent in the young than the adult, (b) Defective sanitary conditions and improper dietary, being more liable to be developed where depressing and vitiating influences co-operate with imperfect nutrition; (c) The existence of previous or actively operating diseases, by which the general force and vitality is lowered.

Immediate or determining influences are to be found in—(a) Direct or local irritation, as contact of acrid materials or mechanical violence, (b) The extension of similar actions from contiguous parts, or disorders of the alimentary tract; (c) Contagion, animate or otherwise, may develop stomatitis. The spores of certain fungi and acari, directly or indirectly implanted, are thus capable of inciting inflammation of the buccal membrane.

1 *Simple or Catarrhal Stomatitis*—This form is chiefly observed in the very young—foals with their dams—although a somewhat similar condition may develop in aged animals from mechanical or other direct irritation. An early symptom of this condition is the appearance of circumscribed red patches on the inner sides of the cheeks and roof of the mouth; these shortly, by death and removal of cell structures, display a raw and excoriated surface, which usually does not remain as patches, but by coalescence extends over the greater part of the buccal membrane. On opening the mouth in advanced cases, the membrane seems swollen, and lightly covered in certain places with a grey, mealy-looking material, collections

38—2

of denuded epithelium ; often there is an accumulation of ropy saliva and a fœtid smell. According to the extent of the excoriation is the difficulty exhibited in sucking. Usually in the foal, and occasionally in the dam, this condition is accompanied with a deranged state of the alimentary canal.

2 *Vesicular Stomatitis* —This modification may be observed in both young and adult animals Appearing sometimes as an accompaniment of the simple form, it more generally starts into existence with its own independent characters of minute round vesicles, situated on the inner sides of the cheeks, around the angles of the mouth, and along the sides and frœnum of the tongue These vesicles both appear and rupture suddenly, their contents being more or less turbid, rarely clear On rupturing they leave a minute ulcer, with slightly elevated margins, and surrounded with a hyperæmic zone. Frequently discrete, they may coalesce and form larger vascular-looking excoriations. In some cases, where the general conditions, intrinsic and extrinsic, are bad, these sores seem indisposed to heal, and have a coating of a plastic material adhering to their raw surfaces ; while in others they seem associated with the mucous follicles, which appear tumefied, and at times plugged with a pasty granular material .

I have observed this form of stomatitis in some developments associated with certain febrile diseases ; more frequently, however, no general disturbance is appreciable

3 *Pustular Stomatitis* —This manifestation of the inflammatory action I have only observed in adult animals. In some instances it appears as the sequel of the preceding The vesicles, remaining unbroken for a longer time, gradually acquire in their contents an opalescent and puriform character, and leave, on rupturing, a rather deeper vascular-looking ulcer More frequently, however, the lesions form as minute indurations or yellowish spots, as if the epithelial elements were being raised from infiltration These excrescences gradually become better defined, develop fluid contents, form distinct pustules, and ultimately rupture, discharging their contents, leaving well-marked, pit-like ulcers

The existence of these pustules, while in many instances dependent on a vitiated state of the blood from previous disease, or contamination with a specific disease element, or some peculiarity of location and diet, are yet, probably more frequently than we have been disposed to believe, to be attributed to parasitic invasion

The existence of the vegetable fungus the *Odium albicans* has long been recognised as connected with some forms of stomatitis, but it is only recently, however previously suspected, that the presence of an acarus has been demonstrated in association with the pustules of equine stomatitis (Mr. Burke, *Veterinary Journal*, July, 1882)

Treatment —The management of all cases of stomatitis resolves itself into—

1. Attention to and strict enforcement of correct hygiene The animals ought to be removed from foul and unwholesome stables, allowed sufficiency of exercise, with fresh air, the food-supply of good quality, and in keeping with the requirements of the system.

2 A consideration of the general state of the animal's health. Here we may, if the indications lead us, require to produce a more pronounced state of tonic sufficiency by the exhibition of medicines If the use of general tonics is only called for in exceptional cases, it will be found that in the greater number some attention to the state of the digestive system is called for In the very young the use of some oleaginous laxative, followed by mild vegetable tonics, will do much to confer healthy tone on the entire digestive tract In some a longer continuance of salines or antacids will be of advantage.

3 Local applications. These are in all instances of benefit. They may be of the mildest form, as good linseed-tea, or a solution of bicarbonate or chlorate of potash, or they may be actively astringent, as a saturated solution of tannic acid or alum The greater number of the commonly observed forms rarely need aught more active than a solution of chlorate of potash or sulphate of soda employed twice or thrice daily Where there is much foetor, a solution of ten grains of permanganate of potash to the ounce of water, or a little carbolic glycerine added to the solution of chlorate of potash, will do well

When the individual sores or ulcerous spots do not appear to heal well, benefit will result from touching these every alternate day with a ten grains to the ounce solution of nitrate of silver

III Glossitis.

Definition —*Simple inflammation of the intimate structure of the tongue*

Apart from direct injury, or the action of irritant substances, simple glossitis in our patients is a rare affection Occasionally it would seem in a mild form to accompany inflammatory action affecting the lining membrane of the mouth, or to follow by extension a similar process in contiguous structures.

When occurring, the body of the organ enlarges from infiltration amongst the muscular tissue, and as much connective-tissue does not exist in association with the lingual structures it shortly becomes tense, painful, and from protrusion dry and brown along the parts exposed, particularly the dorsum With the swelling there is difficulty of swallowing, and retention of tenacious saliva and mucus in the mouth, which shortly smell disagreeably

Treatment —Laxatives, which are usually indicated, not being possible of employment in the usual way, must be introduced by the rectum

The local measures are free scarification, gargling the mouth first with warm water to favour bleeding, afterwards with a mixture of sulphurous acid and water, or a solution of nitrate or chlorate of potash.   Benefit I have also seen follow steady fumigation with medicated vapour from the common nose-bag. Should the swelling not extend and involve the structures of the laryngeal region during the first two or three days, the termination is usually favourable.

IV Parotitis.

Definition —*Inflammation of an acute or subacute character affecting the structure of the parotid gland.*

Nature and Causation.—During attacks of the specific fever of strangles, the parotids are often affected to a greater or less extent. In addition, however, to this, parotitis is often enough encountered either attendant upon some febrile attack, or following as a result of such. In almost all these attacks, with or without catarrh, the inflammatory action is very erratic, in some instances being of an acute type, passing rapidly through its different stages, and terminating in a considerable abscess in the gland-structure ; at other times slow in its progress, affecting only limited portions of structure, and, after a tedious course, issuing in the production of several distinct and circumscribed collections of pus

Symptoms —Those which specially indicate the onset of the inflammatory action are rather insidious, not diagnostic, and of slow development. The horse exhibits a disposition to protrude his nose, with a disinclination to move, or difficulty in turning the head independent of the body. There is pain on manipulation of the throat, with a steady swelling of the parotid structure

This, whenever established, does not necessarily proceed to suppuration, cases often being observed where congestion and tumefaction proceed to a considerable length, and after some days suffer subsidence. When terminating in pus-formation, the skin over one or more points becomes tense, thin, disposed to part with its hair, and inclined to exude a little serous fluid. When not evacuated, or discharging itself externally, the matter may find escape into the pharyngeal pouch, showing itself at the nasal openings.

Treatment.—This consists at first in steady fomentation, with poulticing, while, should the process seem lagging, good will often follow the employment of a smart cantharides liniment, or daily application of common iodine ointment. When the abscess seems matured, a careful incision ought to be made, so as to allow a free escape of the matter. Following its discharge, nothing is needed save attention to cleanliness. If weakness is a marked feature, the horse will require, with good food, some tonic, such as sulphate of iron, either alone or in combination with a vegetable bitter Should any induration remain after recovery, the use, both locally and internally, of some preparation of iodine is indicated.

V Salivation, or Ptyalism.

The condition of the presence in the mouth, and of the discharge from it, of an extra amount of saliva is not unfrequently observed in the horse, and although not a serious may be a troublesome affection.

This annoying symptom of several very different conditions may occur either from an extra secretion of saliva or from an indisposition or inability to swallow it when secreted The discharge, while lasting, is not intermittent, usually continuous, dribbling from the mouth when at rest or work, or forming a pultaceous mass with the food when feeding, it will also, in most instances, be found collected in masses of foam at the angles of the mouth In character this unnatural saliva is a little different from the fluid found in health, particularly when the condition has been established for some time

The causes which seem to operate in the induction of this state are both constitutional and local. It is observed in some cases of tetanus and rabies, also with the continuous reception of certain medicinal agents. It is, however, more as the result of direct or reflected nervous irritation that it is presented to us in the horse. In the former manifestation it may be encountered in some cerebral diseases, and diseases of nerve-structures and cords directly connected with the salivary apparatus. In the latter we observe it in connection with many of those conditions already mentioned of an irritative character, having their seat in the mouth and contiguous structures, also in many affections of the pharynx and throat, or more distant organs and structures Besides association with these obvious disturbances, it may further be seen in what may be regarded as an idiopathic form, or where we are unable to connect it with any appreciable cause.

The symptom of salivation is not likely to be overlooked, but being so varied as to its inducing agencies there is frequently some difficulty experienced in duly appreciating the determining influence operating in each case, conditions of simple local irritation from the presence of foreign bodies or irregular teeth are often enough overlooked in the search for some more serious and hidden condition, it being sometimes difficult to believe that matters so trifling should produce symptoms so persistent and troublesome.

In all cases, ere any attempt at treatment is made, a careful examination ought to be undertaken with the view of discovering whether the disturbance is owing to local and appreciable irritation in connection with the mouth and contiguous structures. It is to the causes of this perversion of function that our attention ought chiefly to be directed, as these must ever be our guide in the selection of remedies and remedial

measures   Often a simple astringent gargle, a smoothing of
trifling dental asperities, or some equally simple measure, will
suffice to confer marked benefit   At other times, however,
when more closely dependent on disturbance of nerve-power
or lesion of nerve-tissue, the progress of the disturbance may
be delayed, and is usually uncertain in its course, still, in
every instance we have to remember that the nervous disturbance upon which it depends, where this can be made out,
demands our attention rather than the mere symptom of
salivation

CHAPTER XXXIV.

DISEASES OF THE THROAT

Diseases of the throat, chiefly of the lining membrane and
immediately associated structures, are common in the horse
at all ages, usually appearing at some part of the course
of epizootic catarrhal fever, and other specific affections in
which the air-passages are involved   It is, however, as independent affections, not as part of the general symptoms of
either influenza or strangles, or any other fever, which we now
speak of them.

1 Acute Pharyngeal Catarrh.—Inflammation of Fauces
and Pharynx.

Definition —*Common inflammation of the textures, chiefly
mucous membrane and submucous tissue of fauces and
pharynx.*

Pathology. *a. Nature* —Under the designation of inflammation of these structures may be grouped many cases of
sore throat, sudden in accession, unattended with fever, and
which in a few days terminate in resolution. The abnormal
action is of a congestive or inflammatory character, with
œdema of the lining membrane of the fauces and pharynx,
the one situation being rarely affected apart from the other.
Following the first conditions of swelling and dryness there is
more than the average amount of secretion, which is more

tenacious than natural, mingled with pus-cells, and disposed to
adhere to the inflamed membrane. There are seldom any
textural changes, although when these do occur they are often
troublesome, as pharyngeal abscesses of different kinds

b. Causation.—Although the larger number of instances of
inflammation of the fauces and pharynx appear as part of the
symptoms of the more general diseased condition known as
catarrh, there are yet many where the state of pharyngeal
catarrh arises independent of association with the more distinctly general disturbance. In these latter, although it is
evident that systemic weakness and atony predispose to the
occurrence of this local disturbance, yet it almost invariably
claims another parentage, such as exposure to depressing atmospheric influences; cold, with damp, following previous
fatigue and general exhaustion, being fruitful sources of the
condition

Direct irritation, resulting from the contact or lodgment of
acrid materials or foreign bodies, will more rarely produce this
state of local inflammation, while it seems not unlikely that
some of the milder instances, in young animals in particular,
are connected with dental disturbance and irregularities of the
digestive organs. Repeated attacks seem in time to confer a
susceptibility under ordinary determining influences to the recurrence of this form of sore throat.

Symptoms—The indications of the existence of this affection are in the pronounced cases unequivocal. Difficulty in
swallowing may be looked upon as the most constantly
present and diagnostic. In bad cases solid food is with difficulty passed along the fauces without inducing coughing,
during which act it is often thrown again into the mouth,
while liquids, after having passed the velum, are discharged
by the nostrils, sometimes coloured with the food materials.
Cough is not a constant feature, unless the laryngeal structures
are involved. The inclination to eat is evident, while the constant inability to swallow, and the presence in the mouth and
trickling from it of ropy saliva, show the irritability and
swelling which exist in the posterior parts.

This condition is distinguished from inflammation of the
laryngeal structures by absence of fever and non-existence of
distinct impairment in respiration. In many, however, it

must be remembered that this pharyngeal catarrh is complicated with laryngeal affection.

Treatment.—Many of the cases of pharyngeal catarrh recover in a few days without any particular attention save resting from work. Whenever the difficulty of swallowing is great, much relief is afforded by fumigating the head with water-vapour, plain or medicated; the medication may be effected through the addition to the material in the nose-bag of some preparation of opium, belladonna, carbolic acid, or iodine. Gargling the mouth with a solution of sulphurous acid, borax, or chlorate of potash is also a means of relieving the irritation, while the free use of compound camphor and belladonna electuary will, without causing any annoyance, often be all that is required.

Heat and moisture, applied externally through the medium of woollen cloths or spongiopiline, ought to be employed continuously for some hours daily.

Rarely will the use of irritant applications, as blisters, be needful in the acute cases, or during the early stages of any; they are better supplanted by the soothing treatment of heat and moisture, unless the restlessness of the patient prevents the steady application of these latter, or when the irritation becomes chronic.

II. Post-, or Retro-pharyngeal Abscess.

Definition.—*Inflammation of the pharynx, resulting in circumscribed collections of pus in the pharyngeal structures.*

Pathology. *a. Nature.*—Pus may in many instances of inflammation of the pharynx form on the exposed surface in diffuse masses, and suffer removal as formed; this condition is not a serious one, differing entirely from that now mentioned. In cases of pharyngeal abscess the collections of pus are situated in the walls of the pouch in connection with the muscular and connective-tissue. They are encountered where simple pharyngeal inflammation has existed; but more frequently where this condition, although not acute, has been associated with some general unhealthy condition, or the advent of a specific fever.

b. Causation.—Although impossible to say exactly upon what these formations of pus are either immediately or remotely dependent, there is evidence to satisfy us that certain

conditions or associations are more than others likely to precede or accompany this, as—(1) A previous general unhealthy
state of the system ; (2) The advent of the pharyngeal inflammation with some of the specific fevers, (3) It may appear as
part of a common pyæmic state ; (4) Certain vitiating influences
seem to have power in determining this pus-formative action
in pharyngeal inflammations.

Symptoms—Although somewhat varying, they may generally
be regarded as—(1) Obvious and audible obstruction in the
acts of breathing and swallowing. (2) Occasional swelling and
tenderness on manipulation externally, general and defined
swelling on examination of the pharynx internally.

Treatment.—When the breathing is much interfered with,
fumigation with the vapour of hot water is indicated, this
removes the tension and hastens the maturation of the abscess.
The smaller abscesses, and those which have developed rapidly,
frequently burst when mature, discharging their contents
through the nose. In cases where suffocation is feared, or
where the abscesses seem tardy in approaching the surface,
and when distinctly felt internally, they may be opened from
within with a guarded knife. In attempting to make this
incision it is better to do so with the animal standing ; in this
way the danger of choking from the rush of pus is considerably
lessened.

CHAPTER XXXV.

DISEASES OF THE ŒSOPHAGUS

THE food-tube, extending from the pharynx to the stomach, is
in the horse a rather rare seat of idiopathic disease. Such as may
be encountered are either—(1) Œsophagitis, or inflammation
of the textures of the tube; (2) Certain functional derangements;
(3) Structural alterations.

1. ŒSOPHAGITIS, OR INFLAMMATION OF THE STRUCTURES COM-
POSING THE TUBE—This is the result—(a) Of direct injury
from irritating liquids administered through mistake ; (b) Of
contact in passing along the tube of hard and too large portions of some food material ; (c) Following the infliction of

injury from without ; (d) More rarely it may follow from the extension of inflammatory action from contiguous parts, or as a part of a general and common catarrhal inflammation of other mucous membranes.

Anatomical Characters.—The entire structures of the œsophagus give the usual indications of inflammatory action, somewhat varied in accordance with the exciting cause. When occurring from the contact of hot water, or irritating fluids, there is generally considerable destruction of tissue, and in all much infiltration of the submucous structure, with the presence of various fluid secretions

Symptoms.—When the morbid action or injury is trifling, the only attractive symptom may be the difficulty in swallowing, variously expressed—sometimes by spasm with ejection of material swallowed, and stamping of the feet , while manipulation over the region affected is accompanied by increase of these. When severe, there is in addition febrile disturbance ; and if the coats are perforated, infiltration of the surrounding tissues will shortly show itself, with additional phenomena

Treatment—Milder cases may be left to recover, with no interference save the exhibition of food of such a character as will not injure the irritated parts. In the more severe cases this will require specially to be attended to , while with a free use of mucilaginous fluids, as linseed-gruel and milk, to which may be added some simple saline, it is better not to attempt the administration of many medicaments. If pain is a marked feature, morphia, used hypodermically, and local medicated fomentations, are likely to be productive of good. The results of severe inflammatory action of the œsophagus, by whatever means induced, are what we have most to dread ; the chief of these, constriction to a greater or less extent, is nearly certain to follow.

2. FUNCTIONAL DERANGEMENTS—Spasm, or œsophagismus, is the only disturbance of this character I have observed in the horse, and this not often. It is of irregular and uncertain occurrence, showing itself on particular occasions without apparent cause, and disappearing in the same erratic manner. Speculation may afford material to account for the phenomenon, but it has not given any satisfactory explanation of it. Local irritation, as circumscribed erosions, and limited textural changes

have in some instances seemed connected with the occurrence
of this disturbance

Symptoms—These are only exhibited when food, chiefly of a
solid character, more rarely liquids, is being swallowed   When
the ingesta has travelled so far along the tube the spasms
develop. and if the material is not ejected immediately, it is
in a short time thrown up   Occasionally it is simply arrested,
the spasm not being sufficiently powerful to cause ejection , in
such instances after a short period it will be passed quietly
along

On the occurrence of spasm the animal seems to feel pain,
there is little, or more probably in the greater number, and the
more active cases, no swelling , the neck is bent in a downward
direction, the nose pointing to the sternum , the muscles of the
œsophageal region seem in active contraction ; there are various
muscular movements of an uncertain character, an extra spasmodic effort, sometimes opening of the mouth, and ejection,
chiefly through the nasal openings, of the lately swallowed
material, mingled with mucus, or slightly tinged with blood.

When not at once ejected or passed on, but retained until
an accumulation occurs, swelling is a distinct symptom, gradually increasing in an upward direction, and slightly painful
when pressed upon   Regurgitation in these instances may
take place with a trifling amount of spasm, less apparently than
in the acute cases, where a smaller amount of food seems to
excite the involuntary action

Treatment—As we are uncertain in the greater number of
cases of the causes which induce this disturbance, anything
which may be attempted is too frequently unsatisfactory; the
only remedy which I have found of much use has been morphia
used in full doses and subcutaneously   Should other indications point to an uncertain state of health, attempts must be
made in the direction of its improvement ; a little laxative
medicine followed by tonics I have believed to be productive of
good   In many it may be needful to introduce the probang,
and ascertain that no obstruction exists , and, above all, food
must be allowed which is not likely to induce local irritation.

3 ORGANIC DISEASE—Of this, the chief manifestation is
stricture with obstruction   This narrowing of the tube may be
the result of—(a) Changes in the walls from previous inflam-

matory or other diseased conditions; (b) The existence of polypi or tumours on the inner structures, (c) The presence of morbid growths in its vicinity When the condition of narrowing of the calibre of the tube is established, certain changes are likely to follow in other parts. above the stricture we will have hypertrophy, with dilatation, from the steady distension which is kept up; below, the opposite conditions are likely to prevail

Symptoms.—These are gradual in their development at first the difficulty in swallowing may not be much, and only shown when certain foods are partaken of, at length obstruction becomes evident and painful, showing itself most distinctly when dry food, or large masses are attempted to be passed along Often food will be retarded at the constricted part, and the upper and dilated portion of the tube become much distended before ejection takes place, the quantity in these cases being considerable

Along with the discharged food there is also much mucus, sometimes blood and purulent matter Careful manipulatory examination from without, and occasional use of the probang, may assist us in determining the causes of the obstruction and the probabilities of recovery; when in certain cases the obstruction is overcome, an altered condition of the œsophagus, consisting of permanent dilatation, is apt to succeed

Treatment—In those cases where the stricture proceeds from textural changes in the walls themselves, little can be done to relieve the animal. When tumours, either within or without the canal, are the constricting agents, there may be some prospect of amendment, their management depending upon their nature and particular situation In all, attention to dieting is particularly called for, so as to secure for the animal what is least likely to irritate the parts, and sufficiently nutritive to support its strength

CHAPTER XXXVI.

OF CERTAIN GASTRIC SYMPTOMS AND FUNCTIONAL DISORDERS.

I VOMITING—EMESIS

Definition —*The act of forcibly ejecting the contents of the stomach through the œsophagus in response to direct disturbance of the brain, or from reflex irritation.*

This condition, common enough in all other animals which engage our attention, is of rather rare occurrence in the horse Why this phenomenon should so seldom exhibit itself in him has from an early period engaged the attention of physiologists and experimenters.

The two chief considerations which have been advanced to account for the rarity of this occurrence in the horse are— (1) The physiological one of the small susceptibility which the animal exhibits to the action of nauseants, and (2) The alleged physical difficulty depending on the anatomical conformation of the viscus, particularly its possession of a constricting or valvular arrangement at the cardiac opening, by which the contents are prevented from escaping into the œsophagus

Without entering into the question of the strength or weakness of the arguments and collections of facts brought forward to prove either of these statements, we may state that—insusceptible as the horse is to the action of emetics, and rare as nausea, the primary inducing factor in the production of emesis, seems to be—vomition, or the forcible ejectment of the contents of the stomach through the œsophagus, is met with under varying conditions The states in which it seems highly probable that such may occur, are not those following the induction of nausea in any marked degree, or when there is direct action upon the nervous system, but are all of them such as pertain to some peculiar state of the organ itself, all seem to have a definite relation to its anatomical characters, particularly to the state of the lining membrane.

I have observed it—

1. When the stomach has been much distended with ingesta, chiefly of a solid nature, and prone to fermentative

changes Some of the most remaikable cases which I have watched were in young horses, and followed feeding upon haws from the hedgerows during the late autumn In some of these animals a fatal result was reached, apparently through gastric and intestinal inflammation. In those which recovered there was much distress, with vomition of considerable quantities of the berries, and well-marked prostration for some days afterwards

2 Where dilatation of the lower extremity of the œsophagus close to the cardiac orifice existed Irregularly occurring but long-continued vomiting I have noticed in a few cases, when, on examination after death, a considerable pouch in the œsophagus existed close to the cardiac opening, and wheie probably this latter was regularly disposed to be dilated

3 Ruptures, partial or complete, of the gastric walls These lesions, when occurring, I am disposed to associate with pressure from within rather than with intrinsic and extensive muscular contraction, and feel satisfied that the vomition occurs subsequent to the rupture, not that the rupture is the result of this functional disturbance

4 Probably, also, in such states as closure of the pyloric opening of the organ, when the contained material is prevented from passing along the duodenum

When the contents of the stomach are regurgitated, they are, of course, chiefly ejected through the nasal apertures. Although always a grave symptom, it is not necessarily indicative of a fatal result, and while symptomatic of gastric rupture, it is not associated with this lesion alone

In the treatment of cases of vomition, when these are the result of merely excessive distension, or at least when structural changes aie not satisfactorily demonstrated, we are always warranted in making attempts to empty the stomach by passing the contents along the canal, and allowing the organ a perfect rest for some days, endeavouiing to support the animal without calling for any, or much, gastric action.

II DYSPEPSIA—INDIGESTION

Definition —*Disturbance of the function of digestion unassociated with perceptible textural change or lesion of the stomach.*

Varieties—Of the different forms in which distuibed diges-

20

tion attracts our attention in the horse, not being immediately attendant on disease of other organs or structural alterations in the stomach itself, the chief are—(*a*) *Indigestion of an acute character*, ordinarily the result of the conveyance into the viscus of an extra amount of material, (*b*) *Chronic indigestion*, proceeding from various causes, chiefly perversion of gastric activities

A ACUTE INDIGESTION—GORGED STOMACH—STOMACH STAGGERS.

Causation—This form of indigestion, more alarming in its symptoms and development than any other, is chiefly, if not entirely, the result of filling the stomach to repletion with food-materials which from their mechanical bulk and physical unfitness for solution or for being sufficiently broken down and converted into a pulp capable of being passed on, or with such as from their special chemical characters, or the chemical changes which they undergo on being taken into the stomach, are rendered similarly unfit for assimilation In both instances the resulting phenomenon is over-repletion or distension of the viscus The chief characteristics of these foods are bulk, indigestibility—not necesssarily innutritiousness—and liability to undergo fermentative changes in the stomach It may also follow the use of any food conveyed into the stomach without sufficient mastication and incorporation with natural secretions.

Brewers' grains, partially damaged wheat, ripe vetches, and cooked food generally, I have found particularly liable to induce this condition

The state of the animal itself, particularly as respects physical exhaustion and period of abstinence from food, also operates materially in determining the existence of acute indigestion. In horses, after prolonged work and an enforced fast, the vital powers generally, and the digestive functions particularly, are much depressed and weakened. Food in such cases may be readily enough taken, and the amount consumed is often in excess of what is usually offered, on the mistaken idea of compensating for the abstinence, and as being needful on account of the extra work done, whereas the opposite is the course which ought to be adopted In such cases, should the food be rather bulky, difficult of digestion, or susceptible of rapid chemical changes, the consequences are likely to be troublesome

Symptoms—These are generally sudden in development, at least they follow immediately as sequels to the condition of impaction, the animal having previously been in his usual state of health   They are not invariably of a similar character, but are capable of being arranged in two groups

1. They may, with trifling modifications, be characterized as *gastric or abdominal.* In these, the earliest indications are those of fugitive abdominal pain, lying down, resting for a little, rising to the feet, and again resuming the recumbent position ; shortly followed by greater restlessness, continued or interrupted pawing with the fore-feet, protruding of the head, and, in some cases, eructations, with, in rarer instances, attempts at vomition and a discharge of liquid matter from the nose.   When the distension of the stomach is considerable, consisting of gas and solid ingesta, the animal may show signs of acute pain, at each eructation straining to vomit ; he will likewise be most careful at first in lying or throwing himself down

In three cases which I had the opportunity of watching, where the animals had eaten a large quantity of haws, there was, during the whole course of the severity of the symptoms, great abdominal pain, dropping at first quietly, and afterwards throwing themselves to the ground, tossing wildly about, occasionally resting on the abdomen, continued eructation with ejection of a sour-smelling brown-coloured fluid from the nose, and persistent attempts to vomit.

2 In numerous instances the evidence of pain and gastric disturbance pure and simple is not great, but the symptoms of cerebral complication are more marked   The horse is dull and semicomatose, stands with his head low and disposed to press the forehead against some resisting body—as the wall or manger, or whatever is most accessible—refuses to eat, is moved with difficulty, and when forced to change his position shows want of control over his movements and an inclination to resume the placing of his head against some fixed object, the breathing being more or less stertorous.

When the abdominal pain is a marked feature the pulse

39—2

and respirations are uniformly increased in frequency and somewhat altered in character, where the condition of coma exists both of these are less frequent, and the pulse is full and of considerable resisting power. These latter are the true stomach staggers of the older writers, and from all accounts it would appear that this form of indigestion and gastric disturbance must in former days have had a more extensive distribution than can be accredited to it in our day

Course and Termination—Mild cases of engorgement of the stomach, many of which are spoken of as colic, even when attended with uneasiness and pain, may of themselves become relieved; this more certainly when the material causing the distension is soft in character and likely to undergo removal rather easily, or in cases where the animals have not been previously debilitated by exhausting work or the organ itself weakened through former attacks of a similar nature. The more severe cases, however, are, if left to themselves, rather disposed to terminate fatally, either by gastritis, rupture of the coats of the stomach, or through cerebral complications. Such fatal cases are often seen where the animal has received the full meal, the direct inducing cause, into a weakened and exhausted stomach, as the last treatment of the day, and is then left to itself for the night. We have found that horses which are habitually greedy feeders, or which have for years been fed on bulky and innutritious food, by which the coats of the stomach have become unnaturally attenuated, are more liable than animals differently circumstanced to become the subjects of fatal distension of the organ

Prevention and Treatment—Amongst the entire class of diseases of the digestive organs which, as a class, may be regarded as eminently capable of being circumscribed by attention to the common rules of dietary, there is probably none so dependent for its existence on neglect of these as this gastric indigestion following engorgement

If those who have the charge of our agricultural and heavier draught horses could only be brought to understand that these creatures are living, not inanimate, machines, that their stomachs have naturally only a limited capacity, and that food may not be received into that organ beyond a certain amount without impairing or destroying its powers of acting upon it, owners of horses would be saved much money, and the animals of which they have the charge much suffering. The stomach of these animals is too often treated as if it were little different from a corn-box, a simple food-receptacle, into which it is advisable to thrust as large a quantity of material, without regard to its character, as possible

Of the truth of these statements I have been abundantly satisfied during a practice of many years in an agricultural district. In this district horses are as hard wrought and as liberally fed as anywhere in Great Britain; in no case is there any stinting of food, or the giving of it of inferior quality for the mere purpose of saving money. At the period of which I speak the usual scale of dietary was oats *ad libitum*, or from eighteen to twenty-three pounds per horse per day, with oat-straw as fodder during two-thirds of the year, and rye-grass hay the remaining third. Four or six nights in the week the evening feed of oats during certain seasons of the year was replaced by a feed of boiled barley; this latter I found was much relished by the horses, but the quantity given was greatly in excess of what any horse ought to receive at one time. This evening feeding with cooked grains I found a most fruitful source of indigestion, it was greedily eaten after a full and often hard day's work, its quantity being in many instances too severe a task for a somewhat exhausted stomach to dispose of ere fermentative and other changes had taken place, and by gaseous elimination further increasing the difficulties

During the season when this system of dieting was most industriously carried out, and amongst those animals that regularly received it, there was invariably a much larger number of cases of illness wholly connected with the digestive organs, and chiefly gastric, than where cooked food was not employed. At this time the loss amongst this class of horses from diseases of the digestive organs was over five per cent. Gradually, in course of years, the same agriculturists have seen cause to alter their views on this matter of horse-feeding, and for some time the use of cooked food has been abandoned, and with its abandonment the sickness and death-rate have fallen fifty per cent.

Horses, for the full and healthy exercise of digestion, do not require their stomachs filled to repletion with material, nutritious or innutritious, while to present them largely with food requiring little or no mastication, from the mistaken idea that this is beneficial to the animals as well as a saving of time by the rapidity with which they may fill their stomach, is the sure way to further gastric derangement from repletion

In the purely medical treatment of these cases of indigestion from engorgement, the first indication to be attended to is restoration of functional power to the organ by removal of the cause of disturbance—the excess of food. Our ordinary method of securing this is by inciting the entire alimentary canal to increased action through the administration of purgatives. In addition to these it is generally needful, at least in all cases where pain is a prominent symptom, that attention be given to relieve this. Our chief reliance for cure is certainly the purgative, which may be either aloes or oil, or both combined. Salines, as the sulphate of soda or magnesia, rarely do so well. For the relief of pain, when it exists, sulphuric ether, from half an ounce to an ounce, may be given in cold gruel every two or three hours until two or three doses have been administered, or from two to four fluid ounces of sweet spirits of nitre with five minims of Fleming's tincture of aconite in a similar vehicle. When liquids, either from choice or difficulty of administration, are objected to, the subcutaneous injection of the solution of the acetate of morphia may be employed with advantage. As a medium dose, forty minims may be injected under the skin in any part of the body, while for the ordinary cases requiring its use the anterior part of the sternum is probably more accessible than any other situation. It may be repeated if considered needful. Should the bowels not respond to the aloes first given, it may be needful to administer a second dose, but not before forty-eight hours have elapsed. When repeating the laxative the aloes had better be combined with one or two drachms of gentian and half a drachm of calomel. Four drachms of aloes with one to one and a half drachms of powdered gentian, and half a drachm of calomel, will generally produce an action equal to six drachms of aloes.

If there is a moderate discharge of material from the bowels, although not fluid in character, it will probably not be requisite to give additional purgatives , but good will result from the daily administration of a ball containing half a drachm to a drachm of aloes, with a drachm each of powdered assafœtida, gentian, and ginger

In those cases where the symptoms of coma and cerebral disturbance are distinct features, where the pulse is full and slow, and the breathing stertorous, the best results attend the early and full abstraction of blood , this bleeding, together with the application to the superior part of the head of woollen cloths kept moist with cold water, and the exhibition of a smart cathartic, followed by treatment somewhat similar to that which has already been indicated, is that which experience recommends as most likely to be productive of good.

In the very young, foals, there is often encountered a form of acute indigestion or derangement of the functions of the stomach, the result of an irregular milk-supply consequent on their removal from the dam for uncertain and lengthened periods, the latter being sent to work, and returned to their foals often in a heated and exhausted condition. Both from the abstinence forced on the young creature, and consequent disposition to take more milk when the opportunity occurs than is compatible with healthy gastric digestion, and also from the somewhat depraved condition of the milk, from not having been removed at proper intervals, it seems in many cases that these long-delayed and irregularly recurring feeding-periods act injuriously.

The curd which is originally formed in the stomach is not redissolved, either from the simple repletion of the organ, or the suddenness after a fast with which conditions are reversed, or other changes entailing impairment of function , or if altered in part, the remainder proves an irritant, undergoing chemical changes, and further disturbing digestion   In this gastric disturbance in these young animals the accompaniment or result is usually diarrhœa, which will be noticed when we come to consider the unnatural conditions more properly intestinal.

B. CHRONIC INDIGESTION.

Causation.—Of the agencies which are in operation to induce chronic dyspepsia in the horse, the greater number may be grouped under—(1) Errors in dieting, (2) Changes in the gastric and other secretions. (3) Abnormalities affecting the movements of the stomach. Of all these it is probable that the first, errors in dieting, may be regarded as paramount, acting primarily in directly disturbing function generally, and secondarily in inducing specific changes in secretion. This may be accomplished apart from another condition, which we will shortly examine, and which may be regarded as a fruitful source of dyspepsia, chronic gastritis. Sometimes it is difficult, if not impossible, to lay our hand on the precise cause dietetically of this form of disordered gastric function, the cases developing so slowly and insidiously. In many it seems merely the direct result of the continuance of some particular kind of food, which, either from its physical or chemical unfitness for the particular animal, at length induces perverted or defective secretion of the gastric fluids. It is a custom with many, in attendance upon horses kept for fast work, to restrict the amount of hay and increase the quantity of grains; of these the leguminous kinds, when given in excess, are very liable to induce dyspepsia with acidity of the stomach.

From experience and observation we are taught that the undue allowance of stimulating food, and its non-admixture with material of a cooling character, inducing undue tension and strain upon the stomach by the excessive and persistent stimulation of the vascular and secreting structures, is apt to be followed by disturbance of function—gastric indigestion.

Even when the food supplied is unexceptionable in quality, its dry and stimulating character is sufficient to induce the disorder of function indicated. When, however, the food is of an inferior quality, either from its inherent innutritious character, or rendered so by some change, chemical or mechanical, which has overtaken material originally good, disturbed gastric function is even more likely to ensue. We observe such results to follow from feeding on hay or grains which have been badly harvested or otherwise manipulated; and with foreign oats which have undergone bleaching to give them an appearance which they would not otherwise possess. The injudicious employment of certain condensed or concentrated foods and condiments is also attended with similar results.

In defective movements and want of expulsive power of the

stomach from impaired muscular or nervous power, in conditions of undue irritability and in imperfect control over the passage of ingesta, we find occasional causes of gastric indigestion of a subacute or chronic type.

Symptoms.—These vary much both as to number and intensity, and are exhibited in direct relation to the length of time the disturbance may have existed, and the severity of the attack : at times the animal affected may only show capricious appetite, with a morbid desire for unnatural materials—he will lick the walls, eat earth, or foul matter of almost any sort. There may be troublesome acid eructations, unnatural thirst, mouth sour-smelling and pasty, skin dry and hard to the touch, bowels irregular, and fæces coated with mucus ; in advanced or severe cases colicky pains.   The pulse is usually not much affected in the ordinary cases, nor yet the respirations

The horse, if put to work, will show an amount of weakness not commensurate with the work done , he is disposed to sweat with little exertion, and will most probably be dull and spiritless both in and out of the stable, while, if not relieved, he will gradually loose flesh, and exhibit a lax state of the entire muscular system   Should he still continue to feed moderately well, the food taken does not seem to be assimilated or productive of healthful results, but rather the opposite ; there is a tendency to develop a further condition of irregularity of function in the intestinal portion of the canal   It is in such instances where the appetite continues, and the function of digestion remains impaired, that abdominal pain is most likely to be a prominent feature   Many of these cases are marked by a non-continuance or an alteration of the symptoms shown, and by intermissions in their severity

Treatment.—In the milder forms of chronic gastric derangement it is often only necessary for the restoration of healthy function that some little attention be paid to the food-supply , this is particularly the case in young animals.   With adult animals suffering from dyspepsia, where there is no engorgement of the stomach, it is always needful to make a careful examination, with a view to discover, if possible, the cause of the derangement.

It may proceed from such simple matters as peculiarities of

dentition, injuries to the mouth, or diseases of the teeth themselves, any of these, if existing, must at once be attended to. When none of these causes seem to exist, and where the bowels are not already in a lax condition, the exhibition of a dose of laxative medicine is generally indicated; following this, should evidence of acidity of the stomach—pyrosis—be shown by the eating of earth, the licking of the walls, or by acid eructations, moderate and repeated doses of some mild alkali, as bicarbonate of soda or potash, are indicated; these may be exhibited in the drinking-water or in the food, or they may be combined with powder, or extract of gentian, or powdered myrrh, and given as a bolus two or three times daily. Glycerine four fluid ounces, with water eight, given twice or three times daily, I have found of advantage in some of these cases.

At the same time it is absolutely needful, whatever the dietary may have been, that a change should be adopted. Should the animal have been receiving dry grains, with hay, this ought to be changed to some soft material, as a little steamed oats with bran, to which a little crushed linseed has been added. If cooked food has been the usual diet, substitute uncooked grain, with dry bran, and add a little linseed-oil. Most animals will take this with a very little education; it is best given in small quantities at first, from a half to two fluid ounces twice daily; and when taken readily, it may be increased. The bran, when added to the oats, is useful as a means of mixing the oil, and in all cases it is better that the quantity of food given be rather restricted, even when the appetite would seem to demand more.

When acidity of the stomach is a troublesome symptom, it is good to place in the manger a large piece of chalk, of which the horse may take as he feels inclined, instead of eating earth.

Tonic medicines, as preparations of iron, are not admissible in all cases; indeed, their indiscriminate use is productive of evil rather than good. It is better to exercise patience for some time, and trust to dietetic management, ere recourse is had to medicine.

I have found good to result in some of these obscure cases from the use of ox-gall, prepared by reducing it to the condition of a soft extract by boiling in a water-bath, and giving it, combined with gentian or a small quantity of nux vomica, in ball, twice daily

At this stage, some of the mineral acid in small doses, much diluted with water, and combined with some preparation of quinine, may be tried, and if found to agree, may be continued. The best of such combinations is probably from half a drachm to a drachm of the dilute nitric acid, with twenty to thirty grains of sulphate of quinine.

In the greater number of cases, however, I have found most benefit from bitter stomachics, as gentian, quassia, or nux vomica, combined with alkalies, as the potash or soda carbonates, particularly during the early stages.

When the more active symptoms are somewhat abated, and food is received without bad results, a course of arsenic will often tend to re-establish the tone of the stomach

This is best administered in the form of liquor arsenicalis, or powdered arsenic with bicarbonate of potash, the former in half-ounce doses twice daily in the food or drinking-water, the latter as two grains of arsenic, with two drachms of the salt twice daily.

CHAPTER XXXVII.

GASTRITIS—INFLAMMATION OF THE STOMACH.

I. ACUTE GASTRITIS.

Definition.—*Inflammatory action of varying intensity affecting the stomach, tending to softening and other textural changes, chiefly involving the pyloric portion.*

Causation.—In the horse, gastritis rarely shows itself as an idiopathic or independent affection, and is only known probably as the result of irritation of the mucous membrane. Of the existence of gastritis *per se* during life, and as independent of gastric impaction or intestinal complication, we may not be certain, seeing that the clinical phenomena which it exhibits are not sufficiently specialized to enable us to regard them as diagnostic of gastric inflammatory action apart from other complications.

The conditions under which irritation is apt to develop this inflammatory action are—(1) Errors of dieting, inducing disturbance of function   That it does show itself in some of the cases of gastric distension from food, and where these have been of repeated occurrence, we have sufficient evidence in those cases which terminate fatally, although during life our knowledge may not have been such as enabled us to connect symptoms with definite morbid changes   (2) Following injury from foreign bodies not articles of food, although possibly contained in the food   (3) The existence at the time, or immediately preceding the lesion, of certain specific fevers or general diseased conditions   This we see well-marked in certain attacks of the epizootic distemper or catarrhal fever of horses (4) Following the introduction into the stomach, or in some instances the body—irrespective of its means of entrance—of certain poisons   The chief mineral irritants we meet with inducing gastritis, or gastritis as a dominant feature amongst somewhat complicated morbid conditions, are arsenic and its compounds, the salts of copper, mercury, and sometimes lead Amongst the vegetable irritants, if we exempt certain medicinal agents which, either from a peculiar individual susceptibility, or the exhibition of an overdose, occasionally culminate in inflammation of the digestive organs, the most largely credited with the production of gastritis is the foliage of certain trees and shrubs, particularly the yew and rhododendron

Anatomical Characters—These are neither uniform as to extent, area of structure involved, nor yet as to the exact nature of the textural changes, much depending upon the nature of the active agent in the production of the irritation When the cause has been repeated gastric disturbance from errors in dieting, the changes, although occupying a considerable space, are rarely of the same character and intensity over the entire portion invaded   The appearance is simply that of hyperæmia, the mucous membrane is cloudy and opaque, somewhat swollen, and it may be in patches undergoing granular degeneration, with changes in the cell-elements of the gastric tubes

When arising from the direct, or even secondary, action of arsenic and other mineral irritants, the discolouration is usually more uniformly spread in patches, not of a punctiform character, often intensely red or dark purple Sometimes we observe minute ulcerous sores and patches, which have suffered denudation by the removal of the membrane from the severity of the local action and molecular change.

Between the gland-structures various changes of textural elements may be observed in different stages of progression. The secretion of gastric juice is disturbed, and the surface of the membrane in part covered with a closely adherent, ropy, blood-coloured mucus entangling numerous cell-growths Appearances of a somewhat similar character are observed in different parts of the intestines in all gastric inflammations resulting from mineral irritants

In those cases which follow the ingestion of the vegetable irritants mentioned, the appearances are tolerably uniform. In the mouth and fauces there is frequently a considerable amount of frothy saliva, with increased secretion in the œsophagus. The stomach is moderately full of ingesta largely composed of the foliage of the plant which has acted deleteriously, the mucous membrane is much congested, pulpy, and swollen from infiltration into the submucous tissue, and from change in the cell-elements of the tubuli, there are patches of stringy tenacious mucus adhering at various points of the membrane, over which the orifices of the gastric follicles are observed open and dilated Sometimes the inflammatory state of the organ is not confined to the mucous membrane ; it extends to the peritoneal covering not merely of the stomach itself, but also to the loose omentum, while effused fluid may be found in the peritoneal cavity of a straw or reddish-brown colour.

Symptoms—Those instances which have come under my own observation, where on examination after death an inflamed state of the gastric membrane was evident, were marked during life by the usual symptoms of abdominal pain of a persistent character, or where the pain was not absolutely continuous, the animal steadily exhibited an anxious and depressed condition, quickened respiration, with a frequent, rather hard, and wiry pulse There were also frequent and partial sweatings over different parts of the body, particularly the sides of the neck and shoulders, and an intermittent turning of the head towards the side

Although in the case of irritant poisons there is a certain

individuality or speciality of action in the gastric inflammation depending upon the specificity of action of these irritants on other organs and functions, as also upon the quantity introduced and the channel of introduction, upon which we do not here enter, the symptoms, in a general sense, are in all much alike. In the case of arsenic, the most common of irritant poisons, we have nausea, with loss of appetite, restlessness, or much abdominal pain, shown by the usually occurring symptoms, an anxious expression of countenance, thirst, and the existence of much frothy saliva in the mouth; the respirations are short and frequent, the pulse, at first simply frequent, rapidly becomes feeble and imperceptible   Usually the bowels are irritable, sometimes violent purging and tenesmus are present, with much borborygmus and a peculiarly offensive smell of the fæcal matter, with coldness of the extremities, and patchy or general perspiration. Very shortly following the development of these symptoms we have great prostration, staggering, paralysis, particularly of the hind extremities, and sometimes coma, preceding death

With mercurial compounds, in addition to the common symptoms of gastric irritation there have occasionally been observed salivation, peculiar soreness, and heightening in colour of the membrane of the mouth   While from excessive doses of the salts of copper, special disturbance of innervation, with general paresis, sometimes muscular spasms of a tetanic nature and great depression of internal temperature, may be expected

In all cases where I have been certain of the poisoning of horses from eating the foliage of the yew, the symptoms have been developed so rapidly that little time has been allowed for the close observation of these   Such as could be observed were closely analogous to what we have mentioned as attendant upon the action of other irritants

Diagnosis —It will often, in all cases of evident gastric disturbance with much abdominal pain and the exhibition of such serious symptoms as we have indicated, materially assist us in our diagnosis to obtain as much information as is possible regarding the previous history and treatment of the animal.

This no doubt is needed, or at least advantageous, in all

cases, even the simplest and where the cause of the disturbance is most patent, but certainly in cases of suspected gastritis, where the probability or possibility of having obtained
deleterious material exists, it is of infinitely greater moment.
In all doubtful cases the mere necroscopic examination must
never of itself be confided in, but chemical analysis be had
recourse to. In cases which terminate fatally from eating
the yew or other foliage, the finding of this in any amount
amongst the ingesta, or even in some cases the characteristic
smell of the vegetable irritant, together with concomitant and
locally coincident inflammation, is proof sufficient to satisfy most
minds of the cause of death. Where metallic irritants are the
suspected agents in the production of the diseased condition,
the only convincing proof that these have acted as the active
and directly inducing agents in the inflammatory process is
their detection and isolation by certain chemical processes.

Treatment.—When inflammation of the stomach is fairly
developed we have good reason to believe that its course is
rapid and its termination a fatal one; for, rarely, even when
we have been fortunate enough to diagnose the chief morbid
condition, are we able, either by medicinal agents or dietetic
treatment, to arrest the progress of the disease. In cases which
have recovered, the re-establishment in health and restoration
of functional activity have been a tedious matter, necessitating
much patience and careful dietetic management. The treatment which, from a consideration of the nature of the diseased
action and the teachings of experience, seems most rational,
and is alike applicable to similar morbid activities occurring
in other parts of the canal, is that which rests upon the recognition of the well-known fact—that any organ or structure
suffering from such perversion of nutrition, and such tissue-
changes as occur in inflammation, have these abnormal conditions aggravated by being called upon to exercise normal function. When we suspect that gastritis exists, all our endeavours
must be directed to soothe the already irritable structure,
and to place it in a condition of rest or repose, or as near
this as possible; while, should we believe that the morbid
action progressing in the stomach is the result of the operation of any special and specific agent, either mineral or vegetable
irritant, we must, in the employment of the antidotes appro-

priate to these several agents, never lose sight of this chief indication, the soothing and rest absolutely needful for restoration of health.

In gastritis, not the result of the action of any specific
poisonous agent, these ends are best attained by the exhibition
of such demulcents as linseed-tea, or well-boiled oatmeal-gruel,
with full doses of some preparation of opium, as the tincture,
or, probably better still, the watery solution or extract. These
ought to be repeated every two or three hours, and while I
should advise the administration of the gruel or linseed-tea as
indicated, and probably with the first draught a dose of opium
in whatever form determined upon, the others, or at least some
of the other administrations of the medicine, might with benefit
be carried out hypodermically

Should an alleviation of symptoms appear, it is advisable,
after an interval of some hours, to administer a little oil, which
will assist in unloading the canal of retained material   When
we believe the cause of the inflammation to be such an irritant
as yew foliage, or where the original morbid action in the viscus
is likely to be complicated with cerebral disturbance, the opium
had better be left out, and belladonna extract employed instead
When mineral irritants are suspected as the operating cause,
such agents as raw eggs well-broken down and mixed with
gruel, or oleaginous materials, or lime-water, ought to be given
every half-hour for some time, not in excessive quantities, it
being better to exhibit a full dose at first, and afterwards follow
it by smaller ones at short intervals. As the horse cannot,
like some animals, rid his stomach of offending material by
the exercise of the act of vomition, our endeavours must, without losing sight of securing quietude and rest for the organ,
be directed to neutralizing or rendering innocuous, and by
causing to pass along the canal, those substances believed to be
operating thus prejudicially   Whether we can manage to
obtain in an emergency a sufficient amount of hydrated per-
oxide of iron, of charcoal, or of albumen, or any other of the
recognised chemical antidotes for arsenic and other mineral
poisons, we ought never to forget that oil and gruel, or mucilage,
are useful, if not essentials, in the treatment of the most of
these cases   The former of these certainly acts more than
merely favouring the passage of the irritant along the canal, it

seems to serve in retarding or lessening the activity of certain of those irritants in a manner not yet perfectly accounted for

When pain is a prominent symptom the application externally of heat and moisture is advisable, and ought to be persevered in for some hours continuously, and when the rugs are removed, a turpentine stupe or mustard cataplasm may be applied. Should the animal not succumb, and at length show a desire for food, great care must be exercised in the giving of it. Milk or good gruel, either oatmeal or linseed, are to be preferred to any solid material for some days, and we ought to be perfectly sure all the time that the bowels are kept in a moist state.

I am aware that many are very sceptical as to the possibility of recovery in cases of gastric inflammation; I feel, however satisfied that in the horse there are more recoveries from inflammation of the stomach than of the intestines. I have encountered several where there seemed little doubt, judging from previous experience, and from comparison with cases as far as I could discover in every way similar both in their ætiology and symptoms—and where after-death examination demonstrated gastric inflammation—that the animals under treatment were similarly affected, and where, after much suffering, they ultimately recovered under treatment such as indicated.

It may be interesting to notice that several of these cases were similar to those narrated by Mr. Percivall in his 'Hippopathology,' as having occurred in the practice of a Mr. Bean. The immediate cause—eating haws—was in operation in both groups of cases, the symptoms were similar, eructations and ejection of fluid and solid matter from mouth and nose, and in those which died the lesions corresponded.

II. CHRONIC GASTRITIS.

· This condition may possibly occur as a sequel of an acute attack, but is in the horse chiefly found in association with— (1) Continued errors in dieting, either with or without impaction; a steady irritation resulting from indigestible or improperly conditioned food. (2) Textural changes of the gland-structures and component parts of the viscus, possibly connected with other and more general diseased conditions. It is in this manner frequently associated with the form of pulmonic disease in the horse known as broken-wind, in which the stomach suffers from changes resulting in attenuation of its walls, it may also exist with the habit of crab-biting, in which somewhat similar changes are observed (3) Distinct textural alterations of the stomach of a malignant character, as cancer and lardaceous disease. (4) Disease of the liver, in which, from interference with the portal circulation, blood is driven back upon the stomach and other organs (5) Mechanical injury to textures from the continued presence of the larvæ of the œstrus.

Anatomical Characters.—These are of necessity as varied as the causes which operate in its induction In some, particularly such as are the effect of malignant disease—as cancer—or where the injury received has resulted in circumscribed erosions from inflammatory action proceeding from parasitic invasion, the tissue-changes are obvious enough, in others, where nerve influence or vascular supply are chiefly at fault, interfering with the process of nutrition, the steps of the process are less obvious, and only recognised, it may be, in their results

Symptoms—The symptoms of this chronic disturbance are somewhat varied, frequently extending over a lengthened period of time, subject to aggravation from certain extrinsic influences, and of much importance as respects the general health of the animal.

In a large number of instances these are what have already been mentioned when treating of chronic dyspepsia, which, although spoken of separately as a functional disorder of the stomach, must in many manifestations be regarded as simply a symptom of, or the outcome of, this state of chronic gastritis In addition to such symptoms as may be looked upon as strictly connected with disturbed gastric function, there are others more obvious which, although overlooked or viewed in a different light, ought to be linked to these as a result, viz, intestinal disturbance. It seems highly probable that many of those troublesome and recurring cases of colic or bowel disorders are to be directly traced to digestion imperfectly carried out in the stomach, because of some manifestation of chronic gastric inflammation In these, food materials only partially broken down are passed along the intestinal canal, the structures of which not being capable of dealing with ingesta in this crude state, there is induced irritation with its attendant phenomena of restricted or widely spread disturbance

Treatment.—This can only be satisfactory when the agencies in its production are sufficiently well made out, where these are inappreciable our chief reliance must be upon the regulation of the dietary, a careful watching of symptoms and of complications as they arise, and an endeavour to combat these, and thereby to obviate unfavourable results which appear imminent Whatever medical treatment we may pursue, it is essential to recollect that rest to the organ is frequently of greater importance than the reception of medicaments, also that there is probably no organ in the body which in this respect we can so accommodate as the stomach—the quality of the food can be changed and the quantity lessened

---

CHAPTER XXXVIII

RUPTURE OF THE STOMACH

Definition—*Rupture of varying character and extent of the walls of the stomach*

History—At one time regarded as a rather rare lesion, it is now recognised as of rather common and increasing occurrence, particularly amongst certain classes of horses acted upon by special influences

Causation—The more numerous and potent influences in operation to produce this lesion are those connected with errors in dieting and work Thus it is that it is encountered chiefly amongst draught animals of the heavier breeds, those most subject to irregularities and errors connected with the food-supply and the apportioning of their work It is most likely to occur when the quantity of food taken into the stomach is great, and when the organ having lost its power of acting on the contained material, this remains largely unchanged, but subject to the action of chemical laws which, in their development, result in the elimination of gases and consequent increased distension of the viscus I have observed that the occurrence of this lesion is more frequent in horses which have been fed on bruised than on whole grains, and in

40—2

them when, after a full meal, they have at once been put to continuous and severe labour · the reason of this seems to be that the steady pressure of the collar over the œsophagus prevents the eructation and escape of the rapidly generated gases arising from the softening and maceration of the contained food   The lesion may take place by steady pressure from within, without much exhibition of uneasiness or pain ; so that when seen by the professional attendant, the rupture having been accomplished, the attractive symptoms of abdominal pain are indicative rather of further peritoneal and visceral inflammation than of rupture of the stomach itself   At other times it occurs during the course of gastric disturbance and bowel complications, the rupture taking place during and in consequence of the violence of the animal's struggles ; in such cases the symptoms already existing are further aggravated or modified

There may, previous to the rupture, have been no inflammatory action, which may only date from and be consequent on the occurrence of the lesion, the antecedent condition being merely that of uneasiness and pain, the result of extreme distension

Although this lesion of rupture of the walls of the stomach may take place with an animal in which the organ is perfectly healthy, there are fair grounds for believing that in many the viscus has, previous to the fatal lesion, been repeatedly the seat of derangement and distension, and where the rupture can only be regarded as a natural sequel of chronic indigestion   In such cases the walls of the organ have become not only attenuated by the continued stretching process to which they have been subjected, but the muscular tissue of which they are made up may have become somewhat altered in its elementary structure

So far, corroboration of the statement that textural alteration is an important item in the production of the lesion is the fact that it rarely takes place in the young animal, that the aged, exhausted, and hard-worked are its most frequent subjects

Symptoms —The indications of this lesion, although in many cases sufficiently well marked, are not in all such as to leave no doubt of its existence on the mind of the observer   Vomition, or attempts at vomition—an act of rare occurrence in the horse—have often been regarded as specially diagnostic of rupture of the stomach, now, although I would not for a moment desire to cast doubt on the value of what I justly appreciate, and which is probably one of the few symptoms sufficiently well marked in the majority of cases of this lesion to cause us to regard it as a valuable diagnostic symptom, still we must not forget that other lesions of a similar character in connection with other viscera—as in the condition of rupture of the colon and diaphragm—have attached to them as symptoms, attempts at vomition, as also that rupture of the walls of the stomach may take place, and this attractive symptom not be developed.

With regard to the relation of the symptom of vomition, or attempts at vomition, to the actual occurrence of the rupture, there has been some considerable speculation and little certainty. Many have regarded the existence of the lesion as incompatible with any action of the organ approaching to what may be looked upon as vomition, that with the walls of the stomach torn there could be no effort made for the ejectment of what material was contained in it, and that consequently the symptom of vomition, where existing, was always a symptom antecedent to the occurrence of the lesion. Of the correctness of this conclusion we are far from being satisfied; it proceeds upon assumptions which we can scarcely admit, such as the necessity of a stomach ere vomition can be accomplished, the impossibility with a rent in its walls of pressure being exercised upon its contained materials, or of relaxation of its cardiac opening. To our mind, these latter conditions will altogether depend upon the nature and extent of the rupture, and the relations of the viscus to other influences, nervous and muscular. The lesion can certainly be conceived of as being of such a character that its interference with forcible contraction of the muscular tissue and lessening of the capacity would not be absolute and complete. While from observations made on many cases shortly previous to death, and immediately afterwards, there appears satisfactory evidence that rupture and escape of ingesta into the peritoneal cavity may exist some time antecedent to the exhibition of attempts at vomition. In some of these there were adhesions, the result of inflammatory action consequent on the escape of contained material into the abdominal cavity, which adhesions could not possibly have occurred under a period of several hours, while not long prior to death we had attempts at vomition, with ejection of material from the nose Again, it is equally certain that actual vomition has occurred during the simple repletion and distension of the stomach without any rupture of its walls, seeing that following the vomition and discharge of ingesta from the nostrils we have had perfect recovery of the animal Thus, while we do not appear to be in a position to give a distinct and incontrovertible opinion as to the exact relationship which the symptom of vomition, or attempted vomition, bears to rupture of the stomach, there is yet ample reason why we should as a general rule, particularly when this symptom is collateral with others, still continue to regard it as one of the most truly diagnostic of this fatal condition

When an animal suffering from gastric engorgement and distension with much abdominal pain, being very uneasy, tossing himself about with violence, suddenly becomes quiet for a short time with a distinct change in the expression of his countenance, in which is now marked great anxiety, with short, quick respirations, regurgitation of fluid or more solid ingesta from the mouth and nose, with attempts at vomition, pulse becoming quicker and more feeble, the probability is that the walls of the stomach have become torn In some instances there are additional symptoms, such as sudden fits of perspiration, a blanched state of the mucous membranes, cold and clammy mouth, tottering or staggering gait on being moved, or a disposition to move feebly around the box with his nose to the ground.

When the lesion has taken place at once, and exists as the primary affection, often occurring while at work, from which he has been removed on account of the exhibition of pain, there may not at first be great uneasiness immediately accompanying the rupture, but very shortly this becomes a prominent symptom, chiefly from the escape of the contained material into the peritoneal cavity and consequent inflammation of the membranes and organs there Rapidly the pulse and respirations become affected, and show the same characters as in the other form—sinking, with anxious expression of the countenance, attempts at vomition, and, it may be, sitting on the haunches As the case advances, the pallid state of the mucous membranes, and the cold, clammy condition of the mouth, become more marked During the progress of the symptoms the feeble and frequent condition of the pulse is persistent; while towards the termination the animal may show little pain, but stand persistently, until he finally drops; at other times he is violent to the last, gradually becoming unconscious.

Course and Termination—When rupture of the walls of the stomach is complete, the course may be rapid or more protracted, but the termination is generally fatal When the rent in the viscus is not great, and the escape of ingesta trifling, with a tardy development of inflammatory action in the organ itself and in the viscera and structures of the abdomen, the horse may linger for forty-eight hours or more. When however, the organ is extensively ruptured, we find a rapid development of symptoms, terminating in collapse in a few hours When life is prolonged there may, previous to death, be much tympany; in other cases, the opposite condition is observed

As in no case we may be able perfectly to satisfy ourselves or others that this lesion has occurred, attempts will generally be made to combat the most prominent features, those of gastric disturbance with abdominal pain. In this it is generally observed that all medicines which may be administered by the mouth seem to aggravate the already distressing symptoms, and that the only relief obtained is by blunting the sensibility through the subcutaneous injection of morphia.

CHAPTER XXXIX

OF CERTAIN INTESTINAL SYMPTOMS AND FUNCTIONAL DISORDERS.

I. CONSTIPATION.

Definition—*A condition of the bowels in which the fæces are unnaturally retained, or, when voided, are less in amount and harder in consistence*

Pathology *a Nature*—This can scarcely in itself be

regarded as a distinct and substantive disease, but rather as a symptom or manifestation of many diseased conditions. It is undoubted that both in amount and character the discharges from the bowels are largely modified by the nature of the dietary upon which the animal is subsisting, and that there exists in health a great range in these features of intestinal excretion perfectly compatible with the healthy exercise of function.

When appearing as a symptom, or in connection with any special disease, it will require individual and special consideration. Sometimes in these conditions it is a matter of much importance.

When existing independent of any recognised or particular diseased condition, but as a disorder *per se*, it rarely proceeds to such an extent as to endanger life, or even to cause alarm.

Even in many instances usually regarded as simple and uncomplicated constipation, it may be discovered that such is not really the case, that it is but the result of certain disturbance or change, either in the alimentary canal or in some other organ more remotely associated with digestion.

Certain disorders of function of the gland-structures immediately or more remotely concerned in the process of digestion, may not unfrequently operate injuriously in thus altering the excretions of the canal, and although thus disturbed, they of themselves may give no direct evidence of the disturbance by pain or other special visceral symptoms. Thus, what we regard as constipation pure and uncomplicated, may be only a manifestation of disorder or disease of a very different organ or structure from the alimentary canal

b. Causation—As a simple and uncomplicated disorder unconnected with structural lesion, constipation is chiefly observed associated with—(1) Mechanical obstruction in some part of the intestinal tube. This will, in its different manifestations, come under notice in another section (2) Want of sufficient peristaltic motion, the result of impaired nervous irritability of the bowel (3) Diminution in the amount of fluid material from defective secretion, or in some instances excessive absorption.

These latter conditions are both very intimately connected

with, or they may spring from, errors in dietary, combined with the adverse operation of other extrinsic influences.

Amongst certain horses under a particular regimen there is observed a distinct tendency to a torpid state of the bowels unconnected with other visceral derangement, and which is removed by an alteration in the food-supply.

These are usually young, ill-cared-for animals, kept and pastured upon bulky, innutritious, rather dry and ligneous food, and where this restriction to, and large consumption of, such coarse and innutritious food has been carried on for some time, the effect being a weakened and atonic state of the bowels in particular, and of the system generally.

A continuance of this dietary is exceedingly apt to be attended with retention and unnatural dryness of the contained material, which is not passed on, partly from its mechanical characters, and partly from an inactive and paralyzed state of the canal itself. These two conditions, the occlusion of the tube with ligneous matter, and the atonic or paralyzed state of the muscular fibres, continue to act reciprocally upon each other. When not relieved early and judiciously, this retention and unnatural dryness of the ingesta is liable to terminate in such serious results as extensive congestion, or inflammatory action; or the animal may sink from exhaustion, hastened possibly by blood-contamination from intestinal absorption.

Symptoms.—The indications of this functional disturbance, unconnected with any particular organic disease, are at first very slight; there may be neither pain nor uneasiness, simply general lassitude and trifling inappetency. In many of the animals treated as we have indicated there is a full and rather distended state of the abdomen—they are what is known as pot-bellied—rarely the opposite condition exists. As the constipation has not as a rule developed itself suddenly, but has been of gradual though steady progress, the condition as to flesh is usually the reverse of plethora; the hair may be unnaturally long, the skin dry, with a disposition to œdema of the extremities, and a general appearance of weakness. Watched carefully for a length of time, the animals will be observed to void fæces with some difficulty and more or less tenesmus; in some the difficulty and straining attendant on the act, together with the congested state of the mucous membrane of the rectum, are apt to produce eversion, and it may be strangulation, of the posterior portion of that gut.

With the continuance of this disturbance and confinement of the bowels for some time, the appetite becomes more impaired, with better-marked symptoms of general weakness, while, if somewhat more narrowly examined, we may observe that in addition to a small, weak, and somewhat accelerated pulse, we have a foul-smelling mouth, the mucous membrane of which, particularly of the tongue, is of a soapy character, and in very bad cases we may even find sordes on the gums and lips.

We require in these cases also to be on our guard not to be misled by the tenesmus and an occasional discharge of fluid matter, for it is not an unfrequent occurrence in such instances of impaction and atony of the intestines that a certain amount of local irritation from the hardened masses may excite a watery or puriform secretion, which, passing between the fæcal matter and the intestinal wall, is discharged in such a manner as to give the appearance of diarrhœa. With some there may be symptoms of abdominal pain — such, however, is not the usual course, all that is attractive being the general weakness, lassitude, exhaustion, and disturbed appetite, with a trifling amount of local irritability. The cases where abdominal pain is chiefly observed are in horses in work, where the condition of intestinal confinement has been rather sudden in development, and in which, as a symptom, added to the simple hardening and retention of the contents, we encounter certain products of the morbid intestinal action, usually voided along with the retained fæces, and appearing as flocculent or more perfectly solidified casts or envelopes of the hardened masses, sometimes mistaken for collections of destroyed intestinal worms

Treatment.—The management of torpidity and confinement of the bowels, to be judicious, must be conducted apart from the use of many purgatives, particularly such as are of an active nature. No doubt drugs of this class must be given; but we require to use them in moderation, and in conjunction with a carefully regulated dietary. If the animal is still disposed to take a certain amount of food we must be careful to see that its character is fairly nutritious, and such as will tend to promote in the first instance removal of the unnaturally retained ingesta. We ought to remove the animal from the rough innutritious pasture, if the case has occurred there, and allow a little well-boiled barley, or well-steamed oats, with a larger proportion of sweet bran, to which may be added either treacle or linseed-oil When inclined to drink we may dissolve in the water, gruel, or linseed-tea, a moderate amount of sulphate of soda or magnesia. Such treatment, with the employment twice or three times daily of enemata of tepid water or oil, will, in the milder cases, be sufficient in the course of a few days to induce the removal of the retained material; while, with a continuance of a suitable dietary, the animal may be speedily restored to health In more severe or prolonged cases it will generally be necessary to exhibit some purgative agent, either a suitable dose of aloes, or where the patient is young, which they often are, a full oleaginous draught is to be preferred; while, where either tenesmus or rectal irritation has been marked, it is always good practice to resort to the repeated employment of enemata After the bowel has responded to this medicinal interference there is almost invariably a disposition to a recurrence of torpidity, thus it is better not to meet with a renewal of simple purgatives, but with a combination of these and certain tonics, or probably with the latter alone, in conjunction with suitable dietary For such cases I have found that the most useful tonic is a combination of aloes, assafœtida and nux vomica made into ball, and given once or twice daily

These medicines must be continued for some time, and while being continued, as also following their cessation, all will be useless unless the dietary is of such a character as will tend both to general restoration and to the recovery of particular functional activity During the entire treatment, unless the weakness and exhaustion forbid it, the animal ought to have daily exercise in the open air, and an unrestricted allowance of pure or medicated water to drink

Another class of cases of simple or uncomplicated confinement of the bowels often engages the attention of the veterinary practitioner in the very young Foals immediately after birth are found to be much disturbed owing to inability to void the meconium, the material which has accumulated in the canal during intra-uterine life This state of confinement and difficulty of discharging the primary contents of the intestines is more frequently found in animals whose dams have been kept at work until an advanced period of gestation, and where they have been liberally fed upon dry and rather concentrated food, or where the period of gestation has been unnaturally prolonged, it may, however, be observed in foals whose dams have been subjected to none of these influences

The young creature suffering from this disturbance is obviously uneasy, it may keep stretching itself as if wanting to urinate, elevating its tail and straining much, while if not relieved, colicky pains are a usual feature, it will lie down and attempt to roll, or persistently turn its head to the flank. A little continuous watching, and an exploration of the rectum with the oiled finger, will usually satisfy us of the true state of the canal and its contents.

The knowledge that such a condition of the foal is possible, or indeed highly probable, is sufficient with the majority of careful men of any experience in attending upon breeding mares, to cause particular attention to be directed to ensure a regular and rather moist state and healthy condition of the alimentary canal of the dam some time antecedent to the period of parturition. While, when the young animal gives indications of this unnatural confinement, an early enema of oil will generally succeed in facilitating the removal of the offending material, this will require to be repeated until it is evident that a natural action has been obtained. In all cases where the material is hard, it is better to remove it with a scoop, or by means of the finger, previous to employing the enema. Some carry out the practice of gently passing a tallow candle into the rectum, and allowing it to remain for some time, which in the milder cases is sufficient, when repeated three or four times daily, to secure all that is needed.

I have in many instances felt satisfied that benefit resulted from keeping the mare for some days almost entirely on sloppy food, and allowing her in the drinking-water a full supply of sulphate of soda or magnesia. In others, when the patient is more disturbed and abdominal pain is considerable, it will be requisite to exhibit an ounce or two of castor or linseed oil, and to apply cloths wrung from warm water around the abdomen, to be supplemented on their removal by friction with a little soap liniment. The pain will, as a rule, disappear when the bowel has begun to act naturally.

II DIARRHŒA

A ORDINARY DIARRHŒA, SPECIALLY OF THE ADULT

Definition.—*An increase, as compared with what is regarded as normal, in amount and fluidity of the alvine discharges, usually exhibiting as anatomical lesions only hyperæmia and turgescence of the mucous membrane, in exceptional instances inflammatory changes*

Pathology. *a Nature*—As with the opposite condition, this may be looked upon as a distinct and peculiar functional disturbance, or as merely a symptom in the course of certain and separable diseases   It is in the former light we now chiefly regard it

In speaking of this fluid state of the alvine discharges it has often been the custom to make distinctions, and to speak of it under different names, according as its appearance has been marked by differing clinical or anatomical features ; in this way such terms have come to be employed as 'bilious diarrhœa,' ' muco-catarrhal diarrhœa,' etc.   However, it is probably perfectly sufficient for us, and equally conducive to the attainment of our object, that we regard all these states of the intestinal canal characterized by an increase in quantity and fluidity of the material voided as cases of ' diarrhœa.'

Indicative most frequently of functional disturbance of very varied character, occasionally of peculiar structural changes, diarrhœa is common enough in all animals, but is, when appearing in these, severally of very varying importance. In some, as the bovines, a continuance of a very lax state of the bowels may be neither indicative of serious disturbance, nor of immediate nor yet remote danger , whereas a similar condition in the horse is usually indicative of perverted function, and if continued is likely to lead to evil consequences.

When occurring in connection with some general and specific diseases it is often critical, and a matter of much moment , when appearing as we now regard it, independent of any systemic disease or extensive local change, as a mere frequent discharge of liquid excrement alone and unmixed with disease-products, it is rarely of such serious import

b. Causation.—Resulting from increased peristaltic action, excessive secretion, or from both combined, the immediate causes which operate in the production of this unnatural condition of the bowels are numerous as well as varied; all, however, may be ranked—(1) As direct irritants, being chiefly brought from without to operate at once on the mucous membrane of the canal; (2) As indirect excitants to increase secretion and muscular activity, chiefly operating from within the animal itself, the intestinal structures being their special field of operation.

Of the former are all such agents as food, water, parasites, mechanical and chemical irritants, together with certain local tissue-changes, which, by their direct contact with the intestinal mucous membrane, produce their effects. Of the latter, the chief are noxious emanations, products of general and specific diseases, and other deleterious agents, which find their way into the circulating fluids through other channels than the alimentary canal, but which in the course of the processes connected with the purification of the economy are determined to the intestinal mucous membrane for elimination; also all such disturbances of the circulation as ensue from functional or structural changes of other and associated organs, as the liver, the spleen, the pancreas, etc. To these may be added the influence resulting from nervous disturbance, often of a reflex character.

Although agencies belonging to both these classes are met with in the horse, it is probably a more frequent occurrence that these are observed to act directly upon the mucous membrane of the canal itself, having been conveyed there from without in the ordinary processes of eating or drinking, than that they enter by other channels, and are directed ultimately to the alimentary canal, or even that they are the result of local congestion following hepatic or other gland disturbance.

Over-feeding, injudicious feeding, feeding with innutritious or hurtful materials, drinking foul water, drinking excessively of wholesome water, particularly when overworked, exhausted, and exposed to cold and damp, are all, either individually or variously combined, fertile sources of irritability and unnatural laxity of the bowels

With the average specimen of the adult horse, the most frequently operating cause of this irritable state of the intestinal canal is probably injudicious and irregular dieting   All sudden changes in the food-supply, particularly if such are made from a dietary moderately dry and concentrated to one rather bulky and moist, are very apt, even with quiet work, and certainly with rapid exertion, to be accompanied, or closely followed, with a lax condition of the bowels. While certain articles, otherwise wholesome enough, when given as food in particular conditions to horses not habituated to these, will tend to produce the same results. It is in this manner that new hay, new oats, or even good, well-seasoned bruised grains, cannot be given with impunity to horses engaged in rapid or severe work without a previous education. Other articles, again, totally unfit for horse-provender, are yet persistently employed as such, although so frequently productive of not only troublesome, but also of serious consequences. Of these we may instance brewers' grains, roots of all kinds, either cooked or raw, especially potatoes.

The existence of a state of plethora in horses, while at the same time highly nutritious food is still continued to be given, together with a want of regular exercise, or too little of it, with an occasional smart burst of work, will, particularly in aged animals, tend to the development of diarrhœa. This it seems to do through disturbance and congestion of the hepatic and portal system reacting on that of the intestine, inducing a state of passive congestion, there being at the same time no increased arterial pressure or engorgement of the submucous tissue.

This state of congestion, attended with watery and serous exudation, is usually not limited or circumscribed, but diffused over a rather extensive surface of the intestinal tube.

Besides this influence, rather indirect, of hepatic disturbance, there is also to be noticed that which is more direct in the action of an increased outpouring of the biliary secretion, which in numerous instances is the cause of augmented intestinal action and a liquid condition of the excreta.

Symptoms—These are what may be termed unequivocal, and sufficiently attractive to direct immediate attention to the condition of the horse.

Most probably when resulting from an immediate error in dieting, either as to quantity or quality, or to water given in excess, the symptoms may develop themselves with much rapidity as relates to the time occupied between the reception of the offending agent and appearance of these. If put to rapid or severe exertion, this is the more certain to be the result

At first there may be little or no constitutional disturbance The ordinary discharges from the bowel are merely increased in amount, not so much at each single evacuation, but from the frequency of these; steadily a more liquid condition of the excrement prevails, and unless the offending ingesta has been potatoes, I have not observed that this softened and liquefied material is marked by much change in its colour or odour, except that when continued, portions of partially softened or digested fodder become more apparent amongst the ejected matter

When raw potatoes have been the offending agents, the character of the constitutional symptoms, as also of the alvine evacuations, is diagnostic. In these cases, from the commencement of the attack the general prostration is great, sometimes abdominal pain is a prominent feature, and the discharged fæces of a pale colour, watery, and of a peculiar and penetrating odour. Somewhat similar symptoms are found to exist even when these roots, if partaken of largely, are given in a cooked form

Apart from potatoes, raw or cooked, the lax condition of the bowels may continue for some time even while the animal is at work, ere obvious disturbance is induced. Indeed, it is only in exceptional instances, and when the dejections are continuous and distinctly watery, or the result of the action of a direct irritant, mechanical, chemical, or medicinal, that constitutional disturbance or local pain and uneasiness are attendant symptoms. In such, nausea and depression are likely to be exhibited, with irregular and patchy perspiration, often rigors, and the peculiar condition of the skin recognised as goose-flesh, indicated by a rising and falling of the hairy covering. In others we have disturbed respiration, with abdominal pain, the animal conducting himself much as in ordinary colic, pawing a little, crouching, striking at his belly with his hind feet, lying down rather carefully, and when down disposed to rest. The pulse is not usually affected unless the nausea is excessive, or during the paroxysms of pain. In the cases resulting from the free use of potatoes there is often a foul breath, with a furred and pasty state of the tongue and buccal membrane—the latter, as well as the membrane of the nose, unnaturally pale—a depressed and nauseated expression of countenance, sometimes stupid, and rather insusceptible of impressions from without.

When diarrhœa appears as the result of causes originating from within the animal, inducing irritation, or more frequently extensive congestion of the intestinal mucous membrane, such as has already been mentioned as likely to follow hepatic or portal disturbance, the symptoms do not vary much from those already noted. In this latter state the dietetic error is not usually a present operating cause so much as it has been for a considerable time antecedent acting as a steadily preparing or predisposing factor, inducing, through excess of nutriment, an enfeebled and diseased condition of important organs and structures. In these cases of much intestinal congestion, the result of hepatic disturbance, we sometimes observe a distinct icteric state of the system, recognised by a yellowish hue of the visible mucous membranes and a changed physical and chemical state of the urine.

The condition of helminthiasis in some of its forms, as exhibited in connection with the alimentary canal, is a source of a troublesome and sometimes intractable diarrhœa. The particular parasite which appears more liable than others to act as an inducing factor in the production of this state is the *Strongylus tetracanthus*, a very small nematode, of a flesh-colour, a true blood-sucker, and found inhabiting the coats of the large intestines, chiefly the colon and cæcum. In addition to other symptoms indicative of its existence in this situation—as marasmus, steady but fitful, an unhealthy state of the skin, irregular appetite, with the occasional appearance of a helminth or two in the fæces—is intestinal irritability, with fitful diarrhœa, not excessively watery, rather of the character of ordinary fæcal matter, having associated with it an extra amount of liquid.

A rather common and sometimes serious form of diarrhœa is encountered in the occasionally excessive or undue response of the bowels to a dose of purgative medicine. We would speak of it as an undue response to an ordinary purgative

41

rather than as the result of an overdose of medicine, seeing such superpurgation may follow the administration of such an amount of any particular cathartic as, if employed at some other time, would not induce such annoying results. The peculiar systemic conditions operating to induce this idiosyncrasy may be, and often are, beyond our means of detection; at other times they are perfectly appreciable.

A horse under the action of an ordinary dose of purgative medicine, if supplied with an unlimited amount of cold water while the medicine is freely operating, if put to work, or unduly exposed to damp or cold, is very liable to suffer from excessive purgation. Over-purgation from the exhibition of a cathartic is always annoying, but need not unduly alarm, unless the animal gives evidence of constitutional disturbance, such as total failure of appetite, continued watery diarrhœa, or painful tenesmus, pulse of increased frequency, weak or small, with rigors and partial sweats, much prostration, and if in a box an inclination to wander.

B. DIARRHŒA OF THE YOUNG.

In adult horses diarrhœa may be regarded as a benign affection, not usually having a fatal termination; in the very young, however, it possesses characters rather unique, and is attended with serious or fatal results; the same holds true to even a greater extent when it appears in the bovine and ovine species. This condition may in all these animals exhibit some diversity in its manifestations in the different species and in individuals of the same species, but in all it seems essentially the same disorder. The great characteristic feature is functional disturbance intimately associated with the process of digestion, together with a specific intestinal catarrh and a perverted condition of the secretion from the gastric and intestinal mucous membrane, apart from any very marked inflammatory or structural changes either in the intestines or organs associated with them. Inflammatory lesions may occur, but they are neither diagnostic nor common.

This form of diarrhœa is said to appear occasionally in some countries as an epizooty, committing great havoc amongst young stock; as such I have often enough encountered it in calves, and with them can testify both as to its apparently contagious and certainly fatal character, amongst solipeds, however, although it may not unfrequently be extensively distributed, it is not apparently contagious nor yet so fatal This mitigation in virulence is probably attributable to the better sanitary conditions and the less crowding of stables as compared with cow-houses, together with the more natural manner in which foals are reared

Causation—From what I have observed of this condition when appearing amongst the young of all animals there seem very cogent reasons to induce us to regard as the chief source of its existence certain unnatural conditions of dietary. That it may, when once developed, be further propagated and intensified by contagion emanating from the diseased seems, at least in bovines, probable; while it is certain that the usual debilitating influences of defective or bad sanitary surroundings are decidedly predisposing and augmentative In foals, amongst which in this country it partakes less of the character of a specific epizooty, its contagious character is not manifested It is highly probable that certain ill-understood determining influences operating on the dam may produce such alterations on the lacteal secretion as to render it inimical to the performance of healthy functional activity in the digestive process in the very young

We know it is found that in many instances successful treatment of this infantile diarrhœa in foals is largely facilitated by operating on the mare The system of separating the foal from the dam during long intervals each day while the latter is engaged in work seems more frequently attended with an occurrence of diarrhœa in the former than when the two are left continuously together. In those instances where the mares are kept at work during the greater part of the day they often return to their foals heated and more or less exhausted and fatigued; in this way it seems possible that a certain character or influence of an unfavourable nature may be imparted to the milk—add to which the disposition the young animal possesses from its enforced abstinence to take more than a natural or wholesome amount At the same time we must not forget to note the influence which the presence of constitutional maladies in the dam, and the recep-

41—2

tion of particular articles of diet, are capable of exercising on the young receiving their principal sustenance from the milk-supply

Anatomical Characters—These are of rather more frequent occurrence than in the ordinary diarrhœa of the adult; they may not be met with in every instance, and when existing are of variable character and intensity. In some there is a moderate amount of dark-coloured serous fluid in the abdominal cavity, with a few spots or patches of ecchymosis on the serous surface of the bowels, while, where the intestine is most involved, the mesenteric glands in connection with the section affected are somewhat enlarged, darkened in colour, and rather softened. The intestines are generally empty, while the mucous membrane in many parts of its tract is merely covered with a catarrhal discharge; while in others the velvety epithelium is removed in patches, leaving what may be regarded as extensive but superficial erosions. In various portions of the canal, particularly where the glandular structures are situated, the mucous membrane is œdematous from infiltration of a gelatinous material; while on examination of the material, which is spread over the membrane of the canal, or in some places collected in greater amount, may be found a large quantity of epithelium with what appears as minute organisms or micro-cocci, mycelium filaments, or bacterial forms; whether these latter are to be regarded as specific or only of adventitious origin does not appear certain. The other viscera of the abdomen are not as a rule much altered in appearance, with the exception of the liver, which may be bloodless and of a pale clay-colour.

Symptoms—These usually make their appearance during the first fortnight of the animal's life, while up to the occurrence of the disturbance the creature may apparently have been in the enjoyment of full health and vigour. The character and frequency of the evacuations are most probably the earliest symptoms attracting attention. In many of the milder cases at first, and even throughout the entire course of the diarrhœa, there is little disturbance or irritation with the repeated dejections of the yellowish-white fœcal matter; in the more seriously affected from the outset, and in the greater number which continue for some time, the fœces, while varying in consistence,

become possessed of an acrid character and fœtid odour, and
their discharge is accompanied with more or less constitutional
disturbance and abdominal pain In some the abdominal
pain is acute and in paroxysms, in others it is of a quieter but
more continuous character, the foal remaining nearly constantly in the recumbent position, head laid flat on the ground,
or occasionally turned anxiously to the abdomen With a
continuance of the pain and diarrhœa little or no milk is
taken, and the foal rapidly exhibits much exhaustion with
muscular atrophy With a continuance of the flux there is
usually tenesmus, and an irritated or excoriated condition of
the anus and contiguous skin Death may result without the
intervention of inflammatory action In some, where the
symptoms have from the beginning been severe, and where
the termination has been fatal, I have observed consecutive
pneumonia and a form of purulent ophthalmia

Prognosis and Treatment—The prognosis in the greater
number of cases of diarrhœa, unless such as occur in the very
young, and that which is induced by eating large quantities of
potatoes, is usually favourable The number of cases which
demand medical treatment, properly so called, is small a
properly regulated dietary being sufficient to ensure restoration
to health

In the diarrhœa of adult horses, a just estimate of those
causes which seem to be in operation for its production is
absolutely needful in framing measures for its treatment.
When proceeding from the action of agencies which are without the animal, as fatigue and undue exposure, or from the
reception into the alimentary canal of materials which, by
their mechanical or other properties, produce irritation, with
undue secretion and muscular activity, the first indication is
that the animal be withdrawn from the influence of the offending agencies While, unless the intestinal action is excessive,
and the pain and general disturbance considerable, it is unadvisable at once by medicinal agents to make an attempt to
arrest the discharge.

When the excessively lax condition of the bowels is attributable to the inordinate action of medicinal agents administered
with the view of inducing only a moderate action, a similar
practice of non-interference is at first to be recommended;

care, however, must be exercised in watching the animal, as there seems in these a tendency for this functional disturbance to induce serious changes in the vascular structures of the feet. When these cases remain unalleviated by the change of dietary and careful managment, or where from the first, as in feeding too liberally upon potatoes, either raw or cooked, a more troublesome and difficult state of matters is presented for our consideration, further treatment is requisite. In these conditions, should the horse still continue to feed a little, while general prostration and abdominal pain are not marked features, it is better simply to depend on a carefully disposed dietary for a little time than at once to have recourse to medicinal agents.

The patient ought not to be disturbed; no cold water, but bland fluids, as wheaten-flour gruel or linseed-tea, be allowed for drink, with a little good hay and a few steamed oats with bran; the surface-temperature of the body being at the same time attended to.

Where abdominal pain is shown, either continuously or only accompanying the evacuations, it will generally be advisable to exhibit some soothing and antispasmodic medicine, for which purpose I have found a draught composed of from two to four fluid ounces of spirits of nitrous æther, one drachm of powdered camphor, and one or two fluid ounces of tincture of opium administered in a quart of wheaten-flour or starch gruel, and repeated, if needful, in one or two hours, serve the purpose well.

When the prostration is considerable, and the dejections watery and irritating, accompanied with pain, it is better to add to this draught from four to eight drachms of prepared chalk and two or three raw eggs well whipped up, while in place of one half of the opium tincture I have found that an equal quantity of chlorodyne has seemed to act better; and where obtainable, and expense is not a matter of consideration, from one-third to one-half of a bottle of port wine is a good adjunct. When abdominal pain is persistent, the application for some hours continuously of woollen rugs wrung from hot water, and, on their removal, smart friction with compound soap liniment, and afterwards clothing the animal, is deserving of a trial.

When, from the restlessness of the horse or any other cause, the exhibition of medicines by the mouth is not admissible or very difficult, recourse ought to be had to the employment of morphia subcutaneously.

When there is reason to believe that the diarrhœa is the result of engorgement and obstruction of the portal system, it is not advisable to employ active means to check the flux, but rather, in addition to resting the animal, allow such light and emollient food and drink as will tend to facilitate the passing of this extra functional activity of the bowels into a normal state. This desired result may be hastened by the administration of moderate and repeated doses of tincture or solution of perchloride of iron, with a little of the tinctures of gentian and nux vomica administered in starch-gruel or linseed-tea with raw eggs; while, when exhaustion is considerable, a moderate amount of an alcoholic stimulant will be useful.

When called to advise regarding the treatment of diarrhœa in the very young, it is well to observe what is the character of the discharges, as these seem somewhat modified both as to colour and consistence by the immediate conditions operating in the production of the excessive discharge from the bowels. I have observed that when these were of a deep yellow colour, irritating and slimy, that the condition of the liver was more at fault than when the excreta was of a paler colour and thin.

In the former condition it will generally be better to begin our treatment with a little laxative medicine, and for this purpose castor-oil, given in quantities proportionate to the age and strength of the foal, is to be prefered to salines; to this may be added a drachm of tincture of opium. Following the action of this—indicated by a change of character in the discharges—and also in those cases where the deep yellow colour does not exist from the outset, I have usually employed agents somewhat similar to those recommended for the adult animal. Solution of acetate of ammonia, spirits of nitrous æther, powdered camphor, tincture of opium, or pure carbolic acid, alone or in combination, have been found useful; while instead of flour-gruel as a vehicle, scalded milk, strong tea, or infusion of camomile, seem in these young animals to serve the purpose better. Other agents I have found useful administered with the laxative, or following it, as tincture of rhubarb, camphorated tincture of opium, carbonate of magnesia, or prepared chalk   With many, a most useful draught is from half a drachm to a drachm of chlorodyne given in strong tea, infusion of camomile, or linseed-tea   When weakness is a prominent feature, which it often is, I have found coffee and port wine, or whisky with raw eggs, exceedingly serviceable.

In the employment of all these agents it is much better to exhibit them in moderate doses and often, rather than in large quantities and at long intervals , while all through the course of the case we must be careful that the action of our medicines does not induce undue confinement of the bowels   When abdominal pain is considerable we can do much good by the external employment of heat, dry or moist, to be followed by soap or turpentine liniment, while, should there be any appearance of amendment, and the foal be inclined again to take to the teat, we must be careful that too large quantities of milk are not ingested at once, seeing that in this way a recurrence of symptoms is apt to ensue

III COLIC

Definition—*A painful abdominal affection, usually of an intermittent character, unassociated with fever and not aggravated by manipulation or pressure from without, arising from functional disturbance of the intestinal canal*

Pathology. *a Nature and Varieties.*—Under the very general terms of *colic, intestinal indigestion, disordered bowels, gripes,* etc.—names which are probably chiefly employed to indicate the existence of the one common feature, abdominal pain — have been, and we fear must still continue to be, grouped a variety of conditions   This mingling of causes often essentially different because of a similarity of cognizable phenomena, is a necessity arising in great measure from the uncertainty of our knowledge in regard to organic change, or functional disturbance of internal structures, and the symptoms by which they are severally indicated

Seeing that the great leading feature or diagnostic symptom, abdominal pain, although in an especial manner associated with derangement of the intestinal portion of the alimentary canal, is yet a not unfrequent accompaniment of many visceral changes and disturbances, it has been proposed to regard *colic*, which in the general or extended sense is recognised as the mere expression of abdominal pain, under the distinctive appellations of *true* and *false* The former of these being restricted to those cases where the exhibition of pain is most surely indicative of intestinal changes and disturbance, the latter, where the exhibitional phenomena are attributable to organic changes or functional disturbance of organs and structures connected more or less intimately either through function or contiguity, or not at all, with the intestinal tube

Again, from regarding what we may consider as the immediate factors in the production of this disturbance, or the modes in which these operate in inducing the usually recognised symptoms, we have come to speak of the condition by such terms as spasmodic colic, flatulent colic, verminous colic, etc

True or intestinal colic, as ordinarily encountered, may safely be regarded as immediately originating, in the greater number of cases, from a spasmodic condition of the intestinal tube, as characterized by exhibiting a tendency to self-relief, as not essentially inflammatory, nor yet largely disposed to run on to inflammatory action of the bowel unless improperly treated Although immediately traceable to interference with the normal functional activity of the intestine, this disturbance of function owes its origin to a variety of causes We say not largely disposed to run on to inflammatory action, because to assert that it never does terminate in this more serious morbid condition would be to state what neither the observation nor experience of the majority can corroborate It has long, with many who have had large experience in the treatment of bowel affections of the horse, been deemed axiomatic that unrelieved colic is a fruitful source of enteric inflammation, the absolute truth of this seems open to doubt

From my own experience I am rather disposed to regard the majority of the cases of fatal intestinal inflammations as having been inflammatory from their origin, and that the greater proportion of functional disturbances of the digestive tube of a spasmodic character continue to maintain this character throughout their course, that many, not the whole certainly, of the bowel affections which terminate by the accession of inflammatory action do so rather from some induced unnatural mechanical condition of the structures than from the identity of the morbid actions, spasm and inflammation, or the natural tendency of the former to terminate in the latter

b *Causation*—The causes which seem to operate in the production of this disturbance are all such as interfere with the healthy and normal functions of the intestines, all which obstruct or arrest the peristaltic motion of the tube by which the contained ingesta is passed along, or which pervert or lessen the usual secretions of the follicular and other structures by which digestion is carried on in the canal Of these the chief are ·

1 *Dietetic Errors*—Over-feeding, irregular feeding, feeding with bad or improper material, and feeding when, from fatigue and exhaustion, food ought to be withheld, or at least given in restricted amount, are certainly the most fruitful sources of colic in the horse. We are well aware that many horses are such ravenous feeders that an attempt to satisfy their appetite at any time is certain to imperil the integrity of their digestive organs no doubt we will meet with others where, from constitutional tendency, together with a habit so far acquired, having always been full fed and kept in high condition, this does not occur ; they will rarely gorge themselves, but will eat from abundance only a sufficiency the majority are, however, not so constituted.

That too large quantities of even good food given to healthy horses are likely to induce disturbance of the bowels and the development of colic, I have had abundant evidence during many years' practice in an agricultural district, where the horses, always well fed, are, with the regularity of the return of the seasons, subjected to a condition of high-pressure, both as respects their powers of work-doing and of food-reception With the recurrence of the spring work, and on until the root-crops are sown, dry, nutritious, stimulating food—oats and beans chiefly—is allowed *ad libitum* I have found some animals consuming close upon thirty pounds of these per day, the consequence of this hard work and over-feeding, this forcing of the animals to take into their digestive organs more food not only than they can appropriate, or is needful for them, but more than the animal machine can destroy and pass through the canal, is to increase very largely the percentage of colic cases

Bad as this excessive feeding is, even when the food is of the best quality and most suitable character, it is infinitely worse when it is of an improper form and inferior quality. Under this description I am disposed to place the greater number of varieties of cooked food, both grains and roots, especially when used as feeding materials for horses in severe and rather rapid work. Such foods are in some districts of the country, and for some varieties of animals, largely employed as an evening meal. That cases of colic and severe gastric disturbance should occur where horses, particularly hard-wrought horses, are treated to heavy evening meals of a character totally unfitted for their digestive apparatus, is not to be wondered at.

If food taken in excessive amount by healthy horses is liable to induce disturbance and arrest of digestion, a similar train of untoward results is more likely to follow where the normal vigour and activity of the digestive organs is impaired by exhausting work or other lowering influences. The vital energies being in abeyance, the process of digestion is so far arrested that the ingesta, instead of yielding its nutritious material to the system and gradually passing out of it, is detained, and in its detention acts as an irritant to those structures with which it may be in contact, in addition to which the disturbance is further aggravated by the changes which take place with this unaltered ingesta through the action of chemical forces. In this manner are produced not only the spasmodic state of the intestinal muscular structure, but also the considerable accumulations of gas which are occasionally so distressing and so dangerous.

Besides ordinary food in excessive quantities, and indifferent, bad, or unsuitable food in any quantity, and the reception of all varieties of food in conditions when the digestive organs are unfit to deal with it for healthy appropriation, we find that certain kinds of food, with particular animals, have a special tendency to induce gastric and intestinal irritation. In such cases of individual idiosyncrasy we ought to be guided by timely warning, and withhold what is evidently antagonistic to the maintenance of healthy digestion

2 *Intestinal Obstruction from Concretions*—Obstructions of a serious nature resulting from mechanical displacement and change of position of different portions of the bowel, or from impaction of concretions, usually, we are aware, in the course of diseased activities give rise to colicky pain, what we now refer to, however, is occasional obstruction or arrest in the normal activities connected with digestion from the presence of concretions in the canal. The existence of these concretions, of whatever materials they may be formed, is not necessarily accompanied by colic; probably they only induce this when, by shifting from the position where they have long remained undisturbed and undisturbing, they may have become temporarily fixed in a situation where, by their obstructive influence, they give rise to intestinal disturbance, arrest of function, retention of excrementitious matter, with other undesirable results culminating in, and evidenced by, the exhibition of abdominal pain.

As a rule it is the smaller calculi, or the concretions of the variety formed largely by the agglutination around some special nucleus of the fine cortical materials of the grains upon which the animal may have been fed, or we should rather say obtained from food largely composed of these inferior materials, which create obstruction evidencing itself in abdominal pain. These concretions—apparently from the facility, owing to their lightness, with which they may be moved from their usual position by any extra peristaltic or other movement of the bowel—are more likely to be offending agents than the larger, or those into which mineral matters enter largely, and which, by their weight, keep their retreat in some pouch of the large intestine, in many instances giving no indications of their existence.

3 *Parasitic Invasion of the Bowels and Contiguous Organs*—Certain varieties of intestinal worms, particularly those which inhabit the walls of the intestines, and any variety when excessively numerous, may produce disturbance and irritation sufficient to develop well-marked symptoms of colic. The disturbance, when originating from this cause, is usually of a recurrent type, attended with an irregular and unequal state of the evacuations, and with general marasmus. Those in which this form of helminthiasis appears are oftener the young than the adult, usually under three years of age, and

such as have been rather indifferently treated in every respect, grazed upon poor, damp, badly conditioned land, and where deficiency of shelter has been a marked feature ; this intestinal disorder and general unthriftiness not usually exhibiting themselves until the animals have been taken in hand, or better treated, receiving more and better food, and having the advantage of comfortable lodgings In some of their forms these cases are rather refractory, requiring much time and attention, and not unfrequently, particularly if their treatment has been delayed until the emaciation is confirmed, terminating unfavourably

The existence of parasites in the large bloodvessels supplying the intestines—the mesenteric arteries—has by certain pathologists on the Continent, particularly in some of the German States, been considered a fruitful source of ordinary colic That these vessels are often the habitat of particular nematoid worms, and that, with the presence of these existences, we find a diseased condition of the vessel in which they are found, as also that many horses have died, having previously exhibited severe symptoms of colic, in which, after death, both this arterial disease and parasitic invasion were manifest, is undoubtedly true. And we will even go further, by saying that in many instances there seems evidence to satisfy that this condition of verminous aneurism of the mesenteric vessels does operate in inducing much functional disturbance of the intestinal canal, and in some fatal results, but that it is a common cause or a usual accompaniment of ordinary colic or other fatal bowel affections in this country, after-death examinations do not bear out

4 *Organic Disease of the Intestines* —Under this we may rank glandular disease of the mesentery, a not unfrequent accompaniment or sequel of strangles in the irregular form ; also chronic disease of the structures entering into the formation of the walls of the tube, usually of a degenerative and atrophic nature , and some rarer instances of change, probably malignant. In such the colicky symptoms are usually persistent ; they may be remittent, or even intermittent, seldom entirely removed, while the termination may be said to be invariably fatal

5 *The Reception of Irritant Poisons.*—These may proceed

no further than the production of functional disturbance, or
they may induce inflammatory changes

6 *The Influence of Cold and Damp on the General Surface
of the Body* may be provocative of intestinal disturbance, indicated by abdominal pain

c *Anatomical Characters* —The number of fatal results from
the occurrence of simple colic, apart from complications—as
mechanical obstruction, entanglement of the bowel, rupture of
its coats, or from the arrest placed on the due performance of
respiration from compression of the thoracic viscera, the result
of tympany, together with the ulterior changes attendant on
these mechanical conditions—is not great In some, constriction
or contraction, more or less distinct, of one or more portions of
the bowel, due apparently to persistent contraction of the
muscular structure, has been noticed. Accompanying this state
of continued spasm there may exist a peculiar degenerative
change of both mucous lining and submucous connective-tissue
of a colloid character, occupying a rather extensive tract of the
tube both in the small and large bowel

When colic has been the result of intestinal helminthiasis
the existence of the parasites is usually attractive   As the
large nematodes they may be found collected in heaps or
bunches in the lumen of the tube, oftener as the small tetracanthus strongyle, we find them embedded in the tissues of
the bowel, chiefly the large—the number of distinct points of
irritation often forming, by coalescing, an extensive tract engorged and hyperæmic, studded with numerous spots or sores
where the worms are coiled up, or from which they have
escaped   Verminous aneurisms of the mesenteric arteries have
also been found to exist, and to these have been attributed the
cause of the muscular spasms ; their presence in the horse,
even in fatal cases of bowel disease, is neither constant nor
common.

Symptoms —Although very many, probably the large majority,
of cases of colic have the symptoms of illness developed
suddenly, there are yet many in which, if the animal were
watched carefully, and we were conversant with his entire
history, it would be found that this suddenness was more
apparent than real ; that some days previous to the attack a
certain amount of indisposition—indigestion it might be—or

other trifling functional impairment existed, and that this only culminated in disturbance sufficient to induce expression of abdominal pain by some, fortuitous circumstance which is usually accredited with the production of this disorder.

The evident symptoms of colic, whether we regard these individually or in the aggregate, are all more or less clearly indicative of abdominal pain. The horse suddenly commences pawing, is restless, stamps, and strikes at his belly with his hind feet, looks anxiously at his sides, attempts to bite himself, he puts his nose to the ground, advances his hind feet under the body, and after one or more ineffectual attempts at last lies or drops down. When down he may turn on his side, or roll from side to side, or when near a wall or in a stall may balance himself on his back, the support enabling him to do this without an effort. After remaining in this position for some time, or having tossed restlessly from side to side, the pain abating he will remain quiet or start to his feet, shake the straw from his body, and probably attempt to eat.

The relief, however, may be short-lived, and with an anxious turn of the head to his flanks, he again becomes restless, pawing is renewed, he wanders round the box if loose, or suddenly draws himself together, he crouches, or quietly or suddenly drops to the ground. Rarely, save during the paroxysms of pain, do we find in uncomplicated colic that either the pulse is disturbed or the temperature elevated.

These recurring paroxysms may continue for some time, gradually becoming less severe and having a longer interval between them, until the pain and restlessness entirely disappear and the horse resumes his normal condition, or the intervening periods of quietude are of shorter duration and the evidence of pain more decided gradually becoming continuous, with an altered state of the pulse and hurried respirations, the brain becoming sympathetically affected, excessive excitement or partial stupor is apt to ensue, and death from pain and exhaustion with varying complications will ordinarily be the termination of unrelieved colic.

Although these are the usually observed symptoms of ordinary colic, we shall, on more carefully regarding animals suffering from this disorder, observe that there is a wonderful variety, not only in the intensity and prominence of several of these, but also that there are numerous minor symptoms and features of disturbance which are no less deserving of our attention. The greater number of cases, except such as owe their existence to the ingestion of green food or roots, are marked by a confined state of the bowels. If fæces are voided at all, as they may be in the early stages repeatedly, they are in small amount, sometimes soft, oftener dry and coated with mucus; and all voided in such a manner as to indicate an irritable condition of the canal.

In all, unless in protracted cases, and such as through complications terminate fatally, the pulse is unaffected save during the height of the paroxysm, when it will increase much in frequency, and become altered in character, not unfrequently showing intermittency; at the same time the respirations are hurried or sighing. Retention of urine, or its discharge in a jerking manner, is a common feature of spasmodic colic; the bladder may be distended, but its muscular structure being similarly affected with that of the bowel, the due performance of function is arrested.

It seems probable that the symptoms of extreme restlessness, frequent pawing, much pain, with anxious turning of the head to the flanks, are indicative of involvement to a greater extent of the small intestine, while stretching of the body as if desirous of urinating, throwing the head upwards with curling of the upper lip, and a disposition to move backwards and press with the posterior parts against some resisting object, as the wall or stall-post, are more particularly indicative of disturbance associated with impaction of the large bowel. In these cases of impaction and decided torpidity of the colon in particular, there is a disposition to strain violently and to resist the introduction of the hand or enema into the posterior bowel, which is itself empty, lax, and dilated, often dry and covered with husky feculent matter or tenacious ill-conditioned mucus.

Independently of the condition of intestinal spasm pure and simple, or of mere accumulation of ingesta, as the result of over-repletion or of feeding on indigestible and bulky material, or of paralysis and incompetency of the canal to act on the material which it may contain, or of a combination of these causes, we have a somewhat different condition with a certain speciality of the symptoms, all, however, essentially indicative of abdominal pain and intestinal disturbance, and usually recognised under the name of

Flatulent or Tympanitic Colic —This condition of distension of the intestines with gas may occur as a distinct unnatural condition of itself, or it may follow or accompany the state of spasm or impaction.

When appearing unassociated with either of these already noted conditions it is generally found to be the result of some acute and extensive disturbance of the digestive function incident to a shortly antecedent speciality in diet, or it may follow as the result of an inveterate habit of crib-biting. Food that is succulent, or which from its mechanical or chemical characters is prone to undergo rapidly fermentative changes, is particularly liable to induce this condition of tympany, specially when received in certain states of the system.

The symptoms in well-marked flatulent colic, although quite distinctive and pronounced, are not so attractive or acute, apparently, as when spasm is the leading feature, they are more constant, and the results in severe cases are more to be dreaded than in the more frequently occurring spasmodic form. When developing unassociated with any other disordered condition the seizure is usually sudden, the horse becomes restless, as in all abdominal disturbance; patchy perspiration may break over the body, shortly to be followed—if these symptoms have not been preceded—by distension of the abdomen, which is tense and resonant on percussion; the breathing is short, catching, and thoracic; the pulse increased in frequency and altered in character. In some animals there may be observed a swollen and everted state of the anus and vulva, which looks very serious, but usually subsides with the subsidence of the more acute conditions of the tympany. In this state of abdominal distension the horse is not disposed to roll or even to lie down, which he seems afraid to do; and when he makes the attempt it is always in a cautious manner—nor can he rest when down.

Should relief not be afforded, the continued distension and thoracic compression is most likely to give rise to further untoward symptoms connected with the circulatory and respiratory functions; while it is not uncommon that a fatal

42

termination more rapidly follows this condition of excessive tympany through the occurrence of such lesions as rupture of the bowel—generally the colon—or of the diaphragm.

Although colic or abdominal pain may be the common bond of union which links together these different forms of disturbed function, spasm of the bowel, accumulation of excrementitious matter, and varying degrees of tympany, it is probable that its most frequent manifestation is in connection with disturbance which is a variable combination of all these individual conditions, the course, progress, and final result of each case depending largely upon the prominence or position of one or more of these individual forms of disturbed activity, as well as on the manner in which this specific disturbance has been induced

Course and Termination—Both as to duration and termination the various disordered states of the bowels recognised by the name of colic are extremely variable. Very many, probably the greater number of seizures, recover with very trifling or no treatment whatever, other cases, again, under recognised methods of management, continue in pain, more or less marked, through a period of two or three days and still recover.

The greater number of animals which in an attack of colic are considered sufficiently ill to be placed under medical treatment can rarely be considered safe or removed from danger as the consequence of the attack within a period less than twelve hours, or until the bowels have responded to the laxative medicine which it is generally safe and needful to exhibit. In all protracted cases, with much restlessness and pain, the danger to be apprehended is largely in the direction of mechanical displacement or entanglement of the intestine, which, when occurring, is all but certain to terminate fatally in inflammatory action. Where tympany is excessive and unrelieved, the chief risk is usually in the direction of the occurrence of rupture of the large bowel or of the diaphragm. The chance of the occurrence of these lesions, as also of fractures, is much augmented when the horse during his sufferings is confined in a stall or any situation where both loins and feet may be made fixed points in his straining and struggles.

That cases of unrelieved and protracted colic, particularly

when following the reception of irritants, either chemical or
specially developed in the food, may terminate in inflammation
of the bowel, may not be questioned; that the ordinary and
greater number of such have this tendency is exceedingly
doubtful As already stated, the weight of evidence seems to
indicate that when cases terminate fatally from inflammatory
action, that this action has not been added to mere functional
disturbance, but has existed from the beginning

Treatment—There is no diseased condition in the horse in
which a greater number, more varied and more opposite
modes of treatment have at different times been advocated
and most vigorously carried out than colic; while it is curious
to note that all these different modes of treatment have had
facts and evidence brought forward in support of their success
sufficient to warrant their trial or adoption

Starting, however, with the belief that by far the greater
number of those cases of illness recognised under the very
general name of colic are directly due to functional disturbance
of the alimentary canal, the result of causes dietetic—that they
are remotely or more closely associated with over-feeding,
irregular feeding, or feeding upon improper material, it seems
that those modes of treatment which have for their end the
restoration of normal functional activity through the removal
of the offending or irritating materials are the most in accordance with the dictates of common-sense and the known laws
of the animal economy, and consequently most deserving of
our favourable consideration and adoption

The simpler forms of intestinal disturbance, indicated by
restlessness or slight abdominal pain, are often corrected for
the time by the adoption of the simplest management or by the
exhibition of the simplest and most common medicaments
Still, because many cases of colic are relieved by these, we
would not, considering the probability of the existing intestinal
disturbance being merely the natural result of some intestinal
irritation, regard these measures alone and of themselves as
the best and most rational possible Indeed, it is often
observed that these originally simple and apparently mild
cases, when thus treated and relieved without further attention
to diet or medicine, are apt shortly to reappear, and that
amongst such recurring cases are found those which terminate

42—2

in inflammatory action. This occurs more frequently than with the primary seizures of a more severe character treated from the outset on a different principle, in which regard is ever had to the earlier and antecedent cause of the pain and disturbance.

The attending to and treatment of the pain, the most characteristic feature in all cases, ought not to be neglected, still, if we go no further than this, the probability is that we shall only have indifferent success. We ought not merely to combat the symptoms, but our efforts ought to reach further; we ought to attack the cause of these, which in the majority of cases consists in the presence in the intestine of some offending body.

That it is unwise, unnecessary or inexpedient in any case to employ such agents as tend merely to alleviate pain, is not meant to be maintained. What is particularly insisted upon is, that upon these alone and of themselves it is unsafe and injudicious in any instance to rely for cure of colic, for perfect restoration of function of the intestines, when this is so largely dependent upon accumulation of offending material.

In all exhibitions of colic except those in which diarrhœa is a prominent symptom, our correct and safe course of treatment is first of all, through the administration of such agents and the employment of such means as are appropriate to that end, to ensure an action of the intestinal canal and a removal of the irritating material therein contained. Certainly where pain exists it is both expedient and needful that attention be directed to the removal of such, which may be accomplished in conjunction with the main object, the evacuation of the bowels. In carrying out these principles of treatment our chief reliance must be placed on the action of those agents recognised as evacuants of the canal, assisted by the use of enemata. Of these the best for our purpose is undoubtedly aloes, oleaginous or saline laxatives are here too uncertain and too slow to satisfy our demands. The beneficial results of the administration of aloes in colic are not to be estimated by, nor do they appear to be dependent merely upon, the evacuant action on the bowel, for it is certain that in infinitely less time than is requisite to secure this may the beneficial influence of the drug be shown. The medicine is best given in bolus, by which its solution, absorption, and entrance into the circulation is secured from the anterior portion of the alimentary canal, those situations where absorption is most rapid, and in this way it is that in colic its earliest effects become appreciable

Amongst the earliest, and certainly the most enthusiastic, advocates for the employment of aloes alone in the treatment of colic, Mr. Gamgee senr strongly expresses his opinion in favour of the use of Cape aloes in preference to the variety generally in use, known as Barbadoes. During a lengthened experience in the use of this drug in bowel affections in the horse, I cannot speak thus favourably of the Cape variety, but must express a partiality for the other, the Barbadoes. It is possible that in my employment of the former I may never have been fortunate enough to secure the correct extract he so highly recommends With the Barbadoes, in its employment here, I have had no reason to complain, either because of its uncertainty of action or its drastic results

The amount to be given must in every instance be regulated by the character of the animal, its breed, age, bulk, as well as by the manner in which it may have been fed for some time previously.

In conjunction with the administration of aloes in relieving the bowels, we ought not to neglect the judicious employment of enemata In the simpler cases these may of themselves prove efficacious, and need only consist of tepid water. Where large masses of ingesta have accumulated in the colon, there seems reason to believe that benefit is derived from the addition to this of a solution of aloes, or some bland mucilage or oil.

In all cases where pain is distressing, we regard it as even more than expedient that in addition to the use of aloes and enemata, attention ought to be directed to the immediate alleviation of this, although anticipating that with the entrance of the aloes into the circulation there will result a mitigation of this most prominent feature This may be accomplished without largely interfering with the action of the aloes, or, where they have not been employed, by the administration once, or twice if necessary, of from one to two fluid ounces of tincture of opium, or the same quantity of an equally strong watery solution, given alone or in combination with from two to four ounces of spirits of nitrous ether in half a pint of tepid water or gruel, or what may serve the purpose equally well, is four ounces of solution of acetate of ammonia, with half a drachm of extract of belladonna, to which is added from four to six minims of Fleming's tincture of aconite For many years I have, in all cases of colic and bowel affections with much pain, found that this, in the large majority of instances, is speedily and permanently removed by the subcutaneous injection of the B P. preparation of morphia This preparation I employed in doses of forty minims, thus conveying into the system with each injection three and one-third grains of the salt This quantity rarely requires to be repeated

The part of the body I have generally chosen for injecting the solution is in front of the sternum, it may be done anywhere, but is most conveniently carried out where the skin is thin, and where it moves freely on the subcutaneous connective-tissue

I have not, save in a very few instances, seen any untoward results from the use of this morphia preparation In these exceptional cases, after the animal's recovery, there existed an indurated nodule, afterwards developing into an abscess at the point where the needle had been introduced In addition to the internal administration of antispasmodics and anodynes, good will often be obtained from the employment of smart friction or of warmth through means of rugs wrung from hot water, with an after-application of soap or turpentine liniment.

In those cases of colic where tympany is an attractive feature, we can less afford to wait patiently until the purgative has acted than where pain alone is predominant

In the control of this condition the whole of those agents which from their supposed chemical or other action have been recommended and employed are extremely uncertain, at one time seeming to be beneficial, and at another—under conditions, as far as we can discover, similar—perfectly inert Those which I have fancied the most useful are carbonate of soda, tincture of assafœtida, common salt, hyposulphite of soda, preparations of ammonia and oil of turpentine The last, when combined with oil, the form in which it has so long and so extensively been used in colic, is probably more beneficial in cases where tympany is a distinct feature than most others

Following the exhibition of any of these agents, it is always desirable to have recourse to smart friction, with warmth, to the abdomen, and where the horse may be moved without much discomfort, to have him walked or trotted smartly for ten or twenty minutes. Should relief not be afforded within an hour from the period of the first administration of the medicine, it ought in some form to be repeated.

In very severe cases in the early stages, and in all where the symptoms of distress continue increasing from the increase of the distension, we are justified in having recourse to puncture of the distended bowel. This operation I have seen performed with varying degrees of success for thirty years; it fell into disuse for long, probably from the little benefit which seemed to attend its employment, and the frequency of fatal results where it had been carried out. That these results were in all cases, or even largely, to be attributed to the performance of this operation I have often had grave doubts. Latterly it seems to have been revived amongst us, and, from what has been published respecting it, with satisfactory results. As the portion of the bowel which is the locality of the tympany is not always exactly the same, it is scarcely possible to indicate the exact spot where this tapping ought to be carried out in every instance.

Usually the distension will be found most prominent on the right side of the horse, and as the great bowel in these cases may be regarded as occupying the greater portion of this side of the abdominal cavity, from the transverse processes of the lumbar vertebræ to the floor of the cavity, in the space comprised between the anterior spines of the ilium and last ribs, we may thus with tolerable safety puncture anywhere between the ilium and margin of the ribs, nearer the former than the latter, extending from the floor of the abdomen to within four inches of the lumbar transverse processes, guided to a certain extent by the prominence of the distension.

The instrument most suitable for the operation is a trocar, with canula of small bore—an eighth of an inch diameter—either round or flat, and is to be preferred of at least six inches in length.

It is not often that ulterior bad results follow this puncturing; it may be, however, that a certain amount of inflammatory action, terminating in an abscess, may take place in connection with the wound of the integuments, and prove a little troublesome. When, however, puncturing of the bowel has been had recourse to either early in the distension or when somewhat advanced, we must not neglect to give attention, by the exhibition of evacuants, to secure the action of the intestines, which here, as in puncture of the rumen in the ox, are disposed after this interference to show unwonted torpidity. Another situation where the distended bowel may with equal success be punctured is from within and through the rectum, here we will find that length of trocar is even more essential than when the operation is carried out by puncturing the abdominal walls.

In the treatment of all cases of acute bowel affections in the horse it will ever be found that a most important element of success is early attendance, obtaining the treatment of the patient before the disturbance has existed for days, or been rendered more complicated by improper management; while, during the progress of any case of colic, it is to be remembered that we are not justified in leaving the animal entirely alone while the symptoms of pain continue, seeing that during the paroxysms there is always the risk that through struggling, while placed in some difficult position, fatal lesions, either of the internal viscera, the limbs, or the back, may occur. To obviate the chances of these dangers, as far as possible, it is always wise to place our patient in a roomy box or open shed, where such is procurable, and, if possible, to prevent his tossing about too much, seeing that with such movements there is always a danger of producing entanglement and strangulation of some portion of the bowels.

CHAPTER XL

INTESTINAL OBSTRUCTION

Definition.—*Obstruction to the passage of the contained material through the intestinal canal.*

Pathology *a Nature*—Obstruction to the passage of the contained material along the alimentary canal is, in the greater number of the forms through which the result is reached, probably not a primary morbid condition, but, as in the instances of entanglement, strangulation, and volvulus, the sequel of some previously existing disturbance, often of colic or enteric inflammation, which during the restlessness and struggling of the animal result in the production of these more fatal lesions   In others, as the cases of obstruction by concretions, the condition is usually independent and of gradual development, often, however, only culminating during the progress of abdominal pain, which has induced during the paroxysms displacement of the concretion, terminating in fatal obstruction

b Causation.—The immediate production of obstruction, the first step in other fatal structural changes, is brought about in various ways, the greater number of which may be grouped under—(1) *Accumulations of matter in the interior of the tube*, (2) *Stricture of the canal from organic disease;* (3) *Mechanical displacement and change in connection with different parts of the bowels.*

1 *Accumulation of Matter in the Intestinal Tube*—(*a*) Masses of stercoraceous material of varying bulk, often adhering to the walls of the tube and allowing portions of the contents to pass along, (*b*) Concretions of variable form and character, the product of particular dietary   Some of these, both such as are composed entirely of vegetable matter, the refuse and indigestible particles of grains, and such as are mainly formed of mineral substances, the phosphates of lime and magnesia, occasionally attain an enormous magnitude and are a source of wonder as to the possibility of their existing in the bowel without inducing painful symptoms.

The position of these larger concretions is usually the great bowel, in the pouches of which they may remain for years without giving evidence of their existence, and are probably only displaced and become impacted in some portion of the canal by spasm of the tube or the tossings of the animal in cases of abdominal pain.   The smaller sized, from the readiness with which they may be moved, are more dangerous than the very large

2. *Stricture of the Bowel from Organic Disease.*—This condition may occur at any portion of the tube, large or small, and

is apparently, when appearing, the result of slow textual changes, often of an inflammatory, occasionally of a degenerative, character affecting the walls of the intestine. Rarely in the horse have we from this condition perfect obstruction of the canal.

3. *Mechanical Entanglement, Alteration of Position, or Displacement of Portions of the Bowels.*—It is here, in some of the many forms of alteration of position, that we meet with the chief causes of perfect obstruction.

(*a*) Strangulation or incarceration of portions of the bowel by adventitious products, as bands of lymph, the result of inflammatory action in connection with the abdominal serous membranes, or more frequently we find the strangulation carried out by a pedunculated fatty or gland tumour of the mesentery, the neck of the tumour being of sufficient length to warp itself around the bowel, the gradual swelling of which tends to tighten the ligature, occluding the canal and strangulating the part.

(*b*) Entanglement of the intestine upon itself. This is ordinarily a condition occupying a good extent of the tube, large or small. In the case of the former the colon is found in its double portion thrown one half or completely around on itself, in this way considerably altering its position in the abdominal cavity. Entanglement of the small intestines is often associated with twisting and laceration of the mesenteric web by which they are attached to the spine, and is carried out by the passage of a double portion through a loop formed upon the bowel.

(*c*) Mesenteric hernia, passage of a portion of the bowel, usually the smaller, through a rent in the peritoneal web, is a common mode of entanglement and strangulation.

(*d*) Incarceration of portions of the intestines in cavities or openings which in perfectly healthy animals usually do not permit of their presence, as in imperfectly closed umbilicus and in excessive dilatation of the inguinal canal.

(*e*) Intussusception, volvulus, or invagination, the passage of one portion of the intestine within the part of the tube continuous with it. This is a cause of obstruction of less frequent occurrence than the varied forms of strangulation. It is said by those who have encountered this lesion in both the human subject and other animals, to be of more frequent occurrence in the very young than with such as have reached maturity. Although commonly it is only a few inches of the bowel which is passed within the continuation of the tube, instances are recorded where the extent of the invagination occupied several feet. Like other states of entanglement, this is in all probability a condition not occurring of itself and apart from some other abnormality, but merely developing as a concurrent symptom or occasional feature during the progress of several disturbances or textural changes

Symptoms—The clinical phenomena indicative of obstruction either from intestinal concretions or mechanical displacement are somewhat varied, not diagnostic, rather, upon the whole, such as are common to many conditions of disturbed function, or to organic change affecting the organs of the abdomen, particularly the bowels One class in particular, developed in connection with accumulations either stercoraceous or of variously-composed concretions, the result of specialities in dieting, are as a rule gradual in growth, or rather the symptoms are of an intermittent character. The others are oftener of sudden occurrence, starting into existence without premonitory warning, or in conjunction with some derangement of abdominal organs associated with pain, as in ordinary colic or states of inflammatory action.

In both classes of cases, but to a greater extent in the former, the history of the case will help us somewhat. Constipation or irregularity in the amount and character of the discharges, with recurring attacks of colic, are characteristic of obstruction from accumulation of adventitious material of whatever sort, while, where entanglement or mechanical displacement is the cause, constipation is not the most attractive feature, rather the violence and continued nature of the abdominal pain indicative of inflammatory action.

In these latter in certain forms, as when the great bowel is twisted upon itself, it is occasionally possible by examination through the rectum to detect the entanglement in the form of a distinct cord, and through the altered position of the double colon With such, also, there is often considerable tympany, borborygmus, and ultimately stupor from disturbed cerebral function

In all cases where there is a probability of external hernia, every care must be exercised that such may not escape detection

Treatment—As it may not be possible in the greater number of instances of obstruction from any of these causes, save where external hernia is evidently the inducing factor—and then the case resolves itself into one of reduction of the hernia by manipulatory interference—to demonstrate to satisfaction their existence, so our management of these is chiefly directed to obtain mitigation of pain, the most distressing symptom, and to relieve the bowel obstruction by favouring the natural discharge of the contained material, or allowing it to retire to the position previously occupied. Where from the previous history of the case, and the intermittent character of the symptoms, concretions are suspected, it is not wise, through the exhibition of active purgatives, to attempt forcible dislodgment of the obstruction The employment of such anodynes as preparations of opium or belladonna, with bland fluids, and the use of enemata, with the steady application, by means of woollen rugs, of heat and moisture, are nearly the extent to which careful treatment may proceed In every instance an examination of the rectum is advisable, seeing many cases occur where obstructing materials there are within reach of the hand, and by judicious manipulation may be removed

If a desire for food still exists, it must be given of such a character as will not aggravate the existing symptoms, and be allowed in moderation When pain is excessive and tympany great, as in many of the cases of strangulation, the same course is to be followed, with the addition probably, under certain circumstances, of the abstraction of blood and tapping the distended bowel, not that these are likely to be of much benefit, but upon the principle that, being uncertain of the exact pathological conditions, we are still warranted in endeavouring to ward off death by relieving the more urgent symptoms, not knowing what may result

Although not operating in inducing obstruction of the bowels, it is under this group of disturbances, change in position of the different parts of the intestine, that we ought to place

Prolapsus or Eversion of the Rectum.

It is chiefly as an accompaniment or sequel of certain cases of colic of a mild and protracted character, accompanied with constipation, or even oftener associated with torpidity of the bowels as a distinct condition, that we encounter eversion or protrusion of the posterior part of the rectum.

In the horse I have more particularly observed this condition in the comparatively young, in animals previous to their being stabled and trained for their special work, usually appearing in these while grazing in pastures where, from certain causes, the herbage is unnaturally dry, and containing an extra amount of woody fibre

In such instances the animals may be observed for some little time to exhibit indications of unthriftiness and want of improvement, but nothing serious is apprehended until bowel-protrusion induces alarm. Others, again, have this state preceded by an attack of colic, with the usual symptoms of abdominal pain.

When the protrusion is inconsiderable, the horse may not exhibit any disturbance save when fæces are voided, at which time there is uneasiness and evident irritation. Sometimes abdominal pain is shown by hurriedly pawing and lying down. On the fæces being passed, he moves away as if nothing had occurred. Should the portion of bowel everted be of great extent, the disturbance and irritation are likely to be continuous. The horse is disposed to lie down, and when raised, moves restlessly from place to place; inappetency is likely to exist, and, with many, occasional or continued straining

If not speedily relieved, the protruded portion, from the continued constriction in which it is held by the anal sphincter, becomes strangulated and gangrenous When once established, it is rarely that this condition of eversion is overcome without manipulatory interference.

Treatment.—When the portion of bowel protruded is not extensive, and when observed early, before its vitality is impaired by strangulation, it is usually successfully dealt with by first removing from the rectum all contained fæces, washing the extruded portion and slightly lubricating it with oil, or what is better, washing it with warm milk and tincture of opium, and smearing it with an ointment of powdered opium and tannic acid; after which, by careful manipulation, replacing it. In order to prevent a recurrence of the protrusion, some recommend and employ a needle or metallic suture passed through the anus, or the application of a properly adjusted truss or bandage. The former may succeed and be admissible in small animals; and the latter, either alone or combined, may be useful in adults, or where they have been subject to being under restraint. With the animals, however, which we are most frequently called upon to treat, unbroken colts or fillies, either of these methods is objectionable. Here we have found that the placing of them upon a soft or rather laxative diet, as steamed bran, with a few oats, to which has been added treacle or linseed-oil, together with a careful watching of them for some days, an occasional enema, and application of the ointment of opium and tannic acid, and replacing of the everted bowel whenever it occurs, is generally sufficient to secure a permanent restoration of parts.

When the protruded portion is much swollen from infiltration, and thus rendered difficult to return, we may expedite the process by free scarification previous to or during the fomentation. Should gangrene have commenced in the everted portion ere we have seen the case, through strangulation by the sphincter, or should it afterwards occur by the repeated protrusions, the removal of the diseased portion will be necessitated. This, although it may be accomplished at once, is, unless the disturbance caused by the eversion be great, better delayed for some time, when, through the gradual death of the structures, hæmorrhage is avoided, and perfect adhesion of the rectum to the anal opening is ensured.

While watching the removal of the strangulated parts, we may facilitate their removal either by freely passing a piece of strong caustic, as chloride of zinc or nitrate of silver, at regular intervals around the line of demarcation, or by the employment of a few interrupted ligatures around the anus, so strangulating circumscribed portions of the texture between the living and the dead, the sphacelated portion in a short time being thrown off.

CHAPTER XLI

RUPTURE OF THE INTESTINAL WALLS

As a result of these different forms of disturbed intestinal function, whether of impaction from ingesta, distension from gases, or both combined, there is occasionally encountered this lesion of ruptured intestinal walls   This is probably oftener observed affecting the colon than the small bowel, and is more likely to follow the existence of degenerative changes in the muscular and other textures of the tube, whereby the integrity and resisting power of these is impaired, as also their natural peristaltic action and other activities interfered with, from which, in all probability, has resulted the impaction or excessive tympany where these have severally existed; the altered textural change in the bowel being thus, in many instances, both the cause of the impaction or distension, and the explanation why the rupture should occur in these particular instances and not in all.

The symptoms which indicate this fatal termination of disturbed function are neither uniform nor diagnostic   In some, the occurrence of the lesion seems to be followed by rapid collapse; in others, it would appear that life may be prolonged for a few days.   With one, we may have mitigation of the distressing features previously existing; with another, on the contrary, all these may suffer aggravation

When occurring in association with impaction or unnatural retention of ingesta in the colon, together with considerable distension from gases in the bowels, in which cases we often have restlessness and much straining, the occurrence of the lesion is usually followed by relief in the symptom of restlessness, and a subsidence of the straining, comparative calm and quietness being the condition succeeding the rupture until death.   In all, with the completion of the rupture, I have observed that exhaustion is a feature rapidly developed; and that although relief from pain seems to have been obtained at once and unexpectedly, there is a haggard, anxious expression of countenance, a frequent and small pulse, steadily becoming more rapid and at last imperceptible, patchy perspiration, short catching respiration, gradually a disinclination and inability to move, the animal balancing itself, as it were, on the limbs until the very last. Whenever cases of colic marked by impaction of the bowels, with or without much distension, accompanied with straining, suddenly exhibit cessation of the pain and straining, together with the appearance of much exhaustion and other symptoms indicated, we have just grounds to fear rupture of some part of the intestinal wall.

In two or three cases of ruptured colon which I watched throughout, the disposition to sit on the haunches, and some attempts at vomition, were particularly persistent. With many there is nothing attractive or diagnostic in the symptoms to differentiate this from ordinary fatal bowel affections in which inflammatory action plays an important part, and the lesion is not even suspected until an after-death examination has been made.

CHAPTER XLII.

ENTERITIS—INFLAMMATORY DISEASE OF THE INTESTINES.

Definition — *Inflammation affecting the intestines generally, or any portion of them individually and in particular.*

Pathology. *a Nature and Varieties* — It has by some been regarded as an established fact that inflammatory disease of the intestinal portion of the alimentary canal is rarely in the horse developed apart from a similar condition of the gastric structures; this, however, does not seem to be confirmed either by clinical or post-mortem observations.

In other of our patients, particularly the smaller ruminants, there seems evidence to induce us to regard the concomitance of these conditions as of more frequent occurrence. Neither are we inclined to regard enteritis, apart from mechanical causes, as such a very common equine disease as many represent it; while, when it does occur, and is fairly developed, there is abundant evidence to satisfy as to its extreme fatality. Like the simple functional disturbances connected with the canal, enteritis, or true inflammatory action, may occur at any period of the animal's life, but is more largely exhibited amongst animals which have reached adult life and are fully under the influence of domestication than with young animals, and such as are roaming at will in the open fields. Rarely, even in the best-marked cases, have we more than a sectional portion of the canal invaded ; in the horse this locality is variable, the large intestine being rather more frequently the seat of the diseased action than the small. Besides this variation as to exact situation, we may also observe that there are certain variations or peculiarities exhibited in the manifestation and results of the unnatural activities In many the progress of events is extremely rapid, the termination fatal, with lesions of a very attractive character; in others, although the clinical phenomena may not be very dissimilar, the course and termination are delayed, while the tissue-changes are less distinctive and sometimes rather occult.

For many years I have been forcibly impressed with the conviction that many cases—the greater number, indeed, which terminate fatally with wonderful rapidity both in towns and rural districts, and which are regularly regarded as enteritis— are in many of their clinical features and post-mortem lesions somewhat different from the conditions which in our day we are inclined to accept as indicative of, or attendant upon, inflammatory action In this opinion I am supported by other observers. These conditions, well enough recognised and regularly encountered by all, particularly by those whose work is in connection with heavy draught animals, have been for such a lengthened period accepted as exhibiting in a characteristic manner the extreme of inflammatory action, that any contrary opinion as to their nature seems to savour largely of heterodoxy. These cases we know develop themselves in horses apparently in the enjoyment of the fullest amount of health and vigour without premonitory warning, and hasten to a fatal termination despite remedial measures in a few hours If truly inflammatory such cases rather stagger us, and seem to refute our preconceived ideas of inflammatory action · first, by the rapidity with which they pass through their several stages and terminate in death , second, when examined as to the effects produced on structures and organs immediately implicated we do not observe the textural changes usually encountered after the development of this unnatural action in other situations Here we have no thickening of membranes which has been gradually progressive,

43

nor any attempt at organization of unnatural or adventitious
products   The whole phenomena appear to partake purely of
obstructive or congestive character, a disturbance of the normal
equilibrium which ought to subsist amongst the various constituent elements of the blood, or an alteration in the conducting
powers of the blood and lymph conduits The very large amount
of gelatiniform material effused would seem to point to distinctive changes in the amount and character of the colloid elements
of the blood, while the largely blood-stained effusion and ingesta
would lead us to suspect rupture of minute bloodvessels   No
doubt we may view these abnormal conditions in somewhat of
another light, and account for both the extent and character
of the exudation from the speciality of structure and function
of the bowel as well as from the nature of the action itself   In
this part of the system we have to recollect the considerable
extent of both lymph and bloodvessels, and the activity of
absorption naturally existing in health

   In other forms of disturbed intestinal activity recognised as
inflammatory the clinical features may be somewhat similar,
more prolonged if somewhat less intense, the tissue-changes
are, however, more in keeping with our ordinary ideas of the
results of inflammation, as these ideas are formed by the nature
of the resulting changes in other situations   In these we have
effusion less extensive in every respect, but better developed
as to its textural characters, and however blood-stained or
coloured it may be, it never presents such resemblances to
anthracoid effusions and congestive states as the former manifestations do

   b *Causation.*—The causes which operate in the induction
of inflammatory action in any part of the alimentary canal are
very similar, if not identical in character with those adverse influences to which have been attributed the occurrence of the
lesser evils, simple disturbance in the functional activities of
the bowel.

   Indigestion, or arrest of those changes which ought naturally
to proceed in the bowel, indicated by expressions of abdominal
pain—colic so-called—may result from influences or agents
precisely similar in character to those which operate in inducing the more serious and destructive inflammatory process
There seems every reason for believing that repeated attacks of

bowel disturbance, associated with expressions of pain, ultimately tend to favour the onset of inflammatory action The causes repeating the bowel disturbance may be similar from first to last, but the parts so disturbed become less able to resist the evil effects of the applied irritation or disturbing agent, and when normal activities are repeatedly perverted, the structures at last refuse to return to their natural condition

All those causes which were enumerated as likely to produce intestinal disturbance with exhibition of pain, as over-feeding, irregular feeding, feeding with improper material, and feeding when fatigued or exhausted, together with injudicious work and exposure to vicissitudes of weather, may with equal propriety be charged with the production of enteritis, particularly of the acute forms Probably the continuous feeding, or feeding for a lengthened period, upon some particular diet may render an animal so treated more susceptible than others when both are similarly acted upon by some disturbing agent. Of the many irregularities in diet likely to act thus detrimentally, none require to be guarded against more carefully than over-feeding, and feeding liberally, previous to active exertion

That ordinary indigestion, or functional disturbance of the bowel, does largely—unless when repeated and remaining long unrelieved—tend to pass on to true inflammatory action is doubtful Rather are we disposed to regard inflammation when occurring as having been such from the first, and more rarely to follow as the natural result of disturbed function which has passed on to the more pronounced change Many cases of enteritis, no doubt, are regularly encountered in which we are totally unable to assign any reason or sufficient cause for their occurrence, still it is equally certain that many apparently sudden attacks, if the animals had been carefully enough observed, would be found to have been preceded by many indications of disturbed health.

Besides all these influences connected with dietary we have others, a smaller number probably, which, although remotely of dietetic origin, can scarcely immediately be regarded in that light ; these are all such as relate to injury done to the intestine, or obstruction produced in any portion of it, the terminations of which are usually inflammatory Also we may place the

43—2

existence of parasites in particular conditions as active inducing factors of enteritis; their presence even in the tube may
be productive of irritation sufficient to terminate in inflammation, much more so when they take possession of the
structures of the walls as their habitat, and there not merely
disturb but become provocative of extensive and dangerous
tissue-changes.

Further, inflammation of the whole or of portions of the
textural elements of the intestinal walls may manifest itself as
part of certain general diseased processes in some fevers and
constitutional diseases

c Anatomical Characters —In those rapidly progressive
and generally fatal forms of enteric disease, marked by much
sero-hæmorrhagic effusion, the lesions observable on after-death
examination are usually of a pronounced character; they are
chiefly located in the large bowel, the colon   Here, in the
submucous tissue of the canal, and in the subserous of the
attached mesentery, are extensive collections of colloid or jelly-
like material in the case of the submucous areas, often extending for several feet, elevating to the extent of two or three
inches the glistening and distended membrane   This gelatiniform material is always more or less coloured, frequently of
a truly hæmorrhagic appearance; while in rarer instances
colouring matter seems to have escaped from the confined
mass, giving a blood-stained appearance to the contained
ingesta   With many of these we observe that much fluid has
found its way into and been mingled with the contents of the
canal, which, although thus semifluid, have remained stationary,
most probably from the paralyzed condition of the muscular
element in the bowel.

In other cases, where the morbid action seems less acute,
more distributed in patches, and occupying a different portion
of the canal, we may observe a disposition to the formation of
fibrinous or coagulable lymph; this would seem to be thrown
out over the surface of the mucous membrane, and is not unfrequently voided with the discharges on cessation of pain
and subsidence of the unnatural action   These portions of
discharged fibrinous lymph, not unlike diphtheritic or croupous
exudation material, are observed as shreds or flakes, or oftener
rolled together in masses, and have been mistaken, as remarked

when speaking of this condition as seen in constipation, for collections of the large ascarides. Occasionally we find the changes not so uniformly diffused, but scattered over isolated portions of the bowels; and although the colour of the parts invaded is not materially altered, the physical characters are somewhat different. The increase in bulk or thickness may not be so great; the tissues are, however, more resistant to the touch, and after some time paler in colour.

In those numerously occurring cases of inflammation of the intestines associated with the varying forms of certain fevers, as influenza, the course and termination of the morbid process is considerably different. In these the action is exceedingly variable, marked in some by extensively distributed sero-hæmorrhagic effusions in the submucous tissue; in others, where less extensive, showing only moderate effusion into the underlying structures, with an occasional patch more distended than the rest, in the centre of which a spot or sore exists, undergoing removal of tissue. Or with a somewhat similar condition of the entire structures pustules may show themselves projected from circumscribed inflammatory patches in the submucous structures. Or the appearance may be that of a very general change and removal of both epithelial covering and limitary membrane, the whole showing a peculiar granular or oatmeal appearance over the surface. Others, again, exhibit in the midst of slightly hyperæmic surroundings, or of tissues perfectly normal, a sharply defined patch or patches of varying size of a coal-black appearance.

Where the morbid action has partaken more of a truly catarrhal character, or where the course has not been marked by symptoms usually indicative of the inflammatory process, and where considerable progress has been made before life seems endangered, another class of changes may present themselves.

In these the changes have evidently been early and continuously associated with the ultimate elements of the tissue invaded. Here the epithelium of the mucous membrane undergoes such changes as disturbs or destroys the cohesion of the cell-elements, which become detached and are shed or thrown off, with the extra liquid existing, as varying forms of pus-cells. Along with these changes on the surface of the

membrane we find somewhat similar changes in the gland-
structures scattered over the bowel, with, in course of time,
particular changes further developed in connection with the
gland-structures from condensation and alteration of the connective-tissue amongst which they are placed. In some we
have distinctly atrophic changes, lessening of the general bulk
of the mucous membrane, with shrinking or disappearance of
the gland-structures proper

Symptoms —In common with simple functional disturbance
of the bowels, known by the generic name of *colic,* the more
serious structural lesions accompanying the peculiar congestions and inflammations which there take place are chiefly
made known to us by the exhibition of those symptoms which
are indicative of abdominal pain   Like simple disturbance
of functional activity, inflammatory action, although usually
said to be developed suddenly, will, if observation has been
carefully exercised, be frequently found to have had a more
gradual development

In differentiating the symptoms of these two conditions
much care is needed, and, even after such has been exercised,
much uncertainty remains

The character of the pain does not, judging from the modes
of its manifestation, seem to differ in either. In ordinary
functional disturbance it may even seem more severe ; it may,
however, in enteritis, as distinct from merely derangement of
the canal, be regarded as being more steadily continuous,
rarely having intervals of remission   In particular instances
of enteric inflammations manipulation or pressure over the
abdomen is not tolerated, but rather tends to aggravate the
distress   The pulse, which in simple disorder of the bowels is
unaltered, save during paroxysms of pain, when it is variously
affected both as to character and frequency, is, in the more
serious textural changes, steadily progressive in disturbance

At first merely increased in frequency, it gradually, in the
earlier stages, acquires a character of tension or resistance, the
volume not perceptibly altered, with no return to its normal
characters , in the latter stages we have increased frequency
with lessened volume but marked resistance, passing on to
feebleness of impulse with rapid and weak cardiac action.

The internal temperature, which in functional disturbance is rarely altered, is in inflammatory action usually elevated, although it may not be distinguished by a great rise

In those instances where the disturbance is more than functional during the continuance of the pain, there is rarely any evacuation from the bowel, with the exception of those where the condition of congestive action is ushered in by the distinct symptom of diarrhœa

In instances of the exhibition of abdominal pain, apart from inflammation, there are ordinarily periods of remission, and the return to normal conditions is accomplished suddenly and at once When pain is the consequence of inflammatory action it is usually continuous, and in cases of recovery, return to health is only reached after a rather tedious process, and through depression or nausea

Of the different modes or phases of physical change of the bowels which result in inflammatory action, there are probably no certain or diagnostic symptoms which may lead us to differentiate the one from the other Occasionally we may be able, by the occurrence of some fortuitous symptoms, to make a happy guess ; the same data, however, not serving us equally well on their next development in some other case. We may be able to indicate whether the disturbance and pain are the results of merely functional derangement, or of more serious inflammatory action , but we are usually unable to determine whether this inflammation is the result of intussusception, strangulation, or some other equally potent but less easily understood operating agency

The tardiness of development and the prolonged existence of symptoms may lead us to recognise the presence of the more occult but steadily progressive morbid changes associated with extensively distributed alterations of the more elementary structures of the intestines, as contrasted with the occurrence of those very destructive sero-sanguineous collections and effusions immediately related to the vascular system. Further, however, we are rarely permitted to go

If the great majority of cases of simple disturbed natural activities of the intestinal canal in the horse rarely terminate fatally, the very opposite may be regarded as true in every form of inflammatory action

In all, or nearly all, which terminate fatally, we often observe previous to death—sometimes several hours before that
event occurs—an apparent improvement in the general appearance of the horse, with a distinct relief from pain. This
relief from actual suffering ought not to deceive us as to ultimate results, did we carefully take into consideration the condition of the symptoms individually and their relations to each
other. Although food in such instances may be partaken of, it
is either in an unconscious manner, or with so much listlessness as may not fail to attract attention, while the haggard
expression of countenance is persistent, or even more marked,
than at an earlier period, the pulse steadily exhibiting less
volume and more irritability, while the respirations become
quicker, more catching, and of less extent

As the termination approaches the animal becomes stupid
and unconscious, stands propped against the wall, or wanders
listlessly around the box or shed when at liberty, the mouth
becomes clammy and cold, the abdomen occasionally tympanitic, and the general surface-temperature lowered. Rarely
is there much struggling previous to death, which is usually
not long delayed after falling to the ground, the animal, in
the latter stages of enteric inflammation, often persisting in
standing

Treatment — Although a very large number of horses,
suffering from inflammation of the bowels, have been some
time previous to their being seen by the professional attendant
beyond the reach of medical treatment as far as recovery is
concerned, or which, if we were aware of the immediate cause of
the morbid action, would be considered alike hopeless from the
outset, still, as we may not be assured of either of these
conditions, and as it may not be denied that recoveries do
occur in some exceedingly doubtful cases, every attention
ought to be directed to overcome the morbid action, or to
guide the animal safely through the different stages of the
process

At one time, probably more than in our day, all cases,
whether believed to be undoubtedly inflammatory or merely
exhibiting abdominal disturbance, were copiously bled. This
idea, however, that indiscriminate blood-letting is likely to be
productive of the greatest amount of good, is not one largely

held by those who, from scientific knowledge or practical experience, are most entitled to give an opinion on the subject. That there are numerous cases where, from inherent conditions and particular surroundings, the abstraction of blood may not only be tolerated, but even indicated as likely to prove of benefit, there seems reasonable grounds for believing.

These are usually seizures where the animals possess sufficient vigour in themselves to warrant us in believing them capable of carrying through the reaction likely to follow, which are not acted upon by immediately depressing influences, and where the vascular disturbance, as indicated by the cardiac and arterial pulse, is of recent origin. Having taken a fair or full amount of blood, it will rarely be needful to repeat the operation. We must be careful not to mistake the cardiac excitement of reaction for increased perversion of normal activities.

The fact that arrest of intestinal action and of discharge of fæcal matter is a prominent symptom, has usually led to the use of some variety of purgative agents in the treatment of enteritis. Now, as I do not believe that a horse in this condition is likely to suffer from the want of discharge from the canal for several days, as also that to solicit the passage of the contained ingesta is likely to induce aggravation of the irritation and already existing morbid action, it seems that the indications of treatment are rather in the opposite direction—that instead of attempts to excite movement of the bowel, we ought to endeavour to secure its repose.

Instead of administering aloes, or large quantities of oil, or even salines, greater benefit, I believe, always results from the employment of some preparation of opium or belladonna, either alone or combined with a camphor mixture, the vehicle being gruel, or gruel with a moderate quantity of oil. When given in a liquid form, the watery solution of opium is to be preferred to the spirituous, and when employed as bolus, is to be exhibited in moderate amount at intervals of a few hours. A very useful mode of employing these medicines, I have found, is first of all to exhibit a draught containing half a drachm of camphor, opium solution equal in strength to half a drachm of the powder, with five minims of Fleming's tincture of aconite in a pint of gruel, with or without a little linseed-oil   Following this, should the pain continue, to inject subcutaneously, at intervals of two hours, forty minims of the B P. solutio morphia hypodermica.

Besides this I have often, and with apparent benefit, had recourse to the exhibition every three hours of a draught containing half a drachm of camphor and four or six fluid ounces of the solution of acetate of ammonia. In addition to the internal administration of such medicines, it is always judicious to employ, as a means of relieving pain, heat and moisture externally   This may be carried out through the medium of woollen rugs wrung from very warm water, and wrapped around the animal's body. These ought to be applied continuously for two or three hours, and when removed, a mixture of equal quantities of oil of turpentine and linseed-oil had better be smartly rubbed over the abdomen   This latter may be repeated in a few hours   Although it may be needful to make an exploration of the rectum to ascertain its condition, it is rarely needful, in the course of inflammatory action, to keep continuously pumping tepid water, plain or medicated, into the bowel

Should the horse during the illness be disposed to drink, allow a sufficiency of oatmeal-gruel or linseed-tea, to which has been added solution of acetate of ammonia or some neutral salt

With abatement of pain within the first six hours there is always hope of recovery. With this remission, however, we should not attempt to force the bowels to action by the exhibition of purgatives   The case ought to be left alone, allowing a sufficiency of gruel, with, if there is a desire for food, a small amount of scalded bran, to which may be added a little treacle or linseed-oil   In some instances an enema of tepid water will be advisable as assisting the natural action of the bowel

The only variation in this treatment which I regard as safe is in the instance of a subacute or chronic character, usually terminating in tissue-changes of the glandular and other integral parts of the bowels   Here it is probable that a more sparing use of the opium preparations, and a more liberal one of the oleaginous and salines, may be carried out; in these I have found that opium is with benefit supplanted, at least in part, if not altogether, by belladonna and camphor Following the subsidence also of the more acute symptoms, these cases seem to improve under the use of mild vegetable tonics, as quinine, gentian, myrrh, etc

CHAPTER XLIII

DYSENTERY—BLOODY FLUX

Definition—*An intestinal inflammatory action of a peculiar or specific character, attended with fever, occasional abdominal pain, and fluid alvine discharges, mingled with blood or albuminous materials, the tissue-changes, which are usually regarded as diagnostic, being situated chiefly in the minute gland-structures and interconnective tissue of the large intestine.*

Pathology *a Nature*—This affection, of less frequent occurrence in the horse than in most other animals, is in several of its features closely linked to diarrhœa, from which, however, it is differentiated by the phenomena of constitutional disturbance, and the existence of local inflammatory action with specific tissue-changes. Whatever may be the immediate or more remote cause in its production, its diagnostic and essential features would appear to reside in elemental tissue-changes of a destructive character, tending to localized gangrene, and ulceration of the mucous membrane and contiguous tissues, chiefly of the large bowels Whether, under particular conditions and influences intrinsic and extrinsic, it is in certain animals capable of extension from the diseased to the healthy, its power of communicability in this way in the horse has not yet been established When appearing in him it is usually in association with agencies which, as a class, are fertile in the production of disturbed assimilation generally In many it may be engrafted on an existing attack of diarrhœa; or, judging from my own experience, it more frequently occurs as a separate and independent affection

It is probable that animals of all ages, and under very varying conditions, may exhibit this disease, but it has chiefly

been encountered in young horses somewhat exposed to adverse
climatic conditions, and in all varieties where indifferent sanitation, defective dietary, and other lowering agencies have been
in operation

   b Causation.—Unlike the practitioner of human medicine,
the veterinary surgeon is not in the position, with respect to
dysentery, to affirm that there are just grounds for attributing
its appearance to direct infection—that is, to the importation
into the healthy of specific disease-germs.

   Both as predisposing and directly inducing factors—when
sufficiently long maintained—we are disposed to place—
(1) All depressing influences, whether of work, exposure, insufficient food, and generally bad sanitation   (2) Noxious
emanations, chiefly animal, resulting from over-crowding, and
tending, by their toxic influence, to induce hæmal contamination   (3) Probably malarial influences, generated in particular
situations where horses may be retained during improper
periods   4 The previous existence of functional disturbance—
diarrhœa—which, from improper treatment or association
with some constitutional cachexia, or already existing diseased
action, as intestinal parasitism, may offer a favourable opportunity for the development of the peculiar textural changes

   That any of these individually may tend to the production
of dysentery is probable ; in practice, however, it is usual to
find that two or more of them have been associated with its
appearance

   c Anatomical Characters—Although in a general sense the
leading anatomical features may be said to be that of inflammation of the bowel, with gangrene and ulceration, when we
come carefully to examine this condition it is found that the
morbid action has certain peculiarities upon which its individuality depends ; also it is to be remembered, that although
possessing in all instances certain great generic features, there
are yet many instances of variation both as to extent and
character   Rarely have we more than portions of the bowel
exhibiting the diagnostic lesions which are irregularly scattered
over the whole extent.   At first, and previous to necrotic
changes and the production of an ulcerous sore, we may observe
small spots or elevations of the membrane projecting from a
somewhat swollen and hyperæmic base; these papules on the

summit, previous to their rupture of structure, may seem somewhat paler in colour than the rest of the elevation. These, when minutely examined, give the idea of increased vascularity and swelling either of the minute glands of the bowels, of the connective-tissue surrounding them, or of both, with, in many cases, the production of a diphtheritic-looking exudate, which may be either a new product, chiefly on the free surface, but as frequently merely the changed and removing covering membrane. There is also an exudation into and amongst the submucous tissue, apparently of the same texture and character with that on the free surface. This new or changed material, usually of a grey colour, is composed of fibrinous material and varying cell-growths, which, after appearing in a tolerably firm state, may undergo degeneration, or in rarer instances more perfect organization When the necrotizing process commences, which it usually does on the summit of the elevation, the rupture extends by inroads, and removal of tissue circumferentially and in depth, the whole extending both by the removal of the newly exuded material as well as by encroaching on the normal structures. When healing, these sores close by rounding of their edges and deposition of new material in their floor, with a greater density of texture and an absence of gland-structure

In those cases which I have encountered in the horse, which have not been numerous, the gland-structures of the mesentery, in connection with the portion of the bowel invaded, seemed swollen, softer in texture and darker coloured In two there was a collection of rather dark-coloured fluid in the abdominal cavity, with some ecchymosis on different portions of the serous covering of the bowel In none have I ever witnessed perforation of the intestine, nor lesion of other viscera of the abdomen, which I could connect with the dysentery

Symptoms —In some, the earliest indications of illness may be taken to represent diarrhœa, the most noticeable feature being the frequent dejection of liquid fæces, in others, from the outset, and usually in all when established, the fever is obtrusive, and general prostration marked. In some, rigors may be observed throughout the entire course of the disease ; in all, the temperature is more or less elevated, with a more frequent and irritable pulse. When advancing insidiously we may not

at first apprehend aught serious until the continued diarrhœa,
with dry unthrifty coat and skin, the general depression and
wasting, with impaired appetite and elevation of internal
temperature, direct our attention to a careful examination of
the discharges from the bowels. Voided with only occasional
and irregularly occurring pain, these on examination will be
found to contain a moderate amount of true fæcal matter, which
is either soft, or more rarely contains, amongst excess of liquid,
hardened masses of ingesta ; the liquid portion is composed
largely of mucus and a jelly-like material mingled with shreds
of membrane or blood, the whole being of a tenacious gluey
character, and emitting a peculiarly offensive smell, which
seems to depend on the amount of necrotized tissue and blood
which are present.

The more severe cases gradually but steadily tend to a fatal
termination. With lessening appetite but increasing thirst,
abdominal pain and more fœtid discharges which no treatment seems to alleviate, marasmus, exhaustion, and fever
of an adynamic type shortly destroy the sufferer. The cases
which have come under my observation have none of them
been of an acute type, all continuing over three weeks.
Although in some the mucous membrane of the mouth was
sodden and pasty, in none did I detect rupture of the buccal
structures ; all exhibited striking marasmus with anxiety of
countenance.

Treatment.—In all cases of disturbed bowels when structural
changes are dreaded, and particularly where symptoms indicate
that such exist, the greatest amount of good is likely to result
from perfect rest, both to the body as a whole and to the
intestinal canal in particular. In addition to good location
and healthful sanitation in every respect, we ought to enforce a
dietary of an essentially moist and emollient character, material
easy of assimilation, fairly nutritious, and not likely from its
physical characters to irritate the tender or abraded membrane ; this I am more disposed to rely upon than extensive
dosing with medicines.

Whenever retention of fæcal matter is feared, a liberal allowance of linseed-oil in the food is to be used so as to facilitate its
removal. From astringents of any class, the most frequently
employed remedies, I have received less benefit than from a

carefully regulated dietary, the ordinary articles of which, when exhaustion is great, are to be supplemented with others, such as milk, raw eggs, beaf-tea, and port wine

When pain is troublesome and the discharges are very fœtid, opium and carbolic acid may be employed with benefit, the acid to be given as carbolized glycerine from two to three drachms, and repeated with the opium every six or four hours. Of the ordinary astringents which in some instances may be given, the best are nitrate of silver in solution, and sulphate of copper, or acetate of lead in combination with opium in bolus. Ipecacuanha, so much employed in dysentery in man, I have tried as powder given with linseed-tea, but have imagined it served the purpose better when combined with opium, one drachm of the former to half a drachm of the latter, made into a ball, and one given two or three times daily. Besides these medicines administered internally, attention ought to be directed, through the use of clothing and friction by hand, to maintain an equable distribution of surface-warmth, and when abdominal pain is troublesome to use turpentine stupes. Moderate cases are fairly hopeful, with the more severe the probabilities of a fatal issue are great.

CHAPTER XLIV

DISEASES CONNECTED WITH THE LIVER, IN WHICH DISTURBED ACTIVITIES OR STRUCTURAL CHANGES, OR BOTH, ARE PROMINENT FEATURES

SOME GENERAL CLINICAL CHARACTERS

HEPATIC disturbance and change, though in no form so frequently occurring, nor yet productive of such serious results in the horse as in man, or even in some other animals which engage our attention, are still with him not to be looked upon as uncommon. Their frequency and severity are here regulated by laws and conditions similar to those which operate in other animals

The liver being an organ which performs rather complex and important functions, it is easy to understand that, like

other organs, it is liable, in proportion to the variety of these
functions, to suffer derangement or textural change.   The
most conspicuous of these functions is the formation of bile, a
material of much importance in the process of digestion ;
besides serving as an eliminatory, it is also of varied and important service in digestion.   On this account many phenomena of an unnatural character connected with digestion and
the alimentary canal and the general depuration of the system,
have been regarded as springing from disturbance of the liver.
There are also activities and functions of other characters, as
the so-called glycogenic function, the disturbance of which has
already been noticed in speaking of 'diabetes,' and the probabilities of its relation to the production of another complex
animal substance—urea.

In both disturbance of its natural functions and in many
textural changes, if not absolutely certain of all the altered
conditions and disease-symptoms to which these give rise we
at least seem to have just grounds in claiming a few as generally connected with these

1. An important group of symptoms connected with disturbed bile-formation, which have been spoken of under the
term of 'jaundice.'   In addition to which are others evidenced
by irregular intestinal action of varying character, according
as bile-production is in excess or deficiency.

2. With many abnormal conditions of the liver there is
obvious local pain, shown by uneasiness and colicky symptoms, which are liable to be increased on local manipulation.

3. A peculiar and often-occurring symptom of hepatic
derangement or of tissue-change is in connection with distant
parts, particularly the right pectoral limb, in which we have
persistent lameness

4. Changes in the hepatic structure and obstruction of the
portal circulation lead to intestinal catarrh, enlargement of
spleen, ascites, and other changes of abdominal structures.

—

CHAPTER XLV.

CONGESTION OF THE LIVER

Definition.—*Engorgement and distension of the liver from over-repletion of the blood or bile conduits.*

Pathology *a Nature and Varieties*—The very extensive and differently distributed vascular relations of the liver render the condition of hyperæmia or excess of blood in its capillary system a rather frequent and to be looked for occurrence. This excess of blood, we find, is probably the earliest and most steadily occurring disturbance connected with the various structural changes to which the viscus is liable

The most commonly appearing form of this is that which is recognised as *passive congestion*, associated with obstructed blood-flow in the hepatic and portal veins, as distinct from turgescence resulting from increased afflux of blood.

This condition seems largely connected with retrocession of blood from external organs and surfaces, and with disease of other viscera, particularly the heart and lungs The state of valvular disease, especially of the right side, and impediments to the blood-flow in the pulmonary artery, intimately related to pulmonary emphysema and collapse, are markedly powerful in inducing this form of hepatic congestion

Another form of turgescence and hyperæmia, known as *active congestion*, arises from an increased or excessive supply of blood to the gland, appearing in the form of distension of the capillaries, probably of the hepatic artery This, as respects the production of hepatic disease, is of itself of rather less importance than the former manifestation. We are aware that active hyperæmia of the liver to some extent accompanies the regular process of digestion, also that over-feeding, or feeding upon highly stimulating materials, together with enforced idleness, tend to intensify this regularly occurring condition

From either or both of these states arises the third form of turgescence, termed *biliary congestion*, in which the minute bile-ducts become loaded and surcharged with the glandular secretion

44

In the first, the secretion of bile being natural, its excretion or outpouring is impeded by the pressure upon the lobules or bile-ducts, exerted by means of the engorged vessels.

In the second, the increased supply of blood on to a certain point provides an increased pabulum for the secreting structures, the product of which the bile-ducts are not at once able to carry away Very shortly, however, this congestion, if continued, or even if frequently repeated, will tend to a result the opposite of augmentation of bile-secretion

Both these conditions of vascular congestion, as far as the liver itself is concerned, may be regarded as passive, while, if kept up for any length of time, they tend to bilious contamination of the blood, and, when repeated, to serious structural changes of the liver, and are the chief source of abdominal dropsy Their attendance upon or preceding such changes as *cirrhosis* may be accounted for by remembering that this continued and repeated constriction of the lobule-cell is likely both to impair its nutrition and power of reproduction, as also that, like other structures, when their natural functions are not duly called into operation they are liable to atrophy and degenerate.

The several conditions of hyperæmia and turgescence of hepatic structure in the horse during life, if we were to judge by clinical history alone, might seem of rather rare occurrence ; but, in the light of after-death examinations, they are evidently of frequent enough existence

In our post-mortem records it is not uncommon to find notices of livers enlarged in every direction, with capsule tightened and distended ; while section of the structure discloses patches and streaks of dark brown, surrounded with tissue of a much lighter colour These are but modifications of the so-called *nutmeg* liver The dark patches are engorged hepatic veins, occupying the centre of the liver lobules, the lighter markings corresponding to the minute ramifications of the portal veins, the pallor probably in some cases owing its existence in part to minute vessels rendered empty by compression, to fatty material in cell-structures, or to increase in amount and alteration in character of the interconnective-tissue

b Causation.—These varied forms of hyperæmia, or congestion, owe their existence to very varied influences, chief of which are, previous pulmonary or cardiac disease, considerable and sudden chills, the advent of certain specific fevers, in which certain noxious materials exist in the blood, errors in dieting or faulty digestion, particularly where an excessive amount of certain rather stimulating foods is taken with less than the natural amount of exercise.

Over-exertion, particularly after a full meal, in plethoric animals, and in warm weather, I have noticed, is occasionally attended with this condition.

Symptoms—The symptoms indicative of either passive or active hyperæmia of the liver can scarcely be said to be pronounced or strictly diagnostic; with careful observation, however, we may often, if not absolutely certain of such, have well-grounded suspicions of its existence. Languor or dulness, probably the most constant, is frequently associated with a visible alteration and change in the membranes of mouth and eyes: a pasty condition and disagreeable smell connected with the former, and a blanched, dull, or icteric appearance of the latter.

There is rarely fever, temperature normal, unless associated with some zymotic disease, as influenza: these same relations largely affect and modify both the pulse and respirations. The appetite is usually impaired, with a rather confined state of the bowels.

In many there may be observed a little uneasiness, occasional turning of the head to the right side, which on being manipulated over the region of the liver produces pain. The extremities are usually cold. To these must be added the existence of disease of other viscera, as heart and lungs, when such are the direct inducing factors; and the frequently existing cause, excess of food to an animal retained unnaturally in an overheated stable, without exercise sufficient to carry off the effete materials and keep the animal machinery in healthy working order.

Hepatic Extravasations and Ruptures—As the result, immediate or more remote, of repeated attacks of congestive and inflammatory action affecting the liver-structure, or as the result of injury, we may not unfrequently, as post-mortem lesions, encounter blood-extravasations and ruptures, either con-

44—2

nected with intimate liver-structure or having their situation
immediately subjacent to the fibrous investing membrane

So long as these ruptures are not extensive, and particularly
so long as they are contained within the proper capsule of the
gland—the Glissonian covering—they are rarely fatal. Such
apoplexies, if not immediately terminating fatally, are exceedingly likely, from the relations and influences of the effused
material, to induce serious textural changes ultimately en-
dangering life

Their occurrence, when of an extensive or serious nature, is
indicated by collapse or sudden evidence of abdominal pain,
with marked alteration in the pulse and the appearance of the
visible mucous membranes. These suddenly appearing symptoms closely connected it may be with some sudden excitation
or disturbance in an animal previously in a plethoric condition,
and in which steady or recurring hepatic congestion has been
a distinct feature

When not extensive and of a serious character, extravasations
of blood, either beneath Glisson's capsule or into the true
hepatic structure, are not to be differentiated from ordinary
congestive attacks, save that their advent is occasionally marked
with symptoms rather more distinctly indicative of abdominal
pain.

Treatment of Hepatic Congestions—When we have reason to
believe that a condition of hyperæmia is being developed in a
manner gradual rather than sudden, the natural course is the
withdrawal of those conditions and influences likely to operate
in the production of the turgescence, lessening of the food-
supply, and allowing more exercise, with the exhibition of a
moderate dose of aloes, to be followed with the liberal use of
such salines as the sulphate of soda or magnesia; these latter
are taken often to a full amount readily enough in food or
drinking-water.

When the horse is otherwise robust, not suffering from some
previous disease, either cardiac or pulmonary, and with no
marked symptoms of syncope, and where the hepatic disturbance has been sudden and is marked by severity, the removal
of blood previous to the exhibition of the purge is indicated
With those cases, however, where the symptoms of involvement
of the liver are only complementary to the existence of some

epizootic fever, or where they appear intimately associated with or dependent on some other well-established visceral disease, the bleeding, and also the aloes, are better left unemployed, and our dependence to remove the congestion thrown entirely on other and less hazardous remedies

Following the employment for some days of these salines, I have often thought that benefit has resulted from alternating them with a moderate quantity of some mineral acid, as the nitro-muriatic; and where pain was unmistakably shown by pressure over the region of the liver, by the assiduous employment of warm-water applications.

CHAPTER XLVI

HEPATITIS—INFLAMMATION OF THE LIVER

Pathology. *a. Varieties of this Morbid Condition.*—Hepatitis, or inflammatory action connected with the liver, seems to occur in more forms than one, and to exhibit rather different textural results. Judging from the extensive alteration of tissue which we often observe in examinations of horses which have died from other affections, there seems little reason to doubt that during life hepatic inflammations of particular characters are not marked by a prominent exhibition of symptoms.

From these post-mortem examinations, and from comparing the structural changes which we observe with corresponding conditions of other organs, and what we know of the development of their morbid states, it seems tolerably certain that inflammatory action may develop itself in connection with two distinct situations, and probably of various degrees of intensity. (1) As inflammation of the investing and penetrating fibrous Glissonian membrane, (2) As inflammation of the true gland-structures throughout the organ.

1. *As Inflammation of an Acute and Circumscribed Character of the Fibrous Covering of the Liver*, we occasionally encounter the diseased action as a concomitant or sequel of pleuritic inflammations, the liver participating in these instances from the contiguity of structures; a similar condition may follow an attack of enteric disease or of peritonitis. From the

circumscribed patches of somewhat thickened and indurated tissue observed over the surface of the gland after death, and the patchy character of the adhesions, extensive and generally diffused inflammation does not appear to be of so common occurrence as circumscribed

This condition when affecting the horse I have not been able to differentiate from the congestive actions already noticed The existence of hepatic disturbance may be certain, to determine whether the gland is congested or superficially inflamed is in the greater number of cases not possible The history of the case may in some instances assist us

2 *Inflammation of the Component Gland-structure*—This form of inflammatory action we know of in the horse chiefly from after-death examination, its existence during life may have been suspected, but positive diagnosis is rendered exceedingly difficult from its intimate association with other diseased conditions more demonstrative and certainly diagnosed As a circumscribed diseased condition resulting in hepatic abscess, it is of much rarer occurrence in the horse than in some other animals In the form of numerous and extensively distributed small and isolated collections of purulent matter it is frequently observed in pyæmia, and particularly so in foals, in association with the very fatal arthritic disease so common in some districts and during certain seasons. Solitary abscesses are rare, small disseminated circumscribed collections of pus are numerous.

CHAPTER XLVII

CHRONIC DISEASES OF THE LIVER.

I. CIRRHOSIS OF THE LIVER

Nature and Anatomical Characters—This condition, which in its purest form may be regarded as a chronic or subacute inflammation of the interconnective hepatic tissue, tending to ulterior and more complex changes, is of more frequent occurrence than either of the forms of acute inflammatory action. In this we observe a peculiar, more or less distinctly granular state of the true hepatic structure, with a marked increase in

amount and density of the fibrous investing membrane which
envelops the gland, surrounding the hepatic vessels and accompanying them all through the hepatic structure. It is rarely
brought under our notice until the changes have made very
considerable advances, often not at all during life, or only when
certain inexplicable or ill-understood conditions and phenomena, associated with some other illness, have drawn attention
to the condition of the liver, which consists essentially in a
fibroid hypertrophy of the enveloping fibrous capsule, passing
also between the true cell-structures. These latter, in the
early stages, may seem swollen—a condition exhibited in
common with the interconnective-tissue, tending to give the
entire structure affected a perceptible increase in volume.
This, however, shortly disappears, the hepatic lobules, from
steady pressure and want of nutrition, gradually shrink, and
ultimately appear as dark-brown spots scattered amongst the
gradually increasing and indurating fibroid connective-tissue.

Over the surface of the organ the capsule assumes a tense,
sometimes almost cartilaginous, character, rough and somewhat
nodulated from the traction exercised upon it by the induration of the attached interconnective-tissue, the edges at
the same time losing their fine attenuation and becoming
rounded. From this extra development of fibroid tissue all
through the gland, very important and serious changes take
place in the vascular and other conduits. The portal and
hepatic vessels are encroached upon, and their lumen materially
altered. This constringing action in the former inducing inani-
tion, atrophy, and pallor, the obstructed portal vessels preventing a free circulation of the blood from the abdominal viscera,
resulting in impairment or stagnation of the blood-flow in the
abdominal veins, tends to prevent absorption, and favours the
accumulation of fluid in the peritoneal cavity.

By the excessive development of the fibroid tissue, the liver-
cells and lobules become much changed, some not at first
destroyed, and appearing as brown spots scattered amongst the
newly-formed tissue, ultimately lose their original character,
and seem to be taken possession of by fatty molecules, while
the minute bile-ducts, by the retention of the secretion, appear
as yellow markings, and give a somewhat jaundiced tinge to
the parts

Causes, etc —In the horse, the agents in operation to produce this fibroid hypertrophy, or chronic inflammation of the liver, are not well made out, any more than are the symptoms by which its existence may be diagnosed

Although I have found it present in aged animals which have succumbed to the last of several attacks of influenza, I cannot believe that, as a rule, its appearance bears any close relation to such fever, or we would hear more of it I am rather disposed to view it as largely dependent upon repeated attacks of congestive or inflammatory action, having a special geminative action on the interlobular connective-tissue, which, steadily proliferating and consolidating, tends by direct pressure to act upon both the vascular supply and the free discharge of bile The healthy condition of the secreting lobule-cell is at the same time interfered with alike by direct pressure as by interference with its source of nutrition

The hypothesis that the true causes are rather to be regarded as the existence of peculiar forms of anæmia, the result of a thoroughly defective and insufficient diet, are, though not contrary to certain experiences, less capable of explaining the state satisfactorily than the occurrence of the conditions just referred to Slow interstitial inflammatory action, extending into the liver-structure, resulting in exudation between the lobules, and by its organization and contraction pressing upon the component textures of the liver, is easily understood as operating in causing destruction of their nutrition

Many cases of anæmia with ascites, in young horses, which have proved fatal, have, on examination after death, shown well-marked cirrhosis of the liver, to which, as the most likely organic change, the abdominal dropsy and general anæmated condition seemed very closely linked But as these have been met with not only where the food-supply was undoubtedly deficient and of bad quality, but also where all this could not be said, the conclusion that the defective food-supply alone was the original factor scarcely seemed substantiated

Symptoms —These chiefly result from the interference with certain functions consequent upon particular textual alterations of hepatic structures 1 There are those which follow the arrest of the free circulation in the viscera of the abdomen consequent on the impeded liver-circulation, and the difficulties offered to the passage of the blood from the portal to the hepatic veins. 2 The entire class of phenomena traceable to disturbed or perverted liver-functions

The former are probably the more extensively distributed and the more important, the latter not always existing, or at least not to such an extent as to be regarded as diagnostic. Of the symptoms indicative of interference with the circulation in the abdominal organs, the most attractive is ascites, which is usually only the most extensive accumulation of fluid in the state of general dropsy.

Owing to this general congestion of the vascular system of the bowels, a state of irritability of the canal may be induced from the amount of fluid thrown upon the mucous membrane; or, in less numerous instances, gastric and intestinal hæmorrhage may be observed Digestion is irregular, and with the settled indications of this we have a state of steadily increasing marasmus, with or without fever, and probably indications of jaundice

In those instances in young horses where the chronic atrophy and contraction of the liver was linked with anæmia, there was noticed capricious appetite, with indigestion and rather unaccountable prostration and languor, in some a disposition to somnolency, a pasty state of the mouth, with rather sour smell, mucous membranes feebly icteric or pallid, marasmus rapid, thirst great, urine variable in amount, but in many of a yellowish colour In few which I have had the opportunity of carefully examining did the thermometer indicate much fever. In two there was an unnaturally dry, thin, and overgrown condition of the coat, with distension of the abdomen and distinct tenderness, on pressure, over the region of the liver

Treatment —It is probable that in all in which this textural change is fully developed—and rarely are any seen until this is the case—treatment is of little avail

When attempted, it is justifiable, with a correct scale of dietary, to make an effort to place the digestive system in as natural a condition as possible by mild laxatives This is to be maintained for some time by repeated exhibitions of soda and potash salts, as the sulphate of the former or the acid tartrate of the latter When the canal is in a fairly healthy condition, such tonics as ox-gall, or nitro-muriatic acid, may be tried. While, when pain over the right side is present, warm-water applications, followed by inunction of iodine ointment, are likely to benefit

The appearance of ascites must be met with the employment of tonic and diuretic medicines, or, when the quantity of fluid is excessive, it may be removed by tapping.

11. FATTY LIVER.

The term 'fatty liver' is often employed to include both the condition of simple fatty infiltration, and that of true fatty degeneration.

In a normal condition the hepatic cells contain a certain amount of oil. In the so-called fatty liver, however, the amount is materially increased, not temporarily, but constantly; this crowding with oil-globules displacing the natural contents, obscuring the nuclei, and impairing their natural activity. This occupation of the cells with fatty material, even when extensive, may not always produce increase of bulk in the liver, although it frequently does so. In appearance it is somewhat changed, being of a light fawn-colour, less clearly thinned at the edges; and when the condition is extensive and well-established, giving to it a rather greasy feeling, with an absence of toughness or resisting power. In specific gravity it may be less than normal, although more bulky, and is always, in this respect, distinctly lower than when affected with albuminoid changes

This condition of fatty change is said in man to be often associated with pulmonary phthisis and other organic changes, in the horse, with the exception of its existence where other fatty infiltrations and changes exist, it does not appear to be intimately related to any particular organic disease or specific fever

It is often enough encountered in animals which have for long periods been kept in a rather artificial and confined state, much pampered with nutritious and rather stimulating food, and which have been used for show or pleasure rather than work. In many horses so circumstanced, stabled in habitually overheated dwellings, fed highly, and only moderately exercised, it seems often associated with periodical attacks of hepatic congestion, and where the organ acquires considerable dimensions it seems largely operative in favouring extravasations and ruptures

Its existence, although not absolutely determined, may often be suspected from the defective manner in which the liver performs its functions, from the history of the animal, and from the recurrence of what are apparently congestive attacks. It is only likely to prove of serious moment when the invasion of the cell-structures with fatty material is such that their normal powers are considerably interfered with

The management of such instances of alteration of structure must proceed upon attempts to remove the causes which are most likely to operate in this abnormal development and deposition of fat. For this object it will be needful to enforce more natural conditions of dietary and location, with a somewhat more active life, and, if need be, by the exhibition of saline aperients

III. ALBUMINOID OR LARDACEOUS LIVER

This condition, known also as amyloid liver, often enough seen in making after-death examinations of the horse, although we may not be able with sufficient accuracy to distinguish the clinical phenomena which accompany it, and to differentiate these from other indications of structural change of the solid organs of the abdomen, may yet not be confounded in these examinations with the altered condition of the same parts just spoken of As in the state of fatty change, the viscus may or may not be enlarged, but when it is so, the enlargement may be distinguished from the increase in bulk of the fatty by its increased specific gravity The colour may not be so markedly different, but the consistence is distinctive. In this albuminoid change the gland possesses much resisting power, is not easily broken down, and when cut with a knife feels firm, while the cut surface is rather glistening and dry The adventitious material deposited, probably appears first around the minute radicles of the hepatic and portal vessels, encroaching upon the cell-elements of the lobules, amongst which, at first, they may still be distinguished Its true chemical characters are not well made out

This condition, although invading the whole or greater portion of the liver-structure, is not everywhere alike uniformly distributed. It may also in many instances be met with combined with fatty changes, and with cirrhosis. Its relations to other general and well-marked diseased conditions is in the horse apparently somewhat different from the human subject, where it is said to be a frequent attendant upon exhaustive and suppurative diseases of many structures. In our patients such is certainly not the case.

Although I have observed this diseased condition in young animals, and in those advanced in years, in none could I say that the clinical features were diagnostic. The most attractive phenomena were persistent disturbance of the functions connected with assimilation, a steady marasmus, and unmistakable declaration of ill-health without an appreciably sufficient cause. While it is also to be observed that in the development of the symptoms, as distinct from what are attendant upon cirrhosis, we rarely find in lardaceous liver the same interference with the portal circulation, and consequently a want of the disturbance in the circulation of the chylo-poietic viscera and the rather rare occurrence of abdominal dropsy, there is also an equally seldom occurrence of the icteric symptoms indicative of infringement of hepatic function, frequently enough seen in the state of chronic hepatic atrophy.

In cases when this peculiar structural change has taken possession of the liver we frequently observe alterations of an analogous character in the other solid organs of the abdomen, the spleen, and the kidneys, in this way adding to and complicating the phenomena attendant on the more extensive hepatic disorder.

IV. HYDATID TUMOURS OF THE LIVER

Cystoid or bladder worms, comparatively rare in the horse, are more frequently represented by the Ecchinococcus veterinorum, the cystic form of the Tænia ecchinococcus, than any other, while it is certain that the liver is more frequently their habitat than any other organ. More rarely they are met with in the kidney, the spleen, or the omentum, in the brain and in the lungs; in the latter situation they are not unfrequently found to have undergone calcification.

In the liver they occur as fibrous sacs enclosing a bladder or cyst of semitransparent elastic material of very variable size and form, within which, floating in a limpid colourless fluid, are numberless minute organisms, immature forms of the Tænia ecchinococcus In size these hydatid tumours vary from the bulk of a hazel-nut to that of an orange, or even larger, while their form is regulated according as they are maternal brood-cysts, secondary, or tertiary productions ; they appear to develop by a multilocular process, both endogenously and exogenously Even when encroaching considerably upon the structure of the liver, which they seem to do chiefly in virtue of their physical bulk, they do not appear to give rise to appreciable disturbance, and rarely is their presence even suspected during life.

That in certain conditions they might prove dangerous is easy to be understood , that they rarely do so is tolerably well established , while we are aware that many of them become abortive, and are found on death filled with a pasty sabulous-looking material, which may have caused the death of the organisms, or have resulted from their arrested vitality.

V Other Changes and Accumulations of Morbid Products in the Liver.

In addition to these retrogressive and destructive changes noticed we occasionally encounter others which are only probably less important and less serious because less commonly occurring. *Pigmentary* changes, *cancerous* and *lymphoid* growths, are to us exceedingly interesting, if only as post-mortem curiosities. The usual form which cancer assumes in the liver of the horse is that of nodules or irregular masses, in consistence between scirrhus and encephaloid; while on appearing on the surface of the organ these growths are disposed to flatten and spread out. The liver itself in such invasions is considerably enlarged and somewhat altered in shape. In conjunction with these growths there is often evidence that accompanying them at some stage of their development, probably on appearing at the surface of the organ, more or less inflammatory action has existed, affecting the covering of the organ and contiguous textures.

In growth and stability these malignant products exhibit great varieties , the softer being disposed to increase with greater rapidity, while the others are more apt to take on retrogressive changes. *Melanotic growths* or deposits seem rather disposed to assume the infiltrated form than that of out-growths; they occasionally occupy a large extent of liver-structure, or they may be scattered in circumscribed patches throughout the gland. *Lymphoid tumours* when appearing are usually numerous, distributed irregularly through the organ, of a smooth, nodulated character and variable size, some of which appear ensheathed in a distinct capsule, and of varying consistence.

The existence of these, although occasionally suspected during life, the suspicion being verified by examination after death, are still, in our present state of knowledge, not sufficiently indicated while developing by either general symptoms or physical signs to enable us to differentiate them. The two latter conditions are probably more within the limits of our diagnostic skill, seeing that with the symptoms of general disturbance, confirmed ill-health, and steady marasmus, unaccounted for by certainly existing and sufficiently enduring factors, may yet in some instances have obscure indications of varying character pointing in the direction of the probable existence of such textural changes.

CHAPTER XLVIII

JAUNDICE—ICTERUS—THE YELLOWS.

ALTHOUGH the condition recognised by these terms can scarcely with propriety be regarded as more than an indication or symptom, still, as it so often occurs without our being able to assign a definite cause for its appearance, or indicate specific textural or organic changes as alone connected with its development, we are content in the meantime to allow it a distinct existence as a substantive disease.

Definition —*It may be regarded as an abnormal condition occurring suddenly, or developing gradually, with or without pyrexia, accompanied with considerable functional disturbance, in which numerous solids and fluids of the animal body acquire a distinct yellow or saffron colour.*

Nature and Causation—Usually grouped with, and regarded

as more properly a disease of the liver, it is certainly known to
occur in connection with structural changes of other organs,.
and unassociated with obvious hepatic alterations

In the exercise of our profession, as practitioners of animal
medicine, we know that the horse is probably less a sufferer
from this affection than other of our patients. While it is
extremely probable that the more frequent exhibitions of this
affection in him, and those, too, which are the most evanescent,
appear as symptoms merely of certain general and febrile disorders, in which we have long and generally been disposed to
link their occurrence with hepatic disturbance. Of the truth
of this, post-mortem examination has often satisfied us ; similar
examinations have also assured us that these icteric symptoms,
in their most severe forms of development, have often been
associated with extensive structural changes of the gland

To account for the phenomena of jaundice, as observed in
association with varying changes and disturbances occurring in
the liver, several hypotheses have been started , the mere fact
of the existence of these indicating that our knowledge of
hepatic function is neither so full nor so exact as we could wish,
nor as we may yet expect it to be, as also the great probability
that the assemblage of symptoms with which we are now dealing may be but the natural expression of several somewhat
dissimilar conditions

Without entering particularly into the consideration of all
the theories propounded to account for the exhibition of the
characteristic symptoms of jaundice, it may be stated that of
these, the most generally accepted by those who are competent
to adjudicate in these matters are—(1) That its appearance is
attributable to the non-elaboration or true hepatic manufacture
of the peculiar liver-secretion bile, the so-called *suppression
theory* , and (2) That it may be attributed rather to the perversion or arrest of its natural outpouring after being manufactured,.
the so-called *absorption theory*.

By the first of these it is sought to be demonstrated that the
arrest of the biliary function preventing the removal from the
blood of certain materials, chiefly cholesterine and bile colouring matters, these are thrown back upon the circulation, this
hæmal impregnation ultimately staining all the tissues which
derive their sustentation from the blood

This condition is probably largely operative in many serious alterations of the liver-structure and in certain specific blood-changes: in the one, the minute secretory elements are at fault; in the other, the material presented to them is not in a condition favourable to carry on the normal exchanges

By the second, the bile, although properly formed, is shown to be unable to reach its natural destination, the alimentary canal, and is in part reabsorbed into the blood from which it. originally came, in this way contaminating it somewhat similarly to the first form.

Regarding the appearance of jaundice as presenting itself to us in the horse, it seems certain that, although it may not unfrequently be seen as associated with some peculiar blood disturbances and diseases of other viscera, that still its most frequent exhibitions and most persistent and serious invasions are as concomitants to disturbance and disease of the liver

It is probably more frequently as connected with disturbed function or actual tissue-change of the liver that jaundice is presented for our consideration, being often present in cases of disturbed circulation, as congestion and varied forms of hepatic inflammation, also in the more serious alterations of structure or adventitious depositions or growths. That it may sometimes be found in alliance with catarrhal states of the bile-ducts, or obstruction to their free discharge of bile, caused by morbid growths and parasitic invasion, is probably true; while its association with hæmal impurities, the result of specific fever, is not improbable.

In treatment it is often of advantage to be able to determine whether this condition, when undoubtedly developed as an accompaniment of hepatic disturbance, is the result of non-elaboration of bile, or of its reabsorption after elaboration. These points have been attempted to be determined by chemical tests. The one ordinarily employed, known as Pettenkofer's, depending upon the manner in which the bile acids comport themselves when strong sulphuric acid is added to urine having a moderate amount of cane-sugar mixed with it, is rather crude and not to be depended upon, seeing there are many conditions operating to modify largely this mode of applying the test.

To be carried out with any degree of certainty the bile acids

require, by a complicated process, to be first separated from
the urine before being acted upon   Notwithstanding this
serious defect, it is, when taken along with other indications, of
a certain amount of value in forming an opinion as to the
origin of the icteric condition

Symptoms—The great diagnostic symptoms of this state are
—(1) The yellow or saffron colour of the several solids and
fluids of the body , (2) The absence of bile in the discharges
from the bowels   The change of colour is very early observed
in the urine, and the visible mucous membranes of the mouth
and eyes, the former having a distinct pasty feeling, and
frequently a disagreeable smell , the urine from these cases,
when treated with strong nitric acid, gives in many, not in all,
a rather pretty iridescent play of colours   From the absence of
bile in the bowel the material voided is drier than natural, of
a light clay colour, and possessed of a peculiarly offensive
odour

In many developments of simple jaundice unassociated with
fever, or other general disturbance, the horse at first shows few
symptoms which may be regarded as unnatural ; there may
be neither pyrexia nor pain, and the pulse will remain long
unaffected, while the appetite may even be good   In those
instances which follow general and febrile disorders there is
usually much constitutional disturbance, marked by elevation
of temperature, and a renewal of the symptoms of the previously
existing disease   When anorexia is a prominent feature there
is, accompanying this, much lassitude and exhaustion, the
animal being spiritless and disinclined to move   In some,
particularly where the disturbance has reached its height, we
may notice a dry scurfy and itchy state of the skin   Even when
these symptoms are well marked and cardiac implication is
manifest, it is rarely, if ever, that we observe in the horse those
very obvious toxic symptoms so conspicuous in man   These
latter are supposed to be owing to the circulation in the blood
either of bile acids, or products resulting from their decomposition, or to some deleterious substance formed in the hepatic
cells, or other products of tissue-change which are undergoing
further alteration previous to their removal from the body by
the kidneys, but which, from the absence of bile, are arrested
in their metamorphosis, and accumulating in the blood, act as

45

poisons. In occasional instances irritability of the bowels exists, and defective movement of the right fore-limb. When these serious symptoms continue unrelieved other organs may become involved, and death result from the addition of such to already existing serious anæmia and exhaustion.

Treatment.—This must in great part be regulated by a consideration of the conditions upon which the assemblage of symptoms, known by the term of jaundice, depend. If these can be discovered, an attempt must be made for their removal; when not possible of immediate removal their untoward results, or the complications which attend them, must be carefully watched and combated, while no endeavour is to be neglected which may promote the general health and special tonic efficiency.

In many of the developments of those symptoms connected with specific fevers, or when not of a severe character and unassociated with any appreciable cause, the abnormal conditions being frequently of an evanescent character, with a disposition on the part of the animal functions to return to their normal conditions, little or no treatment save light diet will be requisite.

When we have reason to suspect congestion and disturbed hepatic action, the use of such agents as are believed to favour the emptying of the canal, and afterwards of those which seem to stimulate the formation of bile or favour its discharge, are indicated. The chief of these are aloes, aloes with moderate quantities of calomel or rhubarb, sulphates of soda and magnesia, or muriatic or nitro-muriatic acid, given alone or alternated with these salines. Many cases will be found to do better with a moderate laxative first, the bowels being afterwards kept soluble with the soda or magnesian sulphate. While, when exhaustion and want of tone are marked, the mineral acid may be used alone or combined with some preparation of quinine.

In many, where weakness is extreme and following particular fevers, I have found good to follow the free use of inspissated ox-bile, given in bolus twice daily, with moderate doses of aromatic spirits of ammonia between. Much of our success in every case will depend on the proper adaptation of the remedies to immediately inducing causes.

CHAPTER XLIX.

DISEASES OF THE SPLEEN

THIS organ, although of considerable bulk and largely supplied with blood, is not when diseased marked by symptoms particularly attractive either in the horse or other of our patients.

This may not be attributed altogether to the rarity of disturbance or textural change, but probably more to the fact that in whatever manner operating in determining the quantity or quality of the blood supplied to other organs, its derangement and change does not appear to be largely productive of phenomena attractive either by their severity or diffusion; it being well known that horses, as well as other animals, will continue to work for years with spleens wonderfully changed and enormously enlarged.

Of the entire diseased conditions affecting this organ we are informed less by any well-ascertained and well-connected clinical history than by the revelations of after-death examinations. That primary and active congestive and inflammatory actions do occur we may believe. Apart, however, from the existence of such in connection with certain manifestations of anthrax, we are probably not able to identify or differentiate these from several somewhat similar conditions of other abdominal organs. Neither are we able to distinguish those secondary congestions and inflammations which we feel tolerably certain take place as the result of embolism and the existence of hæmorrhagic infracts in the organ, the result of the lodgment in the splenic vessels of particles of matter detached from continued abscesses, sloughing sores, or particular forms of structural change of the cardiac valves.

When general congestive and inflammatory changes have occurred, the entire organ or the greater part of it suffers augmentation in bulk, darkening in colour, and loss of cohesion. In the cases of partial plugging of vessels and limited vascular disturbances, which most probably occur during the progress of such diseased conditions as cancer, lymphadenoma, etc., we have circumscribed inflammatory areas extending for a short distance around the infracts and abnormal growths or depositions   Occasionally these centres undergo change, and small or large abscesses occur

Enlargement of the Spleen —In the horse, in this country, true hypertrophy of the spleen apart from the existence of un-natural growth or deposition, is a rather rare condition , as the result of the presence of certain adventitious materials in con-nection with excessive development of pre-existing tissues it is rather common   Particularly well-marked forms of over-growth or enlargement, not of true hypertrophy, are seen in the local manifestations of what are probably general diseased conditions—lymphadenoma and melanosis   The probability that these are only parts of a general diseased condition seems strengthened when we know that similar growths or deposits are found in other organs, as the lungs, the liver, the kidneys, and the lymph-glands

Of both these conditions the pathology, as far as their origin is concerned, is doubtful, it being yet undetermined whether we are to regard them as a general vitiation of the system or as proceeding from a local centre to systemic contamination   In many instances they would seem to start in particular organs, and thence spread to others   Their existence is probably more largely encountered in the old than the young

Of **Lymphadenoma**, when producing enlargement of the spleen or any other organ, its physical characters are not those of a uniform infiltration or diffusion through the organ, but rather of a collection of the particular growth in more or less well-defined rounded masses, some of which appear distinctly encapsuled, giving to the external surface a nodulated appear-ance.

These masses vary in size from a hazel-nut to that of an orange, are of a greyish-white colour and firm consistence, although in this latter character they are variable   Examined more carefully these products or new material seem to differ from cancer, tubercle, and amyloid infiltration, having physical, histological, and clinical features peculiarly their own   They are probably to be regarded rather as hypertrophy of the par-ticular gland-structure with an increase of lymphoid elements

In their origin it is difficult to tell whether the lymph-glands are first diseased, and from them the infective material is conveyed by the lymph-stream to the spleen , or if the disturbance of nutrition is coincident, generally diffused, and appears in these different situations simultaneously, or nearly so. Judging from what we know of the rather numerous exhibitions of this disease in the spleen, it appears to be somewhat slow in development, and to go on for years before producing serious results. As a concomitant of this change of splenic structure, leucocythæmia—white-celled blood—has been said to have been regularly observed; this, however, can only be regarded as true in a limited number of cases, seeing that lymphoid growths have been encountered in the spleen without this peculiar hæmal alteration, as also that this blood-change appears apart from the existence of internal lymphoid tumours.

The symptoms of this enlargement and unnatural condition of the spleen are, as a rule, occult, and with the existence of other abnormal and malignant growths in the same organ, of a negative character. When operating prejudicially, either from their extent in the spleen or their dissemination in other parts, anæmia, irregularly or steadily developed, is probably the earliest and most attractive feature; with this we have blanched membranes, particularly a pale sclerotic, feeble pulse, irregular but rather elevated temperature, capricious appetite; and in two cases which were rather characteristic, there was noted a distinct amount of follicular change of the membrane of the fauces and tonsil cavities, a continued discharge from the mouth of a somewhat frothy and very tenacious saliva, and steady marasmus, with abatement of strength and vigour.

Cancer, Melanosis, and Lardaceous Infiltration.—That these abnormal conditions occur in connection with the spleen, we are aware chiefly by after-death examination. Occasionally, by some visible demonstration of diseased conditions and the co-existence of particular symptoms, a fortunate prediction of their existence may be made. There are, however, no symptoms sufficiently diagnostic by which we may satisfy ourselves of their existence, specially in the spleen, during life; there is nothing in the physical examination to assist us, and only occasionally are the constitutional indications of such a nature as to concentrate attention on the spleen and satisfy us that textural changes of an important character are taking place there.

CHAPTER L

DISEASES CONNECTED WITH THE KIDNEYS AND THEIR FUNCTIONS.

GENERAL CONSIDERATIONS

IN considering even very cursorily the affections of the kidneys, whether manifested by simple disturbance of their normal functions, or partaking of the more serious condition of textural change, it is neither correct nor safe to do so apart from a regard to the condition or character of their peculiar secretion, the urine

This, although in all instances possessed of much similarity, and the secretion of one animal being, to a certain extent, typical of the same secretion in others, is rarely in any individual instance an exact counterpart of its composition at any other period even in the same animal.

Although we are even yet in the dark regarding many agencies and influences which determine the state of this secretion, and of the modes through which changes are produced, we yet know enough to teach us that neither in health nor yet in disease is the urinary secretion at all times, either in similar animals or individual specimens, of uniform amount or character. In health, every change and exchange, vital or purely chemical, occurring in the body influences both the composition and dynamic relations of the blood, and in this way largely determines both the amount and quality of the material eliminated by the kidneys In disease of the intimate structure of these glands, we encounter material alterations in their secretion; but probably these alterations are as extensively and perfectly marked when the textural lesions are not in the kidney, but referable to primary hæmal contamination, or to elementary changes in some other tissue or organ of the body, the results of such changes, in the form of disintegrated plasmic material, finding admission into the blood, and loading or altering it in various ways

Knowing that such changes and alterations of the several activities are ever taking place, and that such disturbances or variations in these exchanges may be perfectly consistent with

health, we must of necessity, in regarding the state of the
urine as an index of disease, allow to it a considerable range or
scope, both as to quantity voided over a determinate period, and
the relative amount of the several materials. Above or below
these points, we may agree to view it as indicative of conditions apart from health.

Without minutely entering into the chemistry of the urine,
as evidenced apart from or even in connection with disease,
we may regard it as exhibiting, in over ninety per cent. of
water, a solution or mixture variously arranged of a rather
important and complex nitrogenous compound, urea: two
acids, uric and hippuric, a considerable amount of inorganic
salts, several organic substances of a nature rather ill understood, known as extractive matter, and certain colouring principles.

These materials represent the various exchanges, or rather
results of the various exchanges, taking place between certain
tissues or elements of the body, and varying extrinsic agents,
together with the regular removal of particular elements which
have served their purpose, or which have been developed in
the course of the activities taking place.

Conditions which Modify the Urinary Secretion—From what
we know of the structure and action of the kidneys, we can
easily understand that any disturbance in the blood-flow
through the capillaries of the malpighian tufts, its increase or
diminution in any given time, as well as any alteration in that
fluid which renders its liquid parts more or less likely to pass
readily through animal membranes, or which confer upon it a
greater solvent power upon materials wherever placed, and
which require removal through the kidneys, must largely
modify the amount and quality of the secretion.

This condition of the blood-channels and quality of their
contents is largely influenced by conditions other than changes
situated in the glands themselves. Such disturbing influences
we observe ever at work in many general congestions originating from apparently extrinsic influences, or through the
development of indwelling morbific agencies. Such are
exemplified in sudden chills or lowering of the surface-tem-
peratures, with disturbance of the circulation in many large
and vascular organs, and as attendant upon hæmal vitiation,

the accompaniment of common and specific fevers   It is
highly probable that both these states, pyrexial accessions and
a toxic condition of the blood, are intimately associated with
phenomena much similar, the degraded or changing plasmic
material in both instances finding its way into the blood.

Wherever we encounter changed germinal matter which
ought to be removed from the system unduly retained, we find
a distinct tendency to systemic disturbance, the result probably more of loading the blood with hurtful material than of
any evil effects which such may exert directly on or through
the nervous system.   This latter, which may exhibit aberrations in pyrexial onsets, is often largely influenced, like other
tissues, through the universal pabulum, the blood   This
changed germinal matter, in whatever form separated, or however broken up on entering the blood, acts with particular
force on the capillary system of those organs by which it
ought naturally to be eliminated ; amongst these the kidneys
hold a prominent place

**Nature of Information to be Gained by Observing the Urinary
Secretion.**—Seeing that in health so many circumstances and
changes alter the character of this secretion, it is very difficult
accurately to determine what ought to be styled diseased as
distinct from normal—how much we should place to some
peculiarity or variation in physiological action which can
scarcely be termed diseased, and how much belongs to processes truly morbid.

The functions of digestion, respiration, and circulation all
materially affect the production in amount and quality of the
matter thrown off by the kidneys, while the state of the secretion of the skin in particular, as also of the liver, if not so
directly connected with the production, are not less closely
related to and influence the quality or character of the
secretion.

Besides deviations from normal character in the kidneys
themselves, and in the extensive mucous tract of the rather
complicated urinary passage, we are aware that many disturbances and changes in distant parts of the body have an intimate connection with the character of the urinary secretion.
By a careful examination of the urine, chemically and opti-
cally, we may not unfrequently be able to diagnose particular

local changes occurring in the kidney or at different parts of the mucous membrane of the urinary tract, while by the exercise of the same means, if not able certainly to determine the existence of disease of other and distant organs, we often find much assistance in forming our opinions and in directing our attention to situations and conditions of disease which otherwise we might not observe

CHAPTER LI

OF CERTAIN ABNORMAL CONDITIONS OF THE URINE

WITHOUT doing violence to the subject, and as likely to include nearly all those abnormal conditions of the urine we may encounter in our particular patient, we shall here regard the unnatural state of the secretion under three considerable groups or varieties   (1) *Characters given to the secretion through excess or deficiency, beyond moderation, of the normal constituents*, (2) *Characters imparted by matters in solution not usually present in health*, (3) *The existence of certain morbid urinary deposits.*

1 **Characters given to the Secretion through Excess or Deficiency of Normal Elements**   *a   Excess of   Water*—Of this unnatural condition we have frequent examples in the horse, notably in the disease recognised by the terms 'Diabetes Insipidus,' or 'Hydruria,' and in other states which, as they do not reach the same extent of discharge of watery urine, have not been dignified with any distinctive appellation

In all these cases of excess of water, although the entire bulk of the urine is largely increased, there may be no very appreciable augmentation of the solid materials of the secretion, no doubt in some, such augmentation does exist, particularly during the earlier stages of the increased secretion   We know that excess of water is favourable to the removal of the products of tissue-waste, as also that with such sudden increase and outpouring of water from the malpighian capillaries, by washing out the uriniferous tubes, there is augmentation for the time of the solid matters in the urine   Usually, however, although we have obvious increase of the water, the solids of the discharge over a complete period of twenty-four hours are not perceptibly augmented.

The greater number of such cases of hydruria in the horse are intimately associated with disturbed digestion and assimilation, with perverted gastric and intestinal function, and more rarely with skin disease; they are attended with great thirst and ingestion of large quantities of liquids. The occurrence of dyspepsia of this form, complicated with increase of the urinary secretion, may in a great proportion of cases be traced to improper food or contaminated drinking-water. Fodder of any kind which has been damaged by exposure to excess of moisture, or otherwise deteriorated by the development in it of certain vegetable organisms, or oats which have, by certain chemical processes, been somewhat bleached or whitened, are very fruitful causes of this unnatural condition of the urine.

b. Deficiency of Water is, when occurring, probably not associated with increase of solids as a whole, or in excess over a definite period, but usually with a distinct increase of these in a given amount of the liquid ; we observe this condition in horses doing rapid and severe work, entailing considerable cutaneous transpiration, and the consumption of much nitrogenized food. Such cases are usually marked by an increase of urea. When the quantity of urine secreted is much diminished, without an obvious means of accounting for the decrease either of water or solid matters, there is reason to fear impairment of secretory power from elementary disease of the kidneys.

c. Excess of Urea. —This, the complex, highly nitrogenized material of urine, believed to be largely dependent for its existence on the changes or disintegration of nitrogenous tissues, and regarded as the medium or combination by which they are removed from the animal body, appears also to be largely influenced as respects the amount present in the urine by the character of the food taken into the body, and the relative amount of other activities taking place. It seems probable that, although part is formed in the blood, a larger amount is the result of changes taking place in the kidneys. With horses enjoying good health, a liberal and rather highly nitrogenized dietary, and in which large quantities of moisture are thrown off by the skin, the urine will be found rich in urea.

In diseases of an acute febrile character it has been found in excess, and has in these instances been ascribed to a process of rapid or excessive oxidation intimately related to heat-production and the pyrexial state. It is, however, highly probable that the elevation of body-temperature, so prominent a feature in fevers, may be accounted for in other ways than as the result of activity of the oxidizing process, while it seems certain that in horses, at least, excess of urea in the urine does occur in conditions rather the opposite of hyperoxidation. In those animals we meet with this condition when after liberal dieting, particularly with albuminous substances and a full amount of work or exercise, there follows a period of enforced idleness

These cases are not, as in man, of gradual development, but rather of sudden occurrence, unattended with premonitory symptoms, and the condition of excess of urea in the secretion is associated with marked alteration of its colour.

The rapid and remarkable changes which occur in the exchanges amongst the various tissues and elements, and the chemistry of these disturbed activities, is ill-understood and requires investigation. The peculiar and extreme nervous disturbance, uræmic poisoning—or uræmia as this condition of the retention or entrance into the blood of excrementitious material is sometimes called—and which so often attends or follows upon certain cases marked by excess of urea in the urine, at one time believed to be due to the conversion of the retained urea into carbonate of ammonia, is probably dependent upon other conditions altogether. It is more likely to follow not the retention in the blood of one material, but many, the result of the breaking up of nitrogenous compounds which, in the processes of the natural exchanges, ought to have been eliminated by the kidneys

It is apparently the result of a disturbance of many changes which are ever occurring in the blood, the proper execution of which is essential to normal nutrition, particularly of nerve-tissue. That there are numerous and different changes always occurring we know from their action and results, but how produced we do not as yet understand.

d Excess of Colouring Matter—The varying shades of colour which occur in urine in disease are probably due to more than one matter; nor are these always the same, nor present in similar proportions. Although not in possession of information sufficiently definite to determine the causes of the change of colour, nor the substances which produce it, or their modes of formation, there is yet evidence enough to satisfy us that the ultimate source of this colouring matter is the blood; and that probably the amount of the chief colouring principle met with—uræmatine—is a not incorrect indication of the amount of change which the blood-globules are undergoing

·We find that in some inflammatory actions, and in certain febrile disorders, as also in special diseases of the liver, this pigment is much increased   From experiments which have been made by Kuhne, it would seem that in the course of the complicated relations which subsist between the liver and the kidneys, there is in the disturbance of the functions of the former a passing of bile acids or products into the blood; that these, acting upon changing blood-corpuscles, convert their colouring matter into a special pigment which escapes by the urine   While of blood-pigment itself, independent of and apart from the blood-globules, we have no doubt that such may be found unchanged in the urine, having passed off from changed blood-corpuscles with the water from the kidneys, or the formed materials may themselves have passed through their vessels, and ultimately undergone disintegration and separation of their colouring matter in the renal tubes

These two latter conditions and causes of colouring of the urine are quite distinct from colouring by either bile or blood-corpuscles themselves

e. Alteration of the other Organic Compounds, the Acid Constituents and Extractive Matters—Both the quantities of the complex animal matters known as extractive, and the special acid, free or combined, of the horse's urine—hippuric —are in disturbed conditions of the system, and in special organic changes, liable to be increased or diminished in amount. Although it is probably quite true that hippuric acid is largely indebted for its formation to the character of the food taken, it seems yet doubtful whether it owes its entire existence to this source, or is not largely manufactured in the liver from the glycocol formed there   Chemical changes occurring amongst the tissues and elements of the body have probably more influence in determining its production than variations of food.

Alterations as respects the matter of these compounds, although not ascertainable by the observation of physical characters, or the employment of physical tests, are yet capable of being determined by appropriate chemical processes Density, as indicated by the urinometer, a most unsatisfactory datum upon which to found any conclusion respecting the character of urine, or the changes which it indicates, tells us nothing The acidity, usually feeble, may be determined to a certain extent, both as to existence and character of stability or otherwise, by litmus-paper and its after-treatment by heat , however, even from its state of perfect solubility, hippuric acid may be separated and demonstrated

f. Excess or Deficiency of the Inorganic Constituents —
Although in the examination of urine as an index of disease much more attention has been given to the consideration of the condition and relative proportions of the constituent organic matters referred to, it seems quite certain that with a greater amount of attention we will find the amount, relative proportion, and combinations of the inorganic constituents not less important and deserving of attention

Of the entire amount of the inorganic materials of the horse's urine, the greater part consists of salts of the alkalies and alkaline earths, chief of which are carbonates, with a small amount of chlorides and sulphates

Considerable variations in the amount of these inorganic compounds as a whole, as also in their relative proportions, are of regular occurrence , this variation depending as much probably on excessive or impeded metamorphosis and disturbance of the normal interchanges occurring in the animal body, as on the amount and character of the food received.

In some constitutional diseases developed in connection with particular localities and under certain dietetic conditions, there seems, from what little we presently know, a distinct change both in amount and relative proportion of several of these inorganic salts. Also in several acute sporadic diseases of an inflammatory type the varying quantities of several of these discoverable in the urine, during particular stages of the disease, is extremely interesting and highly suggestive During disease some of the constituents continue to be thrown off in increased amount , others probably are retained during the progress of certain changes, to be eliminated in greater quantities when such changes are accomplished

2 Substances Present in Solution in Urine not found in Health —In addition to urine in disease holding in solution a greater than normal proportion of its ordinary constituents, we find that certain substances of an accidental and foreign character may also be present

These matters, being soluble, are not detected through their physical appearances or characters, although features possessed by the secretion as a whole may lead us to a chemical examination, by which alone they may be demonstrated   .

Some of these unnatural but soluble materials are occasionally accompanied with matter which, after being discharged with the urine, is deposited, and by its physical or other characters leads us to suspect the existence of some usually accompanying morbid but soluble substance   The chief of those we encounter are *albumen* and *bile constituents*, with probably, in very rare instances, *sugar*

a *Urine containing Albumen* —This condition, known as albuminuria, may in the horse, as in man, exist without the physical character of the secretion being particularly attractive or distinctly diagnostic   In some cases our attention may be directed to make a special examination of the secretion from particular physical appearances presented It may be dark-coloured from mingled blood or blood pigment ; it may be of rather high specific gravity , or there may be present in the deposit thread-like fibrinous elements, probably the result of fibrinogenous material moulded to this form in the uriniferous tubes

As the real pathognomonic importance of the condition consists in the certainty whether albumen exists in solution or not, the determination of this must be carried out by appropriate chemical tests

Those of heat and nitric acid, properly manipulated and conducted with a knowledge of certain eventualities or possibilities, are generally what are relied upon

The existence of albumen in appreciable amount in urine for any length of time, and steadily continuous, cannot be regarded as aught but a serious indication

It may occur from temporary or permanent disturbance, from alterations in the secreting power of the structures of

the kidneys, from congestion and inflammation of the renal
capillaries, from alteration and contamination of the blood
supplied to these structures, and from some other conditions

The gravity of the condition of the discharge of urine containing albumen must of course always be subject to modifications depending upon the cause which appears to operate in
determining those conditions favourable to this state   A
temporary appearance of this material, due to some obvious
irritation inducing hyperæmia and probably active transudation
of blood, being a somewhat different condition to a continued
albuminous discharge, directly the result of textual change
in the renal secreting structures.   In addition it ought not to
be forgotten that in recoveries from many active inflammatory affections, and from some common and specific fevers,
the existence of albumen in the urine is probably less connected with kidney disease than, as we have said, hæmal
contamination.   We are aware that in all these states considerable changes take place in the colloid elements of the
blood, and that materials held in solution in the serum tend
to be eliminated by the kidneys, while at such times a
special aptitude on the part of the blood-fluid to pass through
the containing vessels is not an uncommon feature

  b Urine containing Bile Compounds —The existence in
peculiar states of the system of certain bile compounds, acids,
or simple colouring matter is generally admitted to be
ordinarily evidenced by the more or less yellow or yellowish-
green colour imparted to the secretion   The presence of
these biliary matters in urine is generally held to be
established by the employment of a little nitric acid, which,
when dropped on a white porcelain surface thinly covered by
urine, or added to a little of the secretion in a test-tube to
which heat is afterwards applied, is followed by an iridescent
play of colours.

  The clinical importance of this abnormal constituent is
chiefly in relation to the disease known as jaundice   As to
the manner of its access to the urinary secretion, its mode
of production in relation to either the blood or the urine,
or its significance in connection with hepatic disease, and the
relation of these to jaundice, there is still much uncertainty.
In a general sense, however, the existence of bile compounds

in the urine may be regarded as symptomatic of jaundice, and intimately associated with hepatic disturbance or change

c Urine containing Sugar, the Condition known as Mellituria Glycosuria, or Diabetes Mellitus—Although in the horse, as in other animals, a large proportion of glycogenic material exists and is formed in the liver, and in the course of the normal activities finds its way in some form into the blood, the existence of sugar in the urine, whether the result of increase in the sugar-formative power in the system, or proceeding from diminution in the activity of reduction, is, in the horse, an occurrence of extreme rarity   The only instance in which I am conscious of having encountered such an abnormal condition of the urinary discharge over a long period of observation, was in association with cerebral disturbance   The certainty of its existence may only be determined by appropriate chemical tests.

Besides these abnormal constituents of urine, we have also several other organic materials, which, in addition to being more easily and certainly detected, are not less useful as indices of textural changes occurring chiefly in some part of the extensive efferent urinary channel, viz :

3. **The Existence of Morbid Urinary Deposits.**—The chief of those conditions, usually spoken of under this term from the fact that although suspended in the liquid, the morbid materials are disposed on its settling, when collected in any convenient vessel, to fall to the bottom, are *blood, pus,* and *mucus*

a Blood in the Urine—Hæmaturia may appear in very varied forms, and be indicative of very varied conditions.   It may appear as bright fluid blood, intimately mixed with the urine, or observed immediately succeeding its discharge, or it may evidence its existence by the presence of a brown or dark-coloured deposit, consisting of blood-corpuscles, existing in entirety or undergoing change.   These characters of the urine and its modes of discharge, although not in every case indicating with certainty the seat or nature of the hæmorrhage, are yet of importance in assisting us in forming an opinion and giving a prognosis of the case   When from the kidney, it is usually uniformly mixed with the urine and discharged with it.   There may also, in such instances, be mingled with the blood fibrinous casts of the small uriniferous tubes of the glands or of the great conduits, the ureters. However, the chief points of difference usually observable are not invariably sufficiently diagnostic of the exact seat of the hæmorrhage

The causes of hæmaturia are in the horse largely mechanical, the result of injury received either by direct violence inflicted in the region of the kidney, or following over-exertion or excessive work. It may accompany structural change of the gland, irritation set up by calculi either in the kidney or some other part of the urinary passage, or it may only exhibit itself as a symptom of a general or constitutional disturbance or disease. Regarded as a symptom, hæmaturia may thus be indicative of several very different conditions in which disturbance of normal functions or more serious structural changes are the cause of this alteration in the character of the urine

b Urine Containing Pus and Mucus —Both of these organic substances are met with in the urine of the horse in larger quantities than is imagined. In health the latter material is a common constituent, while the former, even where no disease is suspected, is not uncommon. To urine, after being allowed to settle in some convenient vessel, mucus gives a slightly flocculent but transparent cloud, while pus, settling at the bottom of the vessel, gives an opaque yellowish deposit, liable to be disturbed on slight movement. Both these conditions are determined by microscopic and chemical examination. Although clinically interesting, neither are such serious conditions as some others which we have noticed. It is highly probable that both conditions, particularly the presence of pus, are more common in the female than the male : and although the existence of pus in large quantities is to be regarded with suspicion, and the case watched with care, its presence may be unassociated with much obvious structural change.

Thus it is that, like the discharge of blood with the urine, pus may continue to exist without our being able certainly to determine whether the formed elements of the secretion are passing off from the mucous membrane by some particular change, or are shed steadily from a raw and abraded surface, or the cavity of an abscess.

46

CHAPTER LII

CONGESTIVE AND INFLAMMATORY AFFECTIONS OF THE KIDNEYS

I. RENAL CONGESTION.

Nature and Causation — Hyperæmia or excess of blood in the renal structures, whether of an acute or passive character, is,´like inflammatory action in the same organ, not a common occurrence in the horse When appearing, it is the result of somewhat varying conditions and operating agencies, chief of which are probably—(1) The immediate or previous existence of some common or specific fever; (2) The effect of the ingestion or entrance into the system of some particular irritant, as cantharides or terebinthinate compounds; (3) The action of cold and damp applied to the external surface of the body, causing retrocession of blood upon internal organs; (4) Following external violence and injuries, with other local disturbances of the kidneys following contiguous disease

In those cases of renal congestion, with febrile disturbance and some other systemic changes, there is accumulated in the blood a good amount of excrementitious and effete material which is fitly removed by the kidney This hyper-contamination of the blood very shortly results in hyperæmia of the structure of the kidney The blood, in passing through the vascular secreting structures, owing to its high contamination, is detained a longer time in the vessels, in order that the material to be removed may be separated by the cell-agency; this detention will, supposing the circulation to be only kept up, involve an increased amount of pressure and detention in the vessels behind, which gradually increasing condition of hyperæmia may proceed to transudation of fluid, or in some instances to rupture

Anatomical Characters—When an opportunity is afforded of examining the kidney where congestive action has been in operation, the most attractive feature is a general fulness or excess of blood, and consequent heightening of colour Over any section of the hyperæmic organ there may be seen spots of increased vascularity or ecchymosis corresponding to the distended malpighian tufts In some instances, when carefully examined, the minute urine-tubes show a loosening and discharge of their epithelial lining. Should this state of congestion be protracted or often repeated, changes of a somewhat different nature will develop themselves, chiefly determining the character of the urine-tubes, the amount of intertubular connective-tissue and total bulk of the gland

Symptoms—The arrest of the blood in the vessels which surround the uriniferous tubes, and consequent turgescence of the malpighian capillaries, accounts in numerous instances for many of the symptoms of congestion and inflammation particularly attendant on recoveries from certain fevers and other general disturbances

With few or no constitutional symptoms the only attractive feature may be an alteration in the urinary secretion; this, although usually and in all established cases lessened in amount and of greater density, from the presence of an extra amount of solid materials, with, it may be, albumen and blood or blood-colouring matter, is, in a few of the milder developments and at the commencement, of a more watery character and augmented in bulk. With a continuance of the hyperæmia, or its repetition in close succession and consequent textural changes, the character of the secretion may also vary, and certain tube-casts and particular cell-structures be added

The milder cases, which do not proceed to inflammatory action, or by repetition to serious changes in the gland, usually, after a few days, decline, and the urine assumes its normal characters

Treatment.—When dependent on some general diseased condition the management of the renal congestion must not be undertaken apart from that of the state with which it is so closely linked. When the directly operating agents appear to be food or other material taken into the system by the alimentary canal or otherwise, a removal of the inducing agent is called for; and this in many instances may be expedited by the use of mild laxatives.

When pain, shown by general restlessness or in the employment of local manipulation, is a distinct symptom, this may be alleviated by the employment of heat and moisture to the loins, and the enforcement of perfect rest

46—2

II. NEPHRITIS—INFLAMMATION OF THE KIDNEYS

Inflammatory action having its seat in the kidney may be general and diffuse, or may be confined to particular structures and situations   The term nephritis, in its literal signification, denoting inflammation of the kidneys, has come to include various diseased conditions probably not properly inflammatory.

Usually these numerous morbid conditions have been grouped under the two chief divisions of—(1) Inflammatory action of varying characters attended with dropsy and albuminous urine, (2) Inflammatory action unattended with dropsy or albuminous urine.

Of these morbid conditions, the first of which is usually considered under the generic term of 'Bright's Disease,' and another manifestation, which, from the action being mainly confined to the pelvis and calices of the kidneys, is separately spoken of as 'Pyelitis,' we have fairly well-marked examples in our patients

1 Inflammatory Action of Varying Characters attended with Dropsy and Albuminous Urine   *a. Acute Tubal Nephritis* — Following an acute attack of certain fevers in the horse, as strangles or influenza, and some extensive inflammatory invasions of internal organs, there is, on the subsidence of the more acute stage, and on the first return to normal activity, a large amount of effete and now deleterious matter, with various cell-elements which have suffered death and are undergoing removal, thrown into the blood. In the natural course of exchange these waste materials fall in great part to be eliminated by the kidneys   Upon the cell-elements of the uriniferous tubes a large amount of this work is thrown, while their inability to execute it as rapidly as demanded is the immediately developing agency in the production of congestive and inflammatory action in the capillary system generally. At the same time the action of the empoisoned blood upon the cells of the urine-tubes themselves is destructive to their individual life through impairment of their nutrition, they become detached, undergo change, and collect in the tubes.

From the blood-pressure steadily exercised on the malpighian vessels, both fluid and corpuscular elements are forced through the vessels, partially fibrillating in the tubes and entangling amongst the formed material the changing epithelium of the tubes, in which form these fibrinous and epithelial casts appear in the urine

b. Chronic Tubal Nephritis—Besides this form of acute inflammation of the tubular and vascular structures associated with albuminous urine we sometimes encounter an apparently less alarming, because less pronounced, but steadily progressive and much more destructive diseased action affecting the same and other textures of the kidneys, a subacute or chronic tubal nephritis

This condition may follow an attack of the decidedly acute form, or it may be developed independently of it, it may also be associated with conditions of fatty or lardaceous change in the kidneys, and with arterial capillary fibrosis here and in other important organs

These extensive and serious structural changes in our patients are rarely brought under our notice until considerable inroad has been made in many structures, and until the general health and constitutional vigour is completely undermined

Anatomical Characters—In the one form, where the renal disturbance is rapidly developed and in association with some distinct and recognised blood-contamination, the kidney is enlarged, rather wanting in consistence, and sometimes pale in colour, at others rather darker, when of the former character the cortical structure particularly is, on a clean section being made, seen marked with hæmorrhagic spots. More carefully examined, the capillary system is seen somewhat congested, the urine-tubes are either filled and swollen, or their existence is indistinguishable, several seeming massed together from the amount of adventitious material connected with them, material effused outside the tubes and augmented by increased growth of cell-elements within

In the other and less active form there is a disposition to lessening of size, with a somewhat contracted character of the surface; the main feature, however, being rather a production of interconnective fibroid material existing around the minute tubes and the glomeruli, which by its presence seems to impair the extent and existence of these conduits, rendering in particular the malpighian structures nearly indistinguishable This condition of fibrosis, however occurring, whether from a special development of fibrous tissue, or from degeneration of the tubes themselves and changes in the cell-elements, affects both the vascular and urine-conduits, and seems merely part of a general predisposition, not an accidental local change, seeing that when observed here it may usually be noticed elsewhere in distant and different organs.

Symptoms.—The indications of these disordered renal activities and tissue-changes, which in reality ought not in the first-noted form to be regarded as a disease of the kidneys, but rather as a renal manifestation of a general disturbance or hæmal vitiation, are accession or renewal of the previously existing fever , an elevation of temperature ; an impairment of appetite, which had lately been somewhat improved ; disturbed cardiac and pulmonary action , and a dry, harsh condition of the skin The urine, which shortly antecedently had been voided in good amount, is now restricted, while pain may be shown when urinating ; the secretion itself is increased in density, heightened in colour, and on examination discloses epithelial tube-casts, the existence of albumen and maybe blood

There is in this form of renal disease little or no exhibition of local pain, either on manipulating the loins or in causing movement to be executed

In the more chronic manifestations, when brought under our observation, we have, with failing health and strength, impaired appetite, œdematous limbs, an intermittent or continuous appearance of albumen in the urine—rarely blood—and disturbed pulmonary and cardiac function

Treatment —The milder forms of congestion and inflammation of the tubular structure of the kidney resulting from blood-contamination are, with moderate care, disposed to return in a short time to the previously existing condition of the parts ; when protracted, further and more permanent changes are liable to ensue The horse must be comfortably housed, the action of the skin solicitated by warm clothing and the exhibition of saline febrifuges, as solution of acetate of ammonia with a moderate quantity of spirits of nitric æther and camphor twice daily In some the use of woollen rugs or blankets wrung from warm water and wrapped around the body have been found to be attended with benefit, in combination with the medicines mentioned   No very active diuretic should be given, but the bowels kept in a soluble state through the use of enemata and sulphate of soda, or magnesia given in quantity in the drinking-water   After a few days, when the more pronounced pyrexial symptoms have abated, moderate doses of the solution of the perchloride of iron, or iron in combination with quinine, will be found of much advantage, some of the simple salines being still continued in the drinking-water

2 **Inflammatory Action unattended with Dropsy or Albuminous Urine, Interstitial and Parenchymatous Nephritis with Renal Abscess**—Besides those inflammatory and non-inflammatory changes more properly located in the tubular structures, we occasionally meet with an active form of inflammation in which the diseased processes and tissue-changes, although to a great extent affecting all the elemental parts, yet seem to expend their chief activities on structures other than these   In the former morbid actions it has been noticed that dropsy and albuminuria are marked features, with extensive implication of other organs and structures essential to life, in the latter, albuminuria and dropsical swellings, instead of the rule, are the exception   Such cases seem to arise less from impure blood, the result of systemic disturbance and consequent tissue-change and removal, than from injury or irritation of a more truly local character, induced by external agents or influences, as violence, over-exertion, and probably also the action of irritating materials, which find an entrance into the animal body either by the alimentary canal or otherwise

This form of nephritic disturbance is probably more pronounced and attractive in the development of symptoms than either of the preceding already noticed, and is that which, above others, has been styled nephritis, as exhibiting in a more characteristic form the usually recognised inflammatory features of parenchymatous organs. The extent of structure involved is variable, and upon this largely depends the ultimate physical appearance of the organ

Should the morbid action be trifling in severity, or restricted as to territory invaded, the effusion consequent on the morbid process may be expected to be readily removed, while, where the inflammatory products are large in amount and extensively diffused, cell-proliferation and growth being active, with cell-secretion largely lessened, suppurative inflammation may be established, or other changes of a permanent and degenerative character occur. In the majority of these cases, besides the distinct involvement of the parenchymatous and interstitial structure of the gland, we often observe that the lining membrane of the pelvis gives evidence of the same disturbance.

Causation.—(1) Direct local injury resulting from violence, inflicted as blows, or long-continued and badly-disposed weight ; (2) Laceration, or damage sustained by muscular or other tissue in the lumbar region from excessive or prolonged exertion, the effects of which are propagated from contiguity to the kidneys ; (3) Cold and moisture, in the form of rain, applied directly to the loins, particularly following fatigue and exertion ; (4) The ingestion or absorption of certain irritating materials, as turpentine or cantharides ; (5) The presence of a calculus in the pelvis of the kidney.

Anatomical Characters.—When examined while the action is at its height, and before ulterior changes of either a fatty or fibroid character are established, the kidney is found enlarged, distinctly hyperæmic, with variously distributed hæmorrhagic markings, particularly in the cortical substance. In many instances puriform material exists in connection with the membrane of the pelvis and calices, while there is frequently encountered distinct circumscribed abscesses, sometimes of considerable size, oftener small, and scattered through the structure, but disposed to enlarge by coalescing. These abscesses will in some instances be found to have ruptured probably previous to death, discharging purulent matter and blood into the pelvis of the organ.

Symptoms.—These are usually rapid in development, and so closely linked to the immediately inducing cause, that without any stretch of imagination we at once connect the two in their natural and proper position of cause and effect. As many of the symptoms of colic are present, the marked exhibition of abdominal pain may induce us to suppose that the digestive canal is the seat of the disturbance ; from bowel disturbance, however, this is so far different, that in the affection of the kidneys we have marked pyrexia which, as a rule, does not

exist in ordinary colic. The straining and attempts to urinate
which both affections may exhibit, proceeding from different
causes, may with little trouble be differentiated In nephritis
small quantities of urine may be discharged from a bladder
empty, or nearly so, and when voided it is found much altered
in colour or mingled with blood, in bowel disturbances, although
there may be straining and attempts at urination, the bladder
is more frequently full than otherwise, the urine being discharged when the spasm is relieved In this form of nephritic
disturbance the condition of the urine, when it may be obtained
—it being generally scanty from the failure of the secretion—is
less regularly albuminous, particularly in the earlier stages, than
in those other forms we have noticed

Besides the exhibition of colicky pains and much fever, with
a rather frequent and hard pulse, there is indisposition to move,
with a certain evidence of pain when movement is attempted,
manipulation over the region of the kidneys is badly borne
and provocative of a similar expression of uneasiness.

Suppuration and Abscesses—Although the inflammatory
process, when occurring in an active form in the general structures of the kidney of the horse, appears more likely after a
time to subside, and restoration of normal activity to occur, or
if continued to terminate in fibroid, fatty, or other changes, we
yet occasionally encounter well-marked instances of renal
abscesses, which, when occurring, I have always found terminating fatally; or rather it would be more correct to say, their
existence was only discovered after death

The last case which I had an opportunity of observing was
that of a six-year-old, well bred, good-conditioned gelding He
was left in our infirmary because of urinary disturbance, which
had existed for a week. Sometime previous to this period he
was believed to have sprained his loins by slipping on the
damp pavement, since then he had regularly, during the day,
after frequent attempts, voided a moderate quantity of urine
mingled with blood; his appetite and general health, at first
good enough, were now somewhat affected, and his ability to
do work was evidently impaired. After remaining at rest some
hours, examination indicated a slightly increased cardiac action,
with pulsations at the arteries rather small, temperature
103° F, desire for food and water moderate, particularly the

former Placed under observation at 2 p.m , he twice, between that time and 12 p m , passed a moderate amount of urine, standing stretched both before and after the discharge , on both occasions there would probably be half a pint of pure blood mingled with the discharge, this coagulated nearly entirely on reaching the ground, and was of a rather bright red colour Pressure over the loins and through the rectum, in the direction of the kidneys, was attended with pain. He continued to live and to void urine of the same character for forty-eight hours, when he died without exhibiting much pain The kidneys were the only organs exhibiting structural change. Both externally seemed slightly darker in colour than natural the right, on being laid open in the direction of the long axis, was somewhat congested throughout its entire extent, and blood flowed freely from the cut surfaces , the left, softer and less resistant to the touch, on being cut in the same manner disclosed a considerable abscess, which had either burst immediately before or at the time of death, communicating with the cavity of the renal pelvis No pus had, during life, been observed in the urine

Treatment —The disturbances of function, and the structural changes occurring in the parenchyma of the kidneys, the result of fatigue, exposure, and cold, usually attended with full arterial and cardiac action, stand depletion well, and seem relieved by it ; those directly resulting from outward violence are less favourably acted upon by blood-letting In every instance, however, whether blood is abstracted or not, the indications are undoubtedly in the direction of giving to the structures affected as large a proportion of rest as possible; this is most surely done by throwing the removal of the waste and worn material of the body, ordinarily removed by the kidneys, on the intestinal canal and the skin As the skin in the horse, apart from exercise, is of small service in this direction, the main source of relief is through the bowels.

Moderate purgation, through means of aloes or oil, which, when obtained, is to be kept up by regular quantities of salines given with mucilaginous drinks, is the mode of inducing intestinal action I have found most benefit from When pain is a prominent feature it will be needful to administer repeatedly, in moderate amount, some preparation of opium, either alone or combined with the oil or mucilage used for drinking, or what is probably better, with full doses of solution of acetate of ammonia   With the same object in view I have employed continuous applications of woollen cloths wrung from warm water, or large linseed-meal poultices placed over the loins, persevered with until relief is obtained   The warm water or the poultices will, in many instances, have their beneficial action augmented by being medicated with opium, bella-donna, or digitalis , the latter, it has been repeatedly demon-strated, having a special action in reducing ischuria   When the poultices or warm-water applications are discontinued, either entirely or for a short time, care must be exercised to protect the parts from the injurious effects of the reaction of cold , while, so long as pain continues and the urine is abnormal, the horse should be closely confined to the stable and moderately dieted   On the subsidence of the more active symptoms moderate doses of dilute sulphuric acid with sulphate of iron, or some preparation of quinine and iron, will be found productive of much benefit in restoring functional activity, both local and general.

CHAPTER LIII.

DISEASES OF THE BLADDER

I IRRITABILITY OF THE BLADDER

THIS is a term somewhat abused and rather indefinite , it is usually employed to indicate what is believed to be a disturbed condition of the bladder, exhibited by frequent and continued micturition

Pathology   *a. Causation* —This irritability, or frequency of micturition, may proceed from causes other than are located in the bladder, and therefore ought properly not to be termed irritability of the bladder   It is found associated with renal disease, with changes occurring to the uterus, with disturbance apart from inflammation of the bladder, with similar changes of the urethra, with enlargements of the prostates, and with disease of contiguous organs.   It is sometimes spoken of as

synonymous with the condition observed when the coats
of the bladder have become paralyzed from over-distension,
but from which it is essentially different both in causes and
symptoms In many instances the irritability does not seem
to depend upon structural alterations in the urinary organs,
either primarily or secondarily, but upon impairment or
disorder of organs and functions in some manner related to
the urino-genital system. Certain injuries to muscular structure
in the lumbar region, or possibly to the spinal cord itself,
during the existence of active symptoms, develop this unnatural
functional activity.

b Anatomical Characters—It is only in a limited number of
instances, where the symptoms of this functional disturbance
have been exhibited, that obvious textural alterations may be
discovered In some we may find calculi and structural
changes of varying character in the kidneys and ureters, deposits
of sabulous material in the bladder, or evidence more or less
marked of some antecedent inflammatory action either there
or in some contiguous muscular structure In rarer instances
the cord itself may give evidence of change Such alteration,
although the symptoms may point in this direction, is not so
common as we might expect, judging from the frequency of
disturbed innervation

Symptoms.—These are chiefly the rather sudden development of this repeated desire to urinate, with the ejection of
small quantities of urine In some, particularly when proceeding from errors of a dietetic character, there are other symptoms
which are without difficulty connected with the one common
cause, gastric or intestinal dyspepsia, such as an unthrifty
condition of the skin and coat, sometimes thirst, which, when
present, may or may not be associated with an increased
amount of urine voided. There are no well marked or
distinct indications of pain, merely restlessness and repeated
micturition

Treatment—As the most frequent cause of this irritability is
disturbed digestion, every attention ought to be directed to
correct this, the bowels must be quietly cleared by some
aperient medicine, after which care must be exercised to see
that the food-supply is sufficiently good. The prepuce and
external opening of the urethra in the male will require

examination in order to satisfy ourselves that no irritating and obstructing material has been lodged there, and by soap and water remove the suspicion that disturbed function is the result of want of cleanliness.

The condition of the bladder and prostates should be ascertained as far as possible by examination per rectum, in order to discover if surgical interference may not be needful to remove the inducing cause. While the history of the case as to probable injury of the loins may help us so far.

As the causes which operate in inducing vesical irritability are varied, they may only be successfully met by treatment suited to the different cases.

II CYSTITIS—INFLAMMATION OR CATARRH OF THE BLADDER.

Definition.—*Inflammation of the urinary bladder*

Pathology. *a Causation*—Inflammation of the urinary bladder is in the horse a very rare condition, much rarer than with several other animals which come under our care. The causes which we may chiefly expect to observe operating in inducing the lesion are—(1) Irritation resulting from the presence of foreign bodies, as calculi or morbid growths; (2) From the ingestion of special irritants, as turpentine, cantharides, etc., (3) Ammoniacal urine, existing as the consequence of vesical paralysis following spinal injury and exposure to fatigue, damp, and cold, with bad food.

Anatomical Characters.—Apart from disturbance, the inner lining of the urinary bladder on examination after death gives the impression of a very moderately vascular structure. When suffering from inflammatory action, marked changes occur, and bloodvessels appear where none were previously visible. This morbid action is seldom of a uniform character, intensity, or distribution. It may appear as a catarrhal, adhesive, suppurative, or ulcerative action, and may be largely distributed as to superficial extent, or scattered in circumscribed and small patches. In some the epithelial lining seems little disturbed; in others it is removed in large patches, leaving a smooth abraded surface.

This condition of inflammatory action may not be confounded with the hæmorrhagic spotting which is encountered in many cases of fevers in this and other hollow organs, apparently resulting from hæmal changes and extravasations from the vessels of the submucous tissue. In cases where the cause of the inflammation is mechanical irritation steadily maintained for some time, and not of the most active character, we meet with much increase in the thickness of the walls of the bladder without striking change in colour. This may result from remittent but sustained irritation, or from steadily maintained hyper-activity in efforts to overcome some resistance or urethral obstruction.

Symptoms.—Restlessness referable to abdominal disturbance, a rather peculiar paddling or repeated moving of the hind-feet, and occasional whisking of the tail, repeated micturitions with trifling discharge, pain increased on making attempts to examine the state of the bladder from the rectum; and in cases of some severity or long standing, where the contractile power of the sphincter is lessened, there may be continuous dribbling of urine. In all instances which have come under my observation, except those in which the morbid action was confined to the smallest extent of structure, in addition to symptoms indicative of local changes there existed more or less constitutional disturbance and fever. Rarely have we acute cystitis apparently affecting a large area of the viscus, tending to complete destruction of the contractibility of the structures. Occasionally we meet with a subacute or chronic manifestation not at all favourably influenced by treatment, where well-marked and extensive changes are steadily progressive for a lengthened period; these cases are often indicated by the presence of pus and other cell-structures in the urine, a condition, however, which may be confounded with the more frequent one of chronic pyelitis.

Treatment.—When believing that there exists inflammation of the coats of the bladder, care must be exercised to avoid increased irritation and the chances of ulterior mischief from the presence of large quantities of urine in the organ; and when not naturally evacuated, the urine ought to be withdrawn regularly by the catheter, not, however, unless the inability to void it naturally is decidedly expressed.

With much pain exhibited and marked constitutional excitement, moderate blood-letting, followed with repeated but moderate doses of opium, or opium combined with calomel,

are likely to give relief earlier than any other line of treatment.
Here, also, local soothing, through the employment of blankets
wrung from plain or medicated hot water, may be carried out
with advantage

Although active and severe purgation is not to be recommended in any form of inflammatory action of the urinary
organs, a gentle excitation of the normal intestinal action is
always desirable, and is best secured by a moderate dose of
aloes with a little calomel and gentian, while a soluble condition may be maintained by allowing linseed-oil with the food,
or full doses of sulphate of soda in the water, gruel, or linseed-
tea allowed for drink

Chronic cases of cystic disease, and particularly when of a
catarrhal character, are probably more successfully treated by
a rather tonic system of management Moderate doses of one
of the mineral acids with some preparation of iron, as the
sulphate or carbonate, alternated with sulphate of magnesia
and sulphuric acid, and continued daily for a week or more,
will generally be productive of better results than more active
treatment and the use of lowering remedies Hyoscyamus
extract, copaiba, infusion of buchu and bearberry leaves have,
by those who have tried them, been spoken of as useful agents
in allaying the irritability attendant on chronic catarrhal conditions of the bladder and urinary tract, and of exciting a
healthy action in the diseased membrane

Where irritability of the bladder appears in connection with
such fevers as the epizootic distemper of horses, and where we
fear hæmorrhagic effusions here or in other hollow organs, I
have observed benefit to follow the use of moderate doses of
sulphuric acid and sulphate of iron, alternated with full doses
of salicylic acid

CHAPTER LIV.

DISEASES OF THE CUTANEOUS SYSTEM

GENERAL CONSIDERATIONS AND CLASSIFICATION.

THE importance attaching to diseases of the skin and accessory
structures in the horse, although never likely to reach, even
relatively, the same consideration, compared with those of the

system generally, which attaches to them in man, are yet from various considerations deserving of more attention than has generally been bestowed upon them

Ever since any care or special knowledge has been directed to the consideration of animal diseases, the larger proportion of cutaneous affections have, in the gross, been looked upon as manifestations of scabies or mange; now we know that, as respects this in its genuine manifestations, a very trifling proportion of skin disturbances are traceable to its inroads

That the knowledge of this group of diseases is rather less cultivated and understood than many others, is probably largely owing to the fact that while the general and obvious features of very many are much alike, the separate elemental lesions of these and of distinct and individual diseases are liable to variation, and that for their correct diagnosis there is required a somewhat close attention.

They are certainly common enough, and as to their power of inconveniencing the animal, causing much disfigurement, and entailing monetary loss on owners because of their horses' inability to perform ordinary work, they are highly important In their management, too, there is an inducement held out for their careful study, in the fact that remedial measures when beneficial are patent to all

As a field for the operation of morbid activities, we find that elementary textural changes are here very much like similar processes in other situations and textures of the body, modified probably more by position and relations to the outer world than by anatomical formation

In the history of the causation of skin diseases, although agencies operating from within, either congenital or acquired, may possess the power of independently developing or of intensifying and modifying many affections when appearing, there seems little doubt that the more numerous and more potent factors in their production are agencies and influences acting from without. Thus it is that, although we may be assisted in forming our diagnosis by a knowledge of the history of the disturbance in the animal, and the conditions to which it may have been subjected, still our chief means of information rests with the visible manifestations of diseases as presented for our observation ; and that in their treatment local remedies may never be entirely neglected for the sake of the general and constitutional

Classification of Skin Diseases —In systematizing and rendering available our information, and as assisting us to place in their proper position such disturbances and lesions as we may encounter, different modes of arranging these morbid conditions have been proposed and carried out.

And although in attempting to make a classification or grouping of natural objects or activities, it may be impossible to obtain such absolutely correct, seeing that neither organisms nor functions are separable in classes by sharp lines of demarcation, it is not on that account desirable to abandon all classification whatever, better an indifferent grouping than no grouping at all. With cutaneous affections the arrangement has been carried out chiefly, if not entirely, on two separate bases or lines of consideration. The first, which directs attention entirely to the character of the elementary lesion of the disease, and may be termed the *anatomical*, is probably the simpler and more easily grasped, the second, probably the more rational, aims at telling us more than merely the place in a bald group which a particular disturbance ought to take: it endeavours to analyze diseases in accordance with the nature and causes of morbid action, and may be regarded as the *pathological*, or *clinical*.

In the rather brief consideration which is here proposed to be given to skin affections, an endeavour will be made to view them according to the following modified form of the latter mode of classification

CLASSIFICATION OF SKIN DISEASES

Class I Congestive and Inflammatory Diseases.

a Specific inflammatory,
b Local congestive and inflammatory, or *Erythematous.*
c. Plastic inflammatory, or *Papular.*
d. Catarrhal inflammatory, or *Eczematous.*
e Bullous, or *Herpic* inflammations
f. Suppurative inflammatory, or *Ecthymatous.*
g Scaly inflammatory, or *Squamous*

47

Class II. Diseases of Nutrition, including New Formations.

  a. Hypertrophies.

  b Atrophies.

  c New-formation, or heterologous growths.

Class III. Neuroses.

Class IV. Diseases of Accessory Organs and Structures.

  a. Diseases of sudorific glands.

  b Diseases of sebaceous glands

  c Diseases of hairs and hair-follicles

Class V. Hæmorrhages.

Class VI. Parasitic Diseases.

  a Animal (*dermatozoic*)

  b. Vegetable (*dermatophytic*).

Of these divisions, the 1st, 2nd, and 6th are well defined, and together with the 4th will be found to constitute if not the whole, certainly nearly the whole of the skin diseases which in the practice of equine medicine engage our attention.

CHAPTER LV

DETAILED DESCRIPTION OF THE MORE COMMON FORMS OF SKIN DISEASES IN THE HORSE.

CLASS I. CONGESTIVE AND INFLAMMATORY DISEASES.

UNDER this group of congestive and inflammatory action in its many variations which mark these vascular disturbances, we find a large proportion of the skin diseases of our patients We observe that the pure hyperæmia and congestion in erythema may, by effusion into the dermal textures, pass on to the form of plastic or papular inflammation; by exudation into the catarrhal, or developing the higher grade of action, pustulation may occur; while, as the result of these, we may have the various forms of the scaly. All these manifestations of the inflammatory process may be looked at, as they meet us in daily practice—(1) as acute, and (2) as chronic; these being further subdivided into idiopathic and symptomatic. Under the first of these we place the specific dermal exudations, the purely local hyperæmic or erythematous appearances, the non-contagious dermatoses, and probably the herpie

A SPECIFIC INFLAMMATORY LESIONS OF THE SKIN.

Under this group of the inflammatory class are included the eruptions of the acute contagious dermatoses or specific fevers

To the febrile manifestations of these, including their attendant local phenomena, the term Exanthemata has been applied, by this is intended to be conveyed the idea of a morbid process which attacks the whole system, attended with febrile symptoms hastening through a certain determinate acute course, having certain appearances and conditions attached to the cutaneous surface, which local conditions develop a specific contagious principle

These exanthemata possess certain common features by which they may be recognised—(1) They are all preceded by a fever of a variable duration; (2) The skin appearances when developed show themselves in a regular order and sequence; (3) These skin changes have a definite period of existence, (4) The sympathy of the system with the skin appearances is indicated by certain symptoms seen during the existence of the local lesions and after their decline; (5) These diseases, as a rule, only attack animals once during their life.

As these skin developments and phenomena are not truly local diseases, and as they have been noticed elsewhere, nothing further will be said of them here.

B LOCAL CONGESTIVE AND INFLAMMATORY OR ERYTHEMATOUS DISEASES.

Under this subdivision it is desired to place those local dermal disturbances and lesions associated with or attendant upon hyperæmic or congestive action, active or passive, with simple serous effusion, and which ordinarily exhibit little abnormal activity in the tissue-elements outside the vessels, with the production of new material or so-called inflammatory exudation Those diseased conditions, the acute non-contagious dermatites of an idiopathic character, might be classed here,

47—2

had they not already received a position and designation as distinct diseases

The forms of vascular disturbance of the erythematous type which are seated in the vessels of the papillary layer of the dermis, or alone in the capillaries of the hair-follicles and glandular structures, are in the horse chiefly exhibited as **Erythema** and **Urticaria**. Owing to the pigmented condition of the horse's skin, change of colour is not observed, while the close covering of hair considerably obscures the swelling, which, in some instances, is slight. The course of both these affections is generally acute, or, if chronic, it is by repeated attacks, while the secondary effects are desquamation.

Erythema

Definition — *A condition of vascular turgescence or hyperæmia, usually occurring in patches more or less extensive, with a certain amount of effusion into the deeper layers of the epidermis*

General Characters and Form of Development — It is a non-contagious affection, idiopathic or symptomatic, active or passive

With our patients its usual form is idiopathic and active. The patches are slightly elevated, sometimes with a well-defined margin, at others gradually shading off into the healthy skin, which it has a tendency to invade. These are at first tolerably firm, if not much elevated, but, as they subside, become softer. With its appearance in any form there is little general disturbance; only a trifling amount of itching or exudation, not like eczema. When it declines there may be a greater or less amount of desquamation. In its development several modifications may be noticed, and these have been named sometimes in accordance with their form, and at others from the causes supposed to be operating in their production

Erythema traumaticum vel Paratrimma is the circumscribed hyperæmia, with serous effusion into the skin-tissues, occurring as the result of pressure from badly fitting collars, belts, or saddles. This condition, first showing itself in distinct patches, slightly elevated and tender, may, if the pressure is continued, terminate in more serious changes, as the formation of abscesses

Erythema intertrigo is the congestive blush and condition of irritation imparted to the skin from the friction caused by the rubbing of one portion upon another. This is often largely aggravated by the trickling over the parts at the same time of some irritating fluid, as the urine. This condition is a frequent occurrence with animals in a plethoric condition, perspiring much in warm, dusty weather, and when cleanliness and good stable management are not prominent features.

Erythema exudativum is the form most frequently found attendant upon exposure to wet and cold, or the contact of irritating materials with dermal tissues under vascular excitement, seen particularly affecting the legs of horses of our lighter breeds used for active exertion during the winter season, and when these parts have been denuded of hair by closely clipping, and the skin softened and irritated by much washing These conditions seem extremely liable to induce in the skin so acted upon an erythematous inflammation with excess of exudation

Although not entirely due to aught specific in the clay or mud through which horses may be required to move, seeing it may originate without this direct application of mud, and is often very intimately associated with disturbed functional activities of internal organs, there is no doubt that particular soils and mud impregnated with certain materials have a more actively determining influence in producing this exudative erythema than others From what I have seen of this affection I am disposed to regard it as owing more to the altered state of the skin from the removal of the hair than to the effects of washing with cold water, or even contact with such for lengthened and irregular periods

It chiefly occurs over the skin covering the metacarpal and metatarsal bones, and is in numerous instances attended with general disturbance and more or less pyrexia, as well before its appearance as when fully developed At first the skin over the parts—which are rarely in small patches, being nearly evenly diffused over the cannon-bones, or even higher—becomes slightly rough, warmer than natural, with probably a trifling amount of swelling; no exudation, however, or anything approaching to it for some days, when the scales of the epidermis becoming elevated, and at several points detached, roughness is perceptible, gradually passing on to separation and desquamation of the upper layers in a crust-like manner : there is, however, no raw surface and no weeping All through its course the inflammatory action exhibits the true erythematous type as distinct from the phlegmonous, in which the subdermal structures are often involved—seen in the so-called erythema chronicum exhibited in the persistently inflamed skin of the heels of horses naturally possessed of much hair, but which fashion has doomed to be removed.

This acute exudative erythema seems in many of its features closely allied to the true catarrhal inflammation eczema, only in the latter the layers deeper than the rete, as the papillary and true corium, are undoubtedly much involved, which they are not here.

Erythema Chronicum —This term has been applied to the persistent erythematous condition of the skin of the heels—commonly known as chapped heels, otherwise *dermatitis erythematosa*—so frequently encountered during winter in horses, the heels of which have been denuded of hair, and where there has been much exposure to damp or cold draughts from currents of air while in the stable

Even the milder forms of this persistent erythematous inflammation are troublesome, much more so when deeper-seated tissues become invaded and impetigenous or ulcerative processes supervene

Diagnosis —Erythematous inflammation is individualized by its situation in the superficial layers of the skin, by the non-production of new material in the true dermis, and by the absence of pus-formation There may be exudation, even extensive, and attended with scaling of the epidermis It is distinguished from its companion affection, *urticaria*, by the existence in the latter of evanescent soft swellings or patches ; and from *eczema* by the presence in the latter of distinct vesicles, which in rupturing form crusts on the surface of the skin, and, when removed by itching, leave a weeping raw surface

Treatment —In the successful management of any cases of idiopathic erythema local measures are of the first importance , attention must be given to the removal of all irritants, to secure cleanliness and good sanitary conditions.

In the milder cases such simple agents as a solution of bicarbonate of potash and glycerine, or glycerine with rose-water, for local application, together with simple salines, as magnesium sulphate, given in the drinking-water, will be all that is required When the intertrigo is severe and irritation great, a solution of tannic acid with glycerine, or an ointment of tannic acid and opium, will give relief, or the parts may be painted with a weak solution of nitrate of silver

In the extensively distributed and well-marked forms of exudative erythema, so common on the limbs of hunters, more attention will be required, and much time will elapse ere the epidermic scales are shed, and the hair, which has been killed, is renewed Unless in exceptional cases, when inconvenience from the exudation is considerable, moisture should be kept away from the parts, the skin of which may be kept soft by a daily use of some glycerine mixture, a little oxide of zinc or calamine ointment, or a light application of vaseline. A very useful liniment may be made with soft soap, one part, glycerine, two parts, water, four parts When the use of this is needful for some length of time, the parts to which it is applied should be sponged or washed occasionally, and the liniment re-applied Along with this a moderate dose of laxative medicine will be needful, and the after and occasional exhibition of saline diuretics, if the animal is weak, or in poor condition, it is probable that tonics will be required, as tincture of gentian, or cinchona with a little mineral acid

As a means of preventing the occurrence of this troublesome condition, I would advise that the hair be not removed from the limbs, and when much washing is required to remove the dirt, that, previous to being perfectly dried, a little glycerine and water—equal proportions of each—be rubbed over the heels and those parts of the skin most likely to suffer

Leaving the mud on the legs of hard-wrought horses until perfectly dry, when it may be brushed off, is by many considered the most effectual method of guarding against this erythematous inflammation, as, however, this is not altogether free from objections, the other seems equally applicable, and certainly in most cases efficacious.

Urticaria—Syn Nettle Rash.

Definition—*An eruption over irregularly distributed, frequently symmetrical portions of skin, of slightly elevated, oval, or roundish patches, soft, but possessed of a moderate amount of resistance to the touch, and extremely evanescent.*

Pathology *a. Nature.*—This is an extremely interesting disease; and in the horse, as well as in cattle, it may appear in almost any part of the body, being, however, less frequently seen on the limbs, seeming to have a partiality for the head, neck, and upper parts of the trunk. It appears without premonitory symptoms, and may or may not be accompanied with fever and general disturbance. When appearing in certain parts of the body special symptoms attend such developments.

b. Causation.—The agencies and influences operating in the production of this condition are, like those related to several other cutaneous disorders, various; but probably all turn upon the disturbance of nutrition in the parts invaded, such as— (1) Local irritation to a naturally hypersensitive skin; (2) Reflected irritation from deranged digestive organs; (3) Effete material circulating in the blood—this may be regarded as only another form of direct local irritation.

The exact rationale of the production of the immediate manifestation of the disturbance is not without difficulty of explanation. The anatomical features point to the infiltration of the superficial part of the papillary layer of the corium, and of the layers of the epidermis; while the suddenness of the appearance of the swellings, and their equally sudden disappearance, and the absence of sequelæ, seem to indicate some other cause in operation than impurity of blood. Certain atmospheric and meteorological disturbances have been supposed to be in operation for the production of these phenomena, while there is not wanting evidence to favour the idea of its neurotic origin and intimate connection with disturbed vaso-motor power. It does not, in any animal, seem to be of a catching nature, and inoculation with the blood has failed to produce it.

Symptoms—These are distinctive, and not likely to be mistaken: rapid of development, and scattered over various parts of the body, the wheals or circumscribed swellings resemble whip or thong stripes, varying somewhat according to the locality where situated When over the throat and eyes a certain amount of speciality attends their existence, as impeded respiration, deglutition, and vision.

In many instances the horse is languid, with some general disturbance and moderate fever. It is the sudden and startling character of the appearance of the local manifestations, which may occupy only a few hours, which usually alarms the owner. In a few instances I have noticed the eliminatory organs, bowels and kidneys, somewhat disturbed. The period which the swellings remain prominent varies much, in some cases only a few hours, in others their entire removal will require a week. On their disappearance there is extremely little desquamation, sometimes a slightly open state of the coat may remain for a little. One crop, however, may fade while another starts into existence; itching and irritability of the parts may exist, but are not diagnostic symptoms.

When occurring around the throat and eyes a peculiar appearance is given to the animal, with occasionally distressing symptoms, as embarrassment of breathing and stupor, while, if special attention is not bestowed upon the case, the general œdema of the parts may threaten serious results.

Diagnosis.—The individuality of the symptoms, their rapidity of appearance and evanescent character, connected with the general state and condition of the patients, prevent us from confounding this with any other disease. The local swellings, although when in the region of the throat they may simulate some other affections, as purpura hæmorrhagica or scarlatina, may, with a little care, be differentiated from either of these. Here there has been no previous debility or weakening disease, as with those other œdematous affections; the swellings are also marked by great capriciousness wherever appearing, while occasionally they are easily enough connected with some dietetic error or external irritation.

Treatment—Although in every instance a good amount of attention must be bestowed upon the local phenomena of infiltration and itching, a radical cure can only be effected by a recognition and treatment of the disturbance or irritation upon which these local symptoms depend; this will, of course, in every case demand a special study. Should the cutaneous disturbance arise from contaminated blood, owing to the presence of effete and deleterious matter, the natural emunctories of bowels and kidneys must be placed in conditions favourable for its purification

When the animal is plethoric, moderate purgatives, followed by salines and diuretics, are indicated If systemic weakness is a prominent feature, a too active state of the bowels will have to be guarded against, and probably such tonics as muriate of cinchonine with muriatic acid, or sulphate of iron with sulphuric acid, will serve our purpose better

If we discover disturbance of functional activity of other organs, as liver or uterus, we must, by appropriate means, endeavour to correct such ; while, if improper food or bad stable conditions seem to have been operating, they will require to be altered. Generally a mild evacuation of the bowels, and attention to dietary, guided by the consideration whether the animal is above or below par, followed by the employment of moderate tonics and diuretics, are the constitutional remedies most likely to be attended with good results Locally we will seldom fail to allay the irritation by repeated damping or washing with an alkaline mixture, to which has been added a little glycerine and dilute prussic acid. When the itching is troublesome, either here or in other skin affections, I have found much good from the use, twice daily, of a wash composed of bichloride of mercury, grs xii , dilute hydrocyanic acid, fl ʒiv , glycerine, or almond mixture, fl ʒii ; water, fl ℥x.

C PLASTIC OR PAPULAR INFLAMMATIONS

By the majority of those who have described the skin diseases of our patients it would appear that the forms of cutaneous inflammatory action which I am disposed to place under this division have been regarded either as manifestations of *eczema,* or of true pustular inflammation, *ecthyma* There seems, however, sufficient evidence to satisfy that inflammatory action of a plastic character does occur separate and distinct from the true catarrhal on the one hand, and the pustular on the other

In these cutaneous inflammations of a plastic character there is an effusion of coagulable lymph into the papillary layer and rete, with distinct and circumscribed elevations, which, unless abraded by friction—which they not unfrequently are—owing to existing itching, do not exude even serous fluid. On abrasion, however, there may occur a considerable exudation, which somewhat alters their general appearance. On their natural subsidence a full exfoliation of minute epithelial scales takes place, with sometimes a marked heightening of colour in the freshly developed hairs.

The originally appearing or elementary lesions in the papular inflammation may, in the horse, be fairly well embraced by the two recognised forms of skin papulation, lichen and prurigo. Although retaining these terms of comparative pathology, as representing with tolerable accuracy the papulary or plastic inflammatory action ordinarily met with in the horse, it must not be taken for granted that these equine affections are in every respect the analogue and counterpart of similarly named skin diseases in man. Both these affections are chronic rather than acute; and with *eczema*, in its various developments, may be regarded as representing the pruriginous dermatoses of the horse.

In the former, the irregularly scattered, sometimes roughly symmetrical papules, or irritations of the dermal tissues, are smaller, more distinctly accuminated, and less itchy, than in the latter, with which, in addition to the papulation, there is well-marked infiltration and thickening, with distinct coriaceous characters imparted to the skin, and where the itching is always a prominent symptom.

In Lichen, in the horse, the papules are relatively larger than in man, and more resemble the development of ecthyma, only they do not suppurate. By abrasion, both in this and prurigo, there may be much exudation and crusting. In some individual cases, their character of special invasion of the hair-follicles, and their extension by repetition of the separate follicular inflammations and excessive cell-proliferation, is very well made out.

Their course is usually erratic, or rather prolonged, and their resolution is attended with much shedding of bran-like scales.

In Prurigo, the papules or elevations which result from exudation into the papillary layer and the rete, together with hypertrophy of the epidermis, are more varied in size and less discrete. Amongst a number of smaller elevations scattered

irregularly over the neck and quarters, we may observe larger
and rather flattened projections exactly of the character of
urticaria, probably the result of rubbing

We seem to observe this condition of papulation as a sequel
to the true papular elevations which have been accompanied
with much friction, the itching, however, continuing to increase
with the rubbing, the infiltration and general thickening of the
skin between and amongst the papules depending much upon
the effusion resulting from irritation incident to the rubbing.

These papules which are in larger amount distributed
over the superior parts of the body, become abraded by
rubbing, and may, when a little rest from irritation is
allowed, be found covered over their summits with a dark-
coloured crust of coagulated blood and epidermic scales, while
the entire texture of the skin upon which they are situated
is more distinctly thickened from infiltration, and often denuded
of hair

In the severe and very chronic cases, we have very moderate
elevation or papulation, but well-marked general infiltration
and coriaceous characters, with much exudation, the formation
of fissures, a dry wrinkled state of the skin, separate collections of pus beneath the epidermic crusts, great shedding of
scales, much itching, and sometimes swelling of the lymph-
glands with constitutional disturbance

In addition to this plastic or papular inflammation of the
skin, it must not be forgotten that some other conditions, such
as the presence of the scab acari and pediculi, may be, and often
are, attended with much itching and cutaneous infiltration

Causation —As respects the causes, either remote or immediate, which determine the appearance of these pruriginous
papular affections, we are very often in the dark. It seems
highly probable that those which may more properly be classed
as general or constitutional, as distinguished from local, are of
more importance and general operation

We find them appear both when the animal is above and
below par, certainly many of the most troublesome and intricate cases I have encountered have been connected with
malassimilation and defective nutrition, and were most benefited by a course of treatment which aimed at the re-establishment of healthy functional activity.

I am satisfied, also, that the tendency to contract these affections is transmitted as an inheritance from parent to progeny.

That both nervous disturbance and a loaded condition of the blood, from retention in the system of matters which ought to have been eliminated by ordinary emunctories, may be closely connected with such local disturbances, is highly probable; but at present we do not possess information sufficiently definite in confirmation of the certainty of such, nor of the mode through which their operations are carried out.

Treatment.—Wherever we are satisfied that dyspepsia exists, that effete and waste material is retained in the system, the indication is to correct such unnatural conditions in accordance with rational views of the case and the teachings of experience.

It the animal is weak and debilitated through want of proper food, or as a sequel of some general disease, good food, plenty of fresh air, with moderate but repeated doses of tonics, of which the mineral acids deserve a trial, together with the administration of neutral salines, are likely to be productive of good results. When of full habit of body, a gentle purge, followed by moderate but daily doses of salines, as the sulphate of soda or magnesia, are to be employed early and previous to aught else.

Whenever the irritation and itching are troublesome, soothing washes or ointments will require to be liberally used.

In many cases an alkaline wash, as a saturated solution of bicarbonate of potash or the ordinary liq. amm. acet., with a small quantity of glycerine and dilute hydrocyanic acid applied twice daily, will serve the purpose well, or one grain of the bichloride of mercury to the fluid ounce of liquid, with a little chloroform or tincture of opium or digitalis, with glycerine and water, may be used alternately. With some cases of most determined itching, relief has followed two or three applications of grs. ii. of nitrate of silver, or grs. iii. cyanide of potassium, to the fluid ounce of water. When the condition of the skin has assumed a decidedly chronic character, with much thickening and scaling of the superficial layers, some of the tarry preparations with sulphur and oil will be more likely, by their special stimulating properties, to restore healthy activity to the parts. In the internal treatment of these more chronic cases, I have had good results from the exhibition, twice daily in water, of an ounce of Donovan's solution; this, after a few days, to be alternated with moderate quantities of dilute sulphuric acid and sulphate of iron.

Both general and local treatment require to be persevered with for some time, and will be greatly assisted by a carefully arranged regimen and adaptation of other local conditions favourable to general and local health.

D. CATARRHAL OR ECZEMATOUS INFLAMMATIONS

This form of disturbed activity in the cutaneous textures is admittedly common; but notwithstanding the frequency of its occurrence, when spoken of as a particular manifestation of catarrhal action, much difference of opinion has been expressed with respect to the limiting of the term 'catarrhal.'

Eczema, which may be taken as the true type of cutaneous catarrh, is regarded as an inflammatory action of the dermal tissues, with exudation and cell-production extending into the superficial layer of the true skin, the rete-malpighii, and to the epidermis, accompanied by an eruption of papules, vesicles, or pustules, which rupturing, discharge a fluid disposed to collect in crusts, and cause matting of the hair, attended with much itching; and when these crusts are removed by rubbing, there is a tendency to ichoration and chronicity

In this form of inflammatory action there is not merely hyperæmia with exudation into the rete and epidermic layers, but we have a distinct discharge, an exudation on the surface of the skin with changes in the corium, and a tendency to pus-formation. The eruption, when observed, which it is not in every case, is of small, closely-packed vesicles, which burst, exude a material, agglutinate the hairs and form crusts. This eruption is characterized also by its disposition to appear in successive crops, and by the frequency with which the matter exuded is sero-purulent.

Anatomical Features—The anatomy of this, which seems true catarrh of the skin, consists in swelling and upheaval, from the presence of fluid, of the cells and scales of the epidermis; this fluid has been conveyed to the superficial layer of the epidermis, the elevation of which constitutes the vesicles, by the agency of cell-structures, and is originally the material exuded from the congested vessels of the papillary layer of the true skin When these vesicles rupture, and their contents are dissipated, we may have the deeper-seated structures, as the rete, exposed, and a considerable ichorous discharge

In the severer forms, the cell-proliferation and infiltration is not confined to the rete or epidermis, but extends to the structure of the corium, amongst which the inflammatory exudation may result in new-formations and true hypertrophy of the papillary structures

Of this typical catarrhal inflammation of the skin, four tolerably distinct varieties may be noted, distinguished so far from each other by tolerably well-marked clinical features · (1) *Eczema simplex*, mild, usually localized, and with few or no symptoms of general disturbance (2) *E. rubrum*, more general in distribution, more truly inflammatory, both as to local phenomena and general disturbance (3) *E. impetigenodes*, inflammatory action with pus-formation ; this latter often in excess of apparent inflammatory action. (4) *E. chronicum* or *squamosum*, characterized by an abundant furfuraceous shedding of epidermic scales

Symptoms —Eczema, in all these forms, may occur in any part of the body, but is most frequently observed over the superior parts of the neck and trunk, over the quarters and around some of the natural orifices

Typical cases may exhibit all the changes and gradations from erythematous congestion, papulation, vesiculation, on to pus-formation and shedding of epidermic scales In others, certain of these recognised stages may be missed or left out, and chronicity may be exhibited at any period The condition of vesiculation is not often observed in the horse, unless very carefully looked for, the hairy covering obscuring these early changes. The first indication of disturbance is most probably local irritation and itching, with an open state of the coat, while on passing the hand over the parts affected, the small tear-like masses, in separate clusters or elevations, will give the impression of not uniform and unbroken, but rather of scattered or more closely-set points of concreted exudation These small elevated masses of hardened, serous fluid, when detached by rubbing, leave a slightly excoriated surface, which exudes a serous or sero-purulent fluid itself, hardening into

differently formed and constituted crusts The primary exudation would appear to be largely connected with the hair-
follicles, around which the minute vesicles are grouped; these
follicles seem also usually in the centre of the first-formed and
small pustules

In *Eczema rubrum*, where both general and local symptoms
are tolerably well marked, there is often some gastric derangement with disturbed appetite, sometimes slight fever, and
often obvious external appearances of unthriftiness   Locally
the parts affected feel hot, somewhat tender, and a little
swollen, over extensive areas the hair may be removed, the
skin a little excoriated, weeping from a discharge of ichorous,
blood-stained fluid, or in portions covered with a more or less
perfectly formed brown or yellowish crust.

These conditions are apt to occur when the inflammation
affects the insides of the thighs, and in situations where intertrigo is existing   The discharge from these patches is liable
to irritate the parts yet unaffected with which it may come in
contact, and to cause removal of hair

With *impetigenous eczema*, both in the material discharged
from the vesicles and in that exuded when these and the crusts
are removed, there is mingled a good amount of puriform
material, with probably no more constitutional disturbance
than in the clearly marked inflammatory form of *E rubrum*
With the distinct local irritation we observe that peculiar-
coloured crusts continue to form, and beneath these much
ichorous and purulent matter   This form is rarely general,
while in the horse the usually recognised local development,
popularly known as grease, we prefer considering in the order
to which it more properly belongs—diseases of the gland-
structures of the skin

In addition to these distinctions and forms of manifestation
of eczema, others are occasionally made having reference to the
locality of the primary lesions   Thus *E. facialis vel labialis*,
occurring in certain districts and in particular animals, is eczema
of the impetigenous form occurring in the skin of the face and
lips ; *E mammæ*, eczema confined to the mare, and appearing
around the nipple or over the mammary gland , *E genitale*,
appearing over or upon the genital organs—penis, vulva, and
vagina—and marked with much disturbance and irritation

Causation—In endeavouring to appreciate those agencies and influences which operate in the production of catarrhal inflammation of the skin, it will be found that these bear a not very distant relationship, as to modes of action manifested, to such adverse influences as tend to the development of a similar inflammatory action in internal mucous membranes Regarding eczema in its various manifestations as essentially a disturbance in the nutritive activities of the skin, we observe that this disturbance may, in a general way, be accepted as the result of causes operating from without or from within the animal itself There is amongst dermatologists much difference of opinion as to the relation which subsists between the vascular disturbance in eczema and the observed activity in cell-proliferation, whether the latter ought to be looked at in the light of cause or effect, or if both ought not rather to be regarded as dependent on nerve paresis

Of extrinsic influences we are aware that several chemical or mechanical agents may develop irritation sufficient to be represented by the assemblage of phenomena recognised as eczema, while of influences operating from within, indigestion and perversion of some of the various activities connected with food assimilation seem to bear no unimportant part In secondary digestion we may also have the operation of such disturbing influences as retention in the blood of excrementitious materials, which, circulating in the capillaries of the skin, may not inaptly be regarded as active local irritating agents. In all probability everything, whether of a systemic and general character or merely local influence, which interferes with or disturbs in any way the healthy nutrition of the skin is to be regarded as a source of eczema In those instances where we may be able to appreciate and recognise with tolerable certainty the agencies operating in these perversions of nutritive activity, it will usually be observed that they are in particular of the character which we may designate local, and the phenomena or symptoms of the disturbance are local also When the causes seem to proceed from general or constitutional improprieties, or the existence of loaded or contaminated blood, the eczema is more frequently general than local in its development. As respects the particular local changes, the proliferation and intimate character of the developed cell-elements in the

48

papillary layer of the dermis and in the rete, whether these
are to result in excess of serous effusion or of pus-formation
will depend greatly on the individual tendency or peculiarity
of the particular animal.   Such changes appear not to be
altogether determined by the mere character, or intensity of
the local action

Diagnosis —As eczema is one of the commonest of the skin
affections to which the horse is subject, it is also that which is
encountered in the greatest number of diversified forms, and is
exceedingly apt to be confounded with, or rather mistaken for,
some other skin affection to which, in one or other of its rather
numerous manifestations, it bears much resemblance

In the true typical form—which it does not always exhibit
—as already noticed, it may pass through the different conditions of erythema, papulation, vesiculation, pustulation, and
squamation   Essentially it is to be regarded as an exudative
or moist disease, and, although we may not always see the
vesiculation or ichoration, we may always possess evidence of
its existence by the resulting encrustation of the exuded
material.   From the papular or plastic inflammations it is to
be distinguished by the fact that, unless considerably abraded,
these are not characterized by discharge and formation of
crusts, but rather by the existence of soft, fleshy excrescences,
or papules   From the acute forms of dermatitis, as erysipelas,
it is clearly marked off by the presence in the latter of much
constitutional disturbance and fever, and by the nature of the
local lesions, which in eczema are vesicles, and in erysipelas
phlyctenæ   In the chronic form it may be confounded with
psoriasis, from which, however, it may be distinguished by
the history of the case, the character of the squamation, and
by the existence, at the same time, in other parts of the body
of the eczematous inflammation in a different stage

Treatment —This ought, to a great extent, to be regulated by
the form of the eczema, and the stage or age of its growth in
which we encounter it.   Remembering that in typical cases it
has a regular course—from irregularly distributed erythema to
furfuraceous scaling, through which it is likely to pass—our
endeavour ought always to be to have the last stage reached
as early and with as few complications as possible

In the simpler forms and earlier stages, when vesiculation

is fresh, soothing and calmative treatment is indicated, in the middle and pustular stage, tonics and mild astringents are better, and in the last, stimulants, particularly local ones, are most conducive to favourable results   Thus every case must be treated on its own merits or requirements, directed by the knowledge that individual constitutional states and peculiarities, and such accidental complications as concomitant disturbance of other organs, largely modify the phenomena of the disease In simple eczema, the conditions being chiefly local, the treatment must of necessity partake chiefly of the same character. Here simple applications, as an alkaline wash with a little glycerine and some liquid preparation of opium, or even starch powder or wheaten flour sprinkled over the parts, will do well Constitutionally, at this stage a mild aperient is indicated, followed by a little acid mixture, while the terminal process of desiccation and scaling may be expedited by a mild stimulating wash, in which some of the tarry preparations are the active agents

In the severer cases, and where there is much exudation, as in *eczema rubrum*, the treatment is at first essentially that of allaying local irritation by dressing the parts with fine starch powder mixed with oxide of zinc, or painting the surface with a weak solution of nitrate of silver in glycerine, or a solution of tannic acid and opium to which has been added a little glycerine   When the exudation is a little dried, a liberal use of the ointment of the oxide or carbonate of zinc or lead may be alternated with either of these lotions   In this form aperients and salines may be less liberally employed, and their place taken by such tonics as sulphuric acid and iron, or cinchona, gentian, and acid, with a free use of linseed oil in the food

When the surface-discharge becomes distinctly lessened, and the swelling and puffiness of the skin gone, and squamation is fairly established, somewhat of the same tonic treatment is to be carried out, aperients and diuretics may occasionally be used, but with less frequency, and the iron and acid, with vegetable tonics, may be alternated with some preparations and compounds of arsenic, iodine, or mercury   It is in this scaly stage, whether accompanied with much or little itching, that I have found greatest benefit from the use internally of arsenic, and externally of the tarry preparations.

48—2

These latter may be beneficial at other stages, but they seem most distinctly indicated in this. The arsenic is conveniently administered in powder with bicarbonate of potash, probably two drachms of the alkali to two grains of the acid twice daily, or simply as Fowler's solution, one table-spoonful, morning and evening, in food or drinking-water. Carbolic acid, highly spoken of by many, is good as an external application, but must be used much diluted and with great care, and does not appear to have aught to recommend it over the more common and safer oil of tar, which, used in the proportion of two parts with one of soft soap, and from ten to twenty of linseed oil, will be found a good and cheap dressing. When this or any other preparation is used two or three times in succession, the whole ought to be washed off with soft soap and tepid water, so as to ensure the removal of the crust, should any form, and allow of the immediate and direct application of the dressing to the skin itself

E. BULLOUS OR HERPETIC INFLAMMATIONS

In equine dermatology this subdivision of the inflammatory diseases is a small one, and, with trifling violence to our subject, herpes, the only manifestation of the group in the horse, might have been included in the catarrhal. The bullous or herpetic group of skin diseases is characterized by the presence, as an essential phenomenon, of blebs, bullæ or vesicles, these not being, as in some other conditions, accidental but constant features

The term herpes, we are aware, has been often and extensively employed somewhat loosely. It has been used to designate chronic skin diseases generally, and to indicate in particular acute skin affections, attended with the formation of vesicles in particular parts of the body, also to distinguish a parasitic affection of a scaly nature developing in circular patches, on which are situated small vesicles

Certainly the most characteristic manifestation of this group of the inflammatory skin diseases of the horse is that acute form known as erysipelas, in which large-sized blebs or vesicles are encountered over the affected parts. This, however, as a zymotic disease has been noticed already. The only other form is *herpes*, which term we would restrict to a benign, acute dermatosis, attended with the formation of miliary papules arranged in groups, passing into vesicles, more rarely pustules, and extending over a restricted, usually circular portion of inflamed skin

There is often much difference of opinion respecting the appearance and naming of discrete spots, showing vesicles which fade in a longer or shorter period, and scale off. No doubt the simple inflammatory form, the true herpetic eruption, has been confounded with that which is of parasitic origin, disposed to spread over the body, and capable of passing by transplantation of spores from the diseased to the healthy In the horse, what I would claim as true herpetic inflammation commonly appears in two forms—(1) As an eruption of vesicles, somewhat larger than those of eczema, found in irregular patches at the junction of mucous membrane with ordinary skin, and seemingly symptomatic of irregular digestion or disturbance of some of the complex phenomena of assimilation, it is not unfrequently seen in foals over the face and around the mouth while receiving milk from their dams, and when these latter are not constantly with their young, being kept at work during the day and occasionally heated ; (2) As irregularly distributed patches of a cutaneous eruption, papular, vesicular, or pustular, the true inflammatory herpes of adult animals

In this form the distinct isolated patches of eruption do not, as in man, appear so regularly situated along the course of cutaneous nerves, nor are they found particularly located on one side of the body, but rather scattered irregularly over it, sometimes symmetrically and in spots or patches of a more or less perfectly circular form, inclined for some days to spread at their circumference, and probably not capable of propagation from the diseased to the healthy

I have upon several occasions observed this irregularly distributed and patchy or herpetic inflammation of the skin in horses appearing as a distinct exanthematous fever In these instances the skin eruption was associated with a little catarrh, and it might have been looked upon as merely symptomatic ; still, they were so distinct, so numerous, and so circumscribed by local conditions that they seemed rather independent of it, and only connected as adventitious occurrences

In herpes, as usually observed, the ordinary symptoms are the occurrence of spots irregularly distributed over the trunk of a circular form, upon which the hair is at first open and staring, and from which it shortly falls, the denuded skin exhibiting a slightly scaly condition, with numerous small papules or vesicles closely packed together, which do not often rupture, the fluid which they contain being either absorbed or desiccated. Over these spots there is but slight itching. For the first week they are disposed to extend, the hairs around the margins appearing to die for want of proper nutrition, but reappearing when the epidermic exfoliation is completed, which it usually is in two or three weeks. Rarely during the occurrence of these circumscribed eruptions is there constitutional disturbance sufficient to attract attention. The form recognised as *herpes circinatus*, both from the history of its origin and nonspontaneity of cure, is most probably of parasitic origin

Causation—This, in all animals, is badly made out, and, as with several other morbid conditions and activities, the relations of which to antecedent influences and agents is not comprehended, has been laid to the charge of disturbed innervation. No doubt, in human dermatology, there seems a certain amount of evidence to connect this skin disease with textural changes, sometimes observed in connection with nerve-cords at their spinal origin or their termination. In the horse, such evidence has not yet been forthcoming, but its appearance in association with obvious disturbance of digestive and assimilatory functions and some febrile states, and its departure when these disturbing factors are removed, is so far confirmatory of the intimate dependence of the one upon the other, that we are disposed to regard it in our patient as largely a condition symptomatic of some extensively operating and depressing influence

Treatment—Believing that inflammatory or true herpes is essentially self-limiting, and always exhibits a tendency to a return of normal local functions, little in the way of treatment is needed. Should irritation and itching be troublesome, an alkaline wash with a little dilute prussic acid, tincture of opium or digitalis will be found useful. Or should any tenderness be present, an application occasionally of zinc or lead ointment will be called for, or in cases of evident want of vital activity in the patches which have been denuded of hair, some skin stimulant may be employed Those animals which give evidence of disturbed digestion will require such to be attended to; while it will usually be observed that the greater number of cases give evidence of being below rather than above par, and that general tonics, as sulphate of iron, or quinine with acids, are more likely to be serviceable than repeated doses of purgatives.

F. SUPPURATIVE INFLAMMATORY OR ECTHYMATOUS SKIN DISEASES

By suppurative inflammatory or ecthymatous diseases of the skin it is designed to indicate merely those affections which are marked out and characterized by this phenomenon of pus-formation as a primary lesion.

With our present-day ideas of inflammatory action we can understand that any inflammatory affection of the dermal structures may issue in pus-formation, and practically we are aware, and have noticed, that the catarrhal inflammatory actions of the eczemata may pass from vesicles containing merely serous fluid to the mingling of this with pus-cells Regarding this form of inflammatory action, however, in the former light, as including those in which pus-formation occurs as a primary phenomenon, we have only to deal with ecthyma proper, and probably also furunculus

Ecthyma.

This diseased condition we regard as consisting in distinct, rather large pustules, projected upon an elevated, hard, and tender base, which, when the pus is discharged, become crusted with a dark-coloured scab, rather long in removal, and when detached, resulting in a temporary indented cicatrix. This disease is of rather frequent occurrence in the adult horse, while evidence seems sufficient to satisfy most observers that such distinct pustulation of the dermal textures may occur in at least two forms Accepting the definition of ecthyma already given, these forms may in all essentials be considered identical.

In the one form, the papulation and pustulation may be

earlier and less distinctive, and, in its milder manifestations, may be confounded with impetigenous eczema; it is, however, peculiar and distinct in this, that, under favourable conditions, it is undoubtedly liable to propagate from the diseased to the healthy, and occasionally takes the character of an epizooty. It is also much oftener encountered than the non-contagious ecthyma, and may show a particular tendency to the vesico-purulent character.

Clinical History, etc.—This most frequently encountered form of ecthyma, the contagious, is sometimes spoken of by the name of the 'American skin disease' of horses, from its being largely observed at a period some years since, on the influx of horses from the United States and Canada.

It is more frequently met with in foreign horses, and amongst those which have had close contact with these, than in others differently circumstanced. It is disposed to appear chiefly over the back and along the quarters, where harness and straps come more closely in contact with the skin. The papules or elevations, which appear to spring from the superficial layer of the true skin, take a week or more ere they arrive at maturity. Rarely in any of the papules do we find a well-defined vesicle or bleb; at first, in some, there may be an exudation from the summit of the elevation of a straw-coloured sticky fluid, which, after some days, is mingled with pus-cells. The larger number of these pustules come out during the first week, with occasionally a smaller number following. When matured, the elevations are considerably raised above the general level, round, not running into each other, but separate and distinct, with a well-marked point.

The power of propagation which this form of pustulation undoubtedly possesses, both mediately and immediately, has been conjectured to be dependent upon the existence of a specific organism, plant, or animal. Although, however, fungi have been detected in the pustules, it would seem that these only exist in connection with the crustaceous stage, having been deposited as spores from the air, and retained by the discharges, seeing their existence has not certainly been demonstrated in the pustule or vesicle previous to its rupture.

In both contagious and non-contagious forms, the pustules are distinct and hard, situated on an inflamed and tender base;

both are succeeded by dark-coloured, firmly-adhering crusts, which, on separating, leave temporary indented cicatrices, over which at first darker-coloured hairs are apt to appear The non-contagious form of ecthyma is less common than the other, rarely appearing in such full crops, and although similar in general character, development, and termination, is disposed to exhibit more chronicity than the other.

This only differs from boil or genuine **furunculus** in that the latter springs from and involves the deeper dermal tissues, and on healing, throws out a slough or core.

Causation —The chief developing agencies in these pustular affections of the skin seem to operate through induction of general or systemic disturbance, not disturbance of one particular organ, but of several. They may be generally classed as such as tend to debilitate or depress vital action or general nutrition, and ought probably to be viewed as indicative of general and particular debility. The frequency of one form of ecthyma in imported horses may be owing to the unavoidable disturbance, during transit, of the processes of assimilation, the prevention or arrest of elimination, the retention of waste and used material, and its further development and change into noxious compounds, capable, through transformation in the animal body, of transmitting these deleterious influences to other animals

Treatment.—In the great majority of cases, the treatment is correctly begun by attention to the state of the alimentary canal, by which elimination is most kindly and surely carried out. Following a mild dose of aloes, sulphate of soda or magnesia may be given in two or three drachms twice or thrice daily in the drinking water, while either along with the saline or exhibited separately in draughts, one or two fluid drachms of dilute sulphuric acid will be found useful

After a few days, and when the state of the canal is satisfactory, the salines may be discontinued for a short while, and sulphuric acid and sulphate of iron, with tincture of gentian, substituted

While receiving these tonics, which may be changed or alternated with others, the horse ought to have good food easy of digestion, with a sufficient amount of exercise in the open air. It is also needful to pay particular attention to a thorough cleansing of the clothing, stables, and everything connected with those animals in which the affection appears communicable ⁑ In external treatment, there is nothing better than applications for some hours daily of woollen cloths wrung from warm water, and gentle enunction on their removal with simple ointment or olive oil This to be carried out until the removal of the cicatrices, when the application of some zinc ointment, or a weak solution of sulphate of zinc, to which has been added a little glycerine, will facilitate the healing

G SCALY OR SQUAMOUS INFLAMMATIONS

It is probable that the affections which are usually placed in this group might, with equal propriety, find a place under skin hypertrophies; also we must not forget that a squamous condition of the skin is met with in many and somewhat varied conditions, but, like the state of pustulation, this division is designed to embrace only those affections where the scaly condition is met with, not as a result of previous abnormal dermal actions, but as an essential and primary phenomenon

In other inflammatory actions affecting the dermal tissues, squamation follows as a sequence ; here the hyperæmia, when it does occur, is at once accompanied by an increase of the scales of the epidermis, apart from exudative action

These conditions, hyperæmia and excess of epidermic cell-production, may be local, and chiefly idiopathic, when it is recognised by the term of **psoriasis**, or they may be more general, and often symptomatic, and are then known as **pityriasis**

This latter condition is sometimes encountered chiefly as a symptomatic affair, generally associated with considerable constitutional disturbance and not to be mistaken symptoms of unthriftiness or ill-health Such general hyperæmia and extensive furfuraceous desquamation of epidermic scales, apart from exudative action may appear as itself the chief or only attractive symptom, but is more frequently found in the train of other symptoms, all pointing to some largely operating influence, or considerable organic change

Psoriasis

With this condition of limited disturbance of cell-structures of the epidermis, and local accumulations of these as dry light-coloured scales, we have a larger experience than with the more general condition. The abnormal collections of epidermis —the most obvious symptom—vary in size from small circumscribed areas to considerable extents of skin. The situations on the body where they are mostly observed are the carpal and tarsal flexures, and over the tail, and neck close to the mane In the former situations, as *psoriasis carpi et tarsi*, mallanders and sallenders, we know this affection to be both troublesome and intractable

Pathology.—Although it would appear to be essentially and purely a disease of the skin, and not in any way dependent on general or systemic conditions, seeing it exists in severity when every condition, intrinsic and extrinsic, is favourable to health, we may not shut our eyes to the fact that particular families and animals, with rather lymphatic temperaments and sluggish habits, are more liable to be sufferers than others, and also that it is apparently transmitted as an inheritance from parent to progeny Although classed as an inflammatory condition, there are many manifestations of *psoriasis* in which this morbid activity in cell-proliferation is merely linked to hypertrophy and increase of formative-power in the papillary layer, a condition in many instances disposed to become permanent

Although the essential and distinguishing features are merely an increase in the production of the epidermic cells, and a heaping of these together as scales, we find that in the severer cases the papillary layer of the skin itself undergoes much change, the chief and most marked being of a hypertrophic character, from increased development of tissue and from infiltration In the more chronic forms, in addition, very considerable changes, chiefly of a fibroid character, occur in the corium

Symptoms.—In appearance and development *psoriasis* is not likely to be mistaken for any other affection. It may originate as circumscribed spots; but when observed by us its usual form is that of the diffuse variety. It is disposed to extend, but not rapidly, from the seats of origin, while the collections

of scales are usually deepest in the centre of the portions
diseased When of some time standing, and under certain
conditions, fissures and suppurative action are liable to be
established, causing much irritation and extensive textural
changes in the carpal and tarsal flexures, and also in other
parts of the limbs. This condition is a fruitful source of lameness, not merely from the impediment offered to motion at the
exact situation of the prominent lesion, but also from the
general stiffness connected with dermal infiltration The
entire conditions are liable to exacerbations from various
causes and extrinsic operating agencies, such as accumulations
of dirt, excess of moisture, and sudden atmospheric changes,
while peculiarities of dietary seem also to have a certain
amount of influence on its development Itching, although
existing, is not such a prominent symptom of *psoriasis* in
the horse as of some other forms of inflammatory action.

Treatment —When much local irritation, itching, or congestion exist, the cooling or soothing treatment is particularly
called for. With general and moderate evacuants, such as
ensure an action of the bowels and kidneys, the local employment of glycerine and water, with a little sulphurous acid,
carron oil, or weak carbolized oil, will be found useful The
employment of water liberally or alone, except so far as needful
for cleansing the parts, does not seem to answer well. When
a satisfactory state of the alimentary canal has been obtained,
or in some cases from the first, particularly when debility is a
prominent feature, tonics are indicated, and are best alternated
or given in conjunction with alkaline medicines When the
dry and scaly condition is confirmed, a somewhat stimulant
local treatment is to be preferred Instead of mild glycerine,
lotions, or even zinc ointment, one containing some of the tarry
preparations, or, in some instances, common iodine ointment, is
to be preferred ; while, for internal use, arsenic in combination
with alkalies, and a liberal use of linseed in the food, is always
deserving of trial

CLASS II. DISEASES OF NUTRITION, INCLUDING NEW FORMATIONS.

A. HYPERTROPHIES

These include all those affections in which we have, as primary changes, increase in size or quantity of the normal elements of the skin. With us, the chief are verrucæ, or warts, consisting of hypertrophied papillæ, pedunculated or sessile, distinct in form or collected in masses occasionally reaching a great size; elephantiasis, hypertrophy of the skin and subdermal tissues of some of the extremities, originating from inflammatory changes in the lymph-vessels of the part; and fibroma, a condition of circumscribed hypertrophy, not of the papillary or other particular part, but of all the tissues of the skin.

Verrucæ and fibroma, being conditions more truly requiring manual interference for their treatment and mitigation, scarcely come under our cognizance in speaking of matters more properly pertaining to medicine. The former are exceedingly common, and in certain forms and situations very troublesome, often necessitating surgical interference for their removal

Fibroma—Fibroma Molluscum.

This is a condition much less frequently encountered than simple papillary overgrowth It appears as overgrowths of the entire dermal, and probably subdermal, tissues; at first sessile, these growths shortly take more or less of the perfectly pedunculated character, appearing projected from the level surface like short fingers of a glove, the skin being of the natural colour and covered with hair The tumours, which are scattered over the body and limbs, are soft, and vary in size from a hazel-nut to that of a fig or small orange; when taken between the fingers the inner surfaces of their walls may be rubbed against each other. Proceeding from the base of many of these growths, and extending to others, are cords or corrugations of the skin

In any cases of this disease which I have observed the tumours do not increase rapidly; while occasionally some of the larger become extra vascular, the skin giving way over the summit, and forming an irritable-looking sore not much disposed to heal

Pathology.—The cause of these growths is not known, in structure they consist of an overgrowth of the fibro-cellular elements of the skin, their minute examination disclosing an excess of fibrillated material enclosing cell-elements with excess of a gelatinous material   It is rather an uncommon condition, does not seem to be at all under the control of medicine, and is only partially mitigated through surgical interference.

Elephantiasis

This is a condition of excess of development of dermal and subdermal tissues of a diffuse character, usually involving the larger proportion of these structures of an entire limb, and in the horse is usually the result of repeated attacks of inflammation of the lymphatic vessels of the part affected   It may appear after a primary attack of lymphangitis, but rarely   The first appearance of the disease is a swelling of the subcutaneous tissue, the true dermal becoming involved secondarily   When affected the skin becomes thickened, somewhat hardened and more difficult to move on the subcutaneous tissue   it is dry and coriaceous, occasionally scaly, and falls into folds and fissures which, in cases of long standing, may chap and suppurate   This thickening of dermal and subdermal parts, after a time, causes much alteration of the limb and deformity, with impaired power of motion

Pathology.—The essential characters of this condition, as revealed by morbid anatomy, would appear to be increase of the fibrous subcutaneous tissue and hypertrophic changes of the entire skin, together with infiltration amongst the fibrous tissue of numerous and varied cell-growths, and a large amount of gelatiniform material   These changes would appear to follow the diseased condition of the lymphatics, the immediate result of which is obstruction of their canals, and retention of lymph and lymphoid elements in the tissues, these latter ultimately becoming more or less perfectly organized; all the hyperplastic changes beginning in the subdermal fibrous tissues and extending gradually into the fibrous structures of the corium, the epidermis becoming involved at a later period. With these hypertrophic changes in the fibrous structure of skin and subcutaneous tissue, there may also be noticed atrophic alterations of muscular elements wherever these are included in the area of the disease.

Causation —This condition of steady hypertrophy of skin and other associated structures appears in all instances directly dependent on lymphangitis, the extent and rapidity of the changes being in direct relation to the severity of the inflammation   Although the hyperplastic dermal activities are only set in motion by the inflammatory affection of the lymphatics, and while every fresh attack may give a renewed impetus to the development of particular tissue-elements, the hyperplastic changes, when once started, seem to go on even between these repeated onsets of lymphangitis, only receiving a fresh and more powerful impetus on the occasion of each attack.

Treatment.—This may be palliative ; but seldom, when once established, is the condition reversed   Of all which have been recommended and tried, a judicious combination of purgative and diuretic medicine with a rather liberal use of tonics, vegetable and mineral, together with steady exercise or work, and the employment of daily enunctions with a compound of mercurial and iodine ointment, is more likely to be productive of good than aught else   The more heroic treatment, by the local use of cantharides blisters, issues, or the actual cautery, has in my hands been provocative rather of more serious results.

B. ATROPHIES

True atrophic changes in the horse's skin, apart from such as follow continuous circumscribed pressure, are not often observed   Of the accessory structures, the hairs are found to suffer from this change more than others   This condition, however, will be again noticed under another class.

C. NEW FORMATIONS, OR HETEROLOGOUS GROWTHS.

Under this group are gathered those disordered conditions characterized by the appearance or development locally of adventitious and heterologous material, in connection with or in place of the true dermal tissues   These changes and appearances of new tissue are essentially distinct from hypertrophies, or mere increase of already existing elements.   At first, and in their main and essential characters merely local, they may in process of time become associated with general disturbances and conditions of ill-health, and with the appearance of similar growths in other and different structures of the body This may occur either as part of a general cachexia, as the result of the influence of serious local changes on systemic activity, or from the infective power of the primary local disease

In the horse, diseases of this class are rare, and when seen are usually in the form of some varieties of cancer or sarcoma The growth or development of these malignant conditions is usually slow, but when interfered with they may show un-looked-for activity, with a liability when removed to recur Their description and treatment belong rather to the province of surgery than medicine.

CLASS III   NEUROSES

It is probable that with a more extended and exact dermal pathology many diseases which are presently grouped under other classes may yet be placed under that of disturbed inner-vation.

At present, although satisfied that with many inflammatory affections, disturbance of nerve-function coexists, often as a secondary, but sometimes as a primary condition, still, none are included here as disorders of the nervous element of the skin, which may be differentiated by any distinct elemental change.

The primary affections which may be regarded as comprised under cutaneous neuroses are 'Increased Sensibility,' 'Dimin-ished Sensibility,' 'Perverted Sensibility.'

The latter of these, known as 'Pruritus,' is probably that which most frequently engages our notice.

When remarking upon inflammatory skin diseases, as eczema, prurigo, etc, irritability of the parts and itching were noticed as prominent features   These may also occur in recovery from certain fevers, from the contamination of the blood by the circulation in it of waste materials; in other systemic diseases, as rheumatism; and in certain local affections, as liver and kidney diseases

The more purely nervous character of pruritus, however, is shown apart from the existence of either general or local disease, and where the itching is the only abnormal although attractive symptom.

Pruritus, although in the horse often of a distinctly local character, and the itching confined to particular and limited areas of surface, is sometimes encountered over the greater part of the body, in which conditions the causes in operation for its production will most probably be found in connection with or proceeding from some general disturbance

In all cases except the very mildest, if, on their appearance, no textural changes are observable, such absence of alteration is not likely to continue, seeing excoriations, swellings from congestions and effusions, with papular elevations, corrugations and suppurations, are almost certain to follow the excessive rubbing against walls and other resisting objects, and the tearing with the teeth.

This excessive itching is often developed suddenly without premonitory warning, and is always liable to be aggravated by warmth resulting from work, it seems also capable of being influenced by conditions of the food-supply, and the humidity or otherwise of the atmosphere. Many of these cases of *pruritus* in horses seem to commence as extremely simple matters, but the irritation induced by the rubbing being followed by the formation of lymph-papules or ecthymatous pustules, with no abatement of the itching, gradually developing into changes of an inflammatory character in the deeper-seated structures of the skin, not unfrequently leading to the production of great disfigurement and permanent blemishing of animals

Treatment.—As the causes which operate in the induction of either general or local *pruritus—i e* , excessive itching, as the distinctive and primary phenomenon apart from textural change—are hidden, and often merely matters of speculation, we are necessitated in the management of such to direct our attention and efforts to relieve chiefly in the direction of the symptoms developed Where it may be apprehended that hæmal contamination is largely responsible for the cutaneous irritation, of course attempts must be made to correct this through elimination of noxious materials and general or special restoratives.

If the pruritus is directly resulting from such local causes as the presence of pediculi or other organisms, the destruction of these will generally be followed by subsidence of the itchings. Usually, however, in all typical cases of this disease, it is the alleviation or removal of the distinctive symptom, the itching, which chiefly occupies our attention. This will be found, particularly at first, to be more easily accomplished through the employment of local soothing and anodyne agents than by special stimulants. For this purpose there is nothing which recommends itself more to our favourable consideration on many grounds than an alkaline solution, with a little opium or digitalis tincture or solution; or a mixture of two parts of glycerine, one of medicinal prussic acid, and thirteen of water.

With these local applications a little laxative medicine, followed by the daily use of salines in the water and good wholesome diet, is to be recommended.

When the more active symptoms of irritation and local congestion from rubbing have somewhat subsided, but a considerable amount of itching continues, if cooling and anodyne applications do not seem to induce or hasten the disappearance of the disturbing local irritation, some of the tarry compounds may be used. The employment of these, however, always requires a certain amount of care, in order that their stimulant action be not carried too far; and after two or three applications they ought always to be washed off, and renewed if needed. When the animals affected are weak, or in chronic cases, the internal use of iron and acid, or of arsenic with bicarbonate of potash, or of compounds of iodine, as Donovan's solution, I have found to be productive of good results.

CLASS IV. DISEASES OF ACCESSORY ORGANS AND STRUCTURES OF THE SKIN.

There is no doubt that in various diseases where the entire structure of the skin is invaded, all parts and structures essential and accessory may be involved; here, however, the abnormal conditions which chiefly engage our attention are such as are primarily or in an especial manner connected with the skin gland-structures, and the hairs and hair-follicles.

In the horse, disease of these accessory structures of the skin are almost entirely represented by that condition commonly recognised by the term 'Grease' I have placed this affection here, although perfectly well aware that, as usually seen by us, many and different structures are affected ; that from the character of the morbid action and textures involved, it might with as much propriety be ranked with the impetigenous catarrhal inflammations of true cutaneous tissues, as relegated to disturbance and impairment of function of the sebaceous glands

Still, it seems that at first and early in its appearance the gland-structures, especially the sebaceous, are the parts most distinctly involved After some time the changes which the disordered condition exhibits may in a large measure account for the variations in the names by which it is recognised.

Certainly in the more advanced cases the suppurative action, combined with the extensive involvement of the skin, seem to entitle it not inappropriately to be spoken of as *Erysipelatous Impetigo—Impetigo Erysipelatoides.*

This affection, of a common inflammatory character attacking the gland and cutaneous tissues must not be confounded with the much rarer state of a specific eruptive, inflammatory action in connection with dermal structures in the same situations, viz , the skin of the heels and posterior parts of the fetlocks of the horse's limbs

Pathology *a History*—From an early period suppurative inflammation of the heels of horses has been noted, and much divergence of opinion expressed regarding it. Of one form at least, probably that which we have spoken of as specific, much has been said as to its specificity and close alliance to variola—as being, in fact, equine variola, and of having, when communicated to man, a specific action and influence of a protective nature. This action and influence, if correct as pertaining to a specific eruptive and suppurative disease of the skin of the horse's heels, is certainly not extended to or possessed by any of the products of this common morbid action of which we now speak Experimentation proves this

b Anatomical Characters—In the earlier and mildest

forms of this disease there does not appear any structural change of either the gland-structures or the skin-tissues proper which surround these, the disturbance is purely functional, and consists in an increased amount—*steatorrhœa*—or sometimes an altered character — allosteatodes — of the sebaceous fluid. When increased in amount merely, the secretion is often more watery than natural, while the varieties in character are usually as to consistence, colour, and mode of comporting itself.

When the abnormal conditions proceed beyond mere disturbance of function, alterations in amount or of the character of the secretion, these are shown first by infiltration of inflammatory products about and around the hair-follicles and sheaths, with the formation of pus. With the swelling consequent upon the periglandular inflammation and infiltration, the pus which is developed at length finds its way to the surface, collecting and forming cakes in conjunction with the altered sebum and epidermic cells, the changes taking place in these latter conferring upon the mixed discharges a peculiar and characteristic smell.

The congestion or hyperæmia not being relieved, hypertrophic changes take place in the papillary layer of the skin and in the subcutaneous connective-tissue, the hyperplasia of the papillæ, combined with the perifollicular suppuration and hypertrophy of the underlying fibrous tissue, tending to the production of the well-marked irritable-looking projections bathed in purulent fatty fluid known as 'grapes.'

c. *Causation.*—This is to be looked for as proceeding from influences both general and local, influences operating from within as well as from without the animal.

Steatorrhœa, Seborrhœa, or Erysipelatous Impetigo is always found in situations where activity in the cutaneous glands is expected to be considerable; but this increase in function seems, in direct proportion to their activity, to render them liable to be disturbed by causes affecting the general health as well as by local unfavourable agencies. For its frequent appearance in certain individuals and families it seems largely indebted to constitution and inherited tendency. We find it more frequently in horses of a lymphatic temperament, of sluggish action, with excess of connective-tissue and abundance of coarse hair upon their limbs, all tending to favour local congestions Disturbance of the digestive functions, marked augmentation of nutrition through forced supplies of food, particularly when connected with want of sufficient exercise in animals otherwise disposed through temperament, are liable to be followed by an appearance of 'grease.'

No doubt local changes and adverse influences operate largely in the production of this disease still it does not appear that these are either all-powerful, or even as powerful as others which must ever be regarded as operating from within

Of external influences, we may observe that the heels and fetlocks of horses—particularly the hind ones—the situations where this disease is most common, are very liable to be acted upon unfavourably as to equilibrium of circulation and direct irritation, from their exposure, both within and without the stable, to cold, moisture, and the direct contact of foul and irritating materials In short, whatever tends to sluggishness of circulation, to general or local debility, and all direct irritation, seems to favour the congestive and inflammatory condition of skin-glands and true skin-tissue in the heels of horses, developing into this *erysipelatous impetigo*, ordinarily known as 'grease.'

Symptoms—In the simpler form of merely increased or even perverted secretion, there may be only a trifling amount of swelling of the parts where the follicular disease usually appears—*i e*, in the hollow of the pasterns and posterior parts of the lower extremities of the metacarpus and metatarsus Shortly after this swelling, the characteristic dampness becomes evident, and the hair is somewhat matted, while the parts, when manipulated, impart a soapy feeling and disagreeable smell to the fingers For long this feature of increased and perverted secretion may be the only abnormal feature When, however, it is abundant, and much changed, it will collect in cakes or crusts, beneath which pus accumulates; this crustaceous state causing stiffness in movement, or distinct lameness, particularly in starting from the stable.

Often the perifollicular, suppurative, and cutaneous changes will result in shedding of the hair, leaving a slightly reddened and moist surface; while when the suppuration extends, and the general cutaneous tissues become raw and ulcerated, swelling, with congestion or inflammation of the lymph-vessels, is noticed, extending to the superior parts of the limb.

Treatment—This must vary in accordance with the stage of the affection and the causes believed to be in operation for its production. When evidently associated with some general disturbance of the digestive organs, or when there seems a tendency to plethora, purgatives are called for, together with a proper regulation of diet and attention to needful exercise. This placing of the whole animal functions in a condition as nearly as possible approaching what is recognised as the health-standard, can scarcely be over-estimated; for however much local causes may operate in the production of local disturbance and change, internal agencies have a more powerful and prevailing influence. With some of the milder exhibitions of 'grease,' a moderate dose of medicine and attention to cleanliness, with the non-removal of the long soft hair from the heels, will suffice to give a favourable turn to the disturbed activities. When inflammatory action and pus-formation have proceeded to any extent, particularly when cutaneous fissures and much crusting of discharges have occurred, the necessary removal of the irritation is only well accomplished by local anodyne applications, as poultices. These when the fœtor is considerable, and indeed in most instances, are improved by medication with such agents as charcoal, salicylic, carbolic, or sulphurous acids. Although the removal of hair tends to favour the appearance of this inflammation of the skin, such may be needful, when the disease is once developed, for the proper application of remedies.

Having by poulticing relieved the local tension and pain, it will be found in these instances where the perifollicular inflammation and suppuration have resulted in the production of a raw surface, that some mild astringent is better fitted than aught else to assist in restoration of healthy action. Such washes as chloride or sulpho-carbolate of zinc, from gr. x to gr. xx to the fluid ounce of water, having a little carbolized glycerine added, serve very well in mild cases; for the more chronic, a steady perseverance is needful for some considerable time. When not improving with this or any other treatment, it is better to adopt a change of dressing. In many obstinate cases, I have found a saturated solution of sulphate of copper, with a small proportion of carbolized glycerine, succeed in arresting the foetid discharge and starting a healthy reaction

In those instances where tissue-change and great papillary hypertrophy exist and largely impede the proper application of remedies, the most expeditious and least painful mode of treatment is the removal at once by the actual cautery of the elevated and projecting hyperplastic papillary structures

In all these exhibitions of this chronic skin affection, having obtained a soluble state of the bowels, and given due attention to dietetic and sanitary conditions, we will find benefit from the employment internally of tonic and diuretic medicines Sulphuric acid and sulphate of iron, with vegetable stomachics, are usually alternated with such salines as sulphate of soda or magnesia, or with preparations of arsenic or iodine

B DISEASES OF THE HAIRS AND HAIR-FOLLICLES

When studying the diseases of the skin of the horse, and giving them more than a cursory attention, I have been inclined sometimes to regard this as a rather large class The reason for this being that, in examining the catarrhal inflammatory diseases, I have found that in many instances the early and most distinct pathological changes have occurred in intimate connection with hair-follicles and sheaths, to the exclusion or appearance in a modified form of these in the other skin-textures However, having at present determined to place the eczemata, so called, as examples of catarrhal inflammations of the skin in general, and not as specially attached to the hair-follicles, the affections included under diseases of the hair and hair-follicles—not embracing those of parasitic origin—are few in number. The chief representative is **alopecia** or baldness, known also as **alopecia areata or circumscripta** This, when occurring over limited and circumscribed areas, has been regarded as of parasitic origin, and spoken of as *Tinea decalvaus.*

Regarding the name alopecia as indicating simple baldness or absence of hair, it has been thought, although not certainly proved, that this, as an ultimate result, is reached by two modes of action, one attributable to parasitism, the other to non-parasitic influence As observed in the horse, it has in all cases, or nearly all in my experience, affected animals of adult life, and which were in full work. I have not in them observed that they have been the subjects of any particular disease, or that any marked constitutional disturbance attended this cutaneous affection. They have, however, all been horses subject to sudden spurts of fast work, entailing general vascular excitement, followed by sudden and ill-regulated periods of rest. When occurring, it has only affected the deciduous hairs, not those of the tail or mane, and the removal of these has in every case been accomplished with little or no alteration in the pigmentation.

Symptoms, etc.—It is usually sudden in its development, with little or no cutaneous irritation, itching, appearance of exudation, or even raising of the epidermis.

It is first observed over the back, sides, and neck, where the hair, in the ordinary process of grooming the animal, is detached without the slightest evidence of pain, leaving perfectly smooth and bald patches of varying form and size. With many, the greater part of the entire hairy covering may be detached in flakes or patches, which, when removed, are held together in separate portions by the removal in a planiform manner of the upper layer of the epidermic cells. When the hair has been detached, there is no itching nor perverted sensation of the exposed skin, which is perfectly smooth, soft, and unctuous, having a very light covering of scales.

Pathology—It is extremely difficult, or rather impossible, to account in a clear and definite manner for this sudden and often extensive change. All that we are really able to say is, that it appears as the immediate result of disturbed nutrition and atrophic changes of the epidermis and hair-follicles.

The existence of a vegetable parasite in connection with the hairs or the follicles, as in the different forms of Tinea, has been put forth as the active agent in the death of the hair; this, however, does not seem the true solution of the question. When such organisms have been observed, they are probably an accidental occurrence. The most extensive and destructive exhibitions of *alopecia* which I have encountered have certainly been unconnected with parasitic existences.

Although it is a mistake probably to lay too much stress on the actual appearance and state of the individual hairs, still such is always of so much value   Here they may, when examined, occasionally exhibit a slight change at their root portions, being somewhat compressed and wasted; as often, however, they are unaltered, and throughout their entire extent exhibit none of the brittleness so commonly seen when they are the subjects of parasitic invasion.

In anatomical characters the true skin-structures appear unchanged, and if the hair-follicles and glands are somewhat atrophied it is all that can be detected.

Treatment—As already said, all cases of partial or very extensive baldness have a natural tendency to return to normal conditions, but all seem to be assisted in attaining this by attention to the principles of hygiene

When any weakness is apprehended, general tonics, as iron with gentian or nux vomica, and linseed oil given in the food, seem to benefit much.   While of local means none are more successful than regularly applied stimulation to the skin through the medium of weak cantharides lotions or camphor mixture.   Should the skin become coated or in any measure hardened by the use of these, it ought to be washed with soap and water, and a little glycerine and water applied afterwards.

CLASS V   HÆMORRHAGES.

Cutaneous hæmorrhage, although a rare condition in the horse, is still, from the possibility of its occurrence, deserving of notice   Whether as symptomatic of certain diseased conditions, or resulting from mechanical violence, the seat of the blood-effusion is the same, the superficial vascular layer of the true skin.   In certain fevers, chiefly specific, attended with hæmal changes, we may observe at particular stages of the disease petechiæ or ecchymoses   And probably these would more frequently attract our notice, if observation were not obscured by the hairy covering of our patients.   When occurring in the horse, hæmorrhagic spots are rarely so rapid of development as in man, neither do they comport themselves in the same manner as in him.   The term of their duration does not, as with him, seem to depend on the extent and depth of the hæmorrhage so much as on the progress, favour-

able or unfavourable, of the general disease with which they
are associated, and during their existence, when situated where
their characters may be observed, as on the membrane of the
nose or mouth, the colour is rarely uniform, and they may not
display steady and regular chromatic changes until perceptible
defervescence of the fever upon which they depend is established

Besides petechiæ and ecchymoses accompanying certain
general diseases and resulting from injuries mechanical and
parasitic, the most distinctive exhibitions of cutaneous hæmorrhage seen in our patients are those associated with special
systemic disturbances and changes recognised under the term
of *Purpura hæmorrhagica*   This not being regarded as properly a disease of the skin, has been spoken of under another
class.

In no instance may cutaneous hæmorrhage be regarded as a
diseased condition of itself, but rather as symptomatic of some
other abnormal conditions , most probably in every instance it
is dependent upon some chemical alteration of the blood itself,
upon some disturbance of its dynamic relations, or upon some
textural changes occurring in the capillary vessels

From these considerations we may understand that the successful treatment of this condition depends less upon rectifica-
tion of local changes than upon correction of some general
unnatural state and the establishment of normal systemic
functional activity

CLASS VI.   PARASITIC SKIN DISEASES

Like many other structures of the animal body, the skin is
liable to suffer from disturbance and change, the result of the
association with it of distinct and separable forms of organization, which derive their sustenance from it During the growth
and development of these parasites certain consequences or
results are exhibited which are recognised as diagnostic, as also
other phenomena which can only be looked upon as of an
adventitious character

Cutaneous diseases originating or owing their existence to
parasitic life and development are usually spoken of as *Dermatozoic*, or such as are dependent on animal parasites, and

Dermatophytic, those which are dependent on vegetable existences

A DERMATOZOIC, ECTOZOIC, OR ANIMAL PARASITIC SKIN DISEASES

Of diseases of this group to which the skin of the horse is subject, the chief are, **Scabies** or **Mange, Phthiriasis** or *lousiness,* and the disturbances consequent on the presence in the dermal tissues during certain periods of their life-cycle of such parasites as the **Filaria medinenses** and **Filaria multipapillosa,** etc

Although during a short period of our summer months, and under particular conditions, certain dipterous insects cause our horses considerable annoyance, both when at work and when grazing in the fields, we have in Great Britain really no serious or very troublesome affections attributable to attacks of winged insects

The **Filaria medinenses** or Guinea-worm, so common and troublesome as attacking or chiefly manifesting itself in connection with the skin of man in certain parts of the world has been observed, in those situations where abounding, to locate itself in the subdermal tissues of the horse, and of course inducing there a certain amount of local and circumscribed irritation

Filaria multipapillosa —This nematode, said to be common enough as an irritating visitant of the skin of the horse over considerable parts of Central Europe, is to us chiefly interesting from the circumstance that horses bred there when brought to this country are said in many instances to exhibit, for a lengthened period after their arrival here, symptoms indicative of its presence in the cutaneous tissues   Those which may be regarded as diagnostic are the appearance suddenly and at irregular intervals, chiefly over the neck, the superior scapular region and back, of very minute discharges of red blood, as it the skin had been punctured with a needle

The few in which I have encountered this cutaneous hæmorrhage were Hungarian horses, and they had not been more than twelve months in this country   Knowing that such symptoms had, by Continental observers, been connected with the existence in the skin-tissues of a particular parasite, I was inclined to attribute this hæmorrhage to these intruders, although, by a careful search, I was unable in any case to satisfy myself that such was the cause of the lesions   There were no elevations of the skin—'boutons hémorragiques'—the parts being perfectly smooth, and when carefully denuded of the hair, two or three minute points could be observed from which blood oozed.

As I have only observed this particular hæmorrhage in Hungarian horses, and chiefly in those the first year of their residence in this country, and from what we are told regarding it by observers in Central Europe, where it seems not an uncommon occurrence, also from the fact that it is not kept up but disappears after a residence here, it seems highly probable that it is the direct result of cutaneous parasitism   Still I have been informed by trustworthy observers that a like hæmorrhage is occasionally observed in home-bred animals; this I am unable to corroborate.

In the management of this lesion treatment seems to have little influence, while, with certain reservations, the animal's powers of work-doing do not seem impaired.   When not appearing under the saddle or collar, the small amount of blood which is discharged may be sponged off, and the horse put to his usual work; when the bleeding occurs where the harness rests, if the pressure is continued, there is the liability to the production of an open sore

Phthiriasis—Lousiness

Horses are liable to a disturbed condition of the skin from the residence there of at least three species or varieties of what are ordinarily known as lice.   Two of these are individuals of separate families of the same order of the class Insecta, and the third is an accidental visitant, received from cohabitation with poultry

Of the two former, more commonly recognised as lice, one, the *Hæmatopinus equi,* is the proper pediculus, and a true blood-sucker; the other, the *Trichodectes equi,* lives amongst the hair and on the skin, irritating by its presence, not finding its food-supply from the blood direct, but in the exuvia of the structures   Of these, the former is the more irritating, and is easily enough distinguished from the *Trichodectes* by its narrow and distinct thorax, bearing three pairs of legs, and the triangular head, armed with a tubulous haustellum. The other species, belonging to the *Mallophaga*, mandibular, or biting lice, are entirely different, particularly in their head and thorax, the former being distinctly quadrate, and furnished with mandibles and maxillæ suited to their mode of life. These two species are more apt to be found on horses neglected, or suffering from poverty and privation; while the inroads of the louse of the domestic fowl are regulated largely by the condition of the poultry-houses or roosts and their proximity to stables. They attack horses of all classes, but seem to have a preference for those which are in work and good condition, or probably they have greater facilities for settling on such.

Although horses may harbour in their coats a numerous colony of varying species of lice, it is only in particular instances that much disturbance is witnessed. In some, however, the irritation and itching are most troublesome, proceeding until well-marked traumatic abrasions of the skin or papular and vesicular changes show themselves, the results of this rubbing.

In horses attacked by the poultry-louse, the *Gonioctes Burnetti*, small and scattered spots of depilation occur over a large surface of the body, this depilation being the result of the occurrence over these circumscribed areas of a very minute vesiculation. A similar condition may also show itself in occasional cases of cutaneous irritation, where the insect is of either of the species more common to the horse. As a rule, however, the attack of the former is more sudden, its progress more rapid, and the irritation—probably from the character of the subjects affected—is more marked.

Treatment.—It is easily understood that in those cases, which are certainly not the commonest, where the pediculi are conveyed from poultry, any attempt at the destruction of those on the suffering horses themselves will be unavailing, without the removal of the original cause, the destruction of the lice in the poultry-roosts, or the removal of the larger animals from their influence. In the application of either wash or ointment the difficulty is not that of being able to destroy the insects, but of obtaining at the same time the destruction of their eggs. Usually, the safest mode is that of repeated applications of the parasiticides until the whole are destroyed as they appear. For this purpose infusion of stavesacre, or tobacco, are very efficacious and easy of application. Either of these may be employed in this form, in the proportion of one ounce of the vegetable to twenty or forty of water When prepared it is desirable that the water be kept near the boiling-point for some hours, and then allowed to stand for some time longer before being strained for use

Another very potent parasiticide in these invasions, I have found, is a mixture of creosote, one part; glycerine or spirit, two parts; water, forty parts; while, where great objection is taken to the use of any active or poisonous material, a good dressing of oil, vegetable or animal, and an after-washing with soft soap, will usually destroy the greater number of perfect insects.

Scabies—Mange—Scab.

Definition —*A true dermatozoic skin disease characterized by more or less itching, and occasional eruption of papules, vesicles, or pustules, but diagnosticated by the presence of some variety of acari in or upon the skin*

Pathology *a History, etc*—From very early periods it seems probable that something was known of this skin disease in animals as well as men In the writings of Aristotle there are recognitions of phenomena connected with skin affections which can only be rationally interpreted by believing that the observers were aware of the existence of mites burrowing in the skin, and scattered through the writings of those who took cognizance of matters agricultural during the Roman period and the time of the Saracenic ascendency down to modern times, we may gather information enough to satisfy us that parasitic diseases of the skin, probably scabies in animals as well as men, were not unrecognised.

b Nature.—Affecting the horse we are aware of **scabies** evidencing itself in at least three separate forms, from the existence in or upon the skin of certain *acari*, or mites, of the family Acarida, class Arachnida. Any distinct and particular features these several forms may exhibit are apparently owing to individual peculiarities of the separate and distinct *acari* In two of these forms the habitats of the mites, and the lesions which they produce, are distributed over different parts and varying extents of the body-surface; in the third these are confined, or nearly so, to the limbs

The first of the forms of body-mange is believed to be produced by the burrowing beneath the epidermis of the *acari* known as the *sarcoptes;* the second, and in this country probably the most common variety, depending on the residence upon the skin, of those known as the *psoroptes* or *dermato-dectes*, while the particular mange of the limbs seems to owe its origin to the collection in groups of a third variety of the same family, the *chorioptes* or *symbiotes*.

c Causation.—Although it is undoubted that the essential and immediate factor in the production of mange in any form is the presence of the mange mite, we may not shut our eyes to the teachings of experience, in so far as these tell us that all debilitating and exhausting influences, as exposure, fatigue, want of sufficient food and fitting stabling, render horses more susceptible to the attack and rapid development of the induc-ing parasite, and of course materially influence the progress and termination of the disease The influences of these agencies have been observed and their extent determined by all observers, particularly by those associated with large collections of animals in civil as well as military life. In the latter condition this disease, along with glanders, has ever been the scourge of armies in the field.

No doubt animals of certain temperaments and constitutions would appear more liable to be acted upon by the immediately inducing cause than others, while of all these varieties of scabies, probably that which appears upon the limbs is most disposed to exhibit a tendency to develop in connection with individual peculiarities and dispositions It exhibits, in addition, also a distinct preference for cold over warm weather, there is here apparently existing a close relationship between the *acari* of this variety, and the condition of the skin and its covering at such seasons, peculiarly favourable for its life and pro-pagation

Symptoms.—All the varieties of equine scabies are charac-terized by the appearance of a class of symptoms having much which is common. The truly diagnostic, however, is the detection and recognition of the separate and individual *acari*. In this country the form of scabies resulting from the presence of the *sarcoptic acarus*, which closely resembles the itch insect of man, is rather less common than the other form affecting the general surface of the body, the effect of the residence there of the *Dermatodectes equi*. In both forms the earliest indications of the parasite's existence are itching and irritability of the skin, this in the *dermatodectic* or *psoroptic* variety, when fairly established, being rather more pronounced, and the damage done to the tissues through rubbing is usually greater. The initial and elementary lesions of *sarcoptic* mange in the horse, are said to be vesicular, as those of the *psoroptic* are papular, or papulo-vesicular.

These differences are, however, in many instances rather difficult accurately to determine.

In the former, there is a more uniform distribution of the skin irritation, and a greater disposition to simulate non-parasitic eczema, by the large and general distribution of small elevations of dried serosity   In the latter variety, the papules which exude the serous fluid do not immediately dry up, but continue weeping, and thus render the superincumbent crust more extensive and rather moist; the scabs are consequently larger and less dry than in the *sarcoptic* variety.

The rapidity of the extension of these two varieties in the individual animal, and their powers of propagation, are not exactly alike The more common form, the *psoroptic*, is slower in the distribution of the *acari* over the affected animals, being disposed to continue for variable periods as distinct circumscribed patches, and is less commonly found propagating amongst a number of horses which may have had a certain amount of communication with each other It is also more disposed to be located close to, or in connection with, the permanent hairs of the mane and tail, than the other, which is the result of the activities of the burrowing *acari*.

The *symbiotic* scabies, like the other forms more particularly affecting the body, owes its existence to the activities of the *acari* known as the *Chorioptes vel Symbiotes equi* The mites here are so far like the *Dermatodectes*, that they do not burrow beneath the epidermis or crusts, but live amongst them; and they are particularly tenacious of residence in the localities embraced in the limbs. It is a disease particularly of coarse-bred and hairy-limbed horses, and is most frequently seen, and in greatest severity, during the cold season of the year; not that the creatures upon which it depends depart in the interval, but that they, from some rather ill-understood conditions, seem in greater numbers and activity during cold weather

The symptoms indicating the existence of this condition are, in the early stages, not very attractive; the fetlocks may be somewhat thickened, and an extra amount of scurf may be found over the skin, with a moderate amount of itching, shown by rubbing one leg upon another, by gnawing the parts with the teeth, or by vigorously and repeatedly stamping upon the ground. Commonly the hind limbs are more liable to be invaded by the mites than the anterior extremities. In severe cases, the hair is removed in patches, and a heavy furfuraceous crust exposed which rapidly undergoes change and removal.

In all these manifestations of mange when existing for a lengthened period, we find that considerable changes take place in the tissues of the skin, visibly altering its appearance and the manifestations of symptoms.

Although attention to the form, intensity, and mode of propagation of these symptoms may often be sufficient to give us well-grounded confidence regarding the nature of the malady, none save the detection and identification of the mange mite are to be regarded as certainly diagnostic

Means of Propagation—Seeing that the contagion in every case of scabies is either mature *acari* or their eggs, we can understand that any means which will convey these from diseased to healthy animals are sufficient for the propagation of the diseased condition. This can be accomplished directly by the contact of the suffering with the healthy, also indirectly by the contact of the healthy through use of harness, clothing, or stable-fittings and utensils which have previously been used by the diseased.

As all the forms are not alike contagious, we will find that more liberties may be taken with the *symbiotic* and *dermato-dectic* than with the *sarcoptic* variety.

This last, it may be noticed, is also alone capable—by the transmission of the *acari*—of propagation and a variable tenure of life on the skin of man and other animals.

The retention of vitality by the *acari*, on their removal from

50

the animal on which they may be located, extends to several days, and that of their eggs probably to a longer period.

Management of Cases of Scabies.—The medical treatment of scabies consists, first, in the adoption of strict sanitary measures for the segregation of the diseased from the healthy, the effectual cleansing and disinfection of stables and everything which has been in contact with the diseased, and the keeping of a strict surveillance over the suspected for at least a fortnight. Second, the treatment of the actually suffering. Here a little variation in detail may be needful, when the disease has existed for some time, and when the psoric crusts are abundant. In this latter condition, previous to the application of any remedy, it is always good policy to have as much of these removed by soaking with oil, glycerine and water, or soft soap, as can be obtained, thereby favouring the direct application to the skin of whatever is being used.

In form these applications may be either that of lotion, liniment, or ointment; most probably, in the greater number of cases, the oily preparation is the best.

A very large list of medicinal agents might be given as likely to be productive of good as parasiticides, and the greater number of practitioners have some they value more highly than others.

The more certain, safe, and inexpensive of those employed are sulphur, the terebinthinate or wood-tar preparations, tobacco, white hellebore, stavesacre, and arsenic. A very cheap and efficacious wash may be made by cutting in small pieces an ounce of common roll tobacco, macerating it in water near the boiling-point for six or twelve hours, straining, making the liquid up to twenty-six fluid ounces, and adding from two to four ounces of glycerine. While, if a liniment is preferred, there is nothing better than linseed oil one pint, oil of tar two fluid ounces, *sulphur* two ounces. Whatever dressings are employed ought to be well rubbed into the parts, probably two days in succession, allowed to remain for three or four days, and then washed off with soft soap and tepid water, and reapplied if thought needful.

B DERMATOPHYTIC, EPIPHYTIC, OR VEGETABLE PARASITIC SKIN DISEASES.

The group of vegetable parasitic diseases of the skin in the horse is represented by one, or probably by two, of the so-called *tineæ*

(a) Tinea Tonsurans—Tinea Circinata—Ringworm Proper.

This, in the horse, is the better known and more frequently occurring of the tineæ, and it may be regarded as typical of the entire group.

Definition—*An affection of the hairs, the hair-sheaths and cells of the epidermis over different parts of the body, usually occupying circumscribed circular spots or patches, which start into existence by slight elevations of the superficial cuticular scales, and attended with an altered brittle condition of the hair, slight itching, and the presence of a peculiar cryptogam, the Achorion vel Tricophyton tonsurans*

Pathology *a Nature*—The existence and nature of this affection is evidently closely bound up with the life and development of the peculiar fungus which is inseparably associated with it. This parasite, which consists chiefly of spores or conidia of an oval or round form, often separate and disjoined, but occasionally joined or linked together, and a small amount of elongated tubular matter, apparently invades the interior of the root and shaft of the hair These, when affected, undergo certain recognised changes; they swell or increase in bulk, losing colour, becoming opaque and brittle, ultimately breaking across, and appear frayed at the point of fracture, their interior at the same time becoming more rapidly filled with sporules, granular matter, and mycelium, in this way giving a certain asperity to the surface At the same time the superficial layers of the epidermis become raised from the growth beneath of the fungus; by this raising they possess a clear grey and shining character.

b Causation—The immediate cause of this disturbance is the implantation of the spores or seeds of the fungus into the hair-follicle of the healthy skin. At the same time there seems a certainty that a marked receptivity and accommoda-

50—2

tion is afforded for the growth of these by certain conditions extrinsic as well as intrinsic Youth seems to predispose animals, particularly of certain breeds; and damp, with darkness of location and improper dietary, tend to favour the certainty of the sowing.

Symptoms —The early indications of the disease are an open and altered condition of the hair over circumscribed, more or less perfectly circular patches, with a perceptible elevation of the superficial epidermic scales. As the hairs break off and are cast, the skin may show minute vesicles, papules, or pustules, or there may be simply an extra amount of distinct and separable scales, evenly or with slightly elevated edges spread over the parts

In some, the entire circular patch or patches—for there are generally several—are denuded of hair, and evidently evenly affected—' Tonsurant ,' in others, with a greater circumferential margin, there exists a healthy spot in the centre—' Circinate.' These patches are usually scattered over the upper part of the trunk, and give rise to a trifling amount of itching. Generally disposed to extend, we sometimes meet with cases having a natural disposition to cure themselves, which they seem to do through the death of the *tricophyton*, which evidently perishes from want of sustenance

(b) Tinea Favosa—Favus—Yellow or Honeycomb Ringworm

Definition—*An epiphytic cutaneous disease characterized by the appearance of cup-shaped yellowish-coloured scabs or crusts, sometimes separate and distinct, at others aggregated and confluent; these yellow crusts, consisting of a vegetable fungus—Achorion schonleinii—and capable of transplantation from one animal to another.*

Pathology. a *Nature*—This, it would appear, is dependent upon or consists in the growth and development in the hair-follicles external to the hair proper, and in the epidermic scales of the particular fungus, the *Achorion schonleinii.* This parasite, like the *tricophyton*, is made up of the ordinary fungus elemental structures, chiefly spores or conidiæ, with a small amount of amorphous granular matter, and having occasionally associated with these another and probably distinct

cryptogam, the *Puccinia favi;* this latter is somewhat different
from the tricophyton in the mode in which its cell-elements
are made up and joined together.

Besides the variation in form and colour of the crust, honeycomb differs from ordinary ringworm in that in the former,
when fully developed and of any extent, we recognise a generally constant and peculiar smell, which has been variously
likened to that given off by bruised hemlock, or to the presence
of mice or cat's urine. That the fungi which it would appear
produce this as well as the tonsurant form are one and the
same, only varying as to their manifestations from peculiarities
of soil, the natural consequence of differences in textural
elements in the different species in which these are met with,
seems to me rather doubtful, rendering the explanation of
certain phenomena we observe rather difficult, and not as yet
undoubtedly demonstrated

My own experience as respects this feature of identity of
fungi and varying development of symptoms according to the
species on which it may be implanted, does not corroborate
that of some other observers

I have repeatedly observed the propagation of the common
ringworm of cattle and horses, particularly the former, which
is characterized by the presence of the well-known grey
crusts, to both adult and juvenile human subjects, and in
no instance did the characteristic cup-shaped yellow crusts
of favus appear ; this, I know, is contrary to what such good
observers as Williams and MacGillivray state as having
occurred under their observation in the transmission of the
common ringworm from animals to men

b Causation—This, both as to the immediately acting
agency and the favouring or providing of a suitable habitat for
the reception of the originating parasite, is much similar to
such as have been indicated as operating in the preceding
variety Certainly, it will not appear without the implantation
of the spores of the fungus, but is probably favoured as to
readiness of infection and rapidity of growth by both indwelling and external operating agencies.

Symptoms—These are at first indifferent, not diagnostic
until some progress has been made in the hold upon the skin.
The only cases which have come under my notice in the horse

—and they have been very few—appeared as separate, distinct, and minute spots where the superficial epithelial scales seemed increasing in amount and easy of removal, having the peculiarity of being arranged around individual hairs As these increased, a slightly elevated edge arose of a faint yellow colour, as if developing in the follicle of the hair, which was seen to maintain its position in the central, somewhat depressed portion At last, however, when the separate specks of the follicular invasion extended by coalescence, these seemed to be broken off as in the tonsurant form, they might have shifted from the follicle instead of rupturing

Treatment of Tinea—Both the forms of epiphytic skin disease mentioned, whether we regard them as originating from separate and distinct fungi, or as the result of the modified growth of one, are only successfully combated when recognised as essentially local affections, dependent for their existence upon the life of a certain specific organism

All treatment for their eradication must proceed upon the lines of first destroying the parasites, and second, of rendering the soil in which they grow less fitted for their implantation and development.

The first is achieved through the application to the skin or parts diseased of such agents—parasiticides—as will destroy the vitality of the fungi

Previous, however, to the use of these agents, should a well-marked scaly condition exist, it is advisable to have this removed by soaking and washing with oleaginous, alkaline, or soapy mixtures Following this in well-established cases, there is probably nothing better than a moderate painting with the compound solution or weak tincture of iodine; or a smart enunction with common iodine ointment, or a thorough saturation with a solution of corrosive sublimate, two or four grains to the ounce of water, to which has been added a little glycerine

Following the use two or three times, or even less often, of either of these more active preparations, or when the disease is less active or virulent, merely daily washing with a saturated solution of hypo-sulphite of soda, to which has been added half its volume of the B P solution of sulphurous acid, will be found very serviceable As much, however, depends upon the thoroughness with which the parasiticides are used as upon the special virtue of any

The second indication, particularly when constitutional weakness is a prominent feature, is attained by attention to hygiene, and the exhibition of general or special tonics.

Although often tedious and troublesome, rarely will we find any cases incurable when recognition is made of their parasitic origin and of the modes of attack, and when sufficient attention is given to the proper carrying out of the details of the local treatment

INDEX.

796 INDEX.

THE END

BILLING AND SONS, PRINTERS, GUILDFORD AND LONDON